Drugs and Pharmacology for Nurses

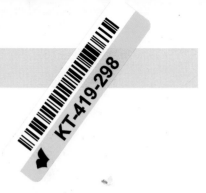
louisa latty

For Churchill Livingstone:

Commissioning Editors: Ellen Green/Alex Mathieson
Head of Project Management: Ewan Halley
Project Development Manager: Valerie Dearing
Design Direction: Judith Wright
Illustrator: Evi Atoniou

Drugs and Pharmacology for Nurses

S J Hopkins PhD FRPharmS
Honorary Consultant Pharmacist, Addenbrooke's Hospital, Cambridge, UK

Assisted by
Jennifer C Kelly MSc RGN RNT
Senior Lecturer in Nursing, Homerton College and Addenbrooke's Hospital, Cambridge, UK

THIRTEENTH EDITION

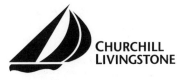
CHURCHILL
LIVINGSTONE

EDINBURGH LONDON NEW YORK OXFORD PHILADELPHIA ST LOUIS SYDNEY TORONTO 1999

CHURCHILL LIVINGSTONE
An imprint of Elsevier Limited

First edition 1963   Ninth edition 1986
Second edition 1965   Tenth edition 1989
Third edition 1966   Eleventh edition 1992
Fourth edition 1968   Reprinted 1993
Fifth edition 1971   Twelfth edition 1995
Sixth edition 1975   Greek translation 1997
Seventh edition 1979   Thirteenth edition 1999
Eighth edition 1983   Reprinted 2000, 2001, 2003, 2004, 2005
                        (twice), 2006, 2007

ISBN-13: 978 0 443 06008 3
ISBN-10: 0 443 06008 8

British Library Cataloguing in Publication Data
A catalogue record for this book is available from the British
Library

Library of Congress Cataloguing in Publication Data
A catalogue record for this book is available from the Library of
Congress

ELSEVIER   your source for books,
            journals and multimedia
            in the health sciences
www.elsevierhealth.com

Working together to grow
libraries in developing countries
www.elsevier.com | www.bookaid.org | www.sabre.org

ELSEVIER   BOOK AID   Sabre Foundation
            International

The
publisher's
policy is to use
**paper manufactured
from sustainable forests**

Printed in China
B/09

Contents

Preface

This 13th edition follows the general pattern of previous editions, and the book remains a nurse-orientated guide to every drug of importance in current use. However, some changes have been made. The position of certain chapters has been altered, and now all those dealing with the cardiovascular system generally are grouped together. The position of references has also been changed, and they are now grouped together at the end of each chapter under the heading 'Further reading'. More importantly, in view of the increasing need for nurses to know more about the pharmacological basis of therapeutics, an extensive revision has been made of the introductory sections of most chapters, and more explanatory figures have been included. In that revisionary work I have been assisted by Jennifer Kelly, who has also drawn all the figures, revised the glossary, and has contributed a new chapter on wound dressings. It is a pleasure to acknowledge her help.

The recent advances in therapeutics are indicated by the wide range of new drugs now available, represented by:

- angiotensin-II receptor antagonists
- potassium channel blocking agents
- atypical antipsychotics and antidepressants
- new cytotoxic agents
- new antidiabetic agents
- new antimigraine drugs
- new drugs for parkinsonism and Alzheimer's disease
- new types of antiviral agents.

It is significant that, although bacterial resistance to antibiotics is increasing generally, no new type of antibiotic has been marketed for some years.

Although the book has been written primarily for nurses, some other health professionals have found it useful, and it has achieved a wider readership. Thanks are again due to those who have kindly commented on the previous edition and made some useful suggestions, most of which have been noted.

Cambridge 1999   S.J.H.

Preliminary notes

Approved and brand names of drugs

British Approved Names are the official names of drugs, and so are used in this book. Such names can be used by any manufacturer, but brand names refer to the products marketed by a single company. So it is possible that the same drug may be available under more than one brand name, which can sometimes be very confusing. British Approved Names will be phased out over the next five years in favour of International Names, but both names will appear on labels for some time. In many cases the differences are slight, such as replacing 'th' with 't', but in a few instances the difference is marked. Adrenaline will be referred to in future as epinephrine. Such different names are given in the book in brackets after the Approved Name. An extensive list of approved and brand names is given in Appendix II.

Mixed products, because of their multiplicity, are referred to only occasionally; however, the official names for certain widely prescribed mixed products have been listed on page 342. The use of mixed products has met with some disapproval, as the dose of each constituent is fixed. For patients on multiple therapy, however, they have the great advantage of reducing the number of tablets to be taken daily, thereby minimizing the risks of confusion.

Dose ranges

When a dose range is given, the lower dose is often an initial dose, to be increased according to need and response.

Dosages given to children and the elderly should be lower than for others. In the young, the ability to metabolize drugs may not be fully developed and overdose may easily occur. In the elderly, impaired renal function may reduce adequate elimination of a drug, so a reduced dose may be necessary to prevent accumulation of the drug to possibly toxic levels.

Side-effects

The references to side-effects are for guidance only, as their nature and frequency vary widely with both drug and patient. An exhaustive list of side-effects, including those rarely encountered, would be more confusing than helpful.

A general warning is given here that many potent drugs will impair car driving and similar activities, and that no drug should be given during pregnancy without consideration of the risks involved. The absence of any such warning later in the book does *not mean* that the drug is free from such risks.

Nurses can play an important role in detecting side-effects, as they are in frequent contact with patients, and any unanticipated side-effect that the nurse might observe should always be reported without delay.

Symbols and abbreviations

New drugs that are currently under surveillance by the Committee on Safety of Medicines for the detection of adverse reactions are distinguished in the text by a black triangle.▼

Drugs that are available only on prescription (the Prescription-Only Medicine, POM, group POM group, which includes most potent drugs) are distinguished in the main references by the sign §; Controlled Drugs (CDs, or drugs of addiction) are identified by a bold star*

The abbreviation BNF refers to the British National Formulary, and BP to the British Pharmacopoeia.

Medical and pharmacological terms

See Appendix V.

Drug dosages and nurse-prescribing

The doses given in this book are for guidance only, as although great care has been taken, the possibility of error remains, and the author does not assume any liability for mistakes. It is the responsibility of the users of the book to obtain confirmation of dose and other information from official publications such as the British National Formulary (BNF) and Martindale's Extra Pharmacopoeia, or from the Data Sheet issued by the manufacturer of the drug concerned. When possible, the information leaflets included in the package inserts of many drugs should be consulted to confirm that there have been no changes in the use and dose of the drug concerned.

Drug administration and nursing responsibilities

The prescriber is responsible for the accuracy of all prescriptions, but in hospital nurses are largely responsible for the day-to-day administration of drugs. Before giving any drug to a patient, every care should be taken to be certain that the right drug is being given in the right dose to the right patient, and that the label on the medicine has been checked against the prescription. The golden rule is simple – READ THE LABEL. Unless the label conveys the required information in full, the product should be rejected until confirmation has been obtained. Drug names can be confusing at times, but even genuine belief that the prescribed drug is being given in the prescribed dose is no substitute for certainty of knowledge. It is sometimes said that safety could be increased by having drug labels and containers distinguishable to some extent by shape and colour, but if conditions make it difficult to check the accuracy of a label, then it is the conditions that require modification, not the label.

Nurses are not always helped by the fact that the amount of drug in an injection or present in a topical preparation may be expressed as a percentage. Many doctors, as well as nurses, have difficulty in translating percentages into the equivalent amount of substance per millilitre, or remembering that a 10 ml ampoule of a 5% solution contains 500 mg of the drug. The following formula can be used:

% concentration × volume(ml) × 10 = dose in mg

but it is worthwhile remembering that a 1% solution contains 10 mg/ml, as with that in mind, the amount in a 0.1% or 10% solution can be calculated without difficulty. In the end, however, nurses must accept the fact that they, like doctors and pharmacists, are responsible for any errors they may make.

Nurse-prescribing

The authority to prescribe has long been restricted to registered medical practitioners. Nurses, however, by the high standard of their training and their close contact with patients are uniquely placed to assess the need for certain drugs for minor illness. There has been increasing pressure for official recognition of the contribution that nurse-prescribing could make to the National Health Service, and that pressure has resulted in the setting up of some Nurse-Prescribing Demonstration Centres to assist Community Nurses to prescribe from an agreed formulary that will include non-opioid analgesics, laxatives, desloughing agents, skin antiseptics and stoma care products. The setting up of these Centres is a long-overdue recognition of the increasingly important part that nurses play in medication and patient care. It may well be that the limited prescribing authority now given to nurses will lead eventually to still wider responsibilities by extending the range of the present limited formulary. Few will doubt the ability of nurses to rise to the new challenge of nurse-prescribing.

Further reading

Baldwin L 1995 Calculating drug doses. British Medical Journal 310: 1154

Rolfe S, Harper N J N 1995 Ability of hospital doctors to calculate drug doses. British Medical Journal 310: 1173

1

Introduction

DRUGS AND PHARMACOLOGY

Drugs or medicines are substances used for the prevention and treatment of disease, and pharmacology is the study of the mode of action of drugs in the body. Medicines of some sort have been used since the dawn of history, and Hippocrates (circa 400BC) who was one of the first medical writers, has been called the 'Father of Medicine'. Treatment was then empirical and directed towards symptomatic relief, and that approach to illness persisted until the latter part of the 19th century, but since then developments have occurred with increasing rapidity, and the physician now has at his command an almost bewildering range of therapeutically active substances. That range includes vegetable drugs, mineral salts, animal products, antibiotics and synthetic drugs.

Crude or vegetable drugs

The main action of a vegetable drug is often due to a single constituent or active principle, which may be an alkaloid such as atropine, or a glycoside such as digoxin. The importance of vegetable drugs has declined with the development of synthetic drugs, but their potential is not yet exhausted, as shown by the introduction of an anticancer agent obtained from the Pacific Yew, and many plant products still await full investigation for medicinal activity.

Mineral salts

These are metallic compounds such as sodium chloride (common salt), potassium chloride, sodium bicarbonate, ferrous sulphate and calcium gluconate. Some are of very great physiological importance, and are constituents of certain intravenous solutions used to restore the electrolyte balance of the body.

1

Animal products

A few animal products remain in use, such as heparin, insulin and some hormones. Bio-engineering techniques now permit the production of certain animal products in quantity, and more importantly, identical with the human product, as for example human insulin.

Synthetic drugs

Synthetic drugs form the most important group of modern therapeutic agents. Representative compounds are antihypertensive agents, antipsychotics (tranquillizers), antidepressants, analgesics, angiotensin-converting enzyme inhibitors and hypoglycaemic agents.

PHARMACOKINETICS

Pharmacokinetics is a wide-ranging term, and includes the study of the actions of drugs, their administration, absorption, onset and duration of action, the metabolic changes that may occur, and the manner and duration of excretion. Before a drug can have any pharmacological action it must reach the receptor site on which it acts, in an active form, and at an effective concentration, but the route of administration, degree of absorption, distribution, metabolism and rate of excretion are important factors in modifying the ultimate response to a drug (Fig. 1.1). The various forms of drug presentation are referred to on page 11, but as most drugs are absorbed from the gastrointestinal tract, the oral route is the most common and convenient form of drug administration. Absorption takes place mainly in the small intestine, where the lining villi offer an enormous area for absorption, but it may be modified by several factors. The presence of food may enhance the absorption of drugs such as propranolol and phenytoin, yet reduce the absorption of isoniazid and the tetracyclines. A few drugs such as captopril, digoxin and rifampicin are better absorbed on an empty stomach. Some drugs, represented by certain antibiotics such as benzyl penicillin and hormones such as insulin, may be broken down by gastric acid or digestive enzymes, and are therefore inactive if given orally.

A few acidic drugs such as aspirin are absorbed from the stomach, but most drugs are absorbed in the small intestine. Absorption largely depends on the ability of the drug to cross the cell membrane, as initially there will be a relatively high concentration

of the drug outside the cell. So in most cases the drug will pass into the cell by passive diffusion to equalize the concentration, but with some drugs lipid solubility is a dominant factor governing absorption. Cell membranes have a lipid or fatty layer, so drugs that are not lipid-soluble will not pass readily across the cell membrane, and absorption may be insufficient for activity to occur. That explains why some water-soluble drugs such as gentamicin must be given by injection. Ionization also plays a part in drug absorption, as only un-ionized compounds are lipid-soluble. Very occasionally, non-absorption may be desirable, as when a drug is required to have a local action, exemplified by the use of salazopyrin in the treatment of ulcerative colitis.

Distribution and metabolism

All drugs taken orally that are absorbed pass by the hepatic portal vein to the liver. Some then pass directly and unaltered into the circulation, but some undergo a degree of metabolic change by the liver enzymes (first-pass metabolism), the main enzyme being cytochrome p450. As a result of that first-pass metabolism, only part of a dose of a drug may eventually reach the tissues to have a therapeutic effect. See Fig. 1.1. With a few drugs, such as glyceryl trinitrate and lignocaine, hepatic metabolism and breakdown is virtually complete, so none of the drug reaches the general circulation. (Glyceryl trinitrate can be taken buccally, as the oral blood vessels do not drain into the portal circulation.) First-pass metabolism also explains to some extent the differences between the oral and injected doses of certain drugs, and why in liver disease larger than normal amounts of a drug may reach the circulation and cause toxic symptoms. However, metabolism does not always inactivate drugs; it can activate. Certain drugs act as 'pro-drugs', as they are inactive when given but are later metabolized into active derivatives. Chloral hydrate is an example of a pro-drug, as it is metabolized after absorption to trichloroethanol, to which the sedative action of chloral is due. Similarly, pivampicillin is metabolized to release the active antibiotic ampicillin. Apart from first-pass metabolism, other metabolic processes may make the drug inactive, or convert it to water-soluble derivatives and so promote more rapid elimination in the urine.

The liver enzymes themselves may be modified by drugs. For example, after an overdose of paracetamol, the enzymes that normally deal with paracetamol metabolism are overwhelmed, and so toxic metabolites accumulate, a state sometimes referred

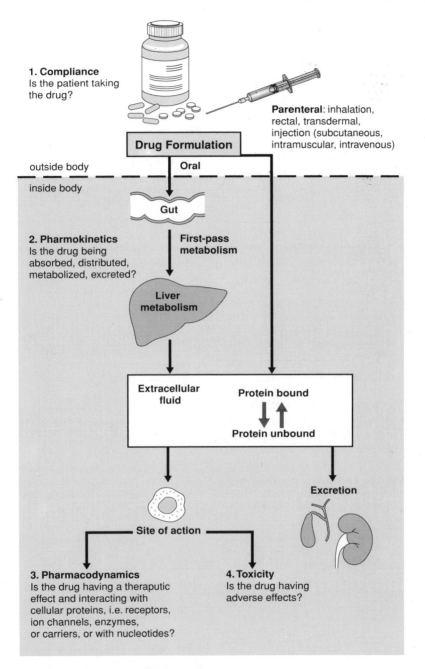

1. Compliance
Is the patient taking
the drug?

Parenteral: inhalation,
rectal, transdermal,
injection (subcutaneous,
intramuscular, intravenous)

Drug Formulation

outside body

Oral

inside body

Gut

2. Pharmokinetics
Is the drug being
absorbed, distributed,
metabolized, excreted?

First-pass
metabolism

**Liver
metabolism**

**Extracellular
fluid**

Protein bound

Protein unbound

Excretion

Site of action

3. Pharmacodynamics
Is the drug having a theraputic
effect and interacting with
cellular proteins, i.e. receptors,
ion channels, enzymes,
or carriers, or with nucleotides?

4. Toxicity
Is the drug having
adverse effects?

Figure 1.1 An overview of pharmacology.

to as dose level saturation. Alternatively, some drugs can stimulate enzyme production (enzyme induction). Such enzyme induction may have a knock-on effect, increasing the breakdown of other drugs that may be given, and requiring an adjustment of dose to maintain the response. Rifampicin is an example of an enzyme-inducing drug, and if used in combination, may lead to a lowering of the plasma levels of propranolol, phenytoin and other drugs. The opposite process of enzyme inhibition may also occur. The antibiotic chloramphenicol inhibits the metabolism of phenytoin and may cause toxic effects.

On the other hand, the combined action of two drugs may be complementary, and so may evoke an increased response. Such a combined action is referred to as synergism, as represented by the combined action of levodopa and carbidopa in parkinsonism (p. 96), and clavulanic acid in association with amoxycillin (p. 65). Very occasionally, drug uptake may be very selective. Iodine, for example, is taken up by the thyroid gland for the production of thyroxine (p. 189), and on that basis radioactive iodine is used for the diagnosis and treatment of thyroid tumours.

Lipid solubility

Lipid solubility not only influences drug absorption generally, but also controls drug penetration into the central nervous system (CNS). Few drugs pass easily into the brain because of the presence of the blood–brain barrier. The capillaries that supply the brain are surrounded by closely packed lipid-containing cells (the glial cells) which, together with the choroid plexus, function as a barrier through which drugs must pass. Lipid-soluble drugs can penetrate the barrier with relative ease, but many others are not sufficiently lipid-soluble to pass through the barrier and exert a central effect. In certain infections, however, such as meningitis, the efficiency of the barrier is reduced, and penicillin, for example, which does not normally reach the CNS, may then pass from the circulation into the brain.

Lipid solubility also influences the duration of action of lipid-soluble drugs such as the intravenous anaesthetic thiopentone. Thiopentone has a short action, not because it is readily metabolized, but because it is rapidly removed from the circulation by temporary storage in body fat and muscle. Lipid solubility may also be linked with side-effects. Propranolol is lipid-soluble and may reach the brain and cause sleep disturbances, whereas atenolol, being poorly soluble in lipids, has little central activity.

Plasma binding

Drugs may be present in the circulation either in the free state or bound to plasma proteins. The strength of such binding is important, as only the free drug is active and can interact with receptors or penetrate cells, and only the free drug is metabolized and excreted. If two drugs are prescribed together which bind to the same plasma protein, the one that binds most strongly will displace the other, resulting in more of the displaced drug remaining available, with a possible increase in toxicity. However, the increased plasma concentration may be in fact transient, as other factors such as increased metabolism and excretion take effect.

Excretion of drugs

The removal or clearance of a drug from the body may be in part by any body secretion, but most drugs are excreted in the urine or the bile, either unchanged or as a conjugated metabolite such as a glucuronide. Renal excretion is closely linked with the glomerular filtration rate, which decreases with age and disease. Drug doses may have to be adjusted accordingly, and in some cases plasma levels of a drug should be monitored to prevent an undesirable rise in the drug plasma level. That is of importance when potentially nephrotoxic drugs such as gentamicin are given.

The carrier transport systems that convey drugs into the tubular lumen also play an important part in renal excretion. Large amounts of penicillin are eliminated in that way, but the process can be slowed down by giving probenecid. Both penicillin and probenecid compete for the same binding site on the carrier, and combined therapy is useful when high and sustained plasma levels of the antibiotic are required, as in infective endocarditis. Probenecid also reduces the re-absorption of urates by the kidney tubules, and so is useful in the treatment of gout (p. 209).

The balance between absorption and excretion determines the half-life of a drug, that is, the time taken for the concentration of a drug in the plasma to fall by 50%. The clinical relevance is that drugs with long half-lives may accumulate and perhaps cause toxic side-effects, and in general drugs with short half-lives are preferred.

Drugs that are excreted in the bile may be re-absorbed to some extent by the enterohepatic circulation, and so have an extended action, which in turn may give rise to unwanted side-effects.

PHARMACODYNAMICS

Pharmacodynamics is the detailed study of the mode of action of drugs in the body, including the pharmacological response at an active site. Some, such as the antacids and laxatives have a direct and localized action, but most drugs have a systemic action mediated by receptors, enzymes, carriers and ionic channels in the tissues.

Receptors

Receptors are proteins present on the cell membrane or within the cell. They are the normal binding sites for hormones and neurotransmitters. Different receptors bind with different types of drugs, but sub-types of receptors are known that have a more selective binding action and so evoke a more specific effect. See Table 1.1.

Receptor binding sets in train a series of changes, many of which are still imperfectly understood, that finally results in a pharmacological response. The general term for receptor-binding substances is 'ligand', and ligands that evoke a response are termed 'agonists'. Ligands that inhibit a response are 'antagonists'. It should be remembered that receptors are not static points, as their number and functional activity vary with drug treatment. Continuous exposure to an agonist may lead to an internalization of receptors, and so reduce their activity, a process known

as 'down-regulation'. That may show up as tolerance to a drug, whereby an increased dose may be required to produce the same effect, although tolerance may sometimes be due to an increased metabolic breakdown of the drug in the body. Many receptors have been identified, as well as some sub-types of receptors, and the closer the relationship between a drug and the receptor it acts upon, the more specific is the subsequent response. The relationship can be compared to some extent with that between a lock and a key, as both receptor and agonist or antagonist must 'fit' together. Adrenaline, for example, has a general action on the adrenoceptors, relaxing bronchial smooth muscle as well as stimulating the heart. Salbutamol, on the other hand, has a selective action on the β_2 receptors, and so is of increased value in asthma with the advantage of reduced side-effects. The position is complicated, as some ligands may have a dual action. Thus although the beta-adrenoceptor blocking agents, represented by propranolol, have as a class a depres-

Table 1.1 Receptors

Type	Sub-type	Agonists	Antagonists
Adrenoceptors	α/β	noradrenaline, adrenaline	labetalol
	α_1	phenylephrine	prazosin
	α_2	clonidine	
	β_1	dopamine, dobutamine	atenolol
	β_2	salbutamol	butoxamine
Cholinoceptors	Muscarinic (M_1, M_2, M_3)	acetylcholine, carbachol, pilocarpine	atropine, hyoscine
	Nicotinic	acetylcholine, nicotine	
Dopamine	D_1, D_2, D_3, D_4, D_5	dopamine, bromocriptine	phenothiazines; haloperidol, domperidone, metoclopramide (D_2); clozapine (D_4)
GABA (γ-amino butyric acid)	$GABA_A$	GABA, benzodiazepines, barbiturates (potentiators)	
	$GABA_B$	GABA, baclofen, tizanidine	
Histamine	H_1	histamine	antihistamines, e.g., promethazine
	H_2	histamine	cimetidine, ranitidine
Opioid	δ, μ, κ	morphine, diamorphine	naloxone;
Serotonin (5-hydroxytryptamine)	5-HT_1, 5-HT_2, 5-HT_3, 5-HT_4	serotonin; sumatriptan (5-HT_{1D}); metoclopramide (5-HT_4)	ergotamine (5-HT_1), methysergide (5-HT_2), ondansetron (5-HT_3)

sant action on cardiac activity, some members of that class may also have limited cardiac stimulant properties, and are referred to as partial agonists. Such beta-blockers have what is described as an 'intrinsic sympathomimetic action'. That difference may sometimes have a clinical advantage, as a partial agonist, whilst exhibiting the main activity of the beta-blockers generally, may cause less bradycardia than the full antagonists represented by propranolol (p. 111).

Very few drugs have in fact a single specific action, and side-effects may be mediated by an action on receptors other than those concerned with the desired clinical response. Thus the tricylic antidepressants, which have a main action on receptors in the central nervous system, may cause dryness of the mouth by inhibiting the action of acetylcholine on the cholinoreceptors. Table 1.1 gives examples of some receptors, agonists and antagonists.

Enzymes

Enzymes are protein catalysts that control many body activities, and are the targets for much drug therapy. Drugs that interact with enzymes may function as inhibitors by binding to the site of action of the enzyme and blocking its access to that point. An example is aspirin, which inhibits cyclo-oxygenase required for prostaglandin production (p. 203).

Ion channels

Ion channels are gaps in cell membranes. They control the movement of electrolytes in and out of cells via electrochemical gradients and ion concentrations. Their opening and closing can be controlled by voltage changes across the membrane, or blocked by drugs attaching to binding sites in the channel. Local anaesthetics act by preventing the movement of sodium ions; others, referred to as modulators, modify the opening or closing of certain other channels. Thus diazepam promotes the opening of specific chloride channels in the brain, inhibits nerve excitation and so has a sedative action.

Carriers

Carriers are proteins involved in moving endogenous substances across cell membranes. They often utilize energy in the form of adenosine triphosphate (ATP) against concentration and electrochemical gradients, and are sometimes referred to as pumps. Some drugs can act as carrier inhibitors, an example being omeprazole, which inhibits the carrier pump system that moves hydrogen ions necessary to form gastric acid (p. 149).

Drug dosage and toxicity

The optimum dose of a drug is high enough to elicit the desired therapeutic effect, yet not high enough to cause unwanted side-effects. The margin between those doses is sometimes referred to as the therapeutic index or window. The index can be calculated as the maximum non-toxic dose divided by the minimum effective dose, and the higher the index the safer the drug (Fig. 1.2). With some drugs the window is narrow and requires careful adjustment of dose, and in such cases a measurement of the plasma level of the drug may be necessary to avoid overdose.

Drugs that have a long half-life, such as digoxin, are sometimes given initially as a loading dose to obtain a high tissue up-take, followed by correspondingly low maintenance doses. The accepted range of dose used clinically is thus a compromise, and the dose prescribed may also vary to some extent with the weight and sex of the patient. The doses of a few very potent drugs are based upon body surface area. Renal or hepatic damage may delay excretion and require a reduction in dose to avoid toxic effects. In other cases, tolerance to a drug may be acquired, and a larger dose may be necessary to obtain the same response. The dose may also vary according to the condition to be treated. Some antipsychotics that have anti-emetic properties are given in much larger doses for psychiatric conditions than when used for the treatment of nausea and vomiting.

The route of administration also influences the size of dose given. Doses by injection are usually smaller than those given orally, and intravenous doses smaller than those given by intramuscular injection. Administration by injection has the advantages of evoking a rapid response and of eliminating the problems of absorption and first-pass loss in the liver. Intravenous injections, however, are not free from risks, as all the injected drug reaches the systemic circulation immediately, and the organs with high blood flows, such as the heart, kidneys, lungs and brain, are exposed to high concentrations of the injected drug, with a corresponding increased risk of toxic effects. As a rule, intravenous injections should be given slowly to reduce the risks of immediate side-effects, and sometimes intravenous infusion of a dilute solution of the drug is preferred.

Whatever the route of administration, the timing and frequency of dose is important, and with long-acting drugs overdosage must be avoided, as otherwise the drug may accumulate in the body and increase the risks of toxicity. In a few cases, an initial high dose may be necessary, but maintenance doses

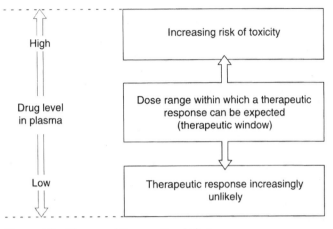

Figure 1.2 Diagram of therapeutic window.

should be at a lower level that strikes a balance between the plasma concentration of the drug and its rate of metabolism and elimination. With corticosteroids used for replacement therapy in Addison's disease, the daily dose should be divided, with about two-thirds taken in the morning and one third in the evening to mimic to some extent the normal pattern of endogenous corticosteroid secretion. If used in other conditions, a single morning dose is preferred to minimize the inhibitory effects on pituitary/corticotrophin secretion and adrenal glucocorticosteroid release.

Doses for infants and children

The assessment of doses of drugs for infants requires care, as their drug detoxifying and excretory systems are not fully developed. The liver lacks some of the enzymes necessary for the conversion of drugs to glucuronides, which is a common method of inactivation, so drugs that are normally excreted as glucuronides will tend to accumulate in infants, even when given in reduced doses; in practice doses must be reduced to even lower levels. The kidneys of infants are also relatively immature, and the renal excretion of drugs may be delayed; so again, doses must be reduced to avoid toxicity, and sometimes monitoring of the drug plasma level may be necessary to control dosage.

Further care is necessary in infants who are seriously ill, as the risk of reactions to drug treatment correspondingly increases. Care is also necessary with locally applied drugs, such as corticosteroids, as the skin of infants is thin and may allow excessive absorption to occur and cause highly undesirable systemic effects.

In general, proportion-to-age-weight doses of drugs that have a wide margin of safety are often used, but doses based on skin surface area are more satisfactory. The problems of dosage are also increased because very young children have a higher metabolic rate than adults, and in some cases they may require higher doses than body weight might suggest. In older children, hepatic metabolism of drugs may sometimes be more rapid than that of adults, as epileptic children, for example, can tolerate relatively high doses of anticonvulsant drugs. Another example of the differences between doses for children and adults is that of the amphetamines. In adults they increase behavioural activity and act as stimulants; in children they increase attention span and decrease disruptive behaviour and so are used to treat 'hyperactive' children.

Doses for the elderly

Increasing age brings about changes in the ability of the body to deal with drugs. Metabolism deteriorates with age as the blood flow to the liver declines by about 40% between the ages of 40 and 80 years, resulting in a reduced first-pass metabolism. Enzyme activity is also reduced and may cause a prolongation of the drug half-life. Metabolism is further reduced by liver disease, which is increasingly common in the elderly. Advancing age also brings with it a deterioration of the glomerular filtration rate, a reduction in renal blood flow and a general loss of renal efficiency. Thus drug accumulation is a major risk in the elderly and dose adjustment may be necessary to minimize possible toxicity. With age the CNS becomes more sensitive to a wide range of drugs, and even small doses of sedatives may cause confusion. Likewise, cardiovascular reflexes become impaired, and the compensatory mechanisms that normally prevent any fall in blood pressure when getting up quickly may fail, so that the elderly may experience dizziness. Postural hypotension may also occur with antihypertensive and diuretic therapy. In general, drug treatment for the elderly should be kept as simple as possible, low doses should be prescribed, and dosage times should be linked with some recurring factor such as mealtimes to improve compliance with drug therapy.

Drugs in pregnancy and lactation

Drugs that cross the placental barrier and damage the fetus are referred to as teratogenic drugs, and their existence was brought to light by the thalidomide disaster. However, in pregnancy many antibiotics and drugs that influence the CNS may pass into the fetal circulation, and as fetal enzymes and renal excretory mechanisms are poorly developed, the metabolism of such drugs is correspondingly slow and their effects may be prolonged.

For many drugs, there is insufficient evidence to be certain that they are harmless to the fetus, especially during the first trimester of pregnancy, and ideally no drug should be given during pregnancy unless its use is essential, and balanced against the risks involved. The absence of such a warning about any drug referred to in the text does not imply, and must not be taken to imply, that the drug can be given during pregnancy.

Similar caution is necessary during lactation, as many drugs appear in breast milk. Although the amount of drug actually received by the breast-fed infant may often be clinically insignificant, that is not always the case (Table 1.2). A few drugs may also affect the milk flow. The dopamine antagonists metoclopramide and domperidone improve lactation by stimulating the production of prolactin, whereas bromocriptine, a dopamine agonist, is used to suppress lactation. The risks of adverse drug reactions in infants can be reduced by avoiding breast feeding when the drug/milk level is likely to be high, usually 2 hours or so after oral administration, by using drugs with short half-lives and avoiding long-acting products.

SIDE-EFFECTS AND ADVERSE REACTIONS

Few drugs have a selective affinity for a single receptor, and a side-effect is an unwanted pharmacological response due to the drug binding to a number of receptors in different tissues. Thus most antihistamines bind not only to peripheral receptors where their effects are required, but also to those present in the brain, and so may have sedative effects. Similarly, morphine depresses the sensory area of the brain but also stimulates the vomiting centre. The incidence of side-effects can be reduced by an adjustment of dose, as with modern low-dose oral contraceptives: the activity is retained but the risks of venous thrombosis have been reduced. Other side-effects are more correctly termed secondary effects, and are linked with the main action of the drug. A patient prescribed an antihypertensive drug may experience postural hypotension as a secondary effect, because the action of the drug on the sympathetic nervous system inhibits the normal compensatory response when the patient stands up quickly. Other common side-effects are dryness of the mouth that may occur with antimuscarinic (anticholinergic) drugs, and the parkinsonism-like symptoms that may follow treatment with antipsychotics of the phenothiazine type.

Adverse reactions are usually more serious, and include neutropenia and agranulocytosis. Haemolytic anaemia, involving the destruction of red blood cells at a greater rate than they are produced, is less common. In most cases these adverse reactions are reversible on withdrawal of the offending drug, but it should never be given again as the patient may have become sensitized to it.

Idiosyncrasy, hypersensitivity and skin reactions

The normal therapeutic response to a drug is known from experience, but as patients do not respond with machine-like precision, some individual variation is not uncommon. However, a patient may occasionally exhibit a markedly unusual response to a drug, referred to as an idiosyncrasy. A special type of idiosyncrasy is hypersensitivity which is usually allergic in nature (p. 229). It involves an antigen–antibody reaction, as the body fails to differentiate between helpful and harmful stimuli, and the drug is treated as a foreign antigen to be attacked. As a result, histamine and other spasmogens are released, which may cause bronchospasm and cardiovascular collapse (anaphylactic shock (p. 90). Nurses should always ask patients about any previous drug reactions before giving any drug for the first time.

Examples of drugs that can cause hypersensitivity reactions include aspirin, which may precipitate a severe asthmatic attack in hypersensitive patients, especially those with a history of allergic disease, and penicillin, which may sometimes evoke anaphylaxis,

Table 1.2 Drugs that should be avoided in breast feeding. The following notes are a general guide only, as in many cases information is scanty. It should be assumed that if a drug of a certain class is listed, related drugs may have a similar pattern of excretion. The omission of any drug does *not* imply that it is suitable for use during breast feeding, as such use remains the responsibility of the prescriber

Drug	Problem
amiodarone	An iodine-containing anti-arrhythmic drug. There is a theoretical risk that it could cause thyroid disturbance
androgens	Could cause masculinization of female and precocious development in male babies; could suppress lactation
aspirin	May cause Rey's syndrome (see p. 54); impairs platelet function in high doses
atropine	Anticholinergic effects
benzodiazepines	Extended use could cause lethargy and weight loss
bromocriptine	May suppress lactation
calcitonin	Best avoided; may inhibit lactation
carbimazole	May depress thyroid function
chloramphenicol	An antibiotic that could cause 'grey baby' syndrome, with vomiting, cyanosis and collapse, as well as bone marrow toxicity
colchicine	Has cytotoxic properties
corticosteroids	Large doses could depress adrenal function
cyclosporin	Best avoided; may appear in breast milk
cytotoxics	Could depress bone marrow function
doxepin	May cause sedation and depress respiration
ergotamine	Could cause ergotism
ethosuximide	Could cause excitability
ganciclovir	Is teratogenic and best avoided
gold	Idiosyncratic reactions and rash
indomethacin	Appreciable amounts in breast milk, risk of neuropathy
isoniazid	Theoretical risk of convulsions
isotretinoin	Is teratogenic and best avoided
lithium	May cause lithium toxicity with cyanosis, neonatal goitre
meprobamate	Appreciable amount in breast milk; may cause drowsiness
metronidazole	Best avoided; may appear in breast milk
nalidixic acid	Avoid in G6PD deficiency
nitrofurantoin	Avoid in G6PD deficiency
oestrogens	May suppress lactation and cause feminization of male infants
phenindione	Risk of haemorrhage in vitamin K deficiency
phenolphthalein	May cause diarrhoea
progestogens	May suppress lactation
sulphonamides	May possibly cause kernicterus in jaundiced infants, and haemolysis in G6PD deficiency
sulphonylureas	Could cause hypoglycaemia
sulpiride	Best avoided; appreciable amounts in breast milk
tetracyclines	Best avoided; theoretical risk of tooth discolouration
thiazide diuretics	Large doses may suppress lactation
vitamins A and D	Best avoided; risk of hypercalcaemia with high doses of vitamin D

a sensitivity that may also occur with the penicillin-related cephalosporins. Other hypersensitivity reactions that may occur include skin reactions, blood dyscrasias and the so-called drug-fever. Drug-induced fever is usually an immunological reaction mediated by drug-induced antibodies, and may occur with many drugs. Blood dyscrasias such as aplastic anaemia, agranulocytosis and haemolysis may also be the result of a drug reaction. Very occasionally, as with penicillin, the hypersensitivity can be reduced by a desensitization process in which initially very small doses of the offending drug are given by injection, but the process is not without risk (p. 230).

Skin reactions

Drug-induced skin reactions may take different forms. Urticaria and erythematous eruptions are relatively common, and appear to be linked with the release of endogenous substances such as histamine. Not all drug-induced skin reactions are serious, but a change in medication is usually necessary. A more severe morbilliform rash may follow treatment with ampicillin and the related amoxycillin, bacampicillin, and pivampicillin. It is more likely to occur in patients with glandular fever (infectious mononucleosis), and chronic lymphatic leukaemia. It is not regarded as a true penicillin allergy in such patients. The Stevens–Johnson syndrome (erythema multiforme) is a much more serious skin reaction with blistering and mucosal lesions.

A few drugs occasionally cause photosensitivity, an abnormal skin reaction associated with exposure to light. Drugs known to cause photosensitivity include the tetracyclines, nalidixic acid, phenothiazines and chloroquine. Care should be taken to avoid sunlight, particularly at midday, and to use a sun-screen preparation that is effective against the entire ultraviolet spectrum (p. 263).

DRUG INTERACTIONS

When patients take more than one drug at a time, there is always a risk that those drugs may interact with each other. Absorption may be inhibited, as when iron salts and antacids form insoluble complexes in the gastrointestinal tract with tetracyclines, and cholestyramine similarly reduces the absorption of digoxin and warfarin by the formation of an insoluble complex. In other cases, the administration of two or more drugs which use the same carrier protein (p. 4) may lead to an increase in effect,

sometimes with potentially serious consequences. The monoamine oxidase inhibitors, by preventing the breakdown of endogenous pressor amines such as noradrenaline, potentiate the action of pressor drugs. They also inhibit the metabolism of tyramine, an amino acid present in cheese, broad beans, yeast and red wine. If taken in quantity, such foods permit larger amounts of tyramine to reach the circulation and stimulate the release of adrenaline and noradrenaline, precipitating a severe hypertensive episode that may be fatal (p. 38).

Very occasionally a drug reaction can be exploited. Disulfiram is sometimes used in the treatment of alcoholism, as if it is given in association with even a small amount of alcohol it causes nausea and vomiting, the so-called disulfiram or Antabuse reaction, which discourages further intake of alcohol. It should be noted that a similar reaction may occur if alcohol is taken with drugs such as metronidazole and cephamandole. A more specific enzyme-associated reaction that is of clinical value is the inhibition of xanthine oxidase by allopurinol, which is used in the treatment of gout (p. 210). It is worth bearing in mind that occasionally a reaction has been traced to a herbal medicine that the patient has been taking in addition to the prescribed drugs or even an illicit drug.

Appendix I gives some notes on drug interactions, but the range is so wide that the list is far from being exhaustive, and some reactions are rare. It should be noted that if a reaction occurs with one type of drug, a similar reaction may occur with other drugs of the same type, e.g. clofibrate potentiates the action of oral anticoagulants, and a similar potentiation may occur with related hypolipidaemic agents.

THE DEVELOPMENT OF NEW DRUGS

The search for new and better drugs is a continuous but very expensive process, as less than 0.05% of new compounds screened for potential activity ever reach the market. In the past, new drugs have been obtained from plants, microorganisms or by chemical synthesis, but with increasing knowledge of molecular biology and computor techniques, drug development is becoming more selective and directed towards the production of drugs designed for more specific purposes.

New drugs that show any potential activity are first studied in animals, following which permission for clinical trials must be obtained from the Committee on Safety of Medicines. Phase I trials involve giving the drug to young male volunteers in initially very small doses, which are slowly increased if tolerated to a level that produces a detectable effect. If Phase I trials are satisfactory, Phase II trials are commenced with a small number of patients to evaluate the potential therapeutic effects, dose range and toxicity. If the results of such trials are acceptable, Phase III trials are set up, involving larger and more varied groups of patients for 6–12 months, during which comparative trials with a placebo or another drug are carried out. Only after those rigorous trials are Phase IV studies carried out when the drug is marketed. Even at that late stage some hitherto unsuspected side-effects may reveal themselves, occasionally severe enough to demand withdrawal of the drug, which explains in part why all new drugs are expensive. In these later-stage trials nurses can play a very important part in reporting any unusual side-effects that may occur, as they are in much closer contact with patients than is the investigating doctor. The Committee on Safety of Medicines keeps most new drugs under very close surveillance for some time, and requires any adverse reactions to be reported on the 'Yellow Cards' provided by that Committee. Those drugs currently under such surveillance are indicated by an inverted black triangle thus ▼.

Presentation of drugs and patient compliance

There are three main stages in the treatment of illness: diagnosis, the supply of drug and compliance by the patient with treatment. Yet patients often fail to collect their prescribed medicines, and some who collect them do not take them; so unless patients comply with treatment, diagnosis and drug supply are virtually an expensive waste of time and money.

Nurses can help by educating patients in the importance of treatment; tactful questioning may reveal non-compliance, and much has been done by manufacturers to increase the acceptability of drugs by improvements in presentation. The main point about drug presentation is that whatever method is used, the activity of the drug must be maintained, and successful formulation requires a wide knowledge of the chemistry, pharmacology, solubility and stability of drugs. Even the choice of a suitable container is of considerable importance in ensuring that a product will retain its stability and therapeutic activity.

The extent to which an active drug reaches the circulation is termed its bio-availability. Bio-availability is linked with drug formulation, and there can be marked differences in the bio-availability between different preparations of the same drug. It must not be assumed that apparently similar medicinal products are interchangeable even though they may contain the same amount of the drug. They are interchangeable sometimes, but if there is any doubt the pharmacist should be consulted.

Many preparations of drugs now on the market exhibit considerable ingenuity in the means employed to increase acceptability or prolong the action of the drug, but basically the preparations of drugs used in therapeutics can be divided into five main groups; i.e. oral preparations, inhalations, injections, rectal preparations and skin applications. Examples of most forms of presentation will be found in the British National Formulary (BNF).

Oral preparations

Tablets. One of the most convenient and acceptable forms of oral medication. They have the great advantage over liquid medicines of affording an accurate dose. A few tablets, notably those containing glyceryl trinitrate, are designed to be placed under the tongue, to promote the absorption and avoid first-pass metabolism. Many tablets are coated to improve stability and appearance, and contain additives to ensure disintegration and absorption in the intestinal tract.

In cases where the drug is a gastric irritant or is broken down by gastric acid, tablets may have an 'enteric' coating. Such coating is designed to permit tablets to pass unchanged into the intestine. Some long-acting tablets contain the drug in the interstices of a porous plastic core, from which the active compound is slowly leached out as the tablet passes along the alimentary tract. It should *not* be assumed that these different sustained-action tablets, although containing the same amount of drug, will all release the drug at the same rate, or that they are interchangeable, as different formulations may be used by different manufacturers.

Nurses should always advise patients to take tablets (and capsules) in a standing or sitting position, and with adequate fluid to avoid delay in oesophageal transit. Such delay may cause oesophageal damage, as has occurred with some non-steroidal anti-inflammatory drugs, with slow-release potassium preparations, and with other drugs including some antibiotics. Nurses should also warn patients that long-acting tablet products should be swallowed whole, not chewed or divided by cutting, otherwise the extended action of the product will be lost. Some standard tablet products, on the other hand, have a 'split line' to facilitate the administration of divided doses. They are also useful on occasions when a tablet to be taken, for example, twice a day causes gastrointestinal or other disturbances. Half a tablet taken four times a day may be better tolerated.

Capsules Small cylindrical containers made of hard gelatin. They are useful as a means of administering bitter drugs, and are popular as containers for orally active antibiotics. Flexible gelatin capsules are also used occasionally, particularly for small doses of unpleasant liquids such as chlormethiazole. Capsules should be swallowed whole, with water, and no attempt should be made to open or split a capsule. Most capsules are sealed to prevent such manipulation.

Mixtures Mixtures are aqueous solutions or suspensions of drugs in water, together with flavouring or suspending agents. Kaolin and Morphine Mixture BNF is a familiar example, and the bottle should be well shaken before measuring a dose to make sure that the contents are well dispersed. Mixtures were once the most popular form of drug presentation, but have been largely replaced by tablets and capsules.

Elixirs and syrups Flavoured and sweetened solutions or suspensions of drugs, often suitable for administration in small doses to children. Some oral antibiotic products are presented as elixirs or syrups.

Emulsion A term applied to mixtures of oils and water, rendered homogeneous by the addition of other substances known as emulsifying agents. Liquid Paraffin Emulsion is an example of an oil-in-water emulsion and contains methyl cellulose as the emulsifying agent.

Linctus A sweet, syrupy preparation of a drug used in the treatment of cough, e.g. Pholcodine Linctus.

Inhalations

The area of lung surface available for drug absorption is so large that the response may be almost as rapid as that following an injection, making this a valuable route for the administration of general anaesthetics and some other drugs.

Modern oral aerosol inhalers contain the drug in a metered-dose pressurized container, with an inert gas as the propellant. The drug is discharged as a very fine spray, which if inhaled orally is carried deep into the lungs. Aerosols allow the administration of drugs such as bronchodilators and corticosteroids in a form that permits fast absorption, allowing the patient to give himself a dose at a time of need when a rapid response is essential. A further

major advantage, especially in the case of corticosteroids, is that the drug is administered directly to where it is needed, reducing dose requirements and minimizing systemic effects.

The effectiveness of aerosols depends on the patient being taught the correct technique, and inadequate control of asthmatic states is often due to poor inhalation technique, including on occasion failure by the patient to remove the cap from the inhaler! Fig. 1.3 demonstrates the technique for one form of inhaler. It is part of the nurse's role to become aware of the different inhalers on the market and teach patients their correct usage. The effectiveness of inhalers can be markedly improved by the combined use of aerosol 'large volume spacers'. These spacers increase the amount of drug reaching the airways and at the same time reduce the dosage lost by systemic absorption. They are particularly useful for children where coordination between the release of a dose and the act of inhalation is poor. A problem with bronchodilator aerosols is overdosage, and possible cardiac stimulation that may occur if repeated doses are inhaled too frequently by over-anxious patients. Nurses must make patients aware of these dangers.

The term 'inhalation' also refers to the steam inhalation of the volatile constituents of such products as Compound Tincture of Benzoin, produced when a small amount of product is mixed with very hot water, as in a Nelson's inhaler. The method is used to relieve nasal congestion and aid expectoration by liquefying sputum. Care must be taken to ensure that patients are protected from burning themselves with the hot water.

Calcitonin and the anti-migraine drug sumatriptan are available as intranasal sprays.

Injections

An injection is a sterile solution or suspension of a drug intended for parenteral administration by intramuscular, subcutaneous or intravenous injection, or less frequently by intra-articular, intrathecal, subconjunctival or intradermal injection. The intramuscular route is employed for most injections, as absorption is fairly rapid and even potentially irritant solutions of drugs may be tolerated by this route.

The rate of response to an injection can sometimes be modified as the addition of adrenaline to local anaesthetic solutions such as lignocaine delays absorption and extends the action by constricting adjacent blood vessels, and an extended action can occasionally be obtained by injecting the drug as an oily solution. (*Oily solutions must always be given by*

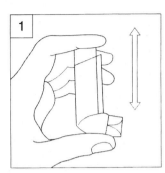

Remove the cover from the mouthpiece and shake the inhaler vigorously.

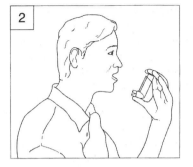

Holding the inhaler as shown, breathe out gently (but not fully) and then immediately...

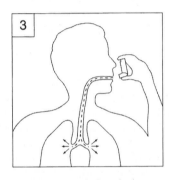

Place the mouthpiece in the mouth and close your lips around it. After starting to breathe in slowly and deeply through your mouth, press the inhaler firmly, as shown, to release Ventolin and continue to breathe in.

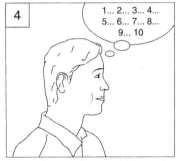

Hold your breath for 10 seconds, or as long as is comfortable, before breathing out slowly.

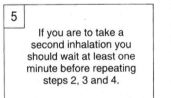

If you are to take a second inhalation you should wait at least one minute before repeating steps 2, 3 and 4.

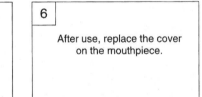

After use, replace the cover on the mouthpiece.

Figure 1.3 Diagram to indicate the use of an aerosol inhaler. (Reproduced by kind permission of Allen and Hanburys Limited, Greenford.)

intramuscular injection.) In other cases, a greatly prolonged action can be obtained from a depot injection containing the drug in a chemically modified and less soluble form. Fluphenazine decanoate, for example, which is used in chronic schizophrenia, has a long action that permits dosing at intervals of 4–6 weeks.

The intravenous route has the advantage of evoking an immediate response, and if there are any side-effects, treatment can be stopped immediately. Drugs that are too irritant to be given by intramuscular injection can often be given in dilute solution by slow intravenous infusion, as with some cytotoxic agents. However, care must be taken not to give any intravenous injection too rapidly as a reaction may be provoked; irritant solutions may cause venous thrombosis, and infection and phlebitis are potential hazards.

Subcutaneous injection has the advantage of being suitable for the self-administration of drugs, insulin being a familiar example. It is less suitable for irritant drugs as the injection may be painful, and in shock the absorption of drugs given subcutaneously is poor. Repeated injections at the same site may cause lipo-atrophy, resulting in erratic absorption. Some vaccines are given by subcutaneous injection. Intrathecal injection is used occasionally when the drug concerned does not pass the blood–brain barrier and direct injection into the cerebrospinal fluid is necessary, as in the treatment of meningitis. Intra-articular injection refers to the injection of a drug into a joint. In ophthalmology, a few drugs are given by subconjunctival injection. Intradermal injection is used mainly for diagnostic purposes.

Injections are best supplied as ampoules, which are sealed glass containers containing a single dose. Multiple-dose containers are also used but are less satisfactory. All solutions supplied in multiple-dose containers must contain a preservative to guard against the risk of accidental bacterial contamination of the contents.

Rectal preparations

The rectal route of administration of drugs remains largely unexploited, although the rectal mucosa has a rich blood supply and first-pass metabolism is largely avoided. The method provides a useful route when oral therapy is not tolerated, as during nausea and vomiting, and also in unconscious patients. However, absorption may be unreliable if the rectum is not empty.

Suppositories   Solid products, torpedo or cone-shaped, for rectal administration. They contain an active drug in a base that melts at body temperature. As absorption from the rectal mucosa is slow, the contained drug has an extended action. Indomethacin suppositories, for example, are used at night to reduce morning stiffness in arthritic patients. Glycerin (glycerol) suppositories on the other hand have a simple laxative action and are used in the treatment of constipation. Pessaries, or vaginal suppositories, are formulated to have a local effect on the vaginal tract. Suppositories are normally inserted via the pointed end, but it has been suggested that retention is more certain if the blunt end is inserted first. Also some patients need to be told to remove the wrapper before insertion.

Enemas   Solutions administered per rectum as laxatives or retention enemas. Laxative enemas include soft soap solution, now used infrequently, and sodium phosphate or magnesium sulphate solutions. These solutions are available as prepacked disposable products, and have a laxative effect by distending the bowel. Oxyphenisatin and docusate sodium enemas are used mainly for bowel clearance before radiological examination or surgery.

Retention enemas include arachis oil for softening impacted faeces; magnesium sulphate is occasionally used to increase the water content of the bowel to produce a temporary lowering of intracranial pressure; prednisolone and salazopyrin are used to reduce inflammation in ulcerative colitis.

Skin preparations

Many preparations for application to the skin have a local or protective action. The skin is not an inert barrier and has a multilayer structure, and some locally applied drugs, such as some anti-inflammatory corticosteroids, are taken up by the stratum corneum, from which slow diffusion of the drug into the lower layers of the skin takes place. Systemic effects from such locally applied steroids are not common, but may occur if large areas of inflamed skin are so treated, or if occlusive dressings are used. In such cases significant amounts of the drug may reach the circulation via the dermal capillaries to cause systemic side-effects, particularly where children are concerned due to their more delicate skin.

On the other hand, the value of the skin as a means of drug administration, which in the past has been largely overlooked, is now being exploited, as shown by the development of skin patches for transdermal medication. Patches are available containing glyceryl trinitrate for the treatment of angina, oestradiol for hormone replacement therapy, fentanyl for pain control, hyoscine for motion sickness, clonidine for hypertension, and nicotine to assist those who wish to give up smoking. These patches usually contain the drug in a reservoir with a rate-controlling membrane (Fig. 1.4) releasing the drug at a steady rate, and so avoiding both gastric breakdown and first-pass metabolism. They are, however, an expensive form of treatment, and suitable only for lipid-soluble drugs of low molecular weight.

Conventional products for application to the skin can be divided into the following main groups.

Creams   These are semi-solid emulsions, and differ from ointments in containing a higher proportion of water, for example Aqueous Cream and Hydrocortisone Cream.

Liniments   Thin creams or oily preparations of drugs intended for application to the skin to relieve

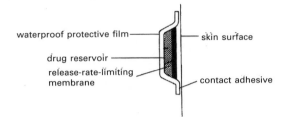

Figure 1.4 Diagram of glyceryl trinitrate skin patch.

mild pain, as pain can be relieved to some extent by rubbing the skin with a mildly irritant product. A number of proprietary products for the relief of rheumatic and other pain are formulated on that basis.

Lotions Solutions or suspensions (shake lotions) of drugs for application to the skin, wounds or mucous membranes, e.g. Calamine Lotion and Aluminium Acetate Lotion.

Ointments Semi-solid preparations mainly used for application to dry skin lesions. Most ointment bases contain soft paraffin, often with other agents such as emulsifying waxes or wool fat. Wool fat, also known as lanolin, may cause a sensitivity reaction in some patients.

Pastes Stiff ointments, often containing a large amount of zinc oxide, e.g. Zinc Oxide and Salicylic Acid Paste.

Liposomes

New or more effective ways of administering drugs are under investigation as alternatives to conventional therapy, and one of these developments is the use of liposomes. These are minute vesicles, bounded by layers of phospholipids or glycolipids and containing small quantities of drugs. When injected, liposomes accumulate at sites of inflammation and infection, in the liver and spleen, as well as in some solid tumours. Liposomes thus provide a method of targeting drug delivery, allowing smaller doses of drug to be used, with decreased toxicity and rapid degradation. Liposome-encapsulated antimony has been used to treat visceral leishmaniasis, while liposomes containing cytotoxic drugs such doxorubicin, cisplatin, and methotrexate are being evaluated in cancer treatment. Liposome-entrapped corticosteroids have been used in intra-articular injection in the treatment of rheumatoid arthritis, and the method has been adopted for the presentation of amphotericin in the treatment of fungal infections (p. 82) resulting in a less nephrotoxic and better tolerated formulation. In the future it may be possible to target liposomes even more specifically by incorporating antibodies against specific tissue antigens onto their surface.

FURTHER READING

Cameron K, Gregor F 1987 Chronic illness and compliance. Journal of Advanced Nursing 12:671–676

Channer K S, Virjee J 1992 Effects of posture and drink volume on the swallowing of capsules. British Medical Journal 285:1702

Corlett A J 1996 Aids to compliance with medication. British Medical Journal 313:926–929

Edwards I R 1997 Adverse drug reactions: finding the needle in the haystack. British Medical Journal 315:500

Ernst M A, Buchanan A, Cox C 1991 Drug errors. Nursing Times 87(14):26–30

George C F 1984 Food, drugs and bioavailability. British Medical Journal 289:1093

Griffith S A 1990 A review of the factors associated with patient compliance and the taking of prescribed medicines. British Journal of General Practice 40:114–116

Jordan S, Torrance C 1995 Bionursing: explaining falls in elderly people. Nursing Standard 9(50):30–32

Kelly J 1994 Understanding transdermal medication. Professional Nurse 10(2):121–125

Kmietowicz Z 1990 Timing of ulcer drug is vital. General Practitioner Mar 2:16

Mathieson A 1986 Old people and drugs. Nursing Times 88(2):22

Nathan A 1992 Interactions between prescribed medicines and over-the-counter medication. Pharmaceutical Journal 246:428–432

Pfister-Minogue K 1993 Enhancing patient compliance: a guide for nurses. Geriatric Nursing May/June:124–132

Rajaei-Dehkordi Z, McPherson G 1997 The effects of multiple medication in the elderly. Nursing Times 93(27):56–58

Smith F, Ross F 1992 Nurse prescribing: principles of drug therapy. Community Outlook 2(2):25–29

Stephenson R P 1956 Receptor theory. British Journal of Pharmacology 11:379–393

Stockwell Morris L, Schulz R 1992 Patient compliance – an overview. Journal of Clinical Pharmacy and Therapeutics 17:283–295

Sundaram B 1995 Tackling the aftermath faced by the daughters of DES. Nursing Times 91(33):34–35

Tettersell M J 1993 Asthma patients' knowledge in relation to compliance with drug therapy. Journal of Advanced Nursing 18:103–113

Torrance C 1989 Intramuscular Injection. Surgical Nurse 2(6):24–27

Torrance C, Jordan S 1995 Bionursing: the role of hepatic enzymes. Nursing Standard 10(8):31–33

Walker R 1992 The correct insertion of rectal suppositories. British Journal of Pharmaceutical Practice 4:8–10

2

Sedatives, hypnotics and anaesthetics

Drugs which depress some part of the central nervous system (CNS) represent one of the largest and most important groups of therapeutic agents. They include hypnotics, sedatives, tranquillizers, antidepressants, anticonvulsants, narcotics, anaesthetics and analgesics. This chapter deals with sedatives, hypnotics and anaesthetics. Other drugs acting on the CNS are dealt with in Chapter 3.

SEDATIVES AND HYPNOTICS

Sedatives, now often referred to as anxiolytics, are drugs that reduce mental activity and thus predispose to sleep, whereas hypnotics are sleep-inducing drugs. The mode of action of drugs that depress the central nervous system, and so have a sedative or hypnotic action, is highly complex and not clearly understood. It is thought that they act on the reticular formation, the limbic system and the cortex, which are in communication (Fig. 2.1). The reticular formation receives information from the limbic system and passes it on to the cortex, which is the highest functional area of the brain and is concerned with the interpretation of sensory information, motor activity and higher mental activity including reasoning, creative thought and memory.

Sedatives and hypnotics are in general unspecific depressants of the CNS although the benzodiazepines appear to act by preventing the limbic system from activating the reticular formation. Some other drugs interact directly with the cerebral cortex via the inhibitory neurotransmitter gamma-aminobutyric acid (GABA, pp. 19, 40). They are widely used in the treatment of insomnia due to anxiety and stress, but before they are given it should be remembered that simple measures, such as adequate physical relaxation and

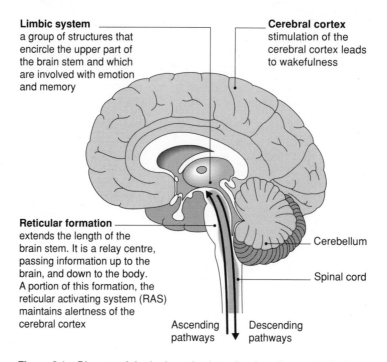

Limbic system — a group of structures that encircle the upper part of the brain stem and which are involved with emotion and memory

Cerebral cortex stimulation of the cerebral cortex leads to wakefulness

Reticular formation — extends the length of the brain stem. It is a relay centre, passing information up to the brain, and down to the body. A portion of this formation, the reticular activating system (RAS) maintains alertness of the cerebral cortex

Cerebellum

Spinal cord

Ascending pathways

Descending pathways

Figure 2.1 Diagram of the brain and points of action of some CNS depressants. Sedatives and hypnotics may act on the reticular activating system, the limbic system and the cerebral cortex.

absence of stimulants will often promote sleep. Many drugs can cause sleep disturbances, for example, most beta-blockers and steroids. In some cases, such side-effects may be reduced by avoiding evening administration. Experienced nurses are often in a better position to assess a patient's need for sedation than is the visiting doctor.

It should be appreciated that although drug-induced sleep may appear to resemble natural sleep, the two are far from being identical, and no currently available drug can induce normal sleep. Natural sleep has two main phases, referred to as the orthodox or slow-wave phase, and the paradoxical or REM (rapid eye movement) phase in which dreaming occurs. Hypnotic drugs may suppress the REM phase, and also influence the orthodox phase. The latter plays an important part in the growth and restoration of body tissues, but the REM phase is linked with the restorative activities of brain tissue.

Both sedatives and hypnotics should be regarded as drugs for short-term treatment only and should not be given indiscriminately. They may cause confusion in the elderly, who are more susceptible to the action of such drugs, and whenever possible the cause of the anxiety and insomnia should be sought.

Insomnia is often associated with depression, and treatment of the depression may indirectly relieve the insomnia. Similarly, when insomnia is due to pain, hypnotics are virtually useless if the pain is not relieved.

Drug dependence

Sedatives and hypnotics may cause drug dependence with extended use. The condition is such that the patient has a strong desire to continue taking the drug, often in increasing doses, and severe withdrawal symptoms occur if treatment is stopped abruptly. Such symptoms include apprehension, anxiety, dizziness, tremor, tachycardia and insomnia. Later symptoms include hallucinations.

BENZODIAZEPINES

The benzodiazepines (BDZs) are a widely used group of drugs as, depending on the particular drug and the dose, they can act as anxiolytics, hypnotics, tranquillizers, anticonvulsants and muscle relaxants (see diazepam, p. 32). As a group, the BDZs have a wide margin of safety with few side-effects, and they

Nursing points about hypnotics

(a) Hypnotics should normally be given about 30 minutes before going to bed to give time for absorption. The exceptions are zolpidem, which has a rapid action and is taken immediately before retiring, and the antihistamines diphenhydramine and promethazine. Their onset of action is slow, and they should be given about 2 hours before retiring.
(b) Low initial doses, especially in the elderly.
(c) Treatment should be limited to 2–3 weeks, and preferably intermittent, as on alternate nights or one night in three.
(d) The onset of drug-induced sleep may be followed by a deterioration of a patient's condition.
(e) If dependence has occurred, withdrawal must be carried out slowly to avoid the sudden onset of withdrawal symptoms.

are regarded as first-choice drugs for the short-term treatment of insomnia.

Benzodiazepines act by interacting with the inhibitory neurotransmitter gamma-aminobutyric acid (GABA), which is found almost exclusively in the CNS. The GABA receptors occur in and are coupled with chloride channels (Fig. 2.2), and when GABA is released from the presynaptic neurone, it binds with receptors, causing the chloride channel to open briefly and allowing an influx of chloride ions into the cell. The postsynaptic neurone is consequently hyperpolarized and unable to fire in response to stimulation from other nervous pathways. The action of GABA at the 'primary receptor' is also linked with the binding of benzodiazepines or barbiturates at 'secondary receptors' on the receptor complex. Binding of benzodiazepines increases the frequency of channel opening in response to a given GABA stimulus, while barbiturates increase channel opening time, both leading to a greater influx of chloride ions and greater inhibition of neuronal response.

Those BDZs listed in Table 2.1 exhibit a range of hypnotic activity, as some have a short action and are therefore of less value when early awakening is a problem, and others have a long action and so may cause some daytime sedation. Car-driving ability and similar activities may be impaired. The BDZs have few side-effects, but they occasionally cause a paradoxical response with varying degrees of excite-

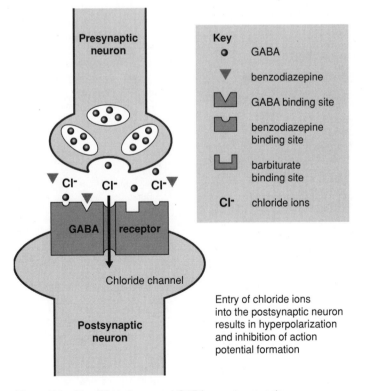

Figure 2.2 Simplified diagram of GABA receptor complex.

Table 2.1 Benzodiazepine hypnotics

Approved name	Brand name	Dose
flunitrazepam[b]	Rohypnol	0.5–1 mg
flurazepam[b]	Dalmane	15–30 mg
loprazolam[a]	Dormonoct	1–2 mg
lormetazepam[a]		0.5–1 mg
nitrazepam[b]	Mogadon	5–10 mg
temazepam	Normisan	10–20 mg

[a] Short-acting hypnotics.
[b] Long-acting hypnotics.

ment and aggression. They do not induce the production of microsomal enzymes in the liver and so interactions with other drugs are less likely. Dependence on the BDZs is a risk and they should not be used continuously for more than four weeks.

Withdrawal symptoms may occur with any BDZ, but they are more common after extended treatment, or after high doses, and they result in a syndrome of rebound insomnia, anxiety, tremor and loss of appetite. Rapid withdrawal should be avoided, as a toxic psychosis with convulsions may be precipitated.

The use of benzodiazepines and other supplementary agents in anxiety and tension states is referred to on page 32.

Nursing points about benzodiazepines

(a) Normally for short-term treatment only.
(b) Drowsiness is a side-effect – warn patients about car-driving.
(c) Alcohol may have additive effects and should be avoided.
(d) Withdrawal of treatment should be slow.

Nitrazepam § (dose: 5–10 mg)

Brand name: Mogadon §
Nitrazepam is a long-acting benzodiazepine hypnotic used mainly when some degree of daytime sedation is tolerated. Induction of sleep begins within 30 minutes, and any subsequent arousal and return to sleep tends to follow a natural pattern. Nitrazepam is given in doses of 5–10 mg, but the smaller doses should be used in the elderly.

Side-effects include hangover, dreaming with nightmares and, paradoxically, agitation and aggression have been noted with some patients. As with all benzodiazepines, care is necessary in respiratory disease and in renal or hepatic impairment.

Temazepam § (dose: 10–30 mg)

Brand name: Normison §
Temazepam is a short-acting benzodiazepine hypnotic of value in the elderly, to whom doses of 5–15 mg should be given. Cumulative effects in standard doses are not common, but some daytime sedation may occur if high doses are given for severe insomnia.

Benzodiazepine antagonist:

Flumazenil § (dose: 100–400 microgram by intravenous infusion)

Brand name: Anexate §
Some benzodiazepines are used for their sedative effects in intensive care units, and also as supplementary agents in anaesthesia. The subsequent reversal of those effects is often desirable, and a benzodiazepine antagonist for that purpose is flumazenil. It acts as a competitive inhibitor at BDZ-receptor binding sites, and following intravenous injection it brings about a rapid reversal of the hypno-sedative effects of the benzodiazepines, and a return of spontaneous respiration and consciousness in anaethesized patients.

The use of flumazenil requires care, as the action of the drug is relatively brief and the sedative effects of the benzodiazepine may return within a few hours, when further flumazenil treatment may be required. Flumazenil is given by slow intravenous injection or infusion in an initial dose of 200 micrograms, followed by 100 microgram doses at 1 minute intervals as required. If drowsiness recurs, further doses of 100–400 micrograms hourly should be given, adjusted to individual need and response. Care should be taken not to arouse patients too rapidly, as they may become agitated. It is contra-indicated in epileptics who have received extended treatment with a benzodiazepine.

OTHER HYPNOTICS AND SEDATIVES
Chloral hydrate § (dose: 0.5–2 g)

Brand name: Noctec §
Chloral hydrate is an old drug that is useful when a mild and safe hypnotic is required. It is rapidly absorbed and metabolized to trichloroethanol, to which the sedative action is finally due. It may be given as Chloral Mixture (500 mg/5 ml) in doses of 5–20 ml, but as chloral hydrate has some gastric irritant properties, the mixture should be well diluted with water. The mixture may be given to children of

6–12 years in doses of 5–10 ml. Chloral is a useful sedative for infants, and may be given as Chloral Elixir Paediatric in doses of 5 ml (well diluted) to infants up to 1 year of age. Chloral hydrate cannot be formulated as a tablet, but it forms a stable complex with betaine, which is present in Welldorm tablets, each equivalent to 414 mg of chloral. The compound breaks down rapidly in the stomach to release the active drug. A derivative of trichloroethanol is also available as Triclofos Elixir (500 mg/5 ml).

Chlormethiazole § (dose: 192–384 mg)

Brand name: Heminevrin §
Chlormethiazole is a short-acting hypnotic of value in the elderly, especially when some agitation is present, as it has little hangover action. It is given in doses of 192–384 mg as capsules or syrup at night, and doses of 192 mg may be given three times a day for restlessness, agitation and confusional states. Dependence may occur with extended treatment.

Chlormethiazole is also used under hospital control to treat acute withdrawal symptoms in alcoholics. Such treatment requires care, and resuscitation facilities must be available, as severe respiratory depression may occur.

Chlormethiazole is also used intravenously in the treatment of status epilepticus (p. 41).

Side-effects of the drug include sneezing, headache and gastrointestinal disturbance.

Paraldehyde (dose: 5–10 ml, well diluted)

Paraldehyde is a colourless liquid with a characteristic odour. It has been used as a hypnotic in doses of 5–10 ml, but it is now used mainly in status epilepticus (p. 42).

Promethazine (dose: 25–75 mg)

Brand names: Phenergan, Sominex
Some antihistamines, of which promethazine is an example, have a sedative action of value in mild insomnia, and are useful in reduced doses for daytime sedation.

Promethazine is given in doses up to 50 mg at night for mild insomnia in adults. It is also useful as a hypnotic for children in doses of 15–20 mg for those of 1–5 years of age, and 20–25 mg for the 5–10 year group.

Side-effects such as dry mouth and blurred vision are those of the antihistamines in general (p. 231). An older antihistamine is diphenhydramine (Nytol) also used for mild sleep disturbances. Dose 25–50 mg.

Trimeprazine § (dose: 3–4.5 mg/kg)

Brand name: Vallergan §
Trimeprazine has an action similar to that of promethazine, although it is used mainly in the relief of pruritus (p. 259). It is also useful as a pre-operative sedative for both adults and children, given $1\frac{1}{2}$–2 hours before operation.

Dose: 3–4.5 mg/kg; children 2–4 mg/kg.

Zolpidem § (dose: 10 mg)

Brand name: Stilnoct §
Zolpidem, although not a benzodiazepine, acts on BDZ-receptors, and so has a BDZ-like action in the treatment of insomnia. It has a rapid action and is given in doses of 10 mg at bedtime; half doses for the elderly.

Side-effects are dizziness and diarrhoea.

Zopiclone § (dose: 7.5–15 mg)

Brand name: Zimovane §
Zopiclone has the actions and uses of zolpidem and is used for the short-term treatment of insomnia, including early awakening, and for the insomnia secondary to psychiatric disturbances. It initiates sleep rapidly, does not reduce REM sleep, and has little residual hangover action. It is given in doses of 7.5–15 mg at night, with initial doses of 3.75 mg for the elderly.

Side-effects of zopiclone are similar to those of many hypnotics, but are usually less common, the most frequent being a bitter or metallic after-taste.

BARBITURATES

The barbiturates were once used extensively as sedatives and hypnotics, but their use has declined markedly with the introduction of the safer benzodiazepines. They are still used to a limited extent in severe and intractable insomnia, although some physicians consider that they have no place in modern therapeutics. Tolerance and dependence may develop quickly, and they should not be given to the elderly. Death has occurred from barbiturate–alcohol induced respiratory depression. Table 2.2 indicates the few in current use; prescriptions must comply with the Misuse of Drugs (CD) Regulations.

MELATONIN

Melatonin is a substance produced by the pineal gland, and may be linked in some way with the

Table 2.2 Barbiturates

Approved name	Brand name	Dose
amylobarbitone	Amytal	100–200 mg
amylobarbitone sodium	Sodium Amytal	100–200 mg
butobarbitone	Soneryl	100–200 mg
quinalbarbitone sodium	Seconal Sodium	100–200 mg
amylobarbitone sodium quinalbarbitone sodium }	Tuinal	100–200 mg

sleep–wake cycle. It is known that the melatonin concentration in the circulation decreases with age, and it has been suggested that there is a relationship between a deficiency of melatonin and an increased prevalence of sleep disorders with advancing age. If that is the case, melatonin replacement therapy may in time prove to be a new approach to the insomnia of age. At present there is no melatonin product marketed in the UK, and it is mentioned here merely as a possible indication of a future development of some interest.

GENERAL ANAESTHETICS

Although general anaesthetics vary chemically from simple gases to complex organic molecules, they can be divided simply into those given by inhalation and those given by intravenous injection. Exactly how they act is not entirely clear, but they depress all excitable tissues including the CNS, cardiac, smooth and striated muscle. Different tissues have different sensitivities to anaesthetics and areas of the brain responsible for consciousness, such as the reticular formation, are among the most sensitive.

The requirements of general anaesthesia for surgical purposes are unconsciousness, analgesia, muscle relaxation, and the maintenance of physiological stability. There is no one anaesthetic agent which will produce all those effects, so anaesthesia usually involves the use of a combination of drugs. In practice anaesthesia is often induced by an intravenous drug, and maintained by an inhalation anaesthetic, together with a muscle relaxant and other supplementary drugs.

When an anaesthetic is given on its own, certain well defined stages are passed through as the concentration of the drug in the blood increases. In Stage I (analgesia) the patient is conscious but drowsy and detached, and the response to painful stimuli is markedly reduced. In Stage II (excitement) consciousness is lost, but the patient may move, talk incoher-

ently, hold his breath or choke. It is a dangerous state but is less common with intravenous anaesthetics. In Stage III (surgical anaesthesia) the irregular breathing of Stage II becomes steady, reflexes are abolished and a progressive muscular relaxation occurs as anaesthesia deepens. The depth of anaesthesia is controlled according to surgical needs.

The speed of induction and elimination of anaesthesia varies with the nature of the anaesthetic. A slow induction occurs when a volatile drug such as either is absorbed into the blood from the alveolar spaces, as subsequent diffusion into the CNS is secondary to the saturation of the blood with anaesthetic. Injected anaesthetics enter the brain by crossing the blood–brain barrier. The ability to cross that barrier is dependent on lipid solubility, and hence the potency of an anaesthetic is linked with its lipid solubility. Recovery from anaesthesia takes place as the concentration of the drug falls as it is temporarily taken up by body tissues, especially fat, for subsequent elimination. Recovery from a highly lipid-soluble anaesthetic such as halothane is correspondingly delayed as the fat acts as a reservoir from which the anaesthetic is slowly released, resulting in hangover effects.

Before the introduction of muscle relaxants, adequate relaxation could be achieved only by full anaesthesia, with undesired toxic side-effects. Now, by suitable premedication and the use of relaxants, a relatively light plane of anaesthesia is often adequate, thus reducing cardiac depression and dysrhythmias and enabling major operations to be carried out in the elderly that were once considered impossible. In all cases, before general anaesthesia is carried out, the effects of any drugs that the patient may already be receiving should be reviewed.

A rare but very serious occurrence during inhalation anaesthesia is malignant hyperthermia or hyperpyrexia. It appears to be triggered off in susceptible patients by anaesthetic drugs, usually halothane and suxamethonium. It is a genetically determined condition, linked with a sudden increase in the concentration of calcium in muscle cells. Early tachycardia with hyperventilation may occur, followed by skeletal muscle rigidity and hyperthermia. Pulmonary oedema and renal failure are later symptoms.

The specific therapy is the intravenous injection of the skeletal muscle relaxant dantrolene, which inhibits calcium movement in muscle cells and brings about muscle relaxation, a reduction of the raised body temperature and a decrease in heart rate. Treatment should be commenced immediately the syndrome is diagnosed with the intravenous injection of dantrolene sodium in a dose of 1 mg/kg, repeated according to response up to an average total dose of 2.5 mg/kg, although total doses of up to 10 mg/kg have been given. Care must be taken to avoid extravasation.

INHALATION ANAESTHETICS

Chloroform

A clear heavy liquid with a characteristic odour. It is of historical interest as one of the first inhalation anaesthetics.

Cyclopropane

Cyclopropane is an inflammable gas supplied in orange-coloured cylinders. It is a non-irritant, volatile anaesthetic, for use in closed-circuit apparatus as it forms an explosive mixture with air and oxygen. It is used mainly for induction. Cyclopropane causes little hypotension, and recovery is rapid.

Ether (diethylether)

A clear, colourless, inflammable liquid. Like chloroform, it is now of historical interest and is rarely used except in those countries where its low cost is an advantage.

Halothane

Brand name: Fluothane
A clear, colourless, liquid volatile anaesthetic of high potency with which induction is smooth and rapid and the incidence of postoperative vomiting low. Severe liver dysfunction and jaundice have occasionally followed halothane anaesthesia, and it should not be given to patients with liver damage. Repeated exposure within 3 months should be avoided, and halothane should never again be given to a patient who has had unexplained jaundice or pyrexia after halothane anaesthesia.

Enflurane

Enflurane is a widely used volatile anaesthetic of the halothane type. It has the advantage of causing less hepatotoxicity, as it largely escapes metabolism, so, unlike halothane, it can be used when repeated anaesthesia is required. It is usually given in association with nitrous oxide–oxygen anaesthesia from a calibrated vaporizer. Enflurane may cause some respiratory depression, but side-effects such as ventricular dysrhythmias are uncommon. Desflurane § (Suprane §), isoflurane § and sevoflurane § have similar properties and uses.

Nitrous oxide

The oldest and safest of the inhalation anaesthetics. It is used for the induction and maintenance of anaesthesia, usually as a 50–70% nitrous oxide–oxygen mixture, often in association with other anaesthetic agents. In weaker concentrations it produces analgesia without anaesthesia, and Entonox, a 50% mixture of nitrous oxide and oxygen, can be given by self-administration from suitable apparatus for obstetric analgesia. Entonox also has applications in changing painful dressings, and in first-aid ambulance work. Theatre nurses should note that prolonged exposure to nitrous oxide may cause a megaloblastic anaemia by an alteration of vitamin B_{12} activity.

INTRAVENOUS ANAESTHETICS

Intravenous anaesthetics are rapidly acting drugs used mainly for induction, although they may be used alone for short operations. They are highly lipid soluble, and cross the blood–brain barrier rapidly, with an arm–brain circulation time of 15–20 seconds. With these agents, the induction phase characteristic of inhalation anaesthesia is absent, and surgical anaesthesia occurs very quickly without excitement. Because of their potency and variations in individual response, overdose with cardiorespiratory depression may occur, and their use requires care.

The sodium salts of some short-acting barbiturates, represented by thiopentone, were the first drugs to be used as intravenous anaesthetics. Aqueous solutions of these drugs are very alkaline, and great care must be taken that none of the intravenous injection solution escapes into the surrounding tissues, as any such leakage may cause severe tissue or nerve damage. If accidentally injected intra-arterially instead of intravenously, severe and extremely painful arterial spasm is caused, followed by thrombosis which may lead to subsequent gangrene.

Thiopentone sodium §

Brand name: Intraval sodium §
Thiopentone sodium is a widely used intravenous anaesthetic. It is given as a freshly prepared 2.5% solution, in doses of 100–150 mg, with further doses at intervals if anaesthesia is to be prolonged. It is sometimes given by continuous intravenous infusion as a 0.2–0.4% solution.

Thiopentone is used mainly for the induction of anaesthesia but it has little muscle relaxant action, and specific muscle relaxants may be required for major surgery and should be given separately. It produces some fall in blood pressure, and care is necessary in patients with hypertension, cardiac disease or impaired liver function. Respiratory depression is common and may be severe. Recovery from thiopentone anaesthesia is usually rapid, as the drug is quickly removed from the circulation by temporary storage in the tissues, but its subsequent metabolism is slow, and some residual sedative action may persist for 24 hours.

Methohexitone sodium §

Brand name: Brietal §
The action of methohexitone sodium is similar to that of thiopentone sodium, but it is less irritant to the tissues, and recovery of consciousness is more rapid. It is useful for minor procedures in out-patient and casualty departments. Dose 50–120 mg initially as a 1–2% solution with maintenance doses of 20–40 mg at intervals of 4–7 minutes, according to response. For more prolonged anaesthesia, combined treatment with other agents is necessary.

Etomidate §

Brand name: Hypnomidate §
Etomidate is a short-acting non-barbiturate intravenous anaesthetic, used chiefly for induction. It is given in a dose of 300 micrograms/kg initially, and supplementary doses can be given at intervals of 6–10 minutes for short operations, or maintained for longer periods by other anaesthetics. Etomidate has no analgesic properties, and premedication is necessary to prevent pain on injection, and undesirable muscle movement during anaesthesia.

Ketamine §

Brand name: Ketalar §
Ketamine has an unusual type of anaesthetic–analgesic activity. It is given by slow intravenous injection in doses of 1–2 mg/kg, repeated according to need and response. A slower onset of action and a longer effect can be obtained by the deep intramuscular injection of the drug in doses of 4–10 mg/kg. It is used mainly for anaesthesia in children, but it is also used for induction of anaesthesia and its analgesic properties are of value in the management of patients with severe burns. The patient should not be disturbed during the recovery period as vivid dreams and hallucinations may occur, which can be

reduced by premedication with droperidol in doses of 0.1 mg/kg by intramuscular injection, or by the intravenous injection of diazepam in doses of 100–200 micrograms/kg. Ketamine is also used as a supplementary analgesic in severe pain that no longer responds adequately to very high doses of opiates.

Midazolam §

Brand name: Hypnovel §
Midazolam has some of the properties of diazepam, but it is used mainly for induction in doses of 200–300 mg/kg intravenously, given over 2.5–3 minutes with the patient in the supine position. Its use requires care, as the full response may be sudden, and respiratory depression and severe hypotension may occur. Continuous control of cardiac and respiratory functions are necessary with Midazolam, and ready access to resuscitation facilities is essential. Midazolam is also given for premedication to produce sedation and amnesia, and is then given in doses of 7–10 micrograms/kg by intramuscular injection.

Propofol §

Brand name: Diprivan §
Propofol has an anaesthetic action similar to that of thiopentone. It is used for the induction and maintenance of anaesthesia for periods of up to 1 hour. Dose by intravenous injection 2–2.5 mg/kg initially, with maintenance doses of 0.1–0.2 mg/kg per minute as required. Recovery is usually rapid.

Side-effects are mild hypotension, transient apnoea and bradycardia. Anaphylactic reactions have followed the use of propofol, and emergency treatment should be available. Convulsions have occurred as a delayed reaction, and an adequate period of recovery must be allowed before any day-patient who has received propofol is permitted to go home.

Propofol is supplied as an emulsion and may cause some pain when injected, but unlike thiopentone, extravascular injection does not cause any local tissue damage.

LOCAL ANAESTHETICS

Local anaesthetics are drugs that reversibly block the transmission of nerve impulses along pain fibres. The drugs penetrate the nerve and once inside the axon they attach themselves to the mouth of the sodium channels, prevent the entrance of sodium into the nerve and so inhibit the generation of an action potential. Small nerve fibres, especially unmyelinated C-fibres which convey painful stimuli, are more easily blocked than large fibres, so sensory impulse conduction is inhibited while larger nerve fibres, in particular motor nerves, remain unaffected unless large doses of drug are used.

As a group local anaesthetics are of considerable importance and can be divided into those compounds which are applied to the mucous membranes and those which are injected. The distinction is not complete as some compounds can be used both topically and by injection into the tissues. Some are used to produce regional anaesthesia by intraspinal and epidural injection.

Most local anaesthetics are used as water-soluble salts and are of little value when applied to the unbroken skin, as they are not absorbed. If the drug's lipid solubility is increased then absorption across the skin occurs, as demonstrated by EMLA, a cream which contains a mixture of lignocaine and prilocaine. It is used to produce local anaesthesia before cannulation or injection in children, and is applied under an occlusive dressing for 1–2 hours. Minimum amounts should be used in infants as methaemoglobinaemia has occurred after repeated daily use.

The addition of adrenaline to local anaesthetics extends their action by constricting adjacent blood vessels and decreasing the rate at which the drug is absorbed into the blood and removed from the injection site.

Lignocaine § (lidocaine)

Brand name: Xylocaine §
Lignocaine is one of the most active and widely used of the local anaesthetics, as it has a rapid, intense and prolonged action. It is widely employed in dentistry as a 2% solution: in infiltration and regional anaesthesia 0.25–0.5% solutions are used, often with a vasoconstrictor such as adrenaline (1–200 000) to localize and extend the action, which may then last for about $1\frac{1}{2}$–2 hours. Such combined solutions should not be used for anaesthesia of fingers or toes, as the vasoconstrictor action may cause local tissue damage.

Side-effects of lignocaine include hypotension and bradycardia; depression of cardiac function may cause cardiac arrest. The central action may cause agitation and convulsions, and care is necessary in

epilepsy. Reduced doses should be given to the elderly and in hepatic impairment.

Lignocaine is well absorbed when applied to mucous membranes and is used topically as ointment (5%), eye drops (2%) and throat spray (4%). A gel containing 2% lignocaine is used as a urethral anaesthetic before instrumentation. (The use of lignocaine in the treatment of cardiac arrhythmias is referred to on p. 101).

Bupivacaine §

Brand name: Marcain §
Bupivacaine is used to obtain a prolonged regional anaesthesia by nerve block. The dose depends on the area to be anaesthetized, the vascularity of the tissues, the number of neural segments to be blocked and the technique of injection. The manufacturer's literature should be consulted for details.

Other local anaesthetics of interest are prilocaine (Citanest 0.5% and 1%), resembling lignocaine in action and uses, and oxybuprocaine (Benoxinate 0.4%), amethocaine 0.5% and proxymetacaine (Ophthaine 0.5%) which are used in ophthalmology.

Nursing points about local anaesthetics

(a) Action may be further localized by adrenaline or noradrenaline.
(b) Such mixed injections should not be used for anaesthesia of the extremities (fingers, toes, ears, nose), as vasoconstriction of end arteries may cause tissue damage and gangrene.

Cocaine*

Cocaine is the alkaloid obtained from coca leaves and is the oldest of the local anaesthetics, but it has now been superseded by safer drugs. It still has a limited place in ophthalmology, as it dilates the pupil of the eye as well as producing anaesthesia (p. 252).

Procaine hydrochloride (novocaine)

Procaine hydrochloride was once the most widely used of the local anaesthetics, but it has now been replaced by lignocaine.

Benzocaine

Benzocaine is insoluble in water and is used for surface anaesthesia by local application as ointment (10%)

or dusting powder. It is the anaesthetic constituent of various antiseptic lozenges. Suppositories of benzocaine (500 mg) are used for painful haemorrhoids.

Spinal and epidural anaesthesia

Bupivacaine and some related drugs are used by intraspinal and epidural injection to produce a localized anaesthesia and for a full consideration of the subject the standard textbooks of anaesthesia should be consulted. Briefly, anaesthesia of the thoracic structures and the lower limbs may be obtained by injecting specially prepared local anaesthetic solutions into the spinal fluid. Such solutions are injected below the first and second lumbar vertebrae to avoid injury to the spinal cord. The area of anaesthesia can be controlled by using solutions that are lighter or heavier than the spinal fluid, and positioning the patient so that the solution flows over the appropriate nerves. Disadvantages of the method include the high risk of infection by bacteria reaching the cerebrospinal fluid, and the fall in blood pressure that often occurs.

Epidural anaesthesia is carried out by injecting the anaesthetic solution into the space outside the dura. It is free from many of the disadvantages of intraspinal anaesthesia, and is often preferred in obstetrics.

FURTHER READING

Anon 1990 The treatment of insomnia. Drug and Therapeutics Bulletin 28:97
Anon 1990 Zoplicone. Lancet 335:507
Bollinger B R 1990 Hypnotics and anxiolytics. British Medical Journal 300:156
Haimov I, Laudon M, Zisapel N et al 1994 Sleep disorders and melatonin rhythms in elderly patients. British Medical Journal 309:167
Lader M 1998 A practical guide to prescribing hypnotic benzodiazepines. British Medical Journal 293:1048
Prinz P N 1990 Sleep disorders and aging. New England Journal of Medicine 323:520

Sanders D L et al 1991 Reversal of benzodiazepine sedation with the antagonist flumazenil. British Journal of Anaesthesia 66:445–453
Speiss L D 1990 Two new pharmacological agents for the 1990s: Flumazenil and Propofol. Journal of Post Anaesthesia Nursing 5(3):186–189
Ward A et al 1986 Dantrolene: a review of its properties and therapeutic use in malignant hyperthermia. Drugs 32:130–186

3

Antipsychotics, antidepressants, anticonvulsants and stimulants

ANTIPSYCHOTIC OR NEUROLEPTIC DRUGS

Antipsychotic/neuroleptic drugs, sometimes referred to as major tranquillizers, are a diverse group of chemically different drugs that function basically as dopamine D_2-receptor antagonists. Many are derivatives of phenothiazine, and can be classified into three main groups, as they differ in their sedative, anticholinergic and extrapyramidal side-effects, as well as their hypotensive properties (Table 3.1). They are used mainly in the treatment of schizophrenia, but are also of value in other psychotic disorders such as mania, severe anxiety and organic psychoses caused by head injuries, alcoholism or other mental disturbances. Table 3.2 indicates the range of drugs available.

The clinical features of schizophrenia are positive symptoms such as delusions, hallucinations and thought disorders, and negative symptoms of apathy, social withdrawal, reduced emotional response and dementia. The cause of schizophrenia is not yet understood, but it involves certain neurotransmitters, and there is strong evidence that the disease is linked with dopamine-receptor overactivity, particularly the D_2-receptors. On that basis antischizophrenic drugs are used that block the effects of dopamine on the mesolimbic and mesocortical pathways, and they may give much symptomatic relief. The response may take days or even weeks to develop fully, and may alleviate the positive symptoms of schizophrenia more than the negative aspects. The benzodiazepines, on the other hand, exert part of their action via 5HT-receptors, which may account for their action in relieving the negative symptoms of schizophrenia.

The side-effects of these powerful neuroleptic drugs are linked with their action on dopamine and

Table 3.1 Classification of neuroleptic drugs

Drug group	Examples	Side-effects			
		Sed	EP	AC	Hypo
Typical neuroleptics					
Phenothiazines					
• Group I	Chlorpromazine, promazine, methotrimeprazine	++	++	++	++
• Group II	Pericyazine, pipothiazine, thioridazine	++	+	++	++
• Group III	Fluphenazine, perphenazine, prochlorperazine, trifluoperazine	+	+++	+	++
Butyrophenones	Haloperidol, droperidol	−	+++	+	+
Thioxanthines	Flupenthixol, zuclopenthixol	+	++	−	+
Atypical neuroleptics*					
Benzamides	Sulpiride	+	+	−	−
Benzisoxoles	Risperidone sertindole	++	++	−	+
Diphenybutylpiperazines	Pimozide	+	+	−	−
Dibenzodiazepines	Clozapine, olanzapine, quetiapine	++	+	+	+

Sed = sedation; EP = extrapyramidal symptoms; AC = anticholinergic side-effects; Hypo = hypotension; the plus symbols give on indication of the relative frequency of the side-effects.
*Atypical drugs are so called because they are generally associated with a lower incidence of movement disorders, and are generally more receptor specific.

other receptors. Their blockade of D_2-receptors in the basal ganglia of the brain leads to a drug-induced reversible form of parkinsonism, which may require a reduction of dose or treatment with an anticholinergic agent such as procyclidine (p. 99). Other effects of D_2-receptor blockade include loss of muscle tone (dystonia), restlessness (akathesia), and a slowly developing tardive dyskinesia. By their action on the D_2-receptors in the pituitary gland they increase the production of prolactin, and may cause galactorrhoea and gynaecomastia.

Other side-effects are linked with the blockade of receptors other than dopamine, particularly acetylcholine receptors, which leads to the anticholinergic symptoms of dry mouth, blurred vision and difficulties with micturition. Effects on alpha-adrenoceptors are the cause of postural hypotension and hypothermia, especially in the elderly, and care is necessary with patients over 70 years of age. Depression of the bone marrow may cause agranulocytosis and other blood dyscrasias. Prolonged high-dose therapy may lead to lens opacity and pigmentation of the cornea. A rare but severe reaction is the development of marked hyperthermia, referred to as a neuroleptic malignant syndrome. It requires immediate withdrawal of the causative drug and treatment with dantrolene (p. 22).

Chlorpromazine was the first phenothiazine used in the treatment of schizophrenia and is described below in some detail as the representative of the group. Other phenothiazines are included in Table 3.2. They all have a basically similar action, but differences in their chemistry manifest themselves in slightly different properties. Thus promazine, for example, is a less potent drug, used mainly for the control of agitation in the elderly; thioridazine is a powerful antipsychotic drug that, unlike chlorpromazine, has no anti-emetic properties; and methotrimeprazine has increased analgesic-enhancing potency, of value in terminal illness. As well as being used in the treatment of schizophrenia and other psychoses, neuroleptics are also used therapeutically to control violent impulsive behaviour, to potentiate the effects of anaesthetics and analgesics, to suppress involuntary movements in Huntingdon's chorea, and occasionally in the treatment of depression (especially sulpiride). They may also appear to bring about a reduction in the perception of and reaction to pain, making them of value in terminal illness, and most members of the group have useful anti-emetic properties.

Chlorpromazine § (dose: 75–300 mg daily; 25–50 mg by *deep* intramuscular injection)

Brand name: Largactil §
Chlorpromazine has a powerful calming action on aggressive schizophrenic patients, and on those exhibiting acute behavioural disturbances. It is also

Table 3.2 Phenothiazine-derived neuroleptics

Approved name	Brand name	Oral daily dose range	Dose by injection
chlorpromazine	Largactil	75–300 mg	25–50 mg i.m., 6–8 hourly
fluphenazine	Moditen	1–20 mg	
fluphenazine	Modecate		12.5–100 mg i.m., monthly
loxapine	Loxopac	20–100 mg	
methotrimeprazine	Nozinan	25–200 mg	12.5–25 mg i.m., or i.v. 6–8 hourly
pericyazine	Neulactil	10–75 mg	
perphenazine	Fentazin	8–24 mg	5–10 mg i.m., 6 hourly
prochlorperazine	Stemetil	15–50 mg	12.5–25 mg i.m., 8–12 hourly
promazine	Sparine	50–400 mg	
thioridazine	Melleril	30–600 mg	
trifluoperazine	Stelazine		1–2 mg i.m., 6–8 hourly

Note: Those phenothiazine derivatives used mainly as anti-emetics are referred to on p. 154

Nursing points about neuroleptic antipsychotic drugs
(a) Warn patients about the sedative effects and the increased risks of driving and machine-related activities.
(b) Tablets to be swallowed whole with water to avoid skin contact.
(c) Avoid over-exposure to direct sunlight.
(d) They may cause hypotension – advise patients not to stand up or get out of bed quickly.
(e) Advise patients of the need to continue treatment, and the consequences of abrupt withdrawal.
(f) Warn patients that parkinsonism-like side-effects may occur, and should be reported.

valuable in the short-term treatment of acute anxiety. Chlorpromazine is also used as a preoperative sedative, as it reduces apprehension, and by potentiating the subsequent response to anaesthesia, it permits the use of a lower dose of anaesthetic. Chlorpromazine is useful in the supplementary treatment of painful terminal disease, as it not only reduces nausea and vomiting, but also brings about an emotional reduction in the awareness of pain, and augments the action of narcotic analgesics. It is occasionally useful for the control of intractable hiccups.

The initial oral dose of chlorpromazine is 75 mg daily, increased as required, with maintenance doses of 75–300 mg daily, but in some severe psychotic conditions larger doses, sometimes up to 1 g daily may be required. In acute conditions, and in emergencies when a rapid action is necessary, the drug may be given by *deep* intramuscular injection in doses of 25–50 mg, repeated as required after 6–8 hours, but transfer to oral therapy should be made as soon as possible. Chlorpromazine may also be given as a 100 mg suppository, and rectal therapy is useful when a slower but more prolonged action is required.

Side-effects of chlorpromazine are those common to many antipsychotic drugs as already indicated (p. 27). Chlorpromazine may also cause skin sensitization and care should be taken to avoid all contact with solutions of the drug.

OTHER POWERFUL ANTIPSYCHOTIC AGENTS

The butyrophenones and pharmacologically related compounds represent another important group of potent antipsychotic agents of value in the treatment of schizophrenia. Although they differ chemically from the phenothiazine derivatives represented by chlorpromazine, they resemble those drugs classified as group III (Table 3.1) in having reduced sedative and anticholinergic side-effects, but being more likely to induce extrapyramidal symptoms. Table 3.3 indicates the range of drugs available, and the following notes refer to some individual compounds.

Table 3.3 Butyrophenones and other powerful neuroleptics.

Approved name	Brand name	Oral daily dose range	Dose by injection
benperidol	Anquil	0.25–1.5 mg	
clozapine	Clozaril	12.5–450 mg	
droperidol	Droleptan	15–100 mg	5–10 mg i.m. or i.v. 4–6 hourly
flupenthixol[a]	Depixol	6–8 mg	
flupenthixol	Depixol Depot		20–400 mg i.m. monthly
haloperidol	Dozic, Haldol, Serenace	4.5–15 mg	2–10 mg i.m 4–6 hourly
haloperidol decanoate	Haldol Decanoate		50–200 mg i.m. monthly
sertindole	Serdolect	4–24 mg	
olanzapine	Zyprexa	6–30 mg	
oxypertine	Integrin	80–100 mg	
pimozide	Orap	2–20 mg	
pipothiazine palmitate	Piportil Depot		50–200 mg i.m. monthly
quetiapine	Seroquel	50–450 mg	
risperidone	Risperdal	2–8 mg	
sulpiride	Dolmatil, Sulpitil	400 mg–2.4 g	
zuclopenthixol	Clopixol	20–150 mg	100–400 mg i.m. monthly

[a]Flupenthixol is also used as an antidepressant (p. 36).

Haloperidol § (dose: 4.5–15 mg daily; 2–10 mg by intramuscular injection)

Brand name : Serenace §, Haldol §, Fortunan §, Dozic §
Haloperidol is a butyrophenone and has some of the actions, uses and side-effects of chlorpromazine, but it is effective in smaller doses. It is used mainly in the control of severe schizophrenia, mania and paranoid psychoses, and in the treatment of behavioural disturbances. Haloperidol is also used in the supplementary short-term treatment of severe anxiety, and in the control of nausea and vomiting.

In psychoses, haloperidol is given in doses of 4.5–15 mg daily, although in very severe and resistant conditions doses of 100 mg daily or more may be required. For the rapid control of acute conditions, haloperidol may be given by intramuscular injection in doses of 2–10 mg or more according to the severity of the condition, with supplementary doses of 4–6 mg hourly as required. Lower doses are usually adequate in elderly and debilitated patients.

Haloperidol Decanoate § is a derivative that is given by deep intramuscular injection when a long-acting depot effect is required. Following a test dose of 6.25–12.5 mg, doses of 50 mg are given at intervals of 4 weeks. The response is variable, and subsequent increases in dose and interval are based on individual need. Haloperidol is also used in the short-term treatment of some non-psychotic emotional distur-

bances such as severe anxiety when other drugs have proved unsatisfactory, and it is then given in doses of 500 micrograms twice daily.

Side-effects of haloperidol are basically similar to those of chlorpromazine, and although extrapyramidal symptoms may be more severe, hypotension is less likely to occur. With long-term treatment, some patients may develop symptoms of tardive dyskinesia, and exhibit involuntary movements of the tongue, mouth, etc.

Benperidol § (dose: 0.25–1.5 mg daily)

Brand name: Anquil §
Benperidol has some of the properties of haloperidol, but it is used only in the management of aberrant sexual and antisocial behaviour.

Clozapine § (dose: 12.5–450 mg daily)

Brand name: Clozaril §
Clozapine has an action that is mediated by a selective blockade of certain dopamine and serotonin receptors in the limbic system, and may bring about an improved balance between dopaminergic and serotoninergic neurotransmission. Clozapine is indicated in schizophrenia resistant or not responding to other neuroleptic drugs, and is given as an initial dose of 12.5 mg once or twice daily, slowly increased over 2–3 weeks up to 300 mg or more daily.

Side-effects   By its selective action, clozapine has a low incidence of extrapyramidal side-effects, but it may cause some initial drowsiness. Clozapine may cause severe neutropenia that may lead to a fatal agranulocytosis, and routine blood monitoring is *essential*. Prompt withdrawal is usually followed by a return of the neutrophil count to a more normal level in about 2 weeks. At present, the use of the drug is restricted to patients registered with the Clozaril Patient Monitoring Service (CPMS), so that treatment may be withdrawn if necessary.

Droperidol § (dose: 15–100 mg daily; 5–10 mg by injection)

Brand name: Droleptan §
Droperidol is of value in the control of agitation in acute psychoses, and of aggression in brain-damaged patients. It is given in doses of 15–100 mg daily, or 5–10 mg by intramuscular or intravenous injection at intervals of 4–6 hours as required. Droperidol is also used for preoperative sedation in doses of 2.5–10 mg by intramuscular injection 30–60 minutes before operation. Droperidol also has some anti-emetic properties and has been used, sometimes by continuous intravenous infusion, during cancer chemotherapy.

In association with a potent narcotic analgesic such as fentanyl or phenoperidine, droperidol is used to induce a state of neuroleptanalgesia, a condition characterized by a detachment from and an indifference to the environment, whilst the ability to communicate is retained. Such a state is desirable when an operative procedure must be carried out during which the patient must be cooperative, yet free from pain and anxiety. For neuroleptanalgesia droperidol is given in doses up to 15 mg by intravenous injection.

Side-effects   of droperidol are similar to those of haloperidol.

Pimozide § (dose: 2–20 mg daily)

Brand name: Orap §
Pimozide is used in the control of both acute and chronic schizophrenia. Treatment is usually commenced with doses of 2–4 mg daily, increased as required at weekly intervals up to a total of 20 mg. In chronic conditions, and when apathy is present, smaller doses may be adequate. Pimozide is also useful for the short-term supplementary treatment of severe anxiety.

Side-effects   of pimozide are similar to those of chlorpromazine. Ventricular arrhythmia is an occasional side-effect, and it is now recommended that an ECG should be carried out before beginning pimozide treatment, and periodically in patients receiving doses of 16 mg or more daily. Care is necessary in depression, epilepsy and parkinsonism, as pimozide may aggravate the symptoms.

Quetiapine § ▼ (dose: 50–450 mg daily)

Brand name: Seroquel § ▼
Quetiapine is a new atypical antipsychotic agent for the treatment of schizophrenia. It interacts with a wide range of neurotransmitter receptors, and has a high affinity for $5HT_2$-receptors. It is given initially in doses of 50 mg daily, rising to 300 mg daily or more according to the response.

Side-effects   include somnolence, dizziness and postural hypotension, but there is no need for routine blood pressure or ECG monitoring.

Risperidone § (dose: 6–10 mg daily)

Brand name: Risperdal §
Risperidone is a recent addition to the range of drugs for the treatment of schizophrenia. It resembles clozapine in its pattern of activity, as it has a high and selective affinity for serotinin $5\text{-}HT_2$ and dopamine D_2-receptors as well as some lower affinity for $alpha_1$-adrenoceptors. Unlike many other antipsychotic agents, risperidone appears to relieve both the positive symptoms of schizophrenia such as hostility and delusions, and the negative symptoms of apathy and withdrawal. It is given in doses of 1 mg twice a day, increased over 2–3 days to 3 mg twice a day, according to response up to 4 mg twice a day. Doses over 10 mg daily are more likely to increase extrapyramidal symptoms than improve the response. Some hypotension may occur, mediated by the alpha-receptor blockade, and require adjustment of dose.

Side-effects   include headache, insomnia, agitation and dizziness, but extrapyramidal effects are usually mild and reversible with adjustment of dose or supplementary treatment with an anticholinergic drug. Unlike clozapine, risperidone does not appear to cause agranulocytosis, and routine blood monitoring is not necessary.

Sertindole § ▼ (dose: 4–24 mg)

Brand name: Serdolect § ▼
Sertindole has a more selective action than clozapine in acute and chronic schizophrenia, and a marked antagonist action on $5\text{-}HT_2$ receptors and D_2-receptors. Dose 4 mg daily initially, rising to 24 mg daily if required.

Side-effects are nasal congestion and dizziness, but it is less liable to cause extrapyramidal symptoms. It reacts with other drugs used in schizophrenia, and combined therapy is inadvisable. Contra-indicated when the QT interval is extended.

Sulpiride § (dose: 400 mg–2.4 g daily)

Brand name: Dolmatil §, Sulpitil §

Sulpiride is unusual in having a bimodal action, as it has both neuroleptic and antidepressant properties. It is used in acute and chronic schizophrenia in doses dependent to some extent on the condition. In chronic states associated with apathy and depression, initial doses of 400 mg twice daily are given, and paradoxically the improved alertness induced by the drug may be increased by a reduction in dose to 200 mg twice daily. In severe conditions with delusions and hallucinations, large doses up to 2.4 g daily may be necessary according to the response. Sulpiride has also been used at low dose levels in neurosis, depression and migraine.

Side-effects of sulpiride are similar to those of other neuroleptic drugs, and galactorrhoea may occur as a result of a rise in the serum prolactin level. Care is necessary in renal disease.

Trifluperidol § (dose: 0.5–8 mg daily)

Brand name: Triperidol §

Trifluperidol has the actions, uses and side-effects of haloperidol but is active in lower doses. It is used mainly in schizophrenia and mania, and is sometimes of value in Huntington's chorea. It is given in initial doses of 500 micrograms daily, increased at intervals of 3–4 days until an adequate response has been obtained up to a maximum dose of 6–8 mg daily.

ANXIOLYTIC AGENTS

The anxiolytic benzodiazepines (BDZs) are represented by diazepam, in contrast to the hypnotic BDZs such as nitrazepam, referred to in Chapter 2. The hypnotic BDZs used to be referred to as minor tranquillizers; the neuroleptics were then referred to as major tranquillizers, but those terms are misleading as the mode of action and side-effects of the two groups are very different. As mentioned on p. 19, BDZs act by modulating the effects of gamma-aminobutyric acid (GABA) at receptor sites in the brain. It is thought that there are two types of BDZ-receptors, Type I being responsible for the anxiolytic actions, and Type II receptors being linked with the hypnotic, anticonvulsant and muscle relaxant actions of the benzodiazepines. It has also been suggested that the central effects of serotonin are mediated by Type I BDZ-receptors in the amygdala, part of the limbic system of the brain.

However they may act, the anxiolytic BDZs reduce emotional reactivity and the somatic responses without marked sedation, but by their pharmacological nature they reduce alertness, and patients should be warned that car-driving ability may be affected, an action that may be intensified if alcohol is also taken. The risks of dependence and the dangers of rapid withdrawal are referred to on p. 20.

These benzodiazepines are of value in the short-term treatment of severe anxiety, but the lowest effective dose should be used and therapy should be withdrawn slowly but without delay. Rapid withdrawal may evoke a rebound response, even after short-term treatment. The BDZs have in general the same type of action, but can be divided into the intermediate-acting and longer-acting drugs. The former include bromazepam, lorazepam and oxazepam, and have the advantage that accumulation of the drug is less likely, although there is a greater risk of withdrawal symptoms. The longer-acting BDZs have a smoother initial action and withdrawal usually causes fewer problems, but the risk of accumulation is greater and the longer-acting BDZs should be avoided in the elderly and in hepatic impairment. Table 3.4 indicates the range of benzodiazepine anxiolytics currently available.

Flumazenil (p. 20) is a competitive antagonist of BDZs and has been used in the treatment of benzodiazepine overdose.

Diazepam § (dose: 5–30 mg daily)

Brand name: Valium §

Diazepam is a benzodiazepine with anxiolytic, muscle relaxant and anticonvulsant properties. It is widely

Table 3.4 Benzodiazepine anxiolytics

Approved name	Brand name	Average daily dose range
alprazolam	Xanax	750–1500 micrograms
bromazepam	Lexotan	3–18 mg
chlordiazepoxide	Librium	30–100 mg
clorazepate	Tranxene	7.5–22.5 mg
diazepam	Valium	5–30 mg
lorazepam[a]	Ativan	1–10 mg
oxazepam[a]		45–120 mg

[a]Intermediate-acting BZs.

used in the treatment of anxiety and tension states, for the relief of anxiety complicating organic and psychosomatic illness, and for the short-term treatment of anxiety-associated insomnia. Diazepam is also given for premedication; and it is sometimes used in dentistry to reduce stress and apprehension. Diazepam has also been used for night terrors in children. It is also of value in the control of acute alcohol withdrawal symptoms. The use of diazepam in status asthmaticus is referred to on p. 41.

In mild anxiety states, diazepam is given in doses of 2 mg three times a day, but in severe conditions doses up to 30 mg daily may be required. In insomnia complicated by anxiety, a dose of 5–15 mg at night may be effective. For the symptomatic treatment of acute alcohol withdrawal, large doses up to 20 mg, repeated 4-hourly, may be necessary.

Diazepam may also be given if required by suppository or rectal solution in doses of 5–15 mg. In severe conditions, and for the control of panic attacks, as well as in alcohol withdrawal, diazepam may be given by *slow* intravenous injection in doses of 5–10 mg, repeated after not less than 4 hours. Intramuscular injection should be avoided, as the response is unreliable, but intravenous injection requires care to avoid respiratory depression, hypotension and thrombophlebitis. (Diazemuls is an emulsified product for intravenous use that is better tolerated.)

Side-effects of diazepam include drowsiness, dizziness and ataxia, especially in the elderly, to whom half-doses should be given. It is not suitable for use with psychotic or depressed patients. The anticonvulsant and muscle relaxant properties of diazepam are referred to on p. 41 and 246.

Alprazolam § (dose: 750 micrograms–1.5 mg daily)

Brand name: Xanax §
Alprazolam is useful for the short-term treatment of anxiety, and of anxiety associated with depression. It is given in doses of 250–500 micrograms three times a day, with half-doses for elderly and debilitated patients. Higher doses may be required when depression is a complicating factor, but a total daily dose of 3 mg should not normally be exceeded.

Chlordiazepoxide § (dose: 30–100 mg daily)

Brand name: Librium §
Chlordiazepoxide has the anxiolytic action, uses and side-effects of diazepam. It is given in doses of 10 mg three times a day, increased if necessary up to 100 mg daily in the short-term treatment of severe anxiety states, with half-doses for elderly patients. It is also used as supplementary treatment in the control of the symptoms of acute alcohol withdrawal in doses of 25–100 mg, repeated at intervals of 2–4 hours according to need.

Lorazepam § (dose: 3–12 mg daily; 25 micrograms/kg by injection)

Brand name: Ativan §
Lorazepam has the actions, uses and side-effects of diazepam, but is effective in lower doses. In anxiety states it is given in doses of 1–4 mg or more three times a day, and as a dose of up to 5 mg at night for insomnia. In acute panic states lorazepam may be given by slow intravenous injection in doses of 25 micrograms/kg 6-hourly according to need. Larger doses of up to 50 micrograms/kg are sometimes given by injection for premedication. Lorazepam is also given intravenously in doses of 4 mg in status asthmaticus, but it may cause respiratory depression (p. 42).

OTHER ANXIOLYTIC DRUGS

Some other compounds, chemically unrelated to the benzodiazepines, have a similar anxiolytic action, and are useful when alternative therapy is required.

Buspirone § (dose: 15–45 mg daily)

Brand name: Buspar §
Buspirone is used for the short-term treatment of anxiety and anxiety associated with depression. It acts on the specific serotonin 5-HT_{1A} receptors, and so lacks the muscle-relaxant properties of the BDZs. Buspirone is given in doses up to 5 mg three times a day, gradually increased according to need, but the full response may not develop for 2 weeks and patients should be warned accordingly. By its action on specific receptors, patients on BDZs cannot be switched directly to buspirone without the risk of a BDZ withdrawal reaction. Buspirone should not be given with a monoamine oxidase inhibitor (MAOI), as the combination may cause a rise in blood pressure.

Side-effects include nausea, dizziness and headache.

Hydroxyzine (Atarax §), dose: 200–400 mg daily; and meprobamate (Equanil §), dose: 1.2–1.6 g daily are other anxiolytic agents, but are used less extensively. The use of some beta-blockers such as propranolol in the control of tremor and apprehension is referred to on p. 111.

ANTIDEPRESSANTS

Depression is a natural reaction to grief and disappointment and is normally self-limiting and relatively brief. However, depression may also occur without apparent cause, and the term depressive illness includes some common but not easily described psychiatric conditions. Depression that appears to come from within is referred to as melancholic or endogenous depression, whereas reactive depression is often an excessive response to stressful circumstances beyond the individual's immediate control, or sometimes a side-effect of drug treatment. The symptoms include feelings of misery, low self esteem, retardation of thought and action, and insomnia, which may vary from mild to severe. It may be accompanied by delusions and mania, sometimes referred to as bipolar depression. The biochemical mechanisms underlying depression are complex, but appear to be linked with an imbalance or deficiency in the brain of certain neurotransmitters such as noradrenaline and serotonin (5-HT), or to a dysfunction of the corresponding receptor sites.

Treatment is aimed at the restoration of the balance of neuroregulating amines by drugs that block their normal neuronal re-uptake in the brain, or those that bring about a similar effect by inhibiting their breakdown by enzymes such as amine oxidase. Attempts have been made to classify to some extent the wide range of antidepressant drugs in current use by their chemical structure, or by their mode of action, but some antidepressants may act at more than one receptor site, their metabolites may not have quite the same action as the parent drug, and classification of antidepressants is correspondingly difficult. Here they will be dealt with basically in separate groups: the tricyclic antidepressants (TCAs), the monoamine oxidase inhibitors (MAOIs), the selective serotonin re-uptake inhibitors (SSRIs), the serotonin/noradrenaline re-uptake inhibitors (SNRIs) and a few non-classified drugs.

TRICYCLIC ANTIDEPRESSANTS (TCAs)

TCAs are so named because of their three-ring chemical structure, although a few of the group have different, but related structures. They are the most widely prescribed antidepressant group, although some 20–30% of patients may not improve with TCA therapy. They are predominantly amine (noradrenaline and serotonin) uptake inhibitors, but exactly how this action is translated into an antidepressant effect is not clearly understood. The fact that TCAs take two to four weeks to show their antidepressant effects suggests an adaptive response within the nervous system, which is believed to involve the down-regulation of receptors. TCAs also block muscarinic (cholinergic) receptors, alpha$_1$- and alpha$_2$-adrenoceptors and H$_1$ and H$_2$ histamine receptors, which accounts for many of their side-effects.

The TCAs all have the same basic action and no individual drug has superior antidepressant activity. Thus choice of drug will partly depend upon its supplementary effects. For example, amitriptyline has some sedative properties that are useful when depression is associated with agitation, anxiety and insomnia, whereas others such as protriptyline have a mild stimulant effect that is of value when depression is linked with apathy and withdrawal.

Drug therapy needs to be tailored to the needs of the individual patient. The dose range of some drugs is wide and the aim of treatment is to obtain effective drug plasma levels with the minimal dose. That optimum dose tends to vary from patient to patient, and careful adjustment may be necessary initially to obtain an adequate response, bearing in mind that full response may take several weeks to months. Small doses should always be given initially to elderly patients as the TCAs may cause postural hypotension due to their effect at alpha-receptors. Caution is also necessary in epilepsy as these drugs may lower the convulsive threshold and precipitate fits. For the same reason, they may modify the action of antihypertensive drugs. They should never be given with a monoamine oxidase inhibitor or within 2 weeks of stopping such treatment.

As well as acting as antidepressants, the TCAs are also effective analgesics in neuropathic pain. This pain results when neurological disease affects the sensory pathways. It occurs in CNS disorders such as stroke and multiple sclerosis, in conditions associated with peripheral nerve damage such as diabetic neuropathy, or herpes zoster infection, and is a component of back and cancer pain. Neuropathic pain is difficult to control with conventional analgesics, and hence the TCAs are particularly valuable, with their analgesic effect being obtained far more rapidly and at lower doses than that required for antidepressant therapy.

Side-effects The side-effects mentioned here should be taken to refer in general to most TCAs, and will not be repeated again when dealing with individual drugs. Many are due to the anticholinergic (antimuscarinic) properties of these drugs, and include dryness of the mouth, blurred vision, and urinary disturbances. Car drivers should be warned that drowsiness may occur. With elderly patients there is a risk of hyponatraemia, possibly linked with the activity of the antidiuretic hormone. Some degree of tolerance to these side-effects may develop with continued treatment. More serious side-effects are those on the cardiovascular system, such as cardiac arrhythmias, heart block and sudden cardiac death, due to their inhibition of Na^+/K^+-ATPase (see Fig. 7.2). Also it must be remembered that TCAs have narrow therapeutic indices and are dangerous in the event of overdose, a real possibility in patients who are depressed.

The following notes refer to some individual drugs, and Table 3.5 indicates the range available.

Amitriptyline § (dose: 50–200 mg daily; 10–20 mg by intramuscular or intravenous injection)

Brand names: Lentizol §, Tryptizol §

Amitriptyline is widely used in the treatment of depression, particularly when some sedative action is also required, as for agitated and anxious patients. It is given in initial doses of 25 mg three times a day, gradually increased up to a maximum dose of 200 mg daily, although maintenance doses of 100 mg daily are usually adequate. Half-doses should be given to elderly patients. If required the full daily dose can be given at night to avoid daytime sedation and at the same time to promote sleep. In severe conditions amitriptyline may be given by injection in doses up

Table 3.5 Tricyclic and similar antidepressants

Approved name	Brand name	Daily dose range
amitriptyline[a]	Lentizol	50–200 mg
	Tryptizol	
amoxapine	Asendis	100–300 mg
clomipramine	Anafranil	10–250 mg
desipramine	Pertofran	75–200 mg
dothiepin[a]	Prothiaden	75–150 mg
doxepin[a]	Sinequan	30–300 mg
imipramine	Tofranil	75–200 mg
lofepramine	Gamanil	70–210 mg
maprotiline[a]	Ludiomil	25–150 mg
mianserin[a,b]		30–90 mg
nortriptyline	Allegron	30–100 mg
protriptyline	Concordin	15–60 mg
trazodone	Molipaxin	150–300 mg
trimipramine	Surmontil	50–300 mg
viloxazine	Vivalan	300–400 mg

[a]These drugs have sedative properties that are of value when depression is complicated by anxiety and insomnia.
[b]Mianserin is a tetracyclic compound.

> **Nursing points about antidepressants**
>
> (a) Onset of action is slow (2–4 weeks).
> (b) Encourage patients to persist with treatment.
> (c) Maintain dose level for at least 1 month after improvement before lowering the dose.
> (d) Drug withdrawal should be carried out slowly.
> (e) Combined treatment with an MAOI is contra-indicated and at least 2 weeks must elapse before commencing MAOI therapy after other treatment.
> (f) Care is necessary in epilepsy, and in any machine-related activities.

to 20 mg four times a day, followed by oral therapy as soon as possible. Following remission of symptoms, dosage should be reduced to a maintenance level, and therapy should be continued for at least 3 months to avoid a relapse, after which the drug should be gradually withdrawn.

By virtue of its anticholinergic action, amitriptyline is sometimes used in the treatment of nocturnal enuresis, and is given in doses of 10–20 mg at night for children aged 7–10 years, and 25–50 mg for children over 11 years. The use of tricyclic antidepressants in children is controversial, not least because of the risk of accidental overdose.

Side-effects of amitriptyline are those of the tricyclic antidepressants generally, referred to on p 34.

Amoxapine § (dose: 100–300 mg daily)

Brand name: Asendis §

One of the disadvantages of the tricyclic antidepressants is the slow onset of action, which may take 2 weeks or more to develop. Amoxapine is a derivative with a more rapid action, as an initial response may occur within 4–7 days. It is given in doses of 25 mg three to four times a day, with maintenance doses between 150 and 250 mg daily, with half-doses for elderly patients. Prolonged treatment is necessary to achieve a full response. Daytime drowsiness can be reduced by administration as a single dose at night. It may cause hormonal disturbances in female patients.

Clomipramine § (dose: 10–250 mg daily)

Brand name: Anafranil §

Clomipramine has the actions and uses of amitriptyline, but with reduced sedative properties. It is given in doses of 10 mg daily initially, subsequently increased according to need. Doses of 150 mg or more daily may be necessary. In severe depression, phobia and other severe conditions, clomipramine has been given by intramuscular injection or by intravenous infusion in daily doses of 100 mg (after a test dose of 25 mg).

Imipramine § (dose: 75–200 mg daily)

Brand name: Tofranil §

Imipramine was one of the first tricyclic antidepressants, and it has been widely used in the treatment of melancholic or endogenous depression. It is given in doses of 25 mg three times a day initially and subsequently increased, although in some cases a single dose of 150 mg at night may be preferred. The onset of action is slow, and may not be apparent for some 2–3 weeks. Extended treatment is necessary for the full remission of symptoms. Lower doses of 10 mg initially should be given to elderly patients. Withdrawal of the drug should be slow, but a course of treatment, including withdrawal, should not exceed 3 months.

Side-effects of imipramine are those of the tricyclic antidepressants in general (p. 34).

Imipramine has also been used for nocturnal enuresis in doses of 25 mg at night for children aged 8–12 years, and of 50 mg for older children.

Desipramine § (dose: 75–200 mg daily)

Brand name: Pertofran §

Desipramine is the active metabolite of imipramine and it has the actions, uses and side-effects of the parent drug. It is used mainly in depressive illness uncomplicated by anxiety and agitation. Desipramine has a long half-life in the body, which permits administration by a single daily dose.

Mianserin § (dose: 30–90 mg)

Mianserin is a tetracyclic derivative with the actions, uses and side-effects of the tricyclic antidepressants. It is given initially in doses of 10 mg three times a day or as a single dose of 30 mg at night, slowly increased according to need.

Side-effects Mianserin is more likely to cause haematological disturbances than the tricyclic drugs, particularly in the elderly, and full blood counts are necessary during treatment. The drug should be withdrawn immediately if any signs of infection occur such as fever, sore throat or stomatitis. An influenza-like syndrome may also develop and hepatic reactions as well as convulsions have also been reported.

Protriptyline § (dose: 15–60 mg daily)

Brand name: Concordin §

Most tricyclic antidepressants have a mild sedative effect, but protriptyline differs in having a stimulant action. It is correspondingly useful in the treatment of depression associated with apathy, and is given in doses of 5–10 mg three times a day. If insomnia is present, the third dose should be given before 4 p.m. Caution is necessary in the elderly, for whom a daily dose of 20 mg should not be exceeded; as is common with other antidepressants, protriptyline may cause hypotension and dizziness. Protriptyline is not suitable for the treatment of depression associated with anxiety as it may aggravate the symptoms.

Side-effects of protriptyline are in general similar to those of amitriptyline, but cardiovascular reactions are more common. Exposure to direct sunlight during treatment should be avoided, as a rash associated with photosensitization to protriptyline may occur.

Flupenthixol § (dose: 1–3 mg daily)

Brand name: Fluanxol §

Flupenthixol is a thioxanthine used in the treatment of schizophrenia (p. 27) but it also has some antidepressant and activating properties. It is sometimes used in the short-term treatment of depression, and it may relieve associated apathy and inertia and may be effective when other depressants are unsatisfactory. It is not suitable for the treatment of severe depression. Flupenthixol is given as a single morning dose of 1 mg initially, increased after 7 days to 1 mg twice a day, with the second dose not later than 4 p.m. Half doses should be given to the elderly.

Flupenthixol has a more rapid action than most antidepressants, but if there is no response to treatment after 7 days, the drug should be withdrawn.

Side-effects include restlessness and insomnia, and care is necessary with excitable patients and in confused states. Paradoxically, it may cause drowsiness initially in a few patients.

Viloxazine § (dose: 300–400 mg daily)

Brand name: Vivalan §

Viloxazine is also used in the treatment of depressive illness, and has the advantage of having less anticholinergic (antimuscarinic) activity and is less likely to cause sedation. It is given in doses of 200 mg in the morning and 100 mg at midday, increased if necessary up to 400 mg daily. The last dose is best taken before 6 p.m.

Tryptophan § (dose: 3–6 g daily)

Brand name: Optimax § ▼

Tryptophan is an amino acid present in food and is a precursor of serotonin. On the basis that depression may be linked with a deficiency of serotonin, tryptophan has become available for the treatment of resistant depression under hospital supervision on a named-patient basis.

SELECTIVE SEROTONIN RE-UPTAKE INHIBITORS (SSRIs)

SSRIs, as their name suggests, inhibit the re-uptake of serotonin at nerve terminals. This more selective action means that they have little effect on the activity of noradrenaline or dopamine, and do not possess significant anticholinergic, antihistamine or α_1-adrenergic blocking properties. SSRIs thus have fewer side-effects than the TCAs, although their antidepressant actions are of similar efficacy and time course. They have a wider therapeutic index than TCAs so the risks of overdose are less. Furthermore, because of their potential to cause nausea, ingestion of large amounts of drug will often produce an emetic response.

Although they have low affinities for histamine receptors, paradoxically sedation can be a problem and care must be taken when driving. Other side-effects include decreased sexual desire and function, tremor, diarrhoea, headache and insomnia. SSRIs must not be used in combination with MAOIs, or within several weeks of stopping such therapy, or with any other drugs that might interfere with serotonin re-uptake. Such combined treatment may lead to a life-threatening syndrome of hyperthermia, muscle rigidity and cardiovascular collapse. SSRIs are highly plasma bound drugs and so may displace other drugs utilizing the plasma protein, and so lead to possible toxicity.

SSRIs are used in a variety of psychiatric conditions other than depression, including anxiety and panic disorders, as well as eating disorders such as bulimia. The following drugs are currently available.

Fluoxetine § (dose: 20 mg daily)

Brand name: Prozac §

Fluoxetine has a longer half-life than some related drugs. In depressive illness it is given in doses of 20 mg daily, but in the treatment of bulimia nervosa larger doses of 60 mg daily are needed. The use of fluoxetine requires care, as it has many **side-effects**, including dizziness, drowsiness, nausea and diarrhoea. It may also cause allergic reactions such as urticaria and anaphylaxis. The development of a rash requires withdrawal of the drug, as it may indicate the onset of a serious systemic reaction. Disturbances of the blood picture may also occur. In the elderly, fluoxetine, in common with many antidepressants, may cause hyponatraemia, possibly because of the abnormal secretion of the antidiuretic hormone. On the other hand, it is less likely to cause cardiotoxicity, which may be an advantage when there is a risk of overdosage.

Fluvoxamine § (dose: 100–300 mg daily)

Brand name: Faverin §

Fluvoxamine is used in depressive illness in initial doses of 100 mg daily, increased as required over 2 weeks or more up to a maximum of 300 mg daily. The tablets should be swallowed whole with water. **Side-effects** include agitation, insomnia, dizziness and tremor. Gastrointestinal disturbances are common. It is contra-indicated in epilepsy, as it may lower the convulsive threshold and precipitate an attack, as may other SSRIs. The plasma levels of warfarin and propanolol may also rise.

Paroxetine § (dose: 20–50 mg daily)

Brand name: Seroxat §

Paroxetine is an antidepressant of the fluoxetine type, and is given in all types of depressive illness, including depression accompanied by anxiety. It is given initially as a morning dose of 20 mg, and slowly increased up to 50 mg daily. The **side-effects** are similar to those of related drugs but extrapyramidal symptoms have been reported more frequently. The combined use of paroxetine and aminophylline/theophylline should be avoided; if such use is essential the doses of those drugs should be halved and their plasma levels monitored.

Sertraline § (dose: 50–200 mg daily)

Brand name: Lustral §

Sertraline is used in the treatment of depressive illness as well as in prevention and recurrence, and is given initially in doses of 50 mg daily with food. The full response may not be noted for 2–4 weeks. When the response is incomplete, the doses may be slowly increased over some weeks, but a daily dose of 150 mg or more should not be continued for more than 8 weeks.

Side-effects   are nausea, diarrhoea and dryness of the mouth. The same precautions about combined therapy and car-driving should be observed with sertraline as with other selective serotonin re-uptake inhibitors (SSRIs).

Citalopram § ▼ (dose: 20–60 mg daily)

Brand name: Cipramil § ▼
Citalopram is a recently introduced SSRI and has the actions and uses of that group of antidepressants. It is given as a single dose of 20 mg, either at night or in the morning, increased if necessary up to 60 mg daily.

SSRI-RELATED ANTIDEPRESSANTS
Mirtazapine § (dose: 15–45 mg daily)

Brand name: Zispin §
Mirtazapine is a presynaptic alpha$_2$-antagonist that increases serotonergic neurotransmission by blocking 5-HT receptors, and so is of value in depressive illness. Dose 15 mg initially at night, slowly rising as required up to 45 mg in divided doses.
   Side-effects   are white blood cell disorders, and care is necessary in cardiac disorders and hepatic and renal insufficiency, epilepsy and glaucoma.

Nefazodone § ▼ (dose: 200–400 mg daily)

Brand name: Dutonin § ▼
Nefazodone has the general properties of the SSRIs, and is given in doses of 100 mg twice a day, increased after 7 days to 200 mg twice a day, rising if necessary to 600 mg daily.

Venlafaxine § ▼ (dose: 75–150 mg daily)

Brand name: Efexor § ▼
Venlafaxine has an antidepressant action linked with an inhibition of serotonin and noradrenaline re-uptake.

Nursing points about SSRIs

(a) Less sedative than the tricyclic antidepressants.
(b) Gastrointestinal side-effects are dose-related.
(c) Do not cause weight gain.
(d) Caution necessary in epilepsy.
(e) A gap of 2–5 weeks must elapse between SSRI and MAOI therapy.
(f) As with tricyclic antidepressants, care is necessary in car-driving and machine-related activities.

Dose 37.5 mg twice a day initially, increased after some weeks to 150 mg daily.
   Side-effects   are allergic in nature, and any rash or urticaria should be reported.

MONOAMINE OXIDASE INHIBITORS (MAOIs)

Monoamine oxidase is a mitochondrial enzyme which catabolizes serotonin and the catecholamines (adrenaline, noradrenaline and dopamine). It is found in two subtypes, namely MAO-A and MAO-B. The former has a substrate preference for serotonin and is the main target for antidepressant therapy, while the latter has a substrate preference for phenylethylamine. Both enzymes act on noradrenaline and dopamine. Type B is selectively inhibited by selegiline (p. 98) which is used in the treatment of Parkinson's disease. The established MAOIs are irreversible, non-selective inhibitors of MAO, while the more recent MAOI moclobemide is reversible and selective for MAO$_A$ and is much safer than the older drugs.

   MAOIs have a general antidepressant action, but they are prescribed mainly for the treatment of depression resistant to other drugs. The onset of action is slow and may take up to a month to reach maximal level, but their main disadvantage is that of interacting with other drugs, reducing the metabolism of barbiturates, opioid analgesics and alcohol. Pethidine is especially dangerous, causing hyperpyrexia, hypotension and coma. Combined treatment with TCAs is hazardous.

   MAOIs directly inhibit first-pass metabolism of tyramine, which is found in a variety of foods including mature cheese, meat and yeast extracts, red wine and broad beans. Consequently, increased concentrations of tyramine reach the systemic circulation and the sympathetic nervous system. Here the tyramine stimulates the release of noradrenaline, producing a syndrome of sympathetic overactivity with severe hypertension, hyperpyrexia, excitement, delirium, and possibly death. In order to prevent these serious effects, patients taking MAOIs must be given extensive information about what they can and cannot eat, and are encouraged to carry a card indicating that they are taking MAOIs. Patients taking MAOIs must also be warned to avoid self-medication as some cough and cold remedies contain small doses of sympathomimetics, and a throbbing headache with MAOI therapy is a warning of a potentially dangerous rise in blood pressure.

Isocarboxazid, dose 30–60 mg daily; phenelzine (Nardil) dose 45–90 mg daily and tranylcypromine (Parnate), dose 20 mg daily before 3 p.m.) are typical MAOIs.

Moclobemide § ▼ (dose: 300–600 mg daily)

Brand name: Manerix § ▼

Moclobemide, sometimes referred to as an RIMA antidepressant (reversible inhibitor of monamine oxidase), brings about a rapid inhibition of MAO activity within a few hours, but the effect fades after about 24 hours as the drug is rapidly metabolized with restoration of enzyme activity, thus permitting single daily doses. Moclobemide is given in severe depression, but other therapy should be withdrawn for 2–3 weeks (5 weeks after fluoxetine), after which the drug is given as an initial dose of 300 mg after food, subsequently increased according to response up to 150–600 mg daily for 2–3 weeks. It should not be given to agitated patients without prior sedation.

Side-effects include nausea, dizziness and sleep disturbances. The same dietary precautions should be taken with moclobemide as with other MAOIs.

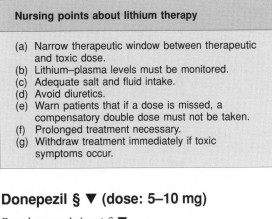

Nursing points about MAOIs
(a) Potentiate the action of many pressor drugs.
(b) Throbbing headache may be a warning symptom of a rise in blood pressure.
(c) Combined treatment with other antidepressants contra-indicated – tranylcypromine with clomipramine is dangerous.
(d) At least 2 weeks must elapse between MAOI therapy and other treatment.
(e) Warn patients not to eat cheese, broad beans, pickled herring, meat or yeast extracts.

Lithium carbonate § (dose: 0.25–1.6 g daily)

Brand names: Camcolit §, Liskonum §, Priadel §

Lithium carbonate is used in the prophylaxis and treatment of mania and recurrent depression, but the mode of action is unknown. It may be linked with changes in the pattern of electrolyte balance between intracellular and extracellular fluid, or with the balance between lithium and sodium ions. Lithium carbonate is given in doses of 250 mg daily initially, slowly increased according to regular laboratory reports to maintain a plasma level of 0.6–1.2 mmol lithium/litre, as the margin between the therapeutic and the toxic doses is narrow. The response is not immediate, and initial treatment is often combined with another antipsychotic drug.

For prophylaxis, extended treatment over 6–12 months may be required to obtain a full response, and continued for 3 years or more to maintain the remission. Such prolonged treatment may cause changes in renal function and require a review of therapy. The same lithium product should be used throughout treatment, as the bio-availability of lithium from different products may vary widely and a change of product requires reassessment of treatment. The anticonvulsant carbamazepine (p. 40) is sometimes used for patients who do not respond to lithium.

Side-effects of lithium therapy include gastro-intestinal disturbances, tremor and polyuria, and it may also induce or exacerbate psoriasis, but toxic side-effects such as coarse tremor, drowsiness, lethargy and ataxia require immediate withdrawal of the drug. Toxicity may be increased by sodium loss induced by thiazide and other diuretics, and care is necessary in other conditions of sodium depletion, as plasma concentrations above 1.5 mmol lithium/litre may be fatal. Lithium citrate (Li-Liquid, Litarex) has similar actions and uses.

Nursing points about lithium therapy
(a) Narrow therapeutic window between therapeutic and toxic dose.
(b) Lithium–plasma levels must be monitored.
(c) Adequate salt and fluid intake.
(d) Avoid diuretics.
(e) Warn patients that if a dose is missed, a compensatory double dose must not be taken.
(f) Prolonged treatment necessary.
(g) Withdraw treatment immediately if toxic symptoms occur.

Donepezil § ▼ (dose: 5–10 mg)

Brand name: Aricept § ▼

Donepezil is a reversible inhibitor of acetyl-cholinesterase. It is used to relieve the mild dementia of Alzheimer's disease, and appears to act by increasing the brain concentration of acetylcholine. Dose 5 mg at night, increased up to 10 mg if necessary Not all patients respond to donepezil treatment. **Side-effects** are diarrhoea and mild muscle cramp.

It is of interest that metriphonate (metrifonate), an old inhibitor of acetylcholine used as an anthelmintic (p. 267), may be introduced in 1999 for the treatment of Alzheimer's disease.

ANTICONVULSANTS OR ANTI-EPILEPTICS (TABLE 3.6)

Epilepsy is a chronic condition characterized by seizures or fits, which affects around 1 in 200 people in western countries. The seizure is caused by an abnormal high frequency discharge of a group of neurons, starting locally and spreading to a varying extent to affect other parts of the brain. The neurochemical basis of the abnormal discharge is not well understood. It may be the result of abnormal electrical properties of the affected cells. However, the finding of raised glutamate levels in areas surrounding an epileptic focus suggests that the cause is enhanced excitory amino acid transmission, while the finding that deficiency of the major inhibitory neurotransmitter GABA (gamma-aminobutyric acid) leads to an excessive response to excitatory factors suggests that the abnormal discharge may result from impaired inhibitory transmission.

Epileptic seizures have been classified as follows:

- generalized tonic–clonic seizures or grand mal, with convulsions and loss of consciousness,
- absence seizures or petit mal, characterized by transient loss of consciousness without convulsions, and
- focal or Jacksonian epilepsy, similar in some ways to the clonic stage of grand mal.

Partial seizures, which are more difficult to control, include those with sensory, motor or autonomic symptoms, as well as the more complex temporal lobe or psychomotor seizures. The atypical seizures of childhood may be associated with retardation or cerebral damage, and may respond poorly to treatment. Status epilepticus is a serious condition in which a series of convulsions may occur without an intervening recovery period.

Table 3.6 lists anticonvulsant drugs that are effective in these different types of seizure. The mode of action of anticonvulsant drugs is not entirely clear, but they are believed to work through one of three mechanisms. They either alter voltage-dependent ion channels involved in action potential propagation, or they interfere with amino acid-mediated excitation at glutamate and N-methyl-D-aspartate (NMDA) receptors, or they augment GABA by mimicking its action or inhibiting its enzymatic breakdown. The successful treatment of epilepsy depends on the maintenance of an adequate plasma level of an effective anticonvulsant drug. Combined therapy with more than one drug may have disadvantages, as some drugs induce

Table 3.6 Anticonvulsants

Approved name	Brand names
Those effective in petit mal:	
phenobarbitone	Luminal
methylphenobarbitone	Prominal
acetazolamide	Diamox
clobezam	Frisium
clonazepam	Rivotril
ethosuximide	Emeside, Zarontin
sodium valproate	Epilim
topiramate	Topamax
vigabatrin	Sabril
Those effective in grand mal and other types of seizure:	
phenobarbitone	Luminal
methylphenobarbitone	Prominal
carbamazepine	Tegretol
chlormethiazole[a]	Heminevrin
clonazepam[a]	Rivotril
diazepam[a]	Valium
gabapentin	Neurontin
lamotrigine	Lamictal
lorazepam[a]	Ativan
phenytoin	Epanutin
primidone	Mysoline
sodium valproate	Epilim
vigabatrin	Sabril

[a]Indicates those drugs used in status epilepticus.

the production of liver enzymes which may both reduce the effective plasma levels and increase toxicity.

In general, dosage must be individually adjusted to need and response, and patient compliance with treatment is essential, as prolonged medication is required. Any change of treatment from one drug to another must be carried out slowly, and withdrawal covered by overlapping doses, as convulsions may be precipitated by the rapid withdrawal of an anti-epileptic drug.

The use of anticonvulsants during pregnancy requires care, as they are potentially teratogenic, and there is an increased risk of neural tube defects with carbamazepine, phenytoin and valproate. The Committee on Safety of Medicines has advised that, where appropriate, women should be informed of the risks and possible consequences, and if necessary offered specialist advice. In addition, during pregnancy the plasma levels of anticonvulsants should be monitored regularly, as the levels may fall, particularly during the later stages.

Carbamazepine § (dose: 0.8–1.2 g daily)

Brand name: Tegretol §

Carbamazepine has an anticonvulsant action that is useful in most forms of epilepsy with the exception of petit mal. It is considered by some to be a first choice drug for the control of partial seizures.

Carbamazepine is given in doses of 200–400 mg daily initially, with food, rising slowly over 7–14 days to maintenance doses of 0.8–1.2 g daily, and control of seizures is usually achieved with a plasma level of the drug of 20–50 micromol/litre. Suppositories of carbamazepine (125 mg and 250 mg) are available for short-term treatment when oral administration is not possible, as postoperatively, or when the patient is unconscious. Carbamazepine is also used occasionally in the treatment of trigeminal neuralgia, mania (p. 40) and diabetes insipidus (p. 176).

Side-effects, especially in the early stages of treatment, are drowsiness and dizziness, and gastro-intestinal disturbances. Double vision may occur as higher plasma levels are reached with continued treatment. A generalized rash occurs in about 3% of patients receiving carbamazepine which may be severe enough to require withdrawal of the drug. Photosensitization and blood disorders have also been reported.

Clonazepam § (dose: 4–8 mg daily)

Brand name: Rivotril §
Clonazepam is chemically related to diazepam and has an anticonvulsant action that is of value in the control of all types of epilepsy. It is given in doses of 1 mg daily initially for a few days, usually at night as it has a sedative action, slowly increased over 2–4 weeks to a maintenance dose of 4–8 mg daily. Clonazepam is also effective in the control of status epilepticus, and is given in doses of 1 mg by slow intravenous injection, repeated as required. Its use requires care, as it may cause apnoea and hypotension requiring intensive treatment.

Side-effects of oral therapy include drowsiness, dizziness, fatigue and irritability. In children, clonazepam may cause respiratory side-effects by increasing bronchial and salivary secretion.

Diazepam § (dose: 10–20 mg intravenously)

Brand names: Diazemuls §, Valium §, Stesolid §
The anxiolytic drug diazepam has valuable anticonvulsant properties when given by intravenous injection, and is the drug of choice in the treatment of status epilepticus. It is given by slow intravenous injection in doses of 10–20 mg, repeated if necessary after 30–60 minutes, with subsequent doses by intravenous infusion after dilution with glucose

5% solution, up to a maximum of 3 mg/kg over 24 hours.

The injection solution frequently causes venous thrombosis, and an emulsified injection product (Diazemuls) is often preferred. Absorption after intramuscular injection is unreliable and when intravenous injection is not possible, diazepam may be given as a rectal solution in doses of 5–10 mg, repeated as required. As with clonazepam, a **side-effect** of intravenous therapy is respiratory depression, and mechanical ventilation apparatus must be readily available.

Ethosuximide § (dose: 500 mg–2 g daily)

Brand names: Emeside §, Zarontin §
Ethosuximide is one of the preferred drugs for the treatment of petit mal (absence seizures). It is given in doses of 500 mg daily initially, slowly increased at weekly intervals up to a maximum of 2 g daily. An optimum response is associated with a plasma level of 300–700 micromol/litre. In mixed seizures, the incidence of grand mal may be increased by ethosuximide, requiring adjustment of other therapy.

Side-effects of ethosuximide are similar to those of related drugs, and include drowsiness, dizziness and gastrointestinal disturbances. Care is necessary in renal and hepatic impairment.

Chlormethiazole §

Brand name: Heminevrin §
Chlormethiazole is used mainly as a hypnotic (p. 21) but it also has some anticonvulsant properties that are useful in status epilepticus. It is then given by intravenous infusion of an 0.8% solution in doses of 40–120 mg/minute up to a total dose of 320–800 mg, continued if necessary with doses of 4–8 mg/minute. The dose must be titrated against response, as the sleep induced by chormethiazole may otherwise easily pass into unconsciousness. It is used mainly when the epileptic state is continuous, or returns after treatment.

Side-effects of chlormethiazole include sneezing, conjunctival irritation, apnoea and hypotension, and resuscitation facilities must be available. Local thrombophlebitis may occur at the injection site.

Gabapentin § ▼ (dose: 300 mg–2.4 g daily)

Brand name: Neurontin § ▼
Gabapentin is a new analogue of GABA and has some useful anticonvulsant properties. The mode of

action is not yet known, as it does not modify the brain level of GABA or inhibit GABA-transaminase activity, or bind to GABA receptors. At present it is used mainly as supplementary treatment in partial seizures not controlled by other drugs. It is given in a dose of 300 mg on the first day of treatment, 300 mg twice on the second day, 300 mg three times on the third day, after which the dose is increased according to need and response up to 1.2 g daily. Exceptionally, doses of up to 2.4 g daily may be required. Care is necessary in mixed seizures, some of which may be exacerbated, and reduced doses are advisable in renal impairment and the elderly.

Side-effects include drowsiness, dizziness, nausea, tremor and weight gain. Withdrawal of treatment should be carried out slowly with tapering-off doses over at least 1 week.

Lamotrigine § ▼ (dose: 100–400 mg daily)

Brand name: Lamictal § ▼

Lamotrigine is an anticonvulsant that is thought to act by inhibiting the release of an excitatory factor such as glutamate. It is used in resistant epilepsy as supplementary treatment with other anticonvulsants, and is given in doses of 50 mg twice a day initially for 14 days, with subsequent adjustment for maintenance doses of 100–200 mg twice a day. Half doses should be given when sodium valproate is being given. Withdrawal, if necessary, should be carried slowly over 2 weeks. Lamotrigine is not recommended for children or the elderly.

Side-effects include rash, fever, blurred vision and dizziness. Renal and hepatic impairment are contraindications, and such functions should be monitored in patients who develop side-effects.

Lorazepam § (dose: 4 mg by injection)

Brand name: Ativan §

Lorazepam is a benzodiazepine with the actions and uses of diazepam that is occasionally used in status epilepticus. It is given by slow intravenous injection in a dose of 4 mg, repeated after 15 minutes if necessary.

Side-effects Apnoea and hypotension may be severe and require resuscitation.

Paraldehyde § (dose: 5–10 ml)

This old hypnotic drug (p. 21) is also of value in status epilepticus. It is given by deep intramuscular injection in doses of 5–10 ml, but not more than 5 ml at one site (with a glass syringe), or rectally in doses of 5 ml as a 10% solution in saline. In specialist centres it has been given by slow intravenous injection in doses of 4–5 ml well diluted with saline, but great care is necessary as intravenous paraldehyde may cause pulmonary oedema and haemorrhage.

Phenobarbitone § (dose: 60–180 mg daily; 50–200 mg by injection)

Phenobarbitone was once the standard drug for the treatment of epilepsy and is still widely used. It has a general sedative as well as an anticonvulsant action, and is of value in all forms of epilepsy with the exception of absence seizures. Phenobarbitone is given in doses of 60–180 mg at night; the dose for children is on the weight basis of 5–8 mg/kg daily. In severe conditions, phenobarbitone may be given by intramuscular or intravenous injection in doses of 50–200 mg.

Side-effects include drowsiness and lethargy, although tolerance may develop, but the elderly may experience confusion and restlessness. In children, who sometimes require relatively high doses, phenobarbitone may have the paradoxical effect of causing hyperactivity. Methylphenobarbitone (Prominal) has similar actions and uses in doses of 100–600 mg daily.

Phenytoin sodium § (dose: 150–300 mg daily)

Brand name: Epanutin §

Phenytoin is used mainly in the control of grand mal and partial seizures, as it is of little value in petit mal. Following initial doses of 150–300 mg daily, maintenance doses range from 300 to 400 mg daily, although occasionally a dose of 600 mg may be required. Dosage must be adjusted in accordance with the drug plasma level to maintain a concentration of 40–80 micromol/litre as there are wide individual variations in the dose required to attain that level. Phenytoin should be taken after food to reduce gastric irritation.

In status epilepticus, phenytoin is given by slow intravenous injection in a loading dose of 15 mg/kg, followed by doses of 100 mg 6-hourly adjusted in accordance with the monitored plasma concentration. Such intravenous injections may cause hypotension and bradycardia, and facilities for resuscitation must be available.

Side-effects of phenytoin are numerous and include dizziness, headache, nausea and insomnia. Skin eruptions, acne and hirsutism may occur as well as overgrowth of the gums, and a megaloblastic anaemia may result from a disturbance of folate metabolism. Slurred speech may be a sign of overdose. The intravenous injection solution is alkaline and may cause local irritation.

Phenytoin binds easily to the plasma proteins, but can be displaced from such binding by a wide range of other drugs. Multiple therapy therefore requires care, as the plasma level of unbound drugs may rise sharply.

It is of interest that phenytoin has some antifolate properties that may play some part in its anticonvulsant activity, and in a search for more potent antifolate agents a drug of value in epilepsy was discovered (see lamotrigine, p. 42).

Primidone § (dose: 0.5–1.5 g daily)

Brand name: Mysoline §
Primidone has some chemical relationship to phenobarbitone, into which it is largely converted in the body. It is chiefly of value as alternative therapy in grand mal and psychomotor epilepsy when the response to other drugs is inadequate. Treatment is initiated with a dose of 125 mg daily at night, increased at intervals of 3 days to a daily dose of 0.5–1.5 g according to need. Children's doses are 10–15 mg/kg twice daily.

Side-effects Primidone occasionally causes drowsiness, nausea, vertigo, fatigue, visual disturbances and skin eruptions, although these reactions may subside as treatment is continued.

Sodium valproate § (dose: 600 mg–2.5 g daily)

Brand names: Epilim §, Epilim Chrono §
Sodium valproate is effective in most types of epilepsy, but is less active against partial seizures. It appears to act by increasing the concentration in the brain of the inhibitory neurotransmitter GABA, possibly by reducing its enzymatic breakdown. It is given in doses of 200 mg three times a day initially, preferably after food, slowly increased as required at 3-day intervals up to a maximum of 2.5 g daily. In conditions where oral therapy is not possible, sodium valproate may be given by intravenous injection or infusion in doses of 400–800 mg, up to the same maximum daily dose of 2.5 g. Children's doses range from 20–40 mg/kg daily. Liver function should be monitored before and during treatment.

Epilim Chrono is a product containing equal parts of sodium valproate and valproic acid. It is claimed that with the mixture there is less variation in the daily plasma levels of the anticonvulsant. Convulex § is a preparation of valproic acid.

Side-effects of sodium valproate are numerous and include nausea, weight gain and occasionally a transient loss of hair. Liver function may be impaired, sometimes severely, and the drug should be withdrawn immediately if vomiting, anorexia or jaundice occurs. Blood platelet function and aggregation may also be disturbed. Care is necessary in pregnancy, as spina bifida has occasionally been associated with valproate therapy. As with phenytoin, interaction with a wide range of other drugs may occur, and multiple treatment requires care.

Vigabatrin § (dose: 2–4 g daily)

Brand name: Sabril §
Vigabatrin is an analogue of GABA and has a highly specific and irreversible inhibitory action on GABA-transaminase, the enzyme concerned with breakdown of GABA. The administration of vigabatrin brings about an extended decline in the activity of GABA-transaminase that results in a rise in the brain level of GABA which is linked with the clinical response to the drug. Vigabatrin is well absorbed orally, it does not induce drug-metabolizing enzymes in the liver, and it is excreted unchanged in the urine. Vigabatrin is used in the treatment of epilepsy not responding to other anticonvulsants, and is given as a supplement to such therapy, which should be continued. It is available as tablets and as sachets containing a sugar-free powder. The powder should be dissolved in water or other drink immediately before administration. Vigabatrin is given in doses of 1 g once or twice a day initially, subsequently adjusted as required, but doses above 4 g daily do not usually evoke an increased response. Reduced doses should be given to the elderly, and to patients with impaired renal function. Children may be given a starting dose of 40 mg/kg daily. Vigabatrin is well tolerated, but withdrawal, if necessary, should be by a gradual reduction of dose over 2 to 4 weeks. Abrupt withdrawal may lead to rebound seizures.

Side-effects of vigabatrin include drowsiness, fatigue, weight gain, dizziness and impairment of car-driving and related abilities. The sedative effects of the drug wane as treatment is prolonged. As with other anti-epileptic drugs, vigabatrin may cause an increase in seizure frequency in some patients, particularly those with myoclonic seizures. Vigabatrin does not become protein bound, so interactions with other drugs are less likely than with some other anti-epileptics.

Nursing points about anti-epileptics

(a) They react variably and unpredictably with many other drugs.
(b) Plasma monitoring of drug level may be required, particularly in late pregnancy (as drug levels may fall).
(c) Mono-anticonvulsant therapy usually preferred.
(d) Change-over from one anti-epileptic to another must be made slowly and with care.
(e) Car-driving may be possible by patients who have had a seizure-free period of not less than 2 years.
(f) Care is necessary in pregnancy, as anti-epileptics are potentially teratogenic. Neural tube defects may occur with carbamazepine, phenytoin and valproate, and patients should be advised accordingly.

CENTRAL STIMULANTS

Many substances are known that have a stimulant effect on the central nervous system and they act by increasing the rate of neuronal discharge or by blocking an inhibitory neurotransmitter, but therapeutically they are of very limited value except in a few specific conditions. There is no pharmacological basis for the use of central stimulants in the treatment of depression, debility or fatigue, and the risks of misuse and dependence are considerable.

Caffeine (dose: 250–500 mg)

Caffeine is the central stimulant constituent of tea and coffee. It acts mainly on the sensory cortex of the brain, increasing mental alertness and postponing drowsiness and fatigue.

Caffeine is present in a number of proprietary analgesic preparations available without prescription, but it adds little or nothing to the pain-relieving properties of such products.

Amphetamine sulphate* (dose: 5–10 mg daily)

The stimulant action of amphetamine is mediated by inhibiting the re-uptake of noradrenaline. It has been abused and now rarely prescribed. The related methylphenidate* (Ritalin*) is an old stimulant which, paradoxically, has been re-introduced for the treatment of hyperactive children.

Dexamphetamine sulphate* (dose: 10–60 mg daily)

Brand name: Dexedrine*
Dexamphetamine has the central stimulant properties of amphetamine, and is used mainly in the treatment of narcolepsy, an uncommon syndrome of recurrent periods of sleep with sudden loss of muscle tone. It is given in doses of 10 mg initially, slowly increased in divided doses up to 60 mg daily. Paradoxically, it has a central sedative action in some cases of brain damage and it is used in the control of hyperkinesia in children. It is then given in initial doses of 5 mg daily, increased slowly according to need and response up to 20 mg daily, although doses up to 40 mg daily have been given. Such use of dexamphetamine requires great care under expert supervision, as it may interfere with growth and development.

Side-effects of dexamphetamine include insomnia, restlessness and agitation, and with large doses personality changes with aggression may occur. Dexamphetamine has some appetite-depressant properties, and it has been used in the treatment of obesity. Dependence is a constant risk, and such use of dexamphetamine is no longer recommended. Phentermine* (Duromine*, Ionamine*) has a similar action and risks of dependence.

FURTHER READING

Anon 1988 Fluvoxamine (Faverin). Drugs and Therapeutics Bulletin 26:33–34
Anon 1990 Fluoxetine, another antidepressant. Drugs and Therapeutics Bulletin 28:95–96
Anon 1990 Vigabatrin – a new anticonvulsant. Drugs and Therapeutics Bulletin 28:95–96
Anon 1990 Zoplicone: another carriage on the tranquilliser train. Lancet 335:507–508

Beasley C M et al 1997 Olazapine versus haloperidol. European Neuropsychopharmacology 7:125–137
Brodie M J 1992 Lamotrigine. Lancet 339:1397–1400
Brodie M J, Dichter M A 1996 Antiepileptic drugs. New England Journal of Medicine 334:168–169
Chadwick D 1988 The modern treatment of epilepsy. British Journal of Hospital Medicine 39:104–110

Edwards J G 1992 Selective serotonin uptake inhibitors. British Medical Journal 304:1644–1645

Glod C A 1996 Recent advances in the pharmacology of major depression. Archieves of Psychiatric Nursing X(6):355–364

Hale A 1997 Depression – a clinical review. British Medical Journal 315:43–45

Jones A L et al 1997 Should methionine be added to every paracetamol tablet? British Medical Journal 315:301–303

Kupecz D 1995 New drugs for the treatment of epilepsy. Nurse Practitioner 20(5):82–85

Lovejoy N C, Matteis M 1996 Pharmacokinetics and pharmacodynamics of mood-altering drugs in patients with cancer. Cancer Nursing 19(6):407–418

Milligan K 1997 Tricyclic antidepressants are also used for the relief of chronic pain. British Medical Journal 314:827–828

Montgomery S 1993 Venlafaxine: A new dimension in antidepressant pharmacotherapy. Journal of Clinical Psychiatry 54:119–126

Pollard A, Friedman T, Aslam M 1994 Tranquillising actions. Nursing Times 90(11):34–36

Rogers S L, Friedhoff L T 1996 The efficacy and safety of donepezil in patients with Alzheimer's disease. Dementia 7:293–303

Sims J 1995 The extrapyramidal effects of phenothiazines on patients. Nursing Times 91(43):30–31

Smith L 1995 Clozapine: indications and implications for treatment. Nursing Times 91(30):40–41

Stewart J E 1992 What can antidepressants tell us about depression? Professional Nurse 7(10):639–642

4

Opioid (narcotic) analgesics and antagonists; non-narcotic analgesics; antimigraine drugs

Pain is a very subjective sensation, so its severity is difficult to assess and therefore difficult to manage. It is more than a purely physical sensation as it is strongly influenced by perception, emotion and the social context. The pain threshold also varies, so that after injury different individuals will experience the pain differently, depending on its meaning for them and the distractions within their environment.

In an attempt to explain the complexities of pain Melzack and Wall developed the Gate Control Theory. This theory suggests that unmyelinated small-diameter C-fibres convey nervous impulses from the site of tissue injury to the substantia gelatinosa in the dorsal horn of the spinal cord. From here the pain signals can be transmitted via the thalamus to the cortex of the brain, where the pain is experienced (Fig. 4.1). The Gate Control Theory suggests that the pain impulses can be modulated in the substantia gelatinosa. Thus nervous impulses entering the spinal cord along rapidly conducting myelinated Aβ fibres (touch afferents) are believed to interact with the pain impulses in the substantia gelatinosa and are able to inhibit their transmission. The substantia gelatinosa is therefore seen as a gate which can be 'closed' to pain impulses by other nervous impulses such as those produced by rubbing the damaged area, or by applying heat or cold. The use of transcutaneous nerve stimulation, i.e. the application of small electrical impulses to the skin, makes use of this concept to successfully control chronic pain.

As well as pain messages being modulated by other physical sensations, they can be moderated by drugs such as morphine. The value of morphine has been known for a long time, but the mechanism of its action is now clearer. In the brain and spinal cord there are receptors for opioids (morphine-like drugs). When the drug binds to the receptor it inhibits the

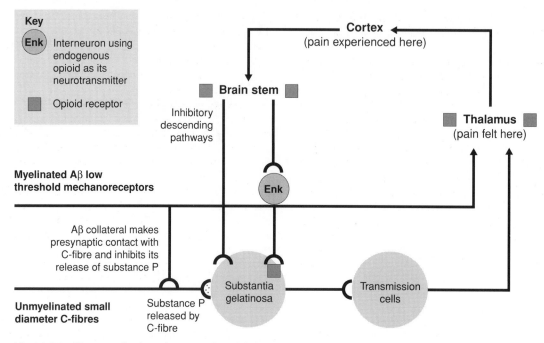

Figure 4.1 Diagram of pain pathways and modulation.

pain message from being relayed on, and so helps to reduce the pain experienced. Why opioid receptors exist became clear a few years ago when researchers found that these receptors are normally used by our own endogenous opioid peptides, i.e. endorphins, enkephalins and dynorphins. These neurotransmitters are released in times of stress, particularly by small interneurons (Fig. 4.1), and help the body escape from danger when pain might otherwise incapacitate it. This perhaps explains why some people become addicted to exercise. The stress of the exercise, for example long distance running, causes endogenous opioids to be released giving the runner a 'high' or 'buzz' similar to taking a dose of morphine.

NARCOTIC ANALGESICS

Narcotic analgesics both relieve pain and induce sleep. The most powerful are the opioids, represented by morphine and diamorphine (heroin), but synthetic opioids are also effective. They act by binding to the opioid receptors (μ, κ, δ) found in the brain and spinal cord, and function mainly as μ agonists. They appear to inhibit the transmission of pain impulses from the relay neurones in the dorsal horn as well as altering the perception of pain in the brain. That

alternation of perception may explain why some surgical patients say that they are aware of the operational pain yet feel that they are in some way detached from it. The opioids are not suitable for treating all types of pain, but are most effective in the control of severe, deep, aching dull pain. Musculoskeletal pain is best treated with non-steroidal anti-inflammatory drugs (NSAIDs) (p. 203), neuralgia with anticonvulsants (p. 41) and muscle cramp pain with skeletal muscle relaxants (p. 246). Some tricyclic antidepressants have useful analgesic properties (p. 34). The opioids also bind to other receptors, as they stimulate the chemoreceptor trigger zone in the brain and cause vomiting; they also cause respiratory depression, and by binding with receptors in the bowel cause constipation. As they produce euphoric responses that can lead to both physical and psychological dependence, they are open to abuse, and so are controlled by the Misuse of Drugs Act 1971 (see Chapter 30).

Opium and papaveretum*

Opium is the dried juice obtained from the seed-capsules of the opium poppy. It contains morphine, papaverine and codeine, and papaveretum is a standardized preparation of those alkaloids. Omnopon* is a proprietary product of similar composition.

Opium as such is rarely used in the UK and papaveretum is used mainly as Papaveretum Injection and as Papaveretum and Hyoscine Injection. They are given by subcutaneous, intramuscular or intravenous injection for preoperative medication and postoperative analgesia, but are now used less frequently. Papaveretum Injection is available in two strengths, 7.7 mg/ml and 15.4 mg/ml, equivalent to 5 mg and 10 mg of morphine. Papaverine and Hyoscine Injection contains 14.4 mg/ml together with hyoscine 400 micrograms/ml.

Both products were formerly widely used for premedication and postoperative analgesia, but their use declined when it was found that a minor constituent (noscopine) was potentially teratogenic. The products have been reformulated and no longer contain noscopine, and may perhaps regain their past usefulness. They are given in standard doses by subcutaneous or intramuscular injection, or by half-dose intravenously.

Morphine* (dose: 10–20 mg)

Morphine is the oldest and most widely used narcotic analgesic. It not only suppresses pain stimuli received from special areas in the limbic system, but also appears to alter subjective reactions to pain. In acute pain it is given in doses of 10 mg by intramuscular or subcutaneous injection, but in shock the former is preferred, as absorption from subcutaneous injection may be delayed because of the intense vasoconstriction that occurs after shock. If necessary, as in acute pulmonary oedema and myocardial infarction, morphine may be given by slow intravenous injection in doses of one quarter to one half of those given intramuscularly. For preoperative use, it is often given with atropine or hyoscine to reduce bronchial secretions. For the relief of chronic pain, morphine is given in oral doses of 5–20 mg 4-hourly, and in terminal illness the dose should be increased according to need; doses of 100 mg or more may be required, if necessary together with an anti-emetic to control any associated nausea. In such cases, the need to relieve pain outweighs the risks of possible dependence. In chronic and severe pain, the frequency of dose may be reduced by the use of long-acting products such as MST Continus. Morphine may also be given as a 15 mg suppository. In severe, chronic intractable pain, morphine has been given by epidural and intrathecal injection. Another method of suppressing severe pain that is now in wider use is patient-controlled analgesia (PCA). This involves the use of an infusion pump that delivers a metered dose of the analgesic by subcutaneous injection. The patient can control the frequency of the injection according to need. The method offers an increased individual control of pain that in itself may improve the response to the analgesic. PCA has also been used to control the painful episodes of sickle-cell disease, even in young children.

Oramorph is a solution of morphine (10 mg/5 ml) for oral use, and the so-called Brompton Cocktail or morphine elixir is a traditional mixture of varying quantities of morphine, cocaine and alcohol (often as gin). Whether the inclusion of cocaine potentiates the analgesia or enhances mood is open to question.

Side-effects Some of the side-effects of morphine are linked with its general action on the central nervous system. It depresses the respiratory centre, and care is necessary in patients with respiratory insufficiency and in asthmatics. Airway resistance may be increased by thickening of bronchial secretions and suppression of cough. Constipation may occur by a reduction in intestinal motility. Occasionally the pain of biliary colic is increased by morphine as it brings about a rise in intrabiliary pressure, and phenazocine is sometimes preferred. Care is necessary in patients with renal or hepatic impairment, and in those receiving antihypertensive therapy.

Children and the aged are particularly susceptible to morphine, and doses should be adjusted to need and response. The toxic dose varies, and in some patients even therapeutic doses may cause vomiting, restlessness and confusion. With larger doses, cyanosis may develop following respiratory depression, with coma and the pin-point pupils typical of opiate poisoning. The use of narcotic antagonists in the treatment of opiate poisoning is referred to on p. 53.

Nursing points about opioid analgesics
(a) Dose and timing are important, as analgesia may be more effective and controllable if given before severe pain develops.
(b) Subsequent doses should be given at suitable intervals to maintain analgesia before pain escapes from control.
(c) Nausea and vomiting are common side-effects, but may subside as opioid treatment is continued.
(d) In terminal analgesia, relief of pain is the primary aim and outweighs any risks of drug-dependence.
(e) Pethidine should not be given to patients receiving MAOI treatment.
(f) Long-acting oral products should be swallowed whole, not chewed or crushed.
(g) Marked respiratory depression may indicate overdose; naloxone is specific treatment (p. 53).

Drug dependence is a problem with all narcotic analgesics and arises from the euphoric side-effects of those drugs. For that reason extended treatment should be avoided, except in terminal illness where the risks of tolerance and drug addiction are much less important than the need to relieve pain.

Diamorphine* (dose: 5–10 mg)

Diamorphine, also known as heroin, is prepared from morphine and has a similar but more powerful analgesic action. It is of great value when increasing doses are required for severe pain in the terminal stages of carcinoma, as its greater solubility permits the use of smaller volumes of injection solution. In chronic pain, diamorphine is given orally or by injection in doses of 5–10 mg which should be repeated according to need and increased as required. Similar doses can be given for the short-term treatment of acute pain, but intravenous doses should be reduced to one quarter to one half of the intramuscular dose. Diamorphine is also given by subcutaneous infusion in the control of the pain of terminal disease.

It is also a powerful cough centre depressant, and is sometimes given as a linctus (3 mg/5 ml) in the severe and intractable cough of terminal disease.

Side-effects of diamorphine are essentially similar to those of morphine.

Alfentanil* (dose: 500 micrograms intravenously initially)

Brand name: Rapifen*
Alfentanil is a potent narcotic analgesic, similar to fentanyl, but mainly used in operative procedures when a rapid onset and short duration of action is required. When used with thiopentone anaesthesia, it permits a reduction in dose of thiopentone, and a more rapid recovery that is useful in out-patient surgery and in poor-risk patients. Doses of 500 micrograms by intravenous injection are given initially, followed by doses of 250 micrograms at intervals of 4–5 minutes according to need. In case of assisted ventilation, an initial dose of 50–100 micrograms/kg is given by intravenous infusion, with supplementary doses of 0.5–1 micrograms/kg/minute as required. Alfentanil may occasionally cause severe respiratory depression which may extend over the postoperative period. It can be reversed by naloxone (p. 53) or doxapram (p. 240).

Buprenorphine* (dose: 200–400 micrograms by injection, 200 micrograms sublingually)

Brand name: Temgesic*
Buprenorphine is a powerful analgesic with a long action that may extend for 8–12 hours, but is less likely to cause dependence. It is given by subcutaneous or intramuscular injection in doses of 200–400 micrograms 6–8-hourly. It is also given orally as sublingual tablets of 200 micrograms. Paradoxically, it also has some of the properties of an opioid antagonist, and may cause withdrawal symptoms in opioid-dependent patients.

Side-effects include drowsiness, vomiting and dizziness, and although buprenorphine has a relatively wide margin of safety, some respiratory depression may occur. The action, which may be prolonged in hepatic disease, is only partly reversed by naloxone.

Dextromoramide* (dose: 5–20 mg)

Brand name: Palfium*
Dextromoramide is a powerful narcotic analgesic that is used mainly in the severe pain of terminal disease. It is less sedating than morphine, but the duration of action is shorter, and may not extend over 3 hours. Dextromoramide is given orally in doses of 5–20 mg, or 10 mg by suppository.

Dihydrocodeine § (dose: 30 mg orally, 50 mg by injection)

Brand name: DF-118 §
A derivative of codeine with increased analgesic potency. It is valuable in the treatment of a variety of moderate to severe painful conditions where the use of more powerful narcotic analgesics is not justified. It also has some cough suppressant properties. Dihydrocodeine is given orally after food in doses of 30 mg up to 4-hourly as necessary, or in doses of 50 mg by intramuscular or deep subcutaneous injection. The injection, but not the oral form, is subject to CD regulation. DHC Continus § is a long-acting oral product containing 60 mg of dihydrocodeine, given twice daily.

Side-effects are similar to those of morphine, but less severe, and dependence is also less likely to occur.

Co-dydramol § (Paramol §) is a mixed product containing dihydrocodeine 10 mg and paracetamol 500 mg.

Dipipanone* (dose: 40–120 mg daily)

Dipipanone is a synthetic narcotic analgesic that is less potent and less sedating than morphine, and less liable to cause respiratory depression. It is used as the mixed product Diconal*, which contains dipipanone 10 mg and cyclizine 30 mg. Cyclizine is added to reduce the **side-effects** of nausea and vomiting, but the mixed product is not suitable for extended use.

Fentanyl* (dose: 50–200 micrograms by intravenous injection)

Brand name: Sublimaze*

Fentanyl is a morphine-like analgesic but of considerably higher potency. It is used mainly as an analgesic during thiopentone anaesthesia, as it permits a reduction in the dose of anaesthetics, and the combination is of value in poor-risk patients. Fentanyl is given by intravenous injection in doses of 50–200 micrograms initially, with subsequent doses of 50 micrograms as required, but if assisted ventilation is used, initial doses of 300–500 micrograms are given. Patches of fentanyl are available for the relief of the chronic intractable pain of cancer as Durogesic*▼, designed to release 25, 50, 75 or 100 micrograms of the drug over 72 hours.

Fentanyl is also used in association with droperidol to promote anaesthesia in children and the aged, and for neuroleptoanalgesia during certain diagnostic procedures.

The main **side-effects** are respiratory depression, nausea and vomiting, but bradycardia and transient hypotension may also occur. Care is necessary in respiratory and liver disease, and in myasthenia gravis.

Meptazinol* (dose: 800 mg–1.6 g daily orally; 100–150 mg by injection)

Brand name: Meptid*

Meptazinol is a potent synthetic analgesic with reduced sedative effects. It is used in the short-term treatment of postoperative and obstetric pain, in renal colic and other conditions of moderate to severe pain in oral doses of 200 mg four to eight times a day. Meptazinol is also given by intramuscular injection in doses of 75–150 mg 2–4-hourly according to need, and in acute pain by slow intravenous injection in doses of 50–100 mg.

Meptazinol is relatively free from opiate side-effects, and is less likely to cause respiratory depression, but nausea and dizziness may occur.

Methadone* (dose: 5–20 mg by injection)

Brand name: Physeptone*

Methadone is a powerful synthetic analgesic resembling morphine in general activity, but with less sedative or euphoric potency, and with an action lasting up to 8 hours. It is given orally or by subcutaneous or intramuscular injection in doses of 5–10 mg three or four times a day according to need, and is useful when adequate analgesia without sedation is required. For extended use, twice daily dosage should not be exceeded in order to avoid accumulation and subsequent overdose.

Methadone also has cough centre depressant properties, and is useful for the control of useless cough in malignant lung conditions. Methadone *linctus* contains 2 mg/5 ml, and is for adult use only. Methadone is also used in the withdrawal and replacement treatment of drug addiction and dependence as methadone *mixture*, which contains 5 mg/5 ml.

Nalbuphine (dose: 10–20 mg by injection)

Brand name: Nubain

Nalbuphine is a synthetic, rapidly acting morphine-like analgesic with reduced side-effects and a lower abuse potential. It is given in moderate to severe pain in doses of 10–20 mg by intramuscular, subcutaneous or intravenous injection at intervals of 3–6 hours according to need.

Nalbuphine is also used to control the pain of myocardial infarction as a dose of 10–30 mg by slow intravenous injection, repeated after 30 minutes if required. When used as a supplementary drug in anaesthesia, it is given in doses of 250–500 micrograms/kg at 30-minute intervals.

Side-effects include respiratory depression and sedation, but nausea and vomiting are less common. Care is necessary in renal and hepatic disease, and in pre-existing respiratory depression.

Pentazocine* (dose: 25–100 mg orally; 30–60 mg by injection)

Brand name: Fortral*

Pentazocine has the general analgesic properties of morphine, but is less likely to cause addiction. Its action is less potent and less prolonged, and after oral administration much of a dose is lost by first-pass liver metabolism. Pentazocine is given orally in doses of 50–100 mg after food, up to a maximum of 600 mg daily, or by injection (subcutaneous, intramuscular or intravenous), according to the severity of the pain, up to 360 mg daily. Pentazocine may also be used as 50 mg suppositories up to four times a day. It may be of value in biliary colic, as it appears to be less likely to cause an increase in biliary pressure than some related analgesics. Care is necessary with patients already receiving an opioid analgesic, as pentazocine, like buprenorphine, may paradoxically increase the pain and bring about withdrawal symptoms.

Side-effects of pentazocine include nausea, dizziness, lightheadedness and hallucinations. As transient hypertension may occur, pentazocine should be avoided in hypertensive states and after myocardial infarction. Convulsions have followed large intravenous doses.

Pethidine* (dose: 50–100 mg orally; 25–100 mg by intramuscular injection; 25–50 mg intravenously)

Pethidine is an old synthetic drug with some of the properties of both morphine and atropine, and has analgesic and antispasmodic actions. Although less potent than morphine, and with a shorter action, it is widely used for the relief of moderate to severe pain, including postoperative pain, in labour, and as a supplementary drug in general anaesthesia. It is not suitable for the treatment of severe and constant pain, as in terminal illness.

Pethidine is given mainly by intramuscular injection in doses of 25–100 mg, repeated 4-hourly as required, or subcutaneously. It may also be given by slow intravenous injection in doses of 25–50 mg (10–25 mg as an adjunct to anaesthesia) but vasodilatation and hypotension may occur. Pethidine may also be given orally in doses of 50–150 mg, but the response is less rapid and less intense. It is also used by injection as an obstetric analgesic, although labour may be prolonged and some neonatal respiratory depression may occur, but to a lesser extent than with other narcotic analgesics.

Side-effects of pethidine are those of the narcotic analgesics generally, but some stimulation of the CNS may occur and convulsions have been reported after high doses. It is less likely to cause constipation, and has no antitussive properties. The prolonged use of pethidine should be avoided, as addiction may result.

Phenazocine* (dose: 5–20 mg)

Brand name: Narphen*

Phenazocine is a synthetic analgesic with the general properties of morphine, but with an increased potency, and effective in lower doses. It is used for the relief of severe painful conditions, including pancreatitis, and in renal colic as it is less likely to increase the biliary pressure. Phenazocine is given orally in doses of 5 mg, repeated 4–6-hourly as required, but single doses up to 20 mg may sometimes be necessary. It may be given sublingually when nausea and vomiting complicate oral treatment.

Side-effects include nausea and vomiting, but phenazocine is less sedating than morphine, and is less likely to cause constipation. Dependence remains a risk with extended use.

Remifentanil §

Brand name: Ultiva §

Opioid analgesics such as alfentanil and flufentanyl are widely used as supplementary drugs during the induction and maintenance of anaesthesia and for analgesia during operation. Their long action may delay recovery. A newer drug of that type is remifentanil which is a potent opioid analgesic, but it differs from related drugs in being rapidly inactivated by blood and tissue esterases. As a result, any postoperative residual analgesic action disappears within 5–10 minutes, and the rapid breakdown of the drug permits its use in renal and hepatic impairment and does not require any adjustment of dose.

For the induction of anaesthesia remifentanil is given as a bolus intravenous infusion in a dose of 1 microgram/kg, followed by the continuous infusion of 0.5–1 microgram/kg. Smaller doses are used with ventilated patients. Smaller doses of anaesthetics such as isoflurane and propofol should be given to avoid excessive depth of anaesthesia, and facilities for dealing with respiratory depression must be available. To avoid postoperative pain, an analgesic should be given before remifentanil is withdrawn.

Tramadol § (dose: 50–100 mg)

Brand names: Tramake § ▼ Zamadol § ▼ Zydol § ▼

Tramadol is a centrally-acting analgesic. The mode of action is not yet clear, but it may act in part on opioid receptors, and in part through an inhibition of the re-uptake of noradrenaline and an increased serotonin release. Tramadol is used in the short-term or intermittent management of moderate to severe pain, and is given in oral doses of 50–100 mg 4–6-hourly. Doses of more than 400 mg daily are seldom required. In severe pain, tramadol may be given in similar doses by intramuscular or intravenous injection. The dosage intervals should be extended in renal and hepatic impairment. Tramadol has a low dependence potential, and cannot suppress morphine-withdrawal symptoms, but prolonged use should be avoided.

Side-effects include drowsiness, dizziness and fatigue.

NARCOTIC ANTAGONISTS

Lofexidine § (dose: 0.4–2.4 mg daily)

Brand name: BritLofex §

It is thought that the symptoms of opiate withdrawal may be linked with an excessive rebound release of noradrenaline in the brain. It is known that clonidine (p. 122) has an inhibitory action on such noradrenaline release, but its value in opiate withdrawal is limited because of its antihypertensive properties. Lofexidine is a related drug with a more selective action on brain noradrenergic activity. It is used in the rapid control of opiate withdrawal symptoms, and may prove useful as transitional treatment before naltrexone therapy is commenced. Lofexidine is given in initial doses of 200 micrograms twice a day, slowly increased according to need and response up to a maximum if required of 2.4 mg daily.

Side-effects are drowsiness, dryness of mouth, hypotension and bradycardia. At the end of treatment the dose should be tapered off over 2–4 days to reduce the risks of rebound hypertension.

Naloxone § (dose: 1.5–3 micrograms/kg by injection)

Brand name: Narcan §

Naloxone is a short-acting specific antagonist of the opioid analgesics, and is used in the treatment of narcotic-induced postoperative respiratory depression and of narcotic overdose. In such respiratory depression, naloxone is given by intravenous injection as an initial dose of 1.5–3 micrograms/kg (or 100–200 micrograms), followed by 100 microgram doses at intervals of 2 minutes as required. For neonates, doses of 10 micrograms/kg, or a single dose of 200 micrograms may be given. It should be noted that naloxone reverses the analgesic action of the opioids as well as their depressant action on respiration, so dosage in the postoperative period must be controlled to avoid the return of pain.

In suspected narcotic overdose or poisoning, naloxone is given intravenously in doses of 0.8–2 mg, repeated at 2-minute intervals according to response, up to a total dose of 10 mg. Alternatively, a dose of 2 mg, after dilution, may be given by continuous intravenous infusion. The absence of a response indicates that the respiratory depression is not due to narcotic overdose.

Naltrexone § (dose: 25–50 mg daily)

Brand name: Nalorex §

Naltrexone is a powerful, long-acting narcotic antagonist that binds selectively with the opioid receptors (p. 47). It is used only to maintain recovery from opioid drug addiction, and prevents re-addiction only while the drug is being taken, so prolonged maintenance therapy is required. It is given in doses of 25 mg initially, later increased to 50 mg daily. Naltrexone must not be given to patients who are still opioid-dependent, as relapse and an acute withdrawal syndrome may be precipitated within minutes. Its use requires care under specialist supervision. Caution is necessary in hepatic and renal dysfunction, as naltrexone is metabolized in the liver and excreted in the urine.

SOME LESS POWERFUL NARCOTIC ANALGESICS

Codeine § (dose: 60–180 mg daily orally; 30 mg by injection)

Codeine is one of the alkaloids present with morphine in opium. It is much less powerful than morphine, and its analgesic value is limited, but it is given in doses of 30–60 mg up to a maximum of 240 mg daily in mild to moderate pain. An increase in dose does not increase the analgesic response. It is occasionally given by intramuscular injection in doses up to 60 mg.

Side-effects include constipation, nausea and sedation. It is contra-indicated in respiratory depression.

Co-codamol § is a mixed product containing codeine 8 mg and paracetamol 500 mg; Co-codaprin § contains codeine 8 mg with aspirin 400 mg, and a number of proprietary mild analgesic products are formulated on a similar basis. The analgesic value of the small doses of codeine in these preparations is open to question. The use of codeine as a cough centre depressant is referred to on p. 242.

Dextropropoxyphene § (dose: 65 mg)

Brand name: Doloxene §

Dextropropoxyphene is an analgesic resembling codeine, but less likely to cause constipation. It is used in the relief of mild to moderate pain in doses of 65 mg three or four times a day, often in association with paracetamol as co-proxamol (Distalgesic §), which contains dextropropoxyphene 32.5 mg with paracetamol 325 mg.

Co-proxamol is used in a wide range of chronic and recurring painful conditions, but the maximum dose of eight tablets daily should not be exceeded. Overdose, especially if taken with alcohol, may cause opioid-induced respiratory depression and collapse, requiring prompt treatment with naloxone. Subsequently, severe paracetamol hepatotoxicity may develop (see p. 313).

NON-NARCOTIC ANALGESICS

Several mild analgesics are available for the relief of the many minor painful and rheumatic conditions that do not call for treatment with more powerful drugs. The more specific antirheumatic drugs, dealt with in Chapter 15, also have useful mild analgesic properties.

Nursing points about mild analgesics

(a) Ask patients about any aspirin hypersensitivity.
(b) Take with food or milk to reduce the risks of gastric irritation.
(c) Soluble aspirin and similar products should be dissolved in water to promote rapid absorption.
(d) In general, alcohol should be avoided, as car-driving and similar abilities may be affected.
(e) Aspirin should not be given to children under 12 years of age as it may cause Reye's syndrome.

Aspirin, acetylsalicylic acid (dose: 2–4 g daily)

Although introduced in 1899, aspirin remains one of the most valuable and widely used of the mild analgesics. It acts mainly by inhibiting the biosynthesis of prostaglandins (p. 203) and is the principal constituent of a variety of popular pain-relieving preparations, often with paracetamol and other drugs.

Aspirin relieves the pain of headache, toothache, neuritis, myalgia and a variety of other conditions requiring mild analgesic therapy. It is given in doses of 300–600 mg five to six times a day, up to a maximum as an analgesic of 4 g daily. In larger doses up to 8 g daily it is given for the treatment of acute and chronic inflammatory conditions such as rheumatoid arthritis.

Aspirin has some antiplatelet activity (see p. 134) and may potentiate the effects of warfarin, and in low doses is used for migraine prophylaxis (p. 56).

Side-effects Aspirin is in general well tolerated, but it can cause nausea, indigestion and gastric irritation with blood loss, and may be the cause of an unsuspected iron-deficiency anaemia when aspirin is taken for prolonged periods.

Idiosyncrasy to aspirin is not uncommon, and in susceptible patients even small doses may precipitate hypersensitivity reactions such as paroxysmal bronchospasm, which may be severe or even fatal.

Some of the gastric side-effects can be reduced by taking the drug after meals, or in association with an alkali, and Dispersible Aspirin Tablets and similar proprietary products are formulated on that basis and contain calcium carbonate.

In high doses, aspirin may cause dizziness, confusion, tinnitus, deafness and hypothrombinaemia. Toxic doses may cause respiratory failure and cardiovascular collapse.

Aspirin may be a causative factor in Reye's syndrome. That syndrome, an acute encephalopathy and fatty degeneration of the liver, is a rare but potentially fatal illness in children. It is now recommended that aspirin should not be given to children under 12 years of age for minor or febrile illness, but be reserved for conditions such as juvenile rheumatoid arthritis (Still's disease).

Benorylate (dose: 4–8 g daily)

Brand name: Benoral

Benorylate is a chemical compound of aspirin and paracetamol and has the anti-inflammatory and analgesic properties of the parent substances but with reduced side-effects. Dose 1.5–2 g three times a day. It should not be given to a patient with a known hypersensitivity to aspirin, or to children under 12 years of age.

Diflunisal § (dose: 500 mg–1 g daily)

Brand name: Dolobid §

Diflunisal is chemically related to aspirin and has a similar pattern of activity, but is less likely to cause gastrointestinal side-effects. It has both analgesic and anti-inflammatory properties and is used in post-traumatic and postoperative pain, in some chronic painful conditions, and in osteoarthritis. Diflunisal is given in initial doses of 500 mg twice daily, preferably after food, later reduced to 250 mg twice daily.

Side-effects are similar to those of aspirin, and diflunisal should not be given to aspirin-sensitive patients, or those with a history of peptic ulcer.

Ibuprofen (dose: 1.2–2.4 g daily)

Brand names: Brufen, Fenbid

Ibuprofen is an analgesic anti-inflammatory drug of the NSAID type (p. 203) used in the treatment of mild to moderate musculoskeletal pain, including the pain of dysmenorrhoea and in mild rheumatoid conditions. It is given in doses of 400–800 mg three times a day, after food. It is also given in doses of 20 mg/kg daily in the treatment of pain and febrile conditions in children.

Side-effects are usually mild, but are basically those common to related drugs and bronchospasm may occur in sensitive patients. Fenoprofen (Progesic, Fenopron), dose 200–400 mg three times a day, has similar actions and uses. Codafen Continus contains ibuprofen 300 mg with codeine phosphate 20 mg.

Ketorolac § (dose: 40 mg daily)

Brand name: Toradol §

Ketorolac is a NSAID (p. 203) with increased analgesic potency, and is used in the short-term treatment of acute postoperative pain. It is given in doses of 10 mg 4–6-hourly up to a maximum of 40 mg daily for up to 7 days. Ketorolac may also be given by deep intragluteal or slow intravenous injection in doses of 10–30 mg at intervals of 4–6 hours, but in the initial postoperative period 2-hourly administration may be required. A transfer to oral therapy should be made within 2 days, but on the day of transfer the total dose given should not normally exceed 90 mg. In elderly patients, lower doses at longer intervals should be given. Ketorolac is a peripherally acting analgesic and does not interfere with opiate-binding receptors, and may be used together with opiate analgesics for the control of severe pain. It has no sedative or anxiolytic action. Ketorolac is contra-indicated in patients sensitive to aspirin or any other NSAID, in active or latent ulcer, or in patients with asthma or coagulation disorders. Ketorolac has many side-effects, and for details the manufacturer's literature should be consulted.

Mefenamic acid § (dose: 1.5 g daily)

Brand name: Ponstan §

Mefenamic acid has analgesic and mild anti-inflammatory properties, and is useful in mild to moderate pain of varied origin, including simple menorrhagia, and in rheumatic states, including Still's disease. The adult dose is 500 mg three times a day after food; children's doses for short-term treatment are 25 mg/kg daily in divided doses.

Side-effects include diarrhoea, which is an indication for withdrawal, as is haemolytic anaemia, hypersensitivity and bronchospasm, rash and jaundice. Blood tests are necessary during prolonged treatment. Overdose may cause convulsions.

Nefopam § (dose: 90–270 mg daily orally; 20 mg by injection)

Brand name: Acupan §

Nefopam is an analgesic with aspirin-like properties, although its mode of action differs, as it has no effect on prostaglandin synthesis. It is used in the relief of moderate and chronic pain in doses of 30–60 mg three times a day up to a maximum of 270 mg daily or more according to need. It is also given in doses of 20 mg up to 6-hourly by intramuscular injection, but some local pain at the injection site may occur. Nefopam has some anticholinergic properties, and may cause dryness of the mouth and urinary retention. Other **side-effects** include nausea, dizziness, tachycardia and confusion. It may give a pink colour to the urine. It is contra-indicated in convulsive disorders and myocardial infarction.

Paracetamol (dose: 1–4 mg daily)

Paracetamol is a very widely used mild analgesic, and is also present in a range of mixed products available under brand names. It has the great advantage over aspirin of being much less likely to cause any gastric irritation but it has no anti-inflammatory action. Paracetamol is given in doses of 0.5–1 g four to six times a day, up to a maximum dose of 4 g daily. In suitable doses, it is useful in febrile conditions in children. In post-immunization pyrexia in infants, paracetamol is given in a dose of 60 mg, followed if necessary by a second dose, administered as Paracetamol Paediatric Elixir (Oral Solution) via an oral syringe. Not more than two doses should be given without medical advice. (Co-codamol is a mixed product containing, unless otherwise prescribed, 8 mg of codeine and 500 mg of paracetamol.)

Paracetamol has few **side-effects**, but excessive and prolonged use may cause liver damage. In acute paracetamol poisoning *early* treatment is essential, as a severe and potentially fatal hepatonecrosis may develop (p. 313).

ANTIMIGRAINE DRUGS

Migraine is an episodic disorder characterized by a pulsating headache, often unilateral at first, which lasts from 4 to 72 hours, accompanied by other symptoms including nausea, vomiting, photophobia and general malaise. An attack is often heralded by an aura of flashing lights, tingling and numbness. Cluster headache, sometimes called migrainous neuralgia, is a short-lived but intense lateral pain that may occur at intervals at the same time of day for some weeks.

The mechanism of a migraine attack is not clear, as an attack may be triggered off by a variety of stimuli including food such as cheese and chocolate, bright lights and even oral contraceptives. The symptoms appear to be due to changes in the cerebral blood vessels that lead to a vasoconstriction and the onset of the aura, followed by an inflammatory reaction causing arterial dilatation and pain. The neurotransmitter serotonin (p. 34) may play an essential part in that process, as the 5-HT_{1D} receptor is found on the cranial vessels and its stimulation causes vasodilatation.

The treatment of an acute attack of migraine may be symptomatic with a mild analgesic or more effectively by targeting the underlying vasodilatation. Ergotamine is a weak 5-HT_{1D} partial agonist and vasoconstrictor, and has long been used in the treatment of migraine, but more powerful agonists such as sumatriptan are now available.

A daily dose of aspirin is useful prophylactic treatment, and methysergide is given for the prophylaxis of severe cluster headaches.

Ergotamine tartrate § (dose: 1–2 mg orally)

Brand name: Lingraine §
Ergotamine is one of the alkaloids of ergot (p. 169) but it is used only for the relief of migraine. The best response is obtained if the drug is taken in adequate dose before an attack has fully developed. It relieves the headache, but may aggravate nausea and vomiting, and combined treatment with an anti-emetic may be required.

The optimum oral dose of ergotamine is best determined by experience, and the initial dose of 2 mg should be taken at the first sign of an attack, preferably sublingually and repeated after 30 minutes. Not more than 6 mg should be taken in any single day, or more than 12 mg in 1 week. Ergotamine may also be given by oral inhalation for a more rapid effect, and the Medihaler-Ergotamine delivers a dose of 360 micrograms, which may be repeated after 5 minutes, but not more than six doses should be taken in 24 hours, or 15 during 1 week. Alternatively, when nausea prevents oral therapy, ergotamine may be given as a 2 mg suppository.

Ergotamine in high doses has a peripheral vasoconstrictor action, and it should be withdrawn immediately if any tingling or numbness in the extremities is noted, as gangrene due to vasoconstriction has occurred. For that reason ergotamine is not used prophylactically.

Side-effects of ergotamine include nausea, vomiting and abdominal pain. Cafergot and Migril are mixed products containing caffeine, which may be better tolerated.

Clonidine § (dose: 100–150 micrograms daily)

Brand name: Dixarit §
Clonidine is used in doses of 50–75 micrograms twice daily in the *prophylaxis* of migraine and other recurring vascular headaches. It appears to act by reducing the sensitivity of the cranial vessels to circulating amines. It has the disadvantage that it may aggravate pre-existing depression and may cause insomnia.

Side-effects include dizziness, dryness of the mouth, nausea and occasional rash. It should be noted that the dose and brand name differ from the clonidine product used in hypertension (p. 122).

Methysergide § (dose: 1–6 mg daily)

Brand name: Deseril §
Methysergide is used under hospital supervision for the long-term prophylaxis of very severe recurrent migraine and cluster headache in doses of 1–2 mg three times a day.

Treatment should not be continued for more than 6 months without a break. Care is necessary in patients with cardiovascular disease and liver or renal damage. Retroperitoneal fibrosis and fibrosis of the heart valves have occasionally followed the prolonged use of methysergide, and the drug is best reserved for those patients not responding to other therapy. Methysergide is also of value in other conditions associated with serotonin release, such as carcinoid disease, where it may give prompt relief of the associated severe diarrhoea. It is then given in doses of 12–20 mg daily.

Pizotifen § (dose: 0.5–3 mg daily)

Brand name: Sanomigran §

Pizotifen is a serotonin and histamine antagonist and is effective in the *prophylaxis* of migraine and cluster headache. It is given initially in doses of 500 micrograms at night (to avoid daytime drowsiness), after which the dose may be increased slowly up to three times a day, or up to a maximum of 3 mg daily.

Side-effects are nausea, drowsiness and weight gain. It has some anticholinergic properties, and caution is necessary in closed-angle glaucoma and renal impairment.

Sumatriptan § (dose: 100 mg)

Brand name: Imigran §

Sumatriptan is a powerful 5-HT_{1D} receptor agonist, with a selective vasoconstrictor action. It is given for the relief of acute migraine as a single dose of 100 mg as soon as an attack occurs, which can be repeated if the attack returns after an initial response up to a total of 300 mg in 24 hours. If no initial relief is obtained, a second dose should not be given. In severe migraine, and in cluster headache, sumatriptan can be given by subcutaneous injection (with an auto-injector) in a dose of 6 mg, repeated after not less than 1 hour if the attack recurs. No more than two doses should be given in 24 hours. Alternatively, sumatriptan may be given by single dose (20 mg) nasal spray, with a repeat dose not less than 2 hours later.

Side-effects include fatigue and dizziness. Chest pain has occurred after injections of sumatriptan. It should not be given intravenously, as angina and coronary vasospasm may be precipitated. It should not be given together with other drugs, or until ergotamine therapy has been withdrawn for at least 24 hours.

Zolmitriptan § ▼ (Zomig §) and naratriptan § ▼ (Naramig §) are newer 5-HT_{1D} receptor agonists effective in doses of 2.5 mg. Tolfenamic acid § (Clotam §) is a NSAID used for migraine. Dose: 200 mg.

Nursing points about migraine treatment

(a) Early treatment advisable before the attack develops.
(b) Mild analgesics helpful, but should be taken with a hot drink to promote absorption.
(c) Ergotamine is more specific in action, side-effects may limit effective dose, and more potent 5-HT_{1D} receptor agonists are often preferred.
(d) Ergotamine treatment should not be repeated for at least 4 days or more than twice a month.
(e) Ergotamine should not be given for prophylaxis.

OTHER ANTIMIGRAINE DRUGS

Other drugs that have a secondary action that may be useful in the prophylaxis of migraine are beta-blockers such as propranolol, metoprolol, nadolol and timolol; tricyclic antidepressants represented by amitriptyline, and calcium channel blocking agents such as nifedipine and verapamil.

The feverfew plant has long had a reputation of being useful as a prophylactic against migraine, but it is not a prescribed product.

FURTHER READING

Bateman D N 1993 Sumatriptan. Lancet 341:221–224
Goadsby P J 1991 Oral sumatriptan in acute migraine. Lancet 338:782–783
Goadsby P J, Olesen J 1996 Diagnosis and management of migraine. British Medical Journal 312:1279–1283
Greenland S 1995 A review of the uses of epidural analgesia. Nursing Standard 9(32):32–35
Grundy R, Howard R, Evans J 1993 Practical management of pain in sickling diseases. Archives of Disease in Childhood 69:256–257

Jordan S 1992 Drugs update – drugs for severe pain. Nursing Times 88(8): 24–26
Lance J W 1992 Treatment of migraine. Lancet 339:1207
Lovett P E et al 1994 Pain relief after major gynaecological surgery. British Journal of Nursing 3(4):159–162
Nelson-Piercy C, De Swiet 1996 Low dose aspirin may be used for prophylaxis of migraine. British Medical Journal 313:691
Reilly R 1994 Acute and prophylactic treatment of migraine. Nursing Times 90(29):35–36

Strang J, Bearn J, Gossop M 1997 Opiate detoxification under anaesthesia. British Medical Journal 315:1249–1250

Southern D A, Read M S 1994 Overdosage of opiate from patient controlled analgesia device. British Medical Journal 309:100–104

Thomas W J, Rose E D 1993 Patient controlled anaesthesia. A new method for old. Advanced Nursing 184:1719–1726

Thomas N 1995 Patient controlled anaesthesia. Nursing Standard 9:31–35

Watchman R J et al 1982 Aspirin as a risk factor in Reye's syndrome. Journal of the American Medical Association 247:3089–3094

5

Antibiotics and other anti-infective chemotherapeutic agents

ANTIBIOTICS AND CHEMOTHERAPY

It was once thought that a substance capable of killing bacteria would by its nature be too toxic for use in the treatment of systemic bacterial infections. The problem was eventually solved when the sulphonamides, the first of the synthetic chemotherapeutic agents, were introduced in 1936. Those drugs were exceptional at the time, as they do not kill bacteria directly but hinder their growth and reproduction, and are now termed bacteriostatic agents. Antibiotics differ, as they are substances produced by some fungi and other branched filamentous organisms.

The development of the antibiotics stems from the chance observation of Alexander Fleming in 1928 that the growth of a staphylococcal culture had been inhibited by the presence of a contaminant mould. It was found that a substance produced by the mould could prevent the growth of some bacteria, and the active substance was eventually extracted and named penicillin, after the name of the contaminant fungus. Penicillin was very difficult to obtain in quantity and did not come into therapeutic use until 1941, but since then many new antibiotics have been discovered, and some semisynthetic derivatives have also been introduced.

Mode of action

Antibiotics differ from antiseptics and disinfectants as they are selectively toxic, because their action depends on differences between prokaryotic bacterial cells and eukaryotic human cells. They target structures that bacteria possess but human cells do not, such as the peptidoglycan nature of the bacterial cell wall. The antibiotics can be divided into two groups, the bacteriostatic and the bactericidal. The former merely inhibit bacterial growth, and the organisms are later eliminated by the normal host-defence system of the body. They are therefore ineffective when that defence system is impaired, as in patients receiving cytotoxic or immunosuppressant drugs. The bactericidal antibiotics have a direct toxic effect on dividing bacteria, which may be mediated by several mechanisms, including interfering with the formation of the bacterial cell walls. The cell walls have a lattice-like structure strengthened by cross linkages. Antibiotics, which must first enter the cells, link with certain penicillin-binding proteins (PBPs) and inhibit cell-wall repair. As the cell wall weakens, it eventually bursts under the osmotic pressure of the cell contents. That explains why antibiotics are mainly active against growing cells, as mature or quiescent organisms are less susceptible to cell-wall breakdown. Antibiotics may also affect the permeability of the cell wall, or interfere with vital processes such as the synthesis of proteins and nucleic acids, or interrupt DNA development and activity.

The antibacterial action of the antibiotics is also influenced by differences in the nature of the cell wall. Some bacteria are readily stained by certain dyes, and are referred to as Gram-positive organisms. Other bacteria have cell walls containing a higher proportion of lipids, and so take up the dye less readily, and are described as Gram-negative bacteria. Those differences in cell wall structure explain to some extent why antibiotics may differ in the pattern of their activity, as some may penetrate the cell wall more readily than others. It should be remembered that as bactericidal agents act mainly against active and dividing cells, they should not be prescribed together with bacteriostatic drugs. The latter may induce dividing cells to change into a dormant condition, against which bactericidal agents have little action.

Therapeutically, antibiotics should be used after the infecting organisms have been identified and their sensitivity to antibiotics has been determined. That is not always possible, and an empirical choice of drug based on experience is often necessary. Table 5.1 indicates the *main* type of activity of most of the antibiotics currently available. They have no antiviral activity.

Bacterial resistance

A resistant microorganism is one that is not inhibited or killed by an antimicrobial agent at concentrations of the agent achievable in the body after normal dosage. That resistance may be natural if the drug is unable to enter the cell, or if it only interferes with a process that is not essential for bacterial survival. Much more important is the problem of acquired resistance, which may be due to a chance mutation. Most staphylococci are now resistant to many antibiotics because they have an enzyme, beta-lactamase, that breaks down the active beta-lactam ring structure of penicillin and related antibiotics. Cross resistance may occur, as such resistance between the penicillins and the cephalosporins is well known.

Table 5.1 Main type of activity of some principal antibiotics

Against Gram-positive organisms	Against Gram-negative organisms	Against Gram-positive and Gram-negative organisms	Antitubercular antibiotics
penicillins	amikacin	amoxycillin	capreomycin
clindamycin	aztreonam	ampicillin	cycloserine
cloxacillin	colistin	azlocillin	rifampicin
erythromycin	gentamicin	bacampicillin	streptomycin
flucloxacillin	kanamycin	carbenicillin	
sodium fusidate	netilmicin	carfecillin	
vancomycin	pivmecillinam	cephalosporins[a]	
	polymyxin	chloramphenicol	
	spectinomycin	ciclacillin	
	ticarcillin	imipenem	
	tobramycin	mezlocillin	
		neomycin	
		piperacillin	
		pivampicillin	
		tetracyclines[b]	

[a]See Table 5.4 on page 67
[b]See Table 5.5 on page 68

Similarly, methicillin-resistant *Staphylococcus aureus* (MRSA) has developed enzymes that permit cell wall synthesis to continue even though the antibiotic is present that would kill non-resistant organisms. Such resistant strains have a selective advantage, as non-resistant organisms will be killed off by the antibiotic, so allowing the survivors to multiply without competition for food or space. It follows that the unwise use of antibiotics can serve to promote the development of drug-resistant bacteria.

Resistance may also be acquired by the transfer of genetic material by bacterial contact. In the process of conjugation one bacterium may transfer a copy of its plasmid (a fragment of genetic material) to another bacterium or even cross species barriers. For example, tetracycline resistance has been transferred from bacteria in the gut of animals to distantly related human intestinal bacteria. Therapeutically, the problem of drug resistance is an increasing one. It has often occurred through the over-use of antibiotics for trivial infections, or the unwise use of broad-spectrum antibiotics before the sensitivity of the invading organism has been confirmed. However, there is now a tendency in hospitals and GP practices to devise an antibiotics policy, and to restrict the use of antibiotics to those infections where they are most likely to be effective. Although some antibiotics are still available that are not inactivated by beta-lactamases or other enzymes, the problem of drug resistance remains unsolved. Unless new antibiotics are found, or new methods of overcoming bacterial resistance are developed, many antibacterial agents now in use will become ever less and less effective.

Supra-infection

Antibiotics alter the patient's normal bacterial population. If this balance is upset some of the patient's harmless commensals may start causing infection. For example, *Candida* infections are common in women after treatment with broad-spectrum antibiotics which kill off the Döderlein's bacillus living in the vagina, thus allowing the *Candida* to multiply out of control.

Diarrhoea is a common side-effect of antibiotic treatment and may be due to a disturbance of the normal balanced bacterial flora of the gut. It may be mild and self-limiting, but a much more serious condition is pseudomembranous colitis, now known as antibiotic-associated colitis (AAC), which may occur occasionally with virtually all antibiotics but most frequently with clindamycin. It is due to the overgrowth of *Clostridium difficile*, the release of diarrhoea-causing toxins, and the superficial necrosis of the bowel mucosa. It occurs most frequently in elderly and debilitated patients, especially after abdominal surgery. Treatment is with metronidazole (p. 72) or vancomycin (p. 73).

Sensitivity reactions

Some degree of sensitivity to antibiotics, particularly the penicillins, is relatively common, and nurses should always enquire about such sensitivity before giving an antibiotic. Most sensitivity reactions are allergic in character, and may be immediate or delayed. Immediate reactions may be itching, flushing and sneezing, but breathing difficulties indicate the possibility of an anaphylactic reaction requiring urgent treatment with adrenaline (see p. 90). Later reactions include urticaria, and delayed reactions are characterized by bullous eruptions and dermatitis. If a reaction does occur the patient's notes should be marked accordingly and the patient should be informed of the name of the drug.

Nursing points about antibiotic therapy

(a) Antibiotics are antibacterial, not antiviral agents.
(b) Whenever possible, the nature of the infective organism and its sensitivity to antibiotics should be determined before treatment is commenced.
(c) Broad-spectrum combinations of antibiotics are not a good substitute for treatment tailored to a particular organism.
(d) Other factors governing choice of antibiotic include previous treatment and hypersensitivity, hepatic and renal efficiency, whether patient is immunocompromised or pregnant.
(e) Route of administration and duration of treatment depends on severity of infection: a simple urinary tract infection may respond to short-term therapy; bone infections require prolonged treatment; serious and life-threatening infections require intravenous high-dose therapy.
(f) The topical use of antibiotics should be avoided.

THE PENICILLINS

The name penicillin formerly referred to benzylpenicillin or penicillin G, but many semisynthetic penicillins have developed that have varying patterns of activity. Some are more resistant to enzymatic breakdown, others are active against the ubiquitous and often resistant *Pseudomonas aeruginosa*. Table 5.2 indicates the range of penicillins now available, and Table 5.3 lists some of the infections against which they are effective.

Table 5.2 Types of penicillins

Approved name	Brand name	Administration
Standard penicillins		
benzylpenicillin	Crystapen	i.m; i.v.
phenoxymethyl penicillin		oral
procaine penicillin	Bicillin	i.m.
Broad-spectrum penicillins		
amoxycillin	Amoxil	oral; i.m; i.v; ivf
ampicillin	Penbritin	oral; i.m; i.v; ivf
ampicillin with cloxacillin	Amplicox	oral; i.m; i.v; ivf
bacampicillin	Ambaxin	oral
co-amoxiclav (amoxycillin with clavulanic acid)	Augmentin	oral; i.m; i.v; ivf
co-fluampicil (ampicillin with flucloxacillin)	Magnapen	i.m; i.v; ivf
pivampicillin	Pondocillin	oral
Penicillinase-resistant penicillins		
cloxacillin	Orbenin	oral; i.m; i.v; ivf
flucloxacillin	Floxapen	oral; i.m; i.v; ivf
temocillin	Temopen	i.m; i.v; ivf
Pencillins active against *Pseudomonas aeruginosa*		
azlocillin	Securopen	i.v; ivf
carbenicillin	Pyopen	i.m; i.v; ivf
piperacillin	Pipril	i.m; i.v; ivf
with tazobactam	Tazocin	i.v; ivf.
ticarcillin	Ticar	i.m; i.v; ivf
with clavulanic acid	Timentin	ivf

i.m. = intramuscular; i.v. = intravenous; ivf = intravenous infusion.

Table 5.3 Infections for which benzylpenicillin is effective

Organism	Disease
β-haemolytic *Streptococcus*	Septicaemia, tonsillitis
Pneumococcus	Pneumonia
Meningococcus	Meningococcal meningitis
Streptococcus viridans	Infective endocarditis
Clostridium tetani	Tetanus
Clostridium welchii	Gas gangrene
Corynebacterium diphtheriae	Diphtheria
Treponema pallidum	Syphilis
Actinomyces	Actinomycosis
Neisseria gonorrhoeae	Gonorrhoea

Benzylpenicillin §, penicillin G §

Brand name: Crystapen §

Penicillin is highly active against many Gram-positive bacteria and against a few Gram-negative and other organisms.

Benzylpenicillin is not effective orally, as it is rapidly broken down by gastric acid, and is given by intra-muscular injection or slow intravenous injection/infusion. The initial dose of 600–1200 mg is followed by maintenance doses of 600 mg two to four times a day. In bacterial endocarditis much larger doses are necessary. In that disease the valves of the heart are infected by *Streptococcus viridans* (although other organisms may also be involved) and become inflamed. In these inflamed tissues large numbers of bacteria are present, and to achieve an adequate cardiac tissue level of penicillin, daily doses of 7.2 g are given by slow intravenous infusion together with gentamicin. Prolonged therapy is necessary to avoid relapse. Penicillin has been used prophylactically against bacterial endocarditis in patients with heart valve lesions, as with such patients a dental extraction may lead to bacteraemia, but oral amoxycillin is now preferred.

In meningitis, penicillin penetrates through the normally resistant blood–brain barrier and is given in doses of 2.4 g by slow intravenous injection or infusion every 4–6 hours.

Procaine-penicillin is a long-acting form given by intramuscular injection. It is used mainly in the treatment of primary syphilis as Bicillin, which contains procaine-penicillin and benzylpenicillin.

Side-effects Although benzylpenicillin and its modifications are relatively non-toxic, allergic reactions and hypersensitivity may occur and are referred to on p. 61.

Phenoxymethylpenicillin § (Penicillin V) § (dose: 1–2 g daily)

Phenoxymethylpenicillin is an acid-stable derivative suitable for oral use. It is used mainly in streptococcal tonsillitis and respiratory infections in children, in doses varying from 62.5 to 250 mg every 6 hours. It is also useful for maintenance therapy after a satisfactory response to penicillin by injection. It is also given prophylactically against reinfection after recovery from streptococcal rheumatic fever in doses of 250 mg twice a day. Phenoxymethylpenicillin is not suitable in any severe condition in which high plasma levels of the antibiotic are required, as absorption is variable.

PENICILLINASE-RESISTANT PENICILLINS

Cloxacillin § (dose: 2 g daily orally)

Brand name: Orbenin §
Although staphylococci were originally largely susceptible to penicillin, most staphylococci are now penicillin-resistant. Some semisynthetic penicillins such as cloxacillin retain their activity, as they are largely immune to enzymatic breakdown, and are of value in the treatment of infections caused by penicillinase-producing staphylococci generally.

Cloxacillin is acid stable, and is active orally as well as by injection. The standard oral dose in staphylococcal infections is 500 mg every 6 hours, 30 minutes to 1 hour before food to secure maximum absorption. In severe infections, it may be given by intramuscular or slow intravenous injection or infusion in doses of 250–500 mg 6-hourly.

Side-effects are those of penicillin generally.

Flucloxacillin § (dose: 1 g daily orally)

Brand names: Floxapen §, Stafoxil §
Flucloxacillin is a beta-lactamase-resistant penicillin very similar to cloxacillin, but is more effective orally. It is given in doses of 250 mg 6-hourly, preferably well before food. In severe conditions it may be given by i.m. or i.v. injection in doses of 250–500 mg or more every 6 hours. Flucloxacillin is used in many conditions associated with

penicillin-resistant *Staphylococcus aureus*, including osteomyelitis, endocarditis and pneumonia. Co-fluampicil (Magnapen) is a mixture of flucloxacillin and ampicillin.

Temocillin § (dose: 2–4 g daily by injection)

Brand name: Temopen §
Temocillin is a penicillin active against many beta-lactamase-producing Gram-negative bacteria, including most enterobacteria. It has little action against Gram-positive cocci or *Pseudomonas aeruginosa*. Temocillin is used mainly in urinary and respiratory tract infections, and in septicaemia associated with susceptible Gram-negative organisms. It is given in doses of 1–2 g every 12 hours by intramuscular or intravenous injection or infusion. As the former may be painful, the antibiotic can be dissolved in 1% lignocaine solution if required. The dose should be adjusted in cases of severe renal impairment. In simple infections of the urinary tract it is given as a single daily dose of 1 g.

Side effects Temocillin is well tolerated, and side-effects are uncommon, but if a rash or other indications of sensitivity develop, the drug should be withdrawn.

PENICILLINS ACTIVE AGAINST *PSEUDOMONAS AERUGINOSA*

Benzylpenicillin and related penicillins are inactive against *Pseudomonas aeruginosa*, but some semisynthetic derivatives have a largely specific action against that ubiquitous and normally resistant organism. The first to be introduced was carbenicillin, now superseded by more powerful antibiotics such as ticarcillin.

Azlocillin § (dose: 6–15 g daily intravenously)

Brand name: Securopen §
Azlocillin is a broad-spectrum antibiotic markedly effective against *Pseudomonas aeruginosa* and *Proteus spp.* It is also active against some anaerobic organisms, including *Bacteroides* and *Clostridium*. In pseudomonal infections of the respiratory and urinary tracts, and in septicaemia, azlocillin is given by intravenous injection in doses of 2 g 8-hourly; in serious infections doses of 5 g 8-hourly by intravenous infusion may be necessary. In renal impairment, the dosage interval should be extended.

Azlocillin may be given in conjunction with an aminoglycoside such as gentamicin in pseudomonal septicaemia, but the drugs must be given separately.

Piperacillin § (dose: 100–300 mg/kg daily by injection)

Brand name: Pipril §

Piperacillin is a more potent derivative of ampicillin and active against a wider range of organisms. It is used mainly in severe infections caused by *Pseudomonas* and associated organisms, including bacterial septicaemia and endocarditis, and is given in divided doses of 100–150 mg/kg daily by intramuscular or slow intravenous injection or infusion, increased in very severe or life-threatening infections up to 16 g or more daily.

In pseudomonal septicaemia piperacillin is given with an aminoglycoside antibiotic, as such combined treatment is synergistic, but the antibiotics should be injected separately. It may also be given with metronidazole in mixed aerobic/anaerobic infections. Piperacillin has also been given by intramuscular injection in doses of 2 g every 12 hours in the extended treatment of uncomplicated urinary tract infections, and a single dose of 2 g has been used in gonorrhoea. In cases of renal impairment the interval between doses should be extended.

The antibacterial potency of piperacillin can be extended to organisms normally resistant to the antibiotic by combined administration with tazobactam as Tazocin. Tazobactam is a potent inhibitor of beta-lactamase, and combined use extends the antibacterial spectrum to include many beta-lactamase-producing bacteria that are normally resistant to piperacillin and other beta-lactam antibiotics. Tazocin is indicated in a wide range of infections, including mixed infections with both aerobic and anaerobic organisms, and is given in doses of 2.25–4.5 g 8-hourly by intravenous injection or slow infusion.

Ticarcillin § (dose: 15–20 g daily by injection)

Brand name: Ticar §

Ticarcillin resembles azlocillin in its general properties, and is used mainly in infections due to *Pseudomonas* and *Proteus spp.* Combined treatment with gentamicin or a related aminoglycoside has a synergistic effect, but the two antibiotics should be given separately.

The dose is 15–20 g daily in divided doses, which may be given by intramuscular or slow intravenous injection or by intravenous infusion. In cases of renal impairment, reduced doses of 2 g every 8–12 hours should be given. In the treatment of acute, uncomplicated urinary tract infections, doses of 3–4 g daily by intramuscular injection may be given, but as such injections may be painful, the antibiotic can be dissolved in 0.5% lignocaine.

Side-effects are few, but skin and mucous membrane haemorrhages have been reported.

Timentin § contains ticarcillin and clavulanic acid. The mixture is active against penicillase-producing bacteria that are otherwise resistant to ticarcillin and is given by intravenous infusion in doses of 3.2 g three or four times a day. Cholestatic jaundice is a late-onset **side-effect** thought to be associated with clavulanic acid.

BROAD-SPECTRUM PENICILLINS

The broad-spectrum semisynthetic penicillins have not only the general action of penicillin, but a range of activity that includes many Gram-negative pathogens, with the exception of *Pseudomonas*. They are not resistant to the penicillinases. Ampicillin is a typical member of the group but some of its derivatives may be better absorbed and give higher plasma levels.

Ampicillin § (dose: 1–4 g daily)

Brand names: Amfipen §, Penbritin §

Ampicillin is widely used in the treatment of respiratory infections such as chronic bronchitis, which is often associated with *Streptococcus pneumoniae* and *Haemophilus influenzae* as well as in ear, nose, throat and urinary infections, including gonorrhoea.

The oral dose of ampicillin is 250 mg–1 g every 6 hours, but in severe infections it is given in doses of 500 mg 4–6-hourly by intramuscular or intravenous injection. Pain after intramuscular injection can be avoided by reconstituting the antibiotic with 0.5% lignocaine solution. In gonorrhoea, a single 2 g oral dose with 1 g of probenecid may be adequate.

Ampicillin should always be given *before* meals, as absorption is incomplete and is further decreased by the presence of food. It is inactivated by penicillinases, and most staphylococci are now resistant to ampicillin, as are many strains of *Escherichia coli*.

Side effects Diarrhoea is a common side-effect, and a reaction of the urticarial type is usually indicative of a penicillin allergy. A macropapular rash is common in patients with infectious mononucleosis or chronic lymphatic leukaemia, but is not usually a penicillin-allergy reaction.

Co-fluampicil (Magnapen) is a mixture of ampicillin and flucloxacillin.

Amoxycillin § (dose: 750 mg–1.5 g daily)

Brand names: Almodan §, Amoxil §
Amoxycillin is a derivative of ampicillin; it has the action and uses of the parent drug, but it is more active when given orally and higher plasma levels are obtained from smaller doses. The standard dose is 250 mg 8-hourly, but double doses may be given in severe infections, or a dose of 500 mg may be given by intramuscular injection, or up to 1 g by intravenous infusion every 6–8 hours. Amoxycillin is of value in bronchial and purulent respiratory infections, in which doses of up to 3 g 12-hourly are given. It is also used in the treatment of typhoid fever, and prophylactically in bacterial endocarditis and dentistry.

Side-effects are similar to those of ampicillin, but diarrhoea is less common.

Co-amoxiclav (Augmentin) is a mixture of amoxycillin and clavulanic acid. That acid is an effective inhibitor of penicillinases, and the mixture extends the action of amoxycillin to include otherwise resistant strains of *Staphylococcus aureus*, *Escherichia coli*, *Haemophilus influenzae* and *Bacteroides*. The dose is one or two tablets 8-hourly.

Care is necessary with co-amoxiclav in hepatic impairment, and cholestatic jaundice has occurred up to 6 weeks after co-amoxiclav treatment.

Other broad-spectrum ampicillin-like antibiotics are bacampicillin § (Ambaxin), dose 800 mg–2.4 g daily, and pivampicillin § (Pondocillin), dose 1–2 g daily.

BETA-LACTAM ANTIBIOTICS (MONOBACTAMS)

A few antibiotics have been developed that are more active against those beta-lactamase-producing organisms that are resistant to other antimicrobial agents. They have valuable but limited therapeutic properties.

Aztreonam § (dose: 3–8 g daily by injection)

Brand name: Azactam §
Aztreonam is active only against Gram-negative organisms, and is an alternative to the aminoglycoside antibiotics and some cephalosporins in infections caused by *Pseudomonas aeruginosa*, *Haemophilus influenzae* and *Neisseria gonorrhoeae*. It is given by deep intramuscular or intravenous injection/infusion in doses of 1–2 g 6-hourly according to the severity of the infection. Doses of 0.5–1 g are given twice daily for urinary infections; in gonorrhoea a single intramuscular dose of 1 g.

Side-effects are gastrointestinal disturbances, hepatitis and blood disorders.

Imipenem § (dose: 1–2 g daily by intravenous infusion)

Imipenem has a wide range of activity against Gram-positive and Gram-negative aerobes and anaerobes, including those resistant to other antibiotics. It is very stable against beta-lactamases, but it is partly inactivated by the renal enzyme dehydropeptidase, with the formation of toxic metabolites, so it is always given with an equal dose of cilastatin, a specific inhibitor of that enzyme (Primaxin).

Imipenem is used in both single and mixed infections, and is given by intravenous infusion in divided doses of 1–2 g daily, increased if necessary to a maximum of 4 g daily. In less severe infections doses of 500–750 mg 12-hourly may be given by deep intramuscular injection. For pre-operative prophylaxis two doses of 1 g by intravenous infusion are given. Care is necessary in known sensitivity to other antibiotics, and in hepatic and renal impairment.

Meropenem § (dose: 1.5–3 g daily by intravenous injection/infusion)

Brand name: Meronem §
Meropenem has the actions and uses of imipenem, but has the advantage of being resistant to breakdown by the renal enzyme that inactivates imipenem and so is given alone.

CEPHALOSPORINS AND ASSOCIATED ANTIBIOTICS

The cephalosporins are a group of semisynthetic antibiotics with some chemical relationships to the penicillins. In general they have a wide range of activity against both Gram-positive and Gram-negative infections, and have an antibacterial action by an interference with cell-wall and crosslink synthesis.

These antibiotics are widely used in a variety of systemic infections not responding to the penicillins, or when alternative therapy is required, and as they are excreted largely unchanged in the urine, they are also used in the treatment of various urinary infections not responding to other drugs.

Some members of the group are largely inactivated by beta-lactamase, and so are not effective against many staphylococcal infections, although others such as cefuroxime and cephamandole, are less susceptible to such inactivation.

Side-effects A wide range of side-effects have been reported with the cephalosporins, some of which occur mainly with the higher doses. Allergic reactions are the most common and include rash, pruritus, urticaria, arthralgia and fever. Cross-sensitivity may occur in 10% of patients sensitive to penicillin. Gastrointestinal disturbances and disturbances of liver enzyme activity may occur, and an interference with blood clotting factors has also been noted. The cephalosporins are excreted mainly in the urine, and may cause renal disturbance in elderly patients. Powerful diuretics such as frusemide, when given in high doses, may increase the risk of renal damage and the dose of cephalosporin may require adjustment.

Nursing points about cephalosporins

(a) Bactericidal antibiotics with a wide range of activity.
(b) Some are less susceptible to inactivation by beta-lactamases.
(c) Cefsulodin and ceftazidime are exceptional in being active against *Pseudomonas*.
(d) Ceftriaxone has a long action that permits single daily doses.
(e) Cefoxitin is active against intestinal organisms.
(f) Main side-effect is hypersensitivity, and 10% of penicillin-sensitive patients are also cephalosporin sensitive.
(g) Exclude such sensitivity before cephalosporin therapy.

Clinically, there is often little difference between many members of the group, although cefsulodin and ceftazidime are exceptional in having a more specific action against *Pseudomonas aeruginosa*. Extended treatment with wide-range cephalosporins carries the risk of supra-infection with resistant organisms. See p. 61.

Those cephalosporins not referred to individually are listed in Table 5.4.

Cefaclor § (dose: 750 mg–4 g daily)

Brand name: Distaclor §
Cefaclor is an orally active cephalosporin effective against a wide range of Gram-positive and Gram-negative bacteria, including *Haemophilus influenzae*. It is often useful in urinary tract infections not responding to other treatment. It is given in doses of 250 mg

8-hourly, with double doses in severe infections. Cefaclor may cause skin reactions in some patients, particularly in children.

Cefadroxil § (dose: 1–2 g daily)

Brand name: Baxan §
Cefadroxil has a longer duration of action than some other oral cephalosporins, and is effective in doses of 500 mg–1 g twice daily. It is used mainly in soft tissue, skin and urinary tract infections. It has little action against *Haemophilus influenzae*.

Cefixime § (dose: 200–400 mg daily)

Brand name: Suprax §
Cefixime is a long-acting and powerful cephalosporin given in doses of 200–400 mg as a single daily dose. At present it is used only in acute infections.

Cefoxitin § (dose: 3–8 g daily by injection)

Brand name: Mefoxin §
Cefoxitin is a cephamycin antibiotic, closely related chemically to the cephalosporins, and having similar actions and uses against a wide range of infections. It is largely resistant to enzymatic breakdown by beta-lactamases, with an increased activity against Gram-negative organisms, and is of value in surgery for the prevention and treatment of intra-abdominal infections associated with *Bacteroides fragilis* and similar organisms, as well as in mixed infections.

Cefoxitin is given in doses of 1–2 g either by deep intramuscular or slow intravenous injection at intervals of 6–8 hours, but in severe infections doses up to 12 g daily may be required. Lower doses are given in renal impairment. The intramuscular injection can be painful, and if necessary the drug may be dissolved in 0.5 or 1% lignocaine solution.

Side-effects are hypersensitivity and occasional gastrointestinal disturbances, but diarrhoea may indicate the development of pseudomembranous colitis (see p. 61).

Cefpodoxime § (dose: 200–400 mg daily)

Brand name: Orelox §
Cefpodoxime is mainly indicated in the treatment of chronic and recurrent respiratory tract infections, and those resistant to other antibiotics, as it is more active than some other oral cephalosporins. It is given in doses of 100–200 mg twice a day with meals, although in sinusitis, double doses are recommended.

Table 5.4 Cephalosporins

Approved name	Brand name	Route of administration	Daily dose	Notes
cefaclor	Distaclor	oral	750 mg–4 g	Typical cephalosporin
cefadroxil	Baxan	oral	1–2 g	Twice daily dose
cefixime	Suprax	oral	200–400 mg	Single daily dose
cefodizime	Timecef	i.m., i.v., ivf	2 g	More active against some Gram-negative organisms
cefotaxime	Claforan	i.m., i.v., ivf	2–12 g	More active against some Gram-negative organisms
cefoxitin	Mefoxin	i.m., i.v., ivf	3–12 g	More active against intestinal bacteria
cefpirome	Cefrom	i.v., ivf	2–4 g	Urinary/respiratory infections
cefpodoxime	Orelox	oral	200–400 mg	Resistant respiratory tract infections
ceftazidime	Fortum	i.m., i.v., ivf	1–6 g	Active against Gram-negative organisms
ceftibuten	Cedax	oral	400 mg	Less active against pneumococci
ceftriaxone	Rocephin	i.m., i.v., ivf	1–4 g	Single daily dose
ceftizoxime	Cefizox	i.m., i.v., ivf	2–8 g	Active against Gram-negative organisms
cefuroxime	Zinacef	i.m., i.v., ivf	2–6 g	Active against *Haemophilius Influenzae* and *Neisseria*
	Zinnat	oral	0.5–1 g	*gonorrhoeae*
cephalexin	Ceporex	oral	2–6 g	Not for severe infections
	Keflex	oral		
cephamandole	Kefadol	i.m., i.v., ivf	2–12 g	Active against *Haemophilus influenzae* and *Neisseria*
cephazolin	Kefzol	i.m., i.v., ivf	2–4 g	Now used less frequently
cephradine	Velosef	oral	1–2 g	Now used less frequently
		i.m., i.v., ivf	2–4 g	

i.m. = intramuscular; i.v. = intravenous; ivf = intravenous infusion.

Side-effects of cefpodoxime are those of the cephalosporins generally.

Ceftriaxone § ▼ (dose: 1–4 g daily by injection)

Brand name: Rocephin § ▼

Ceftriaxone is a representative of the so-called 'third generation' cephalosporins with increased activity against Gram-negative organisms, and is of value in serious infections such as septicaemia, pneumonia and meningitis. It is given by deep intramuscular injection or by intravenous injection/infusion as a single daily dose of 1 g, increased if necessary to 2–4 g daily. The intramuscular injection site should be varied. For pre-surgical prophylaxis a single dose of 1 g may be given. A single dose of 250 mg is used in gonorrhoea. It is excreted mainly via the bile with the possible formation of biliary deposits of the calcium salt.

Cefuroxime § (dose: 2.25–6 g daily by injection; 500 mg daily orally)

Brand names: Zinacef §, Zinnat §

Cefuroxime is a cephalosporin that is active against both Gram-positive and Gram-negative organisms, including *Staphylococcus aureus*, *Haemophilus influenzae* and *Neisseria gonorrhoeae*, and with an increased resistance to enzymatic breakdown by beta-lactamases.

It is used in a wide range of respiratory and urinary tract infections, in bone infections such as osteomyelitis, and in obstetric and gynaecological infections.

Cefuroxime is given by intravenous or intramuscular injection in doses of 750 mg 8-hourly, with double doses by intravenous injection in severe infections. High doses of 3 g intravenously at intervals of 12 hours are given in meningitis. In mixed infections, combined treatment with an aminoglycoside antibiotic may be indicated. In gonorrhoea, in cases where penicillin is unsuitable, a single intramuscular dose of 1.5 g may be given. Reduced doses are necessary in severe renal impairment. Cefuroxime is also used in conjunction with metronidazole for prophylaxis in colonic surgery.

Cefuroxime axetil (Zinnat) is an oral pro-drug form which is hydrolysed after absorption to release the free antibiotic in the circulation. It is given in doses of 250 mg twice a day, doubled in severe infections, but in urinary infections doses of 125 mg twice a day are given. A single dose of 1 g is used in gonorrhoea.

Cephalexin § (dose: 1.5–6 g daily)

Brand names: Ceporex §, Keflex §

Cephalexin is a well absorbed, orally effective antibiotic with a wide range of activity against both Gram-positive and Gram-negative organisms. It is used in acute and chronic infections of the urinary tract, in respiratory, ear, nose and throat infections.

It is given in doses of 500 mg three times a day, but in severe infections doses up to 1.5 g four times a day may be necessary. Reduced doses should be given in renal impairment.

TETRACYCLINES

The mode of action of the tetracyclines differs from that of penicillin, as they interfere with bacterial protein synthesis and so are bacteriostatic and not bactericidal in action. They have a wide range of activity against most Gram-positive and Gram-negative organisms, with the exception of *Pseudomonas aeruginosa* and most strains of *Proteus*, and are active orally as well as by injection. They have been widely used, but drug resistance to the tetracyclines is now common and their importance has declined.

The main therapeutic applications of the tetracyclines include the control of the exacerbations of chronic bronchitis, as they are active against *Haemophilus influenzae*, the treatment of rickettsia, Q-fever and chlamydial infections represented by trachoma, mycoplasmal infections, brucellosis and cholera. They are sometimes useful in infections not responding to other antibiotics, and small doses are used in the long-term treatment of severe acne.

All the tetracyclines have the disadvantage of being taken up and deposited in teeth and growing bones, and should never be given to children under 12 years of age. The tetracyclines are generally well tolerated, and allergic reactions are uncommon, but absorption after oral administration is hindered by antacids, including milk, and by preparations of aluminium, calcium, iron and magnesium. Doxycycline and minocycline are the exceptions, as their absorption is less affected. They are also the only tetracyclines that are not contra-indicated in renal failure.

Table 5.5 indicates the ranges of tetracyclines available, and tetracycline is discussed as a representative member of the group, with short references to doxycycline and minocycline. They should always be taken with adequate fluid and with the patient in a standing or sitting position.

Tetracycline § (dose: 1–2 g daily)

Brand names: Achromycin §, Sustamycin §, Tetrabid §, Tetrachel §
Tetracycline is given orally in doses of 250–500 mg four times a day, but in severe infections it may be given by intramuscular injection in doses of 100 mg

Table 5.5 Tetracyclines

Approved name	Brand name	Average oral dose
demeclocycline	Ledermycin	150 mg 6-hourly
doxycycline	Vibramycin	200 mg initially, then 100 mg daily
lymecycline	Tetralysal	400 mg twice daily
minocycline	Minocin	100 mg twice a day
oxytetracycline	Berkmycen, Terramycin	250–500 mg 6-hourly
tetracycline	Achromycin Sustamycin Tetrabid Tetrachel	250–500 mg 6-hourly

4–8-hourly, or by intravenous infusion in doses not exceeding 500 mg 6-hourly. Oral therapy should be given as soon as possible, and continued for at least 48 hours after the symptoms of infection have subsided.

Side-effects of tetracycline include nausea and diarrhoea, but allergic reactions are uncommon. A more serious side-effect is a 'supra-infection' or staphylococcal enteritis, due to the overgrowth of tetracycline-resistant organisms (see p. 61). Fungal overgrowth with *Candida* may also occur in the same way.

Doxycycline § (dose: 100 mg daily)

Brand name: Vibramycin §
Doxycycline has the general action of the tetracyclines and it has also been used in the treatment of prostatitis associated with *Proteus*, and as an adjunct to amoebicides in the control of acute intestinal amoebiasis. It has the advantage of being effective in low doses, and treatment is commenced with a dose of 200 mg, followed by maintenance doses of 100 mg daily. In the long-term treatment of acne, doses of 50 mg daily are given.

Unlike most tetracyclines, the absorption of doxycycline is not influenced by food, and it may be used with care in patients with renal disease. Some oesophageal ulceration has occurred with doxycycline, and a dose should be given at least 1 hour before bedtime, with a full glass of water, and with the patient in a sitting or standing position.

Minocycline § (dose: 200 mg daily)

Brand name: Minocin §
Minocycline is of value in many tetracycline-sensitive infections, and the standard dose is 200 mg initially, followed by doses of 100 mg twice a day. In

gonorrhoea, single doses of 300 mg are given to adult males, but females require longer treatment. It is also useful in non-gonococcal urethritis and prostatitis. In the prophylactic treatment of meningococcal carriers, minocycline is given in doses of 100 mg twice a day for 5 days. In acne, a dose of 50 mg twice a day is given for at least 6 weeks. Absorption is not influenced to any extent by food.

Minocycline may be given to patients with renal impairment, but reduced doses should be used in cases of severe renal insufficiency.

Side-effects   are those of tetracycline.

Nursing points about tetracyclines

(a) Broad-spectrum antibiotics, value now largely limited by bacterial resistance.
(b) Used mainly in infections caused by chlamydia, rickettsia and mycoplasma.
(c) Tetracyclines bind with calcium and are deposited in teeth, so should not be given to children under 12 years of age or used in pregnancy.
(d) Absorption of most tetracyclines is decreased by milk, food and antacids (except doxycycline and minocycline).
(e) Most tetracyclines may increase renal failure if present, with the same exceptions.

AMINOGLYCOSIDES

The aminoglycosides, of which streptomycin was the first to be discovered, are a group of potent antibiotics which differ from the penicillins and cephalosporins in several respects. They act partly by binding to ribosomes and inhibiting the synthesis of normal proteins, and partly by the production of non-functioning proteins. The aminoglycosides have a wide range of action, and as they are not absorbed orally, for systemic use they must be given by injection. Their use requires care, as they are potentially nephrotoxic and ototoxic, particularly in the elderly, and monitoring of drug serum levels during treatment is advisable, as any renal dysfunction may reduce excretion and increase toxicity. Treatment should not normally be for longer than 7 days.

Care is necessary if potentially ototoxic diuretics such as frusemide are also given. Aminoglycosides should be avoided during pregnancy, as they cross the placenta and may damage the eighth cranial nerve of the fetus. But within those limits they are drugs of exceptional value, as they are active in many infections caused by Gram-negative organisms where other antibiotics may be less effective.

Gentamicin will be considered as a representative member of this valuable group of aminoglycoside antibiotics. The use of streptomycin in tuberculosis is referred to on p. 78.

Nursing points about aminoglycosides

(a) Wide-range bactericidal antibiotics.
(b) Not absorbed orally.
(c) Side-effects are dose-related, and treatment should not exceed 7 days.
(d) Excreted renally; dose should be decreased and dose-interval extended in renal impairment.
(e) Main side-effects are ototoxicity and nephrotoxicity, and may be exacerbated by some potent diuretics.
(f) Plasma levels of aminoglycosides should be monitored.

Gentamicin § (dose: 2.5–5 mg/kg daily by injection)

Brand names: Cidomycin §, Genticin §

Gentamicin is active against a wide range of Gram-negative and Gram-positive organisms, including *Pseudomonas aeruginosa*, and is a valuable drug in septicaemia, meningitis, endocarditis and many other severe systemic infections. In bacterial endocarditis caused by *Streptococcus viridans* or *Strep. faecalis*, combined treatment with penicillin is necessary. It is also effective in the control of biliary and urinary infections, but it is of less value against haemolytic streptococcal infections and is inactive against anaerobes.

The standard dose of gentamicin is 2–5 mg/kg daily, given in divided doses at 8-hourly intervals by intramuscular injection, slow intravenous injection or intravenous infusion. In severe infections, the dose may be doubled and later adjusted according to the serum level findings, as determined 1 hour after injection and again just before the next injection is due. Dosage should be adjusted so that the post-dose level is not greater than 10 mg/l, and the pre-dose level should be less than 2 mg/l. In severe mixed infections, it can be used in association with a penicillin, but injections should be at different sites to avoid inactivation.

Treatment should not normally exceed 7 days, as longer therapy may lead to renal impairment and ototoxicity. Lower doses at longer intervals are essential in renal impairment. In bacterial meningitis, gentamicin has been given by intrathecal injection of 1 mg, increased to 5 mg daily supported by intramuscular therapy, under laboratory control. The use of gentamicin in ocular infections is referred to on page 252.

Early signs of *toxicity* include headache, dizziness, rash and fever. Vestibular damage and nephrotoxicity are later symptoms of toxicity.

Amikacin § (dose: 1 g daily by injection)

Brand name: Amikin §

Amikacin is a semisynthetic aminoglycoside with the actions and uses of gentamicin, and although less potent it is more resistant to enzyme inactivation. Amikacin is effective in many infections caused by Gram-negative organisms, including *Pseudomonas aeruginosa*, as well as some staphylococcal infections, but it is mainly used in severe infections resistant to gentamicin.

Amikacin is given by intramuscular or slow intravenous injection in divided doses of 15 mg/kg daily (average adult dose 500 mg twice daily), adjusted according to the serum levels, up to a maximum total dose of 15 g. Intramuscular doses of 250 mg twice daily may be effective in urinary infections, other than those due to *Pseudomonas*, and the urine should be kept alkaline to increase the antibacterial action.

Side-effects precautions and contra-indications are those of the aminoglycosides generally.

Kanamycin § (dose: 1 g daily by injection)

Brand name: Kannasyn §

Kanamycin has been used in the treatment of severe infections due to Gram-negative organisms, but has been largely replaced by other aminoglycosides. Dose by intramuscular injection 250 mg 6-hourly, or 15–30 mg/kg daily in divided doses by intravenous infusion.

Neomycin § (dose: 6 g daily)

Brand names: Mycifradin §, Nivemycin §

Neomycin is an aminoglycoside antibiotic with a wide range of activity, but it is too toxic for systemic use. It is not absorbed orally and is sometimes given in doses of 1 g 4-hourly for intestinal infections, and for pre-operative preparation for bowel surgery. It is also widely used locally in eye, ear and skin infections (0.5%).

Some skin sensitization may follow extended local application and ototoxicity has occurred following absorption from extensively damaged skin areas.

Netilmicin § (dose: 300 mg daily by injection)

Brand name: Netilin §

Netilmicin is a semisynthetic aminoglycoside with the general action and uses of gentamicin but is less active against *Pseudomonas aeruginosa*. It is active against some infections resistant to gentamicin and related antibiotics, and is used mainly in severe septicaemia and urinary tract infections not responding to the other aminoglycosides. It is given in doses of 4–6 mg/kg daily, but an average adult dose is 100 mg 8-hourly, or 150 mg 12-hourly, by intramuscular injection or intravenous infusion. In very severe infections, netilmicin may be given in doses of 7.5 mg/kg daily in three divided doses, for 48 hours or so, and subsequently reduced to the 4–6 mg/kg daily level. In urinary infections, netilmicin is given in single daily doses of 150 mg for 5 days.

Peak serum concentrations of netilmicin should not exceed 12 mg/1, and the low 'trough' levels should be less than 2 mg/1. If combined treatment with an antipseudomonal penicillin is given, the injections should be made at different sites to avoid inactivation.

Netilmicin has the advantage of having a reduced toxic effect on the eighth cranial nerve, so hearing and vestibular disturbance may be less than with the related drugs and it may be of particular value in the elderly. The dose must be reduced in cases of renal impairment, and the combined use of powerful diuretics, which may also have an ototoxic effect, should be avoided.

Tobramycin § (dose: 200–350 mg daily)

Brand name: Nebcin §

Tobramycin has the action and uses of gentamicin, and is given by intramuscular injection or intravenous infusion in doses of 3–5 mg/kg daily in divided doses. Peak plasma concentrations 1 hour after injection should not exceed 10 mg/1, and should fall below 2 mg/1 before the next dose is given.

MACROLIDES AND LINCOSAMIDE ANTIBIOTICS

The macrolides, of which erythromycin is the oldest member, have a range of activity similar to that of penicillin, but their chemical structure is much more complex. They have a bacteriostatic action by inhibiting bacterial protein synthesis. The lincosamides, represented by clindamycin, have a similar action but are of limited therapeutic value.

Erythromycin § (dose: 1–2 g daily)

Brand names: Erythrocin §, Erymax §, Erythroped §, Ilosone §, Tiloryth §

Erythromycin has a penicillin-like range of activity with the advantage of being active orally, and is suitable for use in penicillin-sensitive patients. It is active against many Gram-positive cocci, and is of value in many respiratory infections including *Mycoplasma pneumoniae* and Legionnaire's disease, which is due to *Legionella pneumophilia*. Those organisms multiply intracellularly, so are more exposed to attack by macrolide antibiotics which enter the phagocytes. Erythromycin is used mainly for short-term therapy, and is given in doses of 250–500 mg four times a day, but in severe infections it may be given by intravenous infusion in doses of 2–4 g daily.

Side-effects of erythromycin include nausea and vomiting, and diarrhoea may occur after large doses. Care is necessary with patients receiving warfarin, as the action of the anticoagulant may be potentiated.

Azithromycin § (dose: 500 mg daily)

Brand name: Zithromax §

Azithromycin is chemically related to erythromycin but it is more acid stable. It is well absorbed after oral administration, giving high tissue levels which decline slowly and so permit single daily doses. It is effective in many soft tissue infections, bronchitis and atypical pneumonia. Such pneumonia, caused by *Mycoplasma* and similar organisms, is becoming more common and resistant to many antibiotics. The invading organisms migrate to the phagocytes, and azithromycin appears to be concentrated in the phagocytes to a greater degree than erythromycin. It is given in single daily doses of 500 mg for 3 days, 1 hour before or after food. Gastrointestinal disturbances are the main **side-effect.** It is contra-indicated in hepatic disease.

Clarithromycin § (dose: 500 mg daily)

Brand name: Klaricid §

Clarithromycin is a derivative of erythromycin with similar actions and uses. It is acid stable, and so has a greater degree of bioavailability. Clarithromycin is given in doses of 250 mg twice a day for 7 days, doubled in severe infections, with treatment continued if necessary for 14 days. It may also be given by intravenous infusion in divided doses of 1 g daily for 5–7 days. Headache, rash and gastrointestinal disturbances are **side-effects.** Care is necessary in renal and hepatic impairment.

Clindamycin § (dose: 600–1200 mg daily)

Brand name: Dalacin C §

Clindamycin is a lincosamide antibiotic that is taken up selectively and concentrated in bone, and is used in the control of staphylococcal bone and joint infections. It is also active against some intestinal anaerobic pathogens, and is used in abdominal sepsis.

Clindamycin is given orally in doses of 150–300 mg (with water) four times a day, and in severe infections by intramuscular injection or intravenous infusion in divided doses of 600 mg–2.4 g daily.

Side-effects A serious and potentially fatal side-effect of clindamycin is the occasional development of a severe pseudomembranous colitis, particularly in elderly patients after abdominal surgery. It may occur with almost any other antibiotic, and is now referred to as antibiotic-associated colitis (AAC) (p. 61). If any diarrhoea occurs, the drug should be withdrawn at once (see vancomycin and metronidazole).

Nursing points about macrolide antibiotics

(a) Penicillin-like range of activity, so useful in penicillin sensitivity and against some penicillin-resistant staphylococci.
(b) Tissue concentrations higher with azithromycin and clarithromycin, with reduced gastrointestinal disturbances.
(c) Combined treatment with astemizole or terfenadine should be avoided (risk of cardiac arrhythmias).

UNCLASSIFIED ANTIBIOTICS

In this section a few unrelated antibiotics are referred to which either have a limited value, or are useful in special circumstances.

Chloramphenicol § (dose: 50 mg/kg daily)

Brand names: Chloromycetin §, Kemecetine §

Chloramphenicol acts by interfering with protein synthesis in bacterial cells, and is highly effective against *Haemophilus influenzae* and many other organisms. It was introduced as a wide-range, orally active antibiotic, but is now considered too toxic for routine use. It remains of value in life-threatening infections due to *H. influenzae* and in typhoid fever and other conditions not responding to conventional therapy. The standard dose orally or by intravenous injection is 50 mg/kg daily in divided doses, which may be doubled in septicaemia and meningitis.

Side-effects The main toxic effect of chloramphenicol is a severe depression of bone marrow activity leading to aplastic anaemia; blood counts should be carried out before and during treatment, with careful monitoring of the plasma levels of the drug. Other side-effects are nausea, vomiting and diarrhoea.

Care is necessary when chloramphenicol is given to neonates, as they may exhibit the 'grey syndrome' of vomiting, respiratory depression, cyanosis and collapse. The condition is associated with a reduced ability of the infant to metabolize and excrete chloramphenicol.

The local use of chloramphenicol in bacterial conjunctivitis is referred to on p. 252.

Metronidazole § (dose: 1.2 g daily)

Brand names: Flagyl §, Metrolyl §, Zadstat §
Most pathogenic organisms can be divided into two groups, those that can develop in the presence or absence of oxygen (aerobes), and the anaerobes, which develop only in the absence of oxygen. Certain anaerobes such as *Bacteroides fragilis* are the cause of some colonic infections, and metronidazole has a selective action against anaerobic organisms by interfering with DNA activity.

In anaerobic infections, which are usually treated for 7 days, metronidazole is given as an initial dose of 800 mg, followed by doses of 400 mg 8-hourly. Alternatively, suppositories of 500 mg may be used three times a day. In severe infections metronidazole is given by intravenous infusion in doses of 500 mg at 8-hourly intervals. In less severe infections such as acute ulcerative gingivitis and in dental infections, doses of 200 mg are given 8-hourly for 3–7 days. Metronidazole is also of value in pre-surgical prophylaxis when given in doses of 400 mg 8-hourly 24 hours before surgery, supported by postoperative intravenous infusion or rectal use in doses of 500 mg 8-hourly until oral treatment can be given. In antibiotic-associated colitis (AAC), (p. 61) it is given in doses of 400 mg three times a day.

Metronidazole has no action against aerobic organisms, so in mixed infections with coliform or other organisms, combined treatment with gentamicin has been used.

Side-effects Metronidazole is in general well tolerated, but nausea, drowsiness and dizziness may occur. Transient convulsions have followed high-dose treatment, and peripheral neuropathy has been reported after prolonged therapy. Nurses should note that metronidazole tablets may cause gastric disturbances, and should be taken with or after food.

Metronidazole mixture, on the other hand, which contains a modified form of the drug, should be given at least 1 hour *before* food. A disulfiram-like reaction may occur if alcohol is taken (p. 10).

Metronidazole also has applications in the oral treatment of infected leg ulcers and pressure sores. It is also used locally as a 0.8% gel (Metrotop) in the control of malodorous fungating tumours associated with anaerobic bacteria, by application to the cleaned area once or twice a day. Metronidazole gel (Elyzol) is used locally for chronic periodontal disease. The use of metronidazole in amoebiasis is referred to on p. 271, in trichomoniasis on p. 173, and in acne rosacea on p. 258.

Tinidazole § (Fasigyn §) has similar actions, uses and side-effects to those of metronidazole, with the advantage of a longer plasma half-life. Dose 2 g initially, followed by 500 mg twice a day.

Spectinomycin §

Brand name: Trobicin §
Spectinomycin is an antibiotic that is used solely in the treatment of gonorrhoea when penicillin is ineffective or otherwise contra-indicated. It is given by deep intramuscular injection as a single dose of 2 g, doubled in severe infections.

Side-effects are nausea, chills, dizziness and urticaria. It is not recommended for use during pregnancy.

Teicoplanin § (dose: 200–400 mg by injection)

Brand name: Targocid §
Teicoplanin is a longer-acting antibiotic with a wide range of activity against aerobic and anaerobic Gram-positive organisms, including resistant staphylococci. It acts by interfering with the biosynthesis of peptidoglycan, which forms the lattice-like structure of the bacterial cell wall. Teicoplanin is used in the treatment of serious staphylococcal infections in patients who have failed to respond to other antibiotics, or where such antibiotics are contra-indicated.

Teicoplanin is given by intravenous injection as a loading dose of 400 mg, followed by single doses of 200 mg daily. In very severe infections, three doses of 400 mg are given at intervals of 12 hours, maintained by single daily doses of 400 mg by intramuscular injection. In severe burns, and in endocarditis due to *Staphylococcus aureus*, intravenous maintenance doses up to 12 mg/kg have been given. Dosage must be adjusted in renal impairment.

Side-effects Gastro-intestinal side-effects, dizziness and anaphylactic reactions may occur with teicoplanin, and blood counts with liver and kidney function tests should be carried out, as it is potentially nephrotoxic.

Vancomycin §

Brand name: Vancocin §

Vancomycin is chemically related to teicoplanin and has a similar pattern of antibacterial activity. It is used for the treatment of severe staphylococcal or streptococcal infections which have not responded to other antibiotics, including staphylococcal endocarditis, osteomyelitis and antibiotic-associated colitis (p. 61). Vancomycin is not suitable for intramuscular injection, and is given intravenously in doses of 500 mg 6-hourly according to need, with monitoring of the plasma concentrations, which should not exceed a peak of 30 mg 1 hour after injection. In staphylococcal endocarditis treatment for 3 weeks or longer may be required.

Vancomycin is the drug of choice for the treatment of the pseudomembranous colitis that may follow the use of clindamycin and other antibiotics, and is then given orally in doses of 125–250 mg four times a day for 7–10 days.

Side-effects Care is necessary with injections, as vancomycin is irritant to the tissues, and other side-effects include nausea, chills, fever, urticaria and rash. Blood counts and renal function tests are advisable. Tinnitus may be an indication of ototoxicity, especially in the elderly, and deafness may be progressive even if treatment is withdrawn.

SULPHONAMIDES AND OTHER ANTIBACTERIAL AGENTS

The sulphonamides have a bacteriostatic action, as they inhibit bacterial growth by preventing the uptake of para-aminobenzoic acid by bacteria that require that amino acid for the synthesis of folic acid. (Bacteria that do not require folic acid for development are resistant to the sulphonamides.) They are active against a wide range of Gram-positive and Gram-negative bacteria, but acquired resistance is now common in many pathogenic organisms. Attempts have been made to extend the action of the sulphonamides by the combined use of trimethoprim, which interrupts bacterial metabolism at a different point, and some resistant infections may

respond to such combined therapy.

Common **side-effects** are nausea, vomiting and malaise, but more serious adverse effects include allergic reactions, cyanosis and agranulocytosis, requiring withdrawal of treatment. Crystalluria may occur, but can be prevented by an adequate fluid intake. The Stevens–Johnson syndrome, a form of erythema multiforme with widespread lesions of the skin and mucous membranes, is more likely to occur with the long-acting sulphonamides and may be fatal.

Nursing points about sulphonamides

(a) High fluid intake is necessary to avoid crystalluria.
(b) Best avoided in the elderly and other patients with a folate deficiency.
(c) Trimethoprim now often preferred for most infections.

Sulphadimidine § (dose: 2–4 g daily)

Sulphadimidine is used mainly in the treatment of infections of the urinary tract. It is given as a loading dose of 2 g, followed by doses of 0.5–1 g every 6–8 hours.

Sulphadiazine § (dose: 1–6 g daily)

Sulphadiazine is now used mainly for the prophylaxis of recurrent rheumatic fever, and is given orally in doses of 1 g daily. It also has a bacteriostatic action on a wide range of Gram-negative and Gram-positive organisms, and in severe systemic infections it has been given by intravenous injection as a loading dose of 2–3 g, followed by 1 g dose four times a day for two days, when oral therapy should be started.

Sulfametopyrazine § (dose: 2 g weekly)

Brand name: Kelfizine W §

Sulfametopyrazine is a long-acting sulphonamide as it binds extensively with plasma proteins. It is used mainly in the treatment of urinary tract infections and in the control of chronic bronchitis in a dose of 2 g weekly. A disadvantage is that if **side-effects** occur, they will be slow in subsiding after the withdrawal of the drug, and the Stevens– Johnson syndrome is more likely to occur with sulfametopyrazine than with more rapidly eliminated sulphonamides.

Sulphamethoxazole §

Sulphamethoxazole has the general properties of the sulphonamides, but is now used as a constituent of co-trimoxazole.

Co-trimoxazole § (dose: 1.92 g daily)

Brand names: Bactrim §, Septrin §
Co-trimoxazole is a mixture of sulphamethoxazole and trimethoprim. The antibacterial range of trimethoprim is similar to that of the sulphonamides, but it interrupts the folic–folinic acid metabolic process at a different point. The mixture thus permits a two-pronged antibacterial attack which increases the activity. Co-trimoxazole has been widely used in the treatment of urinary infections and chronic bronchitis in doses of 960 mg twice daily, but because of **side-effects** it is now a drug of last resort for such conditions. It remains the drug of choice for opportunistic infections such as *Pneumocystis carinii* pneumonia in immunocompromised and AIDS patients in doses of 120 mg/kg daily for 14 days.

When co-trimoxazole is not tolerated, an alternative drug is atovaquone (Wellvone § ▼) which has a different action mediated by the cytochrome enzyme complex. Dose: 750 mg three times a day with food, for 21 days.

Side-effects of co-trimoxazole are similar to those of the sulphonamides, but the trimethoprim component may cause a depression of haemopoiesis. Blood counts are advisable during prolonged treatment, and the drug should be withdrawn immediately if a rash occurs. It is contra-indicated in severe liver damage or marked renal insufficiency.

Trimethoprim § (dose: 400 mg daily)

Brand names: Monotrim §, Trimopan §
Trimethoprim has a wide range of activity and is used in urinary and respiratory tract infections in doses of 200 mg twice a day. In acute infections it may be given by intravenous infusion or slow intravenous injection in doses of 125–250 mg 12-hourly. For chronic infections and prophylaxis, the dose is 100 mg at night. Trimethoprin is suitable for children in age-related doses.

Side-effects are gastro-intestinal disturbances, rash and pruritus. With long-term treatment blood counts are necessary, as depression of haemopoiesis may occur. Severe renal impairment is a contra-indication.

URINARY ANTIBACTERIAL AGENTS

Urine is virtually a culture medium for organisms that gain access to the urinary system, and a high urinary output plays an important part in controlling the incidence of such infections. Before potent urinary antiseptics became available, potassium citrate was widely used to make the urine alkaline, as in some infections the urine becomes distinctly acid. Potassium citrate is still the main constituent of some over-the-counter products for the treatment of cystitis. On the other hand, acidification of the urine may have an antibacterial action (see hexamine p. 76), and interest is being taken in the potential of cranberry juice in urinary infections. It acidifies the urine by forming quinic acid and it has been recommended for prophylactic use in patients prone to urinary infections, such as those with multiple sclerosis and those with stones in the urinary tract. Cranberry juice given in doses of 250 ml twice a day may play a useful part in the prophylaxis of urinary infections as it may augment the activity of other urinary antiseptics.

QUINOLONE ANTIBACTERIAL AGENTS

Urinary infections may initially be confined to the lower urinary tract and cause dysuria and cystitis, or may later reach the pelvis and parenchyma of the kidney and cause pyelonephritis. In the former, a drug is required that is concentrated in the urine, but in kidney infections a drug that also penetrates into the renal tissues is necessary.

Most of the organisms associated with urinary infections are Gram-negative, such as *Escherichia coli*, *Proteus spp.*, but *Streptococcus faecalis* is Gram-positive. Such infections often respond to a suitable antibiotic or a sulphonamide but some unrelated substances also have a place in the treatment of urinary infections. An important group is that described chemically as the 4-quinolones (Table 5.6).

Bactericidal agents of the 4-quinolone group act by inhibiting the enzyme DNA gyrase. That enzyme controls the supercoiling of the long strands of DNA within bacterial cells, and the inhibition of the enzyme by a quinolone brings about irreversible chromosome damage.

The quinolones have many **side-effects**, and they may cause convulsions in patients with or without a history of epilepsy; that risk may increase if a NSAID is also taken. Treatment should be stopped if any neurological disturbances or hypersensitivy reactions occur after the first dose. Most members of the group are used in the treatment of infections of the urinary tract, but ciprofloxacin has a wider therapeutic range.

Table 5.6 4-Quinolones

Approved name	Brand name	Oral Dose
cinoxacin	Cinobac	500 mg twice a day
ciprofloxacin	Ciproxin	250–750 mg twice a day
nalidixic acid	Mictral	1 g four times a day
	Negram	
	Uriben	
norfloxacin	Utinor	400 mg twice a day
ofloxacin	Tarivid	200–400 mg daily

Ciprofloxacin § (dose: 500 mg–1.5 g daily)

Brand name: Ciproxin §

Ciprofloxacin is highly active against Gram-negative organisms, including *Pseudomonas* and *Proteus*, and it is also active against streptococci and other Gram-positive bacteria.

Ciprofloxacin is of value in many systemic infections resistant to other antibacterial agents, in respiratory and urinary tract infections, and in bone and joint infections. In mixed infections, it may be used in association with aminoglycoside or beta-lactam antibiotics, as cross-resistance is uncommon. It is given orally in doses of 250–750 mg twice a day in the treatment of most infections, but in gonorrhoea a single dose of 250 mg may be adequate. In severe infections, ciprofloxacin may be given by intravenous infusion in doses of 200 mg twice a day, reduced to 100 mg twice a day in urinary infections, and to a single 100 mg dose in gonorrhoea. An adequate fluid intake is necessary during ciprofloxacin therapy to avoid crystalluria.

Ciprofloxacin is also given for surgical prophylaxis as a single intravenous dose of 750 mg 60–90 minutes before operation.

Care is necessary in epilepsy, as ciprofloxacin may lower the convulsive threshold. It is not recommended for use in children or adolescents as there is a possible risk of damage to weight-bearing joints. Ciprofloxacin, in common with most other 4-quinolones, may increase the plasma levels of theophylline, and enhance the effects of warfarin.

Side-effects are nausea, diarrhoea, dizziness, rash, pruritus, confusion, visual disturbances and blood disorders. Some local irritation may occur at an injection site.

Nursing points about quinolone antibacterials

(a) Ciprofloxacin has the widest range of activity, being effective against Gram-positive and Gram-negative pathogens.
(b) To be used with caution in epileptic patients, and may cause convulsions in other patients.
(c) Action may increase if NSAIDs are also taken.
(d) Treatment with any quinolone should be withdrawn if neurological or other disturbances occur after the first dose.

Cinoxacin § (dose: 1 g daily)

Brand name: Cinobac §

Cinoxacin is effective in both upper and lower urinary tract infections, and it is also useful as a prophylactic agent in reducing the frequency of recurrent infections.

Cinoxacin is well absorbed orally, and is given in doses of 500 mg twice a day for 7–14 days in acute infections; in prophylaxis, a single nightly dose of 500 mg is used. It is not suitable for use in cases of severe renal impairment.

In general cinoxacin is well tolerated, but **side-effects** include gastrointestinal disturbances and abdominal cramps. *Hypersensitivity* reactions such as rash, itching and urticaria have occurred and anaphylactoid reactions have been reported.

Nalidixic acid § (dose: 2–4 g daily)

Brand names: Mictral §, Negram §, Uriben §

Nalidixic acid has a similar range of antibacterial activity to that of cinoxacin, and is used mainly for treatment of urinary tract infections. The standard dose is 1 g 6-hourly for 7 days, but if longer treatment is required, half doses should be given.

Side-effects include nausea and vomiting, as well as urticaria and other manifestations. Visual disturbances may also occur, but are transient. Patients should avoid strong sunlight as phototoxicity is a possible side-effect. Care is necessary in renal impairment. Nalidixic acid is not suitable for young children, or in epileptics, as it may precipitate convulsions.

Norfloxacin § (dose: 800 mg daily)

Brand name: Utinor §

Norfloxacin is active against many Gram-negative urinary pathogens, and effective in the treatment of acute and chronic infections of the urinary tract. In uncomplicated infections it is given in doses of 400 mg a day, but in more severe infections doses of 400 mg twice a day are required. In chronic infections, doses of 400 mg twice a day may be given for up to 12 weeks, although if a response occurs earlier, the dose may be reduced to 400 mg daily. That lower dose should also be given in cases of renal impairment. In general, single daily doses should be taken in the morning.

Side-effects include nausea, dizziness, abdominal pains and diarrhoea. Photosensitivity and dermatitis have also been reported. Norfloxacin may displace warfarin from serum albumin binding sites, and a rise in plasma levels of theophylline and cyclosporin may occur, and adjustments may be necessary with patients receiving those drugs.

Ofloxacin § (dose: 200–800 mg daily)

Brand name: Tarivid §
Ofloxacin is a fluorinated quinoline with actions and uses similar to those of ciprofloxacin. It is used mainly in urinary and lower respiratory tract infections, and is given as a single dose of up to 400 mg, preferably in the morning with water (larger doses should be taken as two divided doses), for 5–10 days, except in gonorrhoea, where a single dose may be adequate. Absorption may be reduced if iron or antacid preparations are taken within 2 hours of a dose of ofloxacin. In severe infections ofloxacin may be given by intravenous infusion in doses of 200 mg daily.

Side-effects include hypersensitivity reactions, dizziness and other disturbances of the central nervous system. Exposure to strong sunlight should be avoided. Dosage should be reduced in impairment of renal function based on the creatinine clearance rate.

OTHER AGENTS USED IN URINARY INFECTIONS

Fosfomycin § (dose: 3 g)

Brand name: Monuril §
Fosfomycin is a phosphonic acid antibiotic active against a range of Gram-positive and Gram-negative organisms that includes *Staphylococcus aureus* and some enterobacteria. It is given in lower urinary tract infections as a single nightly dose of 3 g after the bladder has been emptied. In urethral investigations a prophylactic dose of 3 g is given 3 hours beforehand, followed by a second dose of 3 g 24 hours later. It is not recommended in patients over 75 years of age, or when marked renal impairment is present, as the necessary urinary concentration may not be obtained.

Side-effects include heartburn, nausea, diarrhoea and rash.

Nitrofurantoin § (dose: 200–600 mg daily)

Brand names: Furadantin §, Macrodantin §, Macrobid §
Nitrofurantoin is a wide-spectrum antibacterial agent that is well absorbed orally, but it is excreted so rapidly in high concentration in the urine that it is of value only in urinary tract infections and after prostatectomy. It is given in doses of 50–100 mg four times a day with food for 7 days. The urine should be kept acid, as nitrofurantoin is inactive in an alkaline urine. As the tissue concentration of the drug is low, it is not suitable in acute pyelonephritis.

Nitrofurantoin is sometimes used in doses of 50–100 mg at night as a suppressive drug in the long-term treatment of urinary infections. It should not be given to infants, or to patients with glucose-6-phosphate dehydrogenase deficiency, as in such patients it may cause haemolytic anaemia.

Side-effects are nausea, vomiting, rash, urticaria and pruritus. Peripheral neuropathy may occur and any tingling is an indication for withdrawal of the drug. Pulmonary infiltration has occasionally been reported, and lung and liver function tests are necessary during long-term treatment. Marked renal impairment is a contra-indication.

Hexamine (dose: 600 mg–2 g)

Hexamine is an old drug that has been used in the treatment of recurrent urinary infections. It is a formaldehyde compound, and in an acid urine it slowly breaks down to release small amounts of formaldehyde, to which the antibacterial action is due. It survives as hexamine hippurate (Hiprex).

Dimethyl sulphoxide

Dimethyl sulphoxide is used mainly as a solvent, but a 50% solution is available as Rimso 50. This product is intended for the symptomatic relief of interstitial cystitis (Hunner's ulcer) and is used by the instillation in the bladder of 50 ml of the product.

ANTITUBERCULAR DRUGS

Tuberculosis is caused by the parasitic bacillus *Mycobacterium tuberculosis,* and may become established in the body before symptoms or other evidence of the disease are detected.

Following the introduction of streptomycin, the first antibiotic to be introduced after penicillin, it was thought that tuberculosis would soon be brought under complete control. In fact, drug resistant *M. tuberculosis* has now become a major problem and the WHO recently declared tuberculosis a 'global emergency'. Treatment of tuberculosis requires multi-drug therapy and when possible antitubercular therapy is given in two stages, an initial stage of triple-drug treatment, and a secondary stage using two drugs. Drug resistance occurs rapidly in tuberculosis if any drug is used alone, and the initial phase of treatment is designed to bring the condition under control as rapidly as possible, and to reduce the risks of drug resistance.

The secondary phase of treatment is initiated after tests have shown which drugs are most active against the strains of organisms of the individual patient, and must be continued for many months. Initial therapy is commenced with any three of the following drugs: isoniazid, rifampicin, pyrazinamide, streptomycin or ethambutol.

Nursing points about antitubercular drugs

(a) Initial or first-phase treatment with three drugs, usually with isoniazid, rifampicin and pyrazinamide.
(b) Continuation phase with two drugs, usually isoniazid and rifampicin.
(c) Compliance with treatment is essential; some patients must be supervised.
(d) Peripheral neuropathy is a side-effect of isoniazid and ethambutol; advise patients to report any numbness or tingling in the extremities or visual disturbances.
(e) Avoid skin contact with streptomycin.

Isoniazid § (dose: 300 mg daily)

Isoniazid is a highly selective antibacterial drug, as although it is active against *Mycobacterium tuberculosis* it has virtually no action against other organisms. It is widely used with other drugs in the primary treatment of pulmonary tuberculosis, as following oral administration isoniazid is rapidly absorbed and penetrates easily into the body tissues and fluids, including the cerebrospinal fluid, and also into caseous areas.

Isoniazid is given in doses of 300 mg daily, orally or by intramuscular injection, but with the slow inactivators (see below), doses of 1 g twice weekly may be given. In tuberculous meningitis, supplementary doses of 25–50 mg have been given by intrathecal injection.

Side-effects Isoniazid is well tolerated and side-effects are not usually serious. Skin reactions may occur, and convulsions and psychotic reactions have also been reported. Persistent nausea and vomiting

may indicate incipient liver damage. Peripheral neuropathy is an occasional hazard with higher doses and pyridoxine in doses of 50–100 mg daily should be given as a prophylactic, as isoniazid may interfere with normal pyridoxine metabolism.

This effect on pyridoxine occurs mainly with the 'slow inactivators'. Isoniazid is inactivated by acetylation in the liver, but the speed of inactivation varies. Patients can be divided into slow-acetylators and rapid-acetylators and a gene factor is involved. As the steady state plasma level of isoniazid is lower with the rapid inactivators, regular and adequate dosing is necessary to maintain the anti-tubercular action, whereas slow acetylators are more likely to develop peripheral neuropathy. The risk is slight when dosage can be controlled.

Rifampicin § (dose: 450–600 mg daily)

Brand names: Rifadin §, Rimactane §

Rifampicin is one of the rifamycin group of antibiotics and it has a wide range of antibacterial activity. It is highly effective against *Mycobacterium tuberculosis* and *Mycobacterium leprae* (leprosy). It penetrates well into the tissues, and reaches intracellular organisms. It is of low toxicity and well tolerated. Rifampicin is a first-line antitubercular drug, and is given as a single daily dose of 450–600 mg, preferably on an empty stomach to obtain maximum absorption.

Side-effects are of varying severity, including nausea, diarrhoea and rash, and it may evoke an influenza-like reaction with chills, fever and respiratory stress, which in some cases may extend to shock and collapse. Thrombocytopenic purpura may also occur.

Rifampicin is mainly excreted in high levels in the bile, but much is reabsorbed by the enterohepatic circulation system and care may be necessary in liver impairment. Jaundice may require a change of treatment. Rifampicin may give a red colour to the urine and sputum, but the colouration is of no significance and may even be useful as a test of compliance with therapy. It may also stain contact lenses.

Combined therapy with other antitubercular drugs, particularly ethambutol or isoniazid, remains essential, and Rifinah and Rimactazid represent products containing both rifampicin and isoniazid. Rifater contains rifampicin, isoniazid and pyrazinamide. Rifampicin is also used with dapsone in the initial treatment of leprosy (p. 271). (Rifampicin has a secondary use in the prophylactic treatment of meningococcal meningitis in doses of 600 mg twice daily for 2 days.)

It should be noted that rifampicin stimulates the hepatic metabolism of many drugs, and adjustment of dose of other therapeutic agents such as warfarin may be required. It also reduces the effectiveness of oral contraceptives and is contra-indicated in pregnancy.

Rifabutin § (dose: 300–600 mg daily)

Brand name: Mycobutin §
Rifabutin is a semi-synthetic derivative of rifampicin, and has a similar range of activity, and in pulmonary tuberculosis it is given as part of combined therapy in doses of 150–450 mg daily for at least 6 months. It is also of value in the prophylaxis and treatment of non- tuberculous mycobacterial disease such as that caused by *Mycobacterium avium–intracellulare* complex (MAC). That organism is the cause of severe opportunistic infections in AIDS patients, and is resistant to many antibacterial agents. Rifabutin is effective against most strains of MAC, and in prophylaxis it is given in doses of 300 mg daily as monotherapy. For treatment, it is given in doses of 450–600 mg daily as part of a multidrug regimen for 6 months after negative cultures have been obtained.

Side-effects of rifabutin are similar in general to those of rifampicin, including the effects on co-administrated drugs mediated by hepatic enzymes such as cytochrome 450 (p. 2). Care is necessary in hepatic insufficiency.

Ethambutol § (dose: 15–25 mg/kg daily)

Brand name: Myambutol §
Ethambutol is sometimes used as part of the primary treatment of tuberculosis, as it is active mainly against young and dividing cells. Its main use is in the early stages of treatment to prevent the emergence of resistance to other drugs. It is given as a single daily dose of 15 mg/kg, although in some cases the higher dose of 25 mg/kg may be necessary. Although generally well tolerated, it is considered less suitable for children or the elderly.

Side-effects include a retrobulbar neuritis with loss of visual acuity and a green–red colour blindness. These ocular toxic effects are more likely in patients with some renal dysfunction who are receiving high doses and usually disappear slowly with a change of treatment. Patients should be warned to report any such visual disturbances without delay.

Streptomycin § (dose: 1 g daily by injection)

Streptomycin, one of first antibiotics to be introduced after penicillin, was once widely used in the treatment of tuberculosis, but ototoxicity limits its use. It survives as part of multiple therapy for use in resistant tuberculosis, and is given in doses of 1 g daily by intramuscular injection.

Side-effects Permanent deafness has followed the prolonged use of the drug because of its toxic effects on the eighth cranial nerve. Other reactions include paraesthesia of the lips, and hypersensitivity reactions may occur. Care is necessary in renal insufficiency and liver dysfunction. Great care should be taken when handling streptomycin, as skin sensitization with dermatitis may occur.

SUPPLEMENTARY ANTITUBERCULAR DRUGS

These drugs are used mainly as alternative therapy in cases of intolerance to conventional drugs, or where resistance requires a change of therapy.

Capreomycin § (dose: 1 g daily by injection)

Brand name: Capastat §
Capreomycin is an antibiotic used in tuberculosis resistant to first-line drugs. It is given in doses of 1 g daily by deep intramuscular injection.

Side-effects include urticaria, renal damage, tinnitus and vertigo. It should not be used with streptomycin or other ototoxic drugs.

Pyrazinamide § (dose: 20–30 mg/kg daily)

Brand name: Zinamide §
Pyrazinamide is active against the intracellular dividing forms of the tubercle bacillus. It is of value in tuberculous meningitis as it penetrates well into the CSF. Pyrazinamide is given in divided doses of 20–30 mg/kg daily or 2 g three times a week. As it is most effective during the early stages of treatment, it should not be given for longer than 2 months.

Side-effects The main disadvantage of pyrazinamide is its *hepatotoxicity*, which can be serious and lead to liver failure, and liver function should be checked during treatment. Care is also necessary in renal impairment and diabetes. Other side-effects are nausea, arthralgia and urticaria.

Cycloserine § (dose: 500 mg–1 g daily)

Cycloserine is used occasionally in tuberculosis resistant to conventional first-line drugs in doses of 250–500 mg twice a day. It diffuses well into the tissues, but it is slowly excreted, and it may cause **side-effects** such as drowsiness, twitching and convulsive seizures, indicative of central nervous system involvement. Epilepsy and psychotic states are contra-indications.

ANTIVIRAL DRUGS

Viruses are minute non-cellular organisms that can replicate only within the living cells of a host to which they have gained access. They are therefore obligate intracellular parasites. They consist essentially of a core of nucleic acid (DNA/RNA) with a protein coating, which may be enclosed in a lipoprotein envelope. Viruses replicate by binding to the receptor proteins on the surface of the host cell, after which the genetic core passes into the cell and makes use of the cell's metabolic processes to produce new viral DNA/RNA and viral proteins for assembly into new virus particles and the development of a new viral infection. When, for example, the virus particles enter the mucosal cells of the nasopharynx, the infection causes the development of antibodies and lymphokines such as interferon, followed by the death and shedding of the infected cells, giving rise to the catarrh and other symptoms of the common cold. New, non-infected cells are formed, so the viral infection is normally short-lived. In some cases, however, an infection does not result in cell death, and the infective virus particles may remain dormant but potentially infective within the host cell (a latent infection). Reactivation of the virus in later life may occur, and give rise to chickenpox or shingles. Others, such as the human papilloma virus, may cause the host cell to undergo malignant changes and cause genital cancer. It is also considered that some viruses with exceptionally long incubation or latent periods may be the cause of Alzheimer's disease and other degenerative disorders.

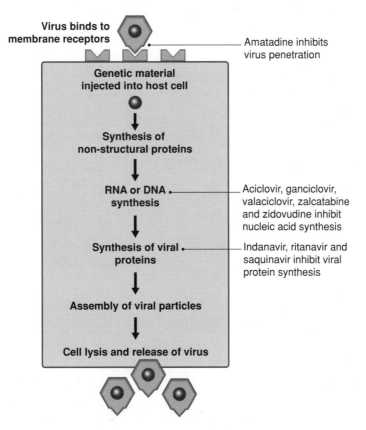

Figure 5.1 Diagram of viral replication and sites of action of antiviral drugs.

The search for antiviral drugs is hampered because viral replication is so closely linked with the metabolic processes of the host cells, and an antiviral drug must have a highly selective action if damage to the host cell is to be avoided. In addition, some viruses mutate very rapidly, and changes in the nature of the viral proteins may also be frequent; receptor sites that would be vulnerable points for antiviral attack may also change. Nonetheless, some advances in antiviral therapy are being made. Some antiviral agents now in use act by inhibiting viral nucleic acid formation via the enzyme nucleoside reverse transcriptase. More recently, a newer class of antiviral agents has been introduced, the protease inhibitors, which act at a later stage and prevent the final development of infectious viral particles. In some viral infections combined treatment may evoke an improved response.

Aciclovir §

Brand name: Zovirax §
Aciclovir is given orally in doses of 200 mg five times a day in the early treatment of herpes virus infections of the skin and mucous membranes, but it is effective only when given in the early stages of infection. It also reduces the acute pain, and the risk of post-herpetic neuralgia. Similar doses can be given in the prophylaxis of immunocompromised patients.

In systemic herpes infection early treatment is also essential, and aciclovir is given by intravenous infusion in doses of 5 mg/kg 8-hourly, increased to 10 mg/kg in immunocompromised patients with varicella zoster infections.

Aciclovir has many **side-effects**, including rash, gastrointestinal and neurological disturbances. Care must be taken to avoid extravasation, as severe local inflammation may occur. Caution is necessary in renal impairment, as the drug is excreted by the kidneys, and monitoring of renal function is advisable. For the treatment of herpes simplex conjunctivitis, aciclovir is used as a 3% ointment to be applied to the infected eye five times a day.

Amantadine § (dose: 200 mg daily)

Brand name: Symmetrel §
Amantadine, used in the treatment of parkinsonism (p. 96) also has some antiviral properties, and is used in the treatment of *Herpes zoster*. It is given in doses of 100 mg twice daily for 14 days, and treatment may be continued for a further 14 days if post-herpetic pain persists. It is also used in doses of 100 mg daily for six weeks in the prophylactic treatment of influenza A infections, but only in unimmunized patients considered to be at risk.

Side-effects include dizziness, gastro-intestinal disturbances and insomnia. Skin discolouration has been reported occasionally. Amantadine should not be given to patients with a history of epilepsy or duodenal ulceration.

Cidovir § ▼ (dose: 5 mg/kg)

Brand name: Vistide § ▼
Cidovir is a new antiviral agent with the actions and uses of ganciclovir. It is used in cytomegalovirus (CMV) retinitis in patients resistant to other drugs in doses of 5 mg/kg once weekly, followed by similar doses every two weeks.

Didanosine § (dose: 250–400 mg daily)

Brand name: Videx §
Didanosine is an antiviral agent chemically related to zidovudine (p. 82) and is used similarly in the symptomatic treatment of human immunodeficiency virus (HIV) infections. Its action is virostatic, not virucidal, so while it inhibits the spread of the virus, it does not eradicate an established infection. Didanosine is used mainly in the treatment of HIV infections no longer responding to zidovudine and is given orally in doses of 200 mg twice a day (250 mg daily for patients weighing less than 60 kg). It is rapidly broken down by gastric acid, and absorption is reduced in the presence of food. Didanosine should therefore be given at least 30 minutes before a meal, or in the fasting state. Didanosine tablets contain antacids to reduce gastric acid hydrolysis, and must be chewed, crushed, or dispersed in water for administration.

Side-effects include diarrhoea (occasionally severe), nausea, vomiting, fever, peripheral neuropathy and hyperuricaemia. Pancreatitis is a complication of HIV infection and should be excluded before starting didanosine treatment.

Famciclovir § ▼ (dose: 750 mg daily)

Brand name: Famvir § ▼
Famciclovir has the general action of aciclovir, and is used similarly in the treatment of herpes zoster (shingles). Like aciclovir, it is phosphorylated in the herpes virus-infected cells, but persists longer and is effective in doses of 250 mg three times a day. The usual course of treatment is 7 days. Reduced doses may be required in renal impairment.

Ganciclovir § (dose: 5–10 mg/kg daily by injection)

Brand name: Cymevene §

Ganciclovir is chemically related to aciclovir, but is more active and effective against cytomegalovirus (CMV). CMV is a major pathogen in immuno-compromised patients and is a common cause of death in AIDS. It also causes a progressive retinitis that may be sight-threatening. Ganciclovir is indicated in the treatment of life- and sight-threatening CMV infections in immunocompromised patients, and in drug-induced immunosuppression associated with organ transplants. It is given by intravenous infusion in doses of 5 mg/kg every 12 hours for 14–21 days, followed by maintenance doses of 5 mg/kg daily for 5 days a week. When stabilized, oral maintenance doses of 1 g three times a day with food may be given. Solutions of ganciclovir are very alkaline, so the administration of the drug requires care. Protective glasses and gloves should be worn when preparing the injection solution.

Ganciclovir has many **side-effects**, and neutropenia may be severe, so regular blood counts are essential. Zidovudine and other drugs affecting bone marrow function should not be used with ganciclovir.

Foscarnet §

Brand name: (Foscavir §)

Foscarnet is an antiviral agent for the treatment of CMV retinitis in AIDS patients when ganciclovir is contra-indicated or unsuitable. It is given initially in doses of 60 mg/kg 8-hourly for 2–3 weeks, followed by maintenance doses of 60 mg/kg daily. Higher doses of 90–120 mg/kg daily may sometimes be required. In mucocutaneous herpes simplex infections, doses of 40 mg/kg are given 8-hourly until the lesions heal.

Side-effects are nausea and hypocalcaemia. Adequate fluids are essential, as foscarnet may cause renal impairment, and monitoring of the creatinine levels should be carried out every second day.

Idoxuridine §

Brand names: Herpid §, Iduridin §

Idoxuridine is an old antiviral agent, but it is still used as 5% solution in dimethylsulphoxide for the local treatment of herpes simplex infections. A stronger solution (40%) is used for *severe* cutaneous herpes zoster infections. If used early and regularly for 4 days, the lesions are soon checked, and there is less post-herpetic neuralgia. The 40% solution is *not* suitable for the treatment of herpes labialis.

Inosine pranobex § (dose: 4 g daily)

Brand name: Imunovir §

Inosine pranobex differs from other antiviral agents as it acts indirectly by stimulating the immune system of the body. That stimulation results in an increase in the proliferation of T and B cells (p. 275) which is depressed by viral infection.

Inosine pranobex is used in the treatment of muco-cutaneous herpes simplex infections, and is given orally in doses of 1 g four times a day for 7–14 days. It is also used as supplementary treatment for genital warts in doses of 3 g three times a day for 14–28 days. It is well tolerated but care is necessary in gout and renal impairment, as it increases uric acid levels.

Interferon

The interferons (alpha, beta and gamma) are glyco-proteins produced in mammalian cells after infection by viruses, and are part of the natural defence system of the body. They not only inhibit viral growth in infected cells, but also protect surrounding cells from attack. Although they have potential value as antiviral agents, at present they are used mainly for their antitumour activity (p. 225).

Lamivudine § ▼ (dose: 300 mg daily)

Brand name: Epivir § ▼

Lamivudine inhibits an enzyme involved in the replication of viral RNA, and is used with other drugs to inhibit HIV infections. It must be used before the immune system is permanently damaged. Dose 150 mg twice a day between meals. **Side-effects** are numerous.

Stavudine § ▼ (dose: 60–80 mg daily)

Brand name: Zerit § ▼

Stavudine resembles some other antiviral agents in being used to delay the progressive deterioration of HIV infections. Dose 30–40 mg twice a day. Peripheral neuropathy requiring withdrawal is one of many **side-effects**.

Tribavarin §

Brand name: Virazid §

Tribavarin is a synthetic antiviral agent indicated in the treatment of young children with severe respiratory syncytial virus (RSV) infections. The virus infects most children up to 3 years of age, and the infection is usually mild, but severe infections require hospital treatment by nebulization of a 2% solution of tribavarin for 12–18 hours daily for at least 3 days, if necessary with assisted ventilation.

Zalcatabine § ▼ (dose: 1.5 mg daily)

Brand name: Hivid § ▼
Zalcatabine has the actions and uses of related drugs used in severe HIV infections. Dose 750 micrograms three times a day.

Side-effects are numerous and severe; peripheral neuropathy, pancreatitis and hepatotoxicity require immediate withdrawal.

Zidovudine § (dose: 1.2–1.8 g daily)

Brand name: Retrovir §
Zidovudine, also known as azidothymidine or AZT, is an antiviral agent used in the suppressive treatment of acquired immuno deficiency syndrome (AIDS) and the control of secondary conditions referred to as AIDS-related complex. The disease is due to the human immunodeficiency virus (HIV) which has an affinity for T-cells that play an essential part in the defence of the body against infection. The synthesis of viral RNA requires thymidine, and zidovudine, which has a chemical relationship with thymidine, functions as a 'false' thymidine and blocks the formation of viral RNA, and so inhibits further viral development. The action is virustatic and suppressive, and the drug is not able to eliminate an established infection.

Zidovudine is used in the treatment of the more severe manifestations of AIDS, and various dosage schemes are in use, such as oral doses of 200–300 mg 4-hourly day and night, and continued as long as necessary, as extended treatment is usually required. Lower doses of 500 mg daily are given in the treatment of asymptomatic patients. It may also be given by intravenous infusion in doses of 2.5 mg/kg every 4 hours in patients unable to cope with oral therapy, but such infusion treatment should not be given for more than 2 weeks.

Side-effects are numerous and anaemia, neutropenia and leucopenia are common and severe, and may be increased if paracetamol is taken. Regular blood counts are essential. Other side-effects are nausea, rash, anorexia, fever, insomnia and myalgia. Liver disorders require immediate suspension of treatment.

Nursing points about antiviral agents

(a) Mainly virustatic, not virucidal in action.
(b) Early treatment necessary.
(c) Some are inactivated by gastric acid and should be given fasting or between meals.
(d) Some of those given by injection are skin irritants – avoid direct skin contact.

PROTEASE INHIBITORS

Most of the antiviral drugs already referred to for HIV infections prevent viral replication by inhibiting the synthesis of viral nucleic acid and DNA/RNA. A small group of newer antiviral agents, termed protease inhibitors, act at a later stage, as they inhibit key enzymes concerned with the formation of functional viral proteins. The subsequent development of infectious virus particles is thus prevented. Antiviral therapy based on the use of different types of antiviral agents would permit antiviral attack at two different points, and may result in an improved clinical response. The protease inhibitors currently available are indinavir, dose 2.4 g daily (Crixivan); ritonavir, dose 1.2 g daily (Norvir), and saquinavir, dose 1.8 g daily (Invirase), given in divided doses between meals. They have many **side-effects** in common, and the Data Sheets should be consulted for details.

Recently, a warning has been given that reports have been received of hyperglycaemia, new-onset diabetes mellitus and exacerbation of existing diabetes in HIV patients receiving protease inhibitors.

ANTIFUNGAL AGENTS

Fungi are saprophytic organisms, as they lack the chlorophyll present in green plants. They take the form of a thread-like branching filamant (mycelium), often referred to as a mould, and as single-celled organisms termed yeasts. Human fungal infections (mycoses) are usually local infections of the skin and mucous membranes, but with the development of invasive surgery, the wider use of immunosuppressive drugs and the spread of AIDS, systemic fungal infections involving deeper tissues have become more common. Some of these systemic infections are opportunistic, and are caused by organisms that are normally harmless but gain a hold when the normal defence mechanisms of the body are impaired, as by viral attack.

Superficial fungal infections are the dermatoses such as the various forms of *Tinea*, and candidiasis (thrush) due to *Candida albicans*. Systemic fungal infections are cryptococcosis, aspergillosis and histoplasmosis.

The drugs used in fungal infections fall into two main groups, the polyene antibiotics amphotericin and nystatin, and the synthetic antifungal agents. Amphotericin acts by binding selectively with cell transport mechanisms, causing a loss of potassium and cell breakdown. It also has an affinity for ergosterol, the principal fungal sterol, with little affinity for the human sterol cholesterol. Nystatin has a similar action, but as it is not absorbed orally it has only a local action. Most of the synthetic antifungal agents are described chemically as azoles, and act by blocking the conversion of fungal lanosterol to ergosterol by inhibiting the enzyme P450. By that action various intermediate substances accumulate in the fungal cells, causing damage and eventual lysis. A few other antifungal agents act by interfering with fungal DNA synthesis.

ANTIFUNGAL ANTIBIOTICS

Amphotericin § (dose: 250 micrograms/kg daily by injection; 400–800 mg daily orally)

Brand names: Ambelcet §, AmBisome §, Amphocil §, Fungilin §, Fungisone §
Amphotericin is not active orally, but when given intravenously it is effective against many yeast-like and filamentous fungi. It is of value in the treatment of deep fungal infections such as cryptococcosis, histoplasmosis and systemic candidiasis, and is given in doses of 250 micrograms/kg daily by slow intravenous injection, often preceded by a test dose of 1 mg, as there is a risk of an anaphylactic reaction. The injection solution should be freshly prepared, and protected from light during administration. The dose is slowly increased up to 1 mg/kg daily, but treatment for some months may be required, with frequent change of the injection site, as amphotericin is an irritant and may cause local pain and thrombophlebitis.

The dose of amphotericin is normally limited by the nephrotoxic effects of the drug and the development of renal insufficiency. The risk of toxicity has recently been reduced with the introduction of new presentations of amphotericin for intravenous infusion. Abelcet and AmBisome are liposome-encapsu-

lated preparations of amphotericin, from which the drug is slowly released; Amphocil is a complex of amphotericin with sodium cholesteryl sulphate. When the complex is reconstituted for intravenous infusion, it forms a colloidal dispersion. With these products the toxicity of amphotericin has been markedly reduced, permitting daily doses of 1 mg/kg to be given initially, increasing as required to 3–4 mg/kg daily.

Amphotericin is not absorbed orally, and so is correspondingly useful in oral and intestinal candidiasis. It is given in doses of 100–200 mg 6-hourly.

Side-effects of standard therapy are numerous and may be dose-limiting, and include nausea, malaise, chills and rash, as well as blood and neurological disorders. Disturbances of liver function require immediate withdrawal and renal function tests are necessary during amphotericin therapy. If treatment is withdrawn for more than 7 days, dosage should be recommenced at the low initial level.

Griseofulvin § (dose: 0.5–1 g daily)

Brand names: Fulcin §, Grisovin §
Griseofulvin is an antibiotic that is effective in ringworm and other fungal infections of the keratin-containing tissues, i.e. hair, skin and nails. Griseofulvin is taken up selectively by such tissues and prevents further penetration by the fungus. The new tissues formed are therefore free from infection, but response to treatment is correspondingly slow and complete elimination of the fungus awaits the natural shedding of infected hair or nails. It is not effective in systemic infections, and is of no value by local application. Griseofulvin is given orally in doses of 125–250 mg four times a day for some months.

Side-effects In general it is well tolerated, but headache, allergic reactions and gastro-intestinal disturbances may occur. Care is necessary in liver damage. Griseofulvin may increase the effects of alcohol on driving skills.

Nystatin § (dose: 2 million units daily)

Brand name: Nystan §
Nystatin is an antifungal antibiotic that is not absorbed orally and is too toxic for systemic therapy; it is used in the treatment of oral, intestinal and vaginal candidiasis. For oral candidiasis it may be given as pastilles containing 100 000 units, to be chewed four times a day, or in similar doses as a suspension to be used as a mouthwash. In intestinal candidiasis, doses of 500 000 units are given four

times a day, a dose that can be doubled in severe infections. In the treatment of vaginal candidiasis, nystatin pessaries of 100 000 units, and vaginal cream are available (p. 175).

Side-effects are nausea and vomiting, with diarrhoea after high doses. Allergic contact dermatitis has been reported as occurring after the topical application of nystatin.

SYNTHETIC ANTIFUNGAL AGENTS

Fluconazole § (dose: 50–150 mg daily)

Brand name: Diflucan §
Fluconazole has a triazole structure and has a selective action on the fungal cytochrome P450 enzyme system; it inhibits fungal development by interrupting the biosynthesis of ergosterol. In mucosal candidiasis it is given in doses of 50 mg daily for 7–14 days, but in vaginal candidiasis fluconazole is given as a single dose of 150 mg. For fungal infections of the skin, such as tinea, similar doses are given but continued for 2–4 weeks or more.

Fluconazole is also given prophylactically in immunocompromised patients in doses of 50–100 mg daily. It is also given by intravenous infusion in systemic fungal infections such as cryptococcosis, cryptococcal meningitis and systemic candidiasis. In such infections, fluconazole is given as an initial intravenous dose of 400 mg, followed by doses of 200 mg daily. Duration of treatment depends on response, and may have to be continued for 6–8 weeks. Dosage must be modified in renal impairment. Combined treatment with astemizole, terfenadine or cisapride should be avoided (risk of cardiac arrhythmias).

Side-effects include nausea and abdominal discomfort. Treatment should be discontinued if a rash develops.

Flucytosine § (dose: 200 mg/kg daily by injection)

Brand name: Alcobon §
Flucytosine has a selective action on yeast-like fungi mediated by interfering with nucleic acid synthesis. It is used in systemic infections such as cryptococcosis and candidiasis, often as an adjunct to amphotericin. It is usually given by intravenous infusion in doses of 200 mg/kg daily for not more than seven days, but cryptococcal meningitis may require extended treatment for at least 4 months. Regular plasma level tests are necessary. It has occasionally

been given orally in doses of 200 mg daily.

It is usually well tolerated, but nausea, diarrhoea, rash and blood disturbances may occur, so blood counts should be taken. Resistance to flucytosine is common, and may develop during treatment, and sensitivity tests may be required before and during the use of the drug. Flucytosine is excreted in the urine, and lower doses are necessary in renal impairment.

Itraconazole § (dose: 100–200 mg daily)

Brand name: Sporanox §
Itraconazole becomes bound to the keratinocytes in the basal layer of the epidermis, and has a sustained antifungal action that is terminated by the natural shedding of the skin. In tinea infections, it is given in doses of 100 mg daily for 15–30 days, but in pityriasis versicolor a 7-day course of 200 mg daily is usually adequate. Itraconazole is also used for the 1-day treatment of vulvo-vaginal candidiasis as two doses of 100 mg. The **side-effects** include headache, nausea and abdominal pain. It is metabolized in the liver, and care is necessary in hepatic disease. Combined use with astemizole, cisapride or terfenadine should be avoided.

Ketoconazole § (dose: 200–400 mg daily)

Brand name: Nizoral §
Ketoconazole is one of the imidazole group of antifungal agents. It is well absorbed orally, and effective in systemic and resistant mycoses, as well as in vaginal candidiasis. It has also been used in the prophylactic treatment of immunocompromised patients.

The standard dose is 200 mg daily with food, increased if necessary to 400 mg in deep-seated and systemic infections. It is also given in resistant and chronic vaginal candidiasis in doses of 400 mg daily for 5 days.

Side-effects include nausea and pruritus, but jaundice and fatal liver damage have followed ketoconazole therapy. It is not recommended for superficial fungal infections. If treatment is continued for more than 14 days, liver function tests should be carried out regularly. Hepatic impairment is a contra-indication. Combined use with astemizole, cisapride or terfenadine should be avoided.

Miconazole § (dose: 0.5–1 g daily)

Brand name: Daktarin §
Miconazole is a systemic antifungal agent with antibacterial properties. It is given orally for mucosal

and intestinal fungal infections in doses of 250 mg four times a day for 10 days. It is also of value in the prophylactic treatment of patients at risk, such as transplant and cancer patients receiving immuno-suppressive treatment.

Side-effects include nausea, fever, pruritus and rash. Combined treatment with astemizole, cisapride and terfenadine should be avoided. The use of miconazole in trichomonal infections is referred to on p. 173.

Terbinafine § (dose: 250 mg daily)

Brand name: Lamisil §

Terbinafine resembles the azole antifungal agents in blocking the synthesis of ergosterol, but differs in acting on another fungal enzyme, squalene epoxi-dase. In fungal infections of the skin it is given in doses of 250 mg daily for 2–3 weeks, but infections of the nails may require treatment for up to 3 months. In athlete's foot terbinafine is used as a 1% cream, applied to the affected areas once or twice a day for 1–2 weeks.

Side-effects of oral therapy are headache, myalgia and gastrointestinal disturbances. Care is necessary in hepatic dysfunction, and any combined treatment that may affect liver enzyme activity.

Other antifungal agents used in candidiasis and dermatophyte infections include clotrimazole (Canestan), econazole (Ecostatin, Pevaryl), isoconazole (Travogyn) and metronidazole (Flagyl)

Nursing points about systemic antifungal agents

(a) When used for oral fungal infections, any dentures should be removed.
(b) In dermatophyte infections of the hair, as much infected hair as possible should be removed.
(c) Special care is needed with ketoconazole; there is a risk of hepatotoxicity, and treatment should be limited to 14 days.
(d) Combined use of azole antifungal agents and astemizole, cisapride and terbinafine should be avoided as there is a risk of cardiac arrhythmias.
(e) They should not be used for superficial fungal infections.

FURTHER READING

Aronson J K, Reynolds D J M 1992 Aminoglycoside antibiotics. British Medical Journal 305:1421–1424

Ayliffe G A et al (eds) 1992 Control of hospital infection: a practical handbook, 3rd edn. Chapman & Hall, London, p 253–273

Bartlett J G 1982 Anti-anaerobic antibacterial agents. Lancet ii:478–481

Brogden R N, Heal R C 1986 Aztreonam: a review of its properties and therapeutic uses. Drugs 31:96–130

Busuttil R 1996 Cranberry Juice. Professional Nurse 11(8):525–526

Cahill J 1994 Applying pharmokinetic data to gentamicin. Professional Nurse 9(11):735–738

Cooksey S 1995 Managing chemotherapy for tuberculosis. Nursing Times 91(35):32–33

Ellis R, Pillay D 1996 Antimicrobial therapy: towards the future. British Journal of Hospital Medicine 56(4):145–150

Fekety R et al 1984 Treatment of antibiotic-associated colitis with vancomycin. Journal of Antimicrobial Chemotherapy 14 (suppl D):97–102

Hampson J P 1996 The use of metronidazole in the treatment of malodorous wounds. Journal of Wound Care 5(9):421–426

Hooper D C, Wolfson J S 1991 Fluoquinolone antibacterial agents. New England Journal of Medicine 324:384–394

Kedzierski M 1991 Understanding virology. Professional Nurse 6(11):99–102

Kelly J, Chivers G 1996 Built-in resistance. Nursing Times 92(2):50–54

Leaver R B 1996 Cranberry juice. Professional Nurse 11(8):525–526

Ramsay J et al 1989 Biofilms, bacteria and bladder catheters. British Journal of Urology 64:395–398

Walters J 1988 How antibiotics work. Professional Nurse 3(7):251–254

Walters J 1989 How antibiotics work: the cell membrane. Professional Nurse 4(10):508–510

Walters J 1990 How antibiotics work: nucleic acid synthesis. Professional Nurse 5(12):641–643

Walters J 1993 How antibiotics work: protein synthesis. Professional Nurse 8(12):788–791

6

Drugs acting on the autonomic nervous system

The nervous system can be divided anatomically into the central nervous system (the cerebral hemispheres, cerebellum, brain stem and spinal cord) and the peripheral nervous system (cranial nerves and spinal nerves). Alternatively, the nervous system can be divided functionally into the somatic or voluntary nervous and the autonomic or involuntary nervous systems. The former is associated with impulses to the limbs and body wall, the latter with impulses to the smooth muscles of the viscera, blood vessels, eyes and exocrine glands. The autonomic nervous system maintains the physiological equilibrium of the body, yet at the same time it is not completely independent of the central nervous system (CNS), as factors which affect higher centres may also influence some physiological functions. The effect of fear and anger on the pulse rate is an example of that interdependence.

SYMPATHETIC AND PARASYMPATHETIC NERVOUS SYSTEMS

The autonomic nervous system has two branches, the sympathetic and parasympathetic nerves. Generally, both branches serve the same organs but cause essentially opposite effects, counterbalancing each other to keep the body systems running smoothly. The sympathetic nerves leave the thoraco-lumbar region of the spinal cord (T1–13) and synapse either in the paravertebral or prevertebral ganglia (collections of nerve cell bodies outside the CNS), and with plexuses in the abdominal cavity. As these ganglia are near the vertebral column, the preganglionic fibres are short, but branch extensively. The post-ganglionic fibres that run out to the smooth muscle are correspondingly long. The parasympathetic fibres originate in the midbrain, medulla and sacral areas of the spinal cord. They leave the CNS as cranial nerves 3, 7 and 9 (the vagus nerve) and as spinal nerves 3 and 4, and are termed the craniosacral outflow. The ganglia are close to the visceral organ concerned, so the post-ganglionic fibres are short.

Transmitters and receptors

Communication within the nervous system is via electrical impulses and neurotransmitters. In the case of the autonomic nervous system, when an impulse is generated in the CNS it passes along the preganglionic fibre until it reaches a ganglion, where it synapses or meets another nerve. There is a small gap between the two nerves (the synaptic cleft), and in the cleft the afferent nerve releases the neurotransmitter acetylcholine (Fig. 6.1). Acetylcholine diffuses across the gap and stimulates the postganglionic fibre to generate a new nerve impulse. The released acetylcholine is immediately inactivated by the enzyme cholinesterase.

The impulse continues along the post-ganglionic fibre and, in the case of the parasympathetic nerves, acetylcholine is again released when the nerve synapses at the myoneural junction. The acetylcholine then binds to receptors on the innervated organ and stimulates the necessary response. The response is limited both in duration and intensity, as the acetylcholine is rapidly destroyed by the tissue enzymes, as it is when released by the ganglia.

Noradrenaline

In the case of the sympathetic nervous system, the post-ganglionic fibres release noradrenaline to act on the adrenoceptors (the exception being those that supply the sweat glands, which release acetylcholine). This release of noradrenaline from sympathetic nerve fibres is also linked with the release of adrenaline from the adrenal medulla in response to stress. Because sympathetic nerves release noradrenaline they have been termed adrenergic nerves, whereas the parasympathetic nerves are sometimes referred to as cholinergic nerves because they release acetylcholine.

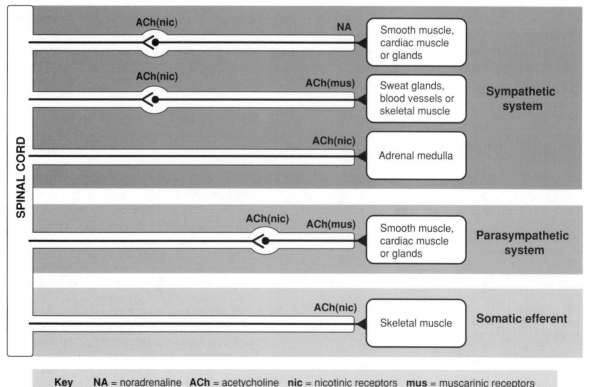

Key **NA** = noradrenaline **ACh** = acetycholine **nic** = nicotinic receptors **mus** = muscarinic receptors

Figure 6.1 Neurotransmitter systems.

Adrenaline and noradrenaline, together with dopamine (a precursor of noradrenaline that functions as a neurotransmitter in the CNS (p. 96) are sometimes referred to as catecholamines (an allusion to their chemical structure). Unlike acetylcholine, the catecholamines are not rapidly inactivated by local enzymes. Some of the released noradrenaline re-enters the noradrenergic nerve terminal by a re-uptake mechanism, and the catecholamines present in the circulation are metabolized by monoamine oxidases and other enzymes.

Physiological balance

The activities of the two parts of the autonomic nervous system are of great physiological importance. In general, both parts of the system act on the same organs, but they act at different sites and produce opposite effects. In health, the two parts are in dynamic balance, constantly changing in response to physiological needs, and can be compared with the accelerator and brakes of a car.

In general, the effects of stimulation of the sympathetic nervous system are more widespread, as a single ganglion may serve many post-ganglionic nerves, whereas the ganglia of the parasympathetic system are usually much closer to the organs they control, and are less extensively innervated. The sympathetic nervous system has been described as the 'fight or flight' system, as it prepares the body to cope with emergencies and intense muscular activity, while the parasympathetic nervous system is the 'digesting and resting' system, as it conserves and stores energy.

The autonomic nervous system can be influenced by drugs at several points, and it will be appreciated that the depression of one part of the system will produce an end-result comparable with that of stimulating the opposite part. Some of the main effects of the two systems are summarized in Table 6.1.

Table 6.1 Main effects

Organ	Sympathetic stimulation	Parasympathetic stimulation
Heart	Rate increased	Rate slowed
Blood vessels	Constricted	Dilated
Lungs (bronchial muscles)	Relaxed	Contracted
Gastro-intestinal tract	Activity decreased	Increased
Urinary system:		
Bladder	Relaxed	Contracted
Sphincter	Contracted	Relaxed
Eye	Pupil dilated	Constricted

SYMPATHOMIMETIC DRUGS

Drugs that interact with the autonomic nervous system are usually targeted at neurotransmitter receptors. Thus sympathomimetic drugs are those that act on the adrenoceptors and elicit a response similar in some ways to that produced by the natural messenger substance noradrenaline. They may act directly on the adrenoceptor or indirectly by releasing stored noradrenaline from nerve endings. Those receptors are of two main types, the alpha-adrenoceptors and the beta-adrenoceptors, and an organ may possess both types. Some sympathomometic drugs may therefore have more than one type of action.

The alpha-receptors have been divided into two groups: α_1 and α_2-receptors. They were originally classified depending on whether their location was on the presynaptic nerve (α_2-receptors) or on the more usual postsynaptic nerve (α_1-receptors). The value of presynaptic receptors is that stimulation of these receptors by noradrenaline released into the synapse provides a negative feedback mechanism, limiting the amount of noradrenaline released. Alpha-receptors as a group are concerned mainly with peripheral and visceral blood vessels, and stimulation leads to vasoconstriction of the vessels to the skin and viscera, thus increasing the amount of blood available to the other organs. The α_1-receptors are also found on a variety of other tissues, in particular the iris of the eye where their stimulation results in contraction of the radial muscle.

The beta-receptors have also been divided into two groups: β_1 and β_2-receptors. The β_1-receptors occur mainly in heart muscle and when stimulated bring about an increase in cardiac force and rate. The β_2-receptors have a wider distribution, as they are found in vascular, bronchial and uterine smooth muscle. Stimulation of these receptors results in relaxation, with vasodilatation and bronchodilation.

Sympathomimetic drugs that have an affinity for and act on adrenoceptors are referred to as agonists, but drugs that have an affinity for but no action upon receptor sites are known as antagonists, or adrenoceptor blocking agents (see Table 6.2). Beta-adrenoceptor agonists are used as bronchodilators and are discussed in Chapter 18, while beta-adrenoceptor blocking agents play an important part in the control of hypertension and angina, and are discussed in Chapter 7.

Table 6.2 Some adrenoceptor agonists and antagonists, and an indication of their range of adrenoceptor affinity at different adrenoceptor subtypes

	Adrenoceptor			
Agonists	α_1	α_2	β_1	β_2
noradrenaline	+++	+++	++	+
adrenaline	++	++	+++	+++
phenylephrine, methoxamine	++	−	−	−
clonidine	−	+++	−	−
isoprenaline	−	−	+++	+++
salbutamol, terbutaline, orciprenaline	−	−	+	+++
Antagonists				
phenoxybenzamine	+++	+++	−	−
indoramin, phentolamine, prazosin	+++	+	−	−
labetalol	+	+	++	++
pindolol, propranolol, sotalol, timolol	−	−	+++	+++
oxprenolol	−	−	+++PA	+++
acebutolol, atenolol, metoprolol	−	−	+++	+

Key: + = small effect; ++ = moderate effect; +++ = large effect; − = no effect; PA = partial agonist

---

Nursing points about sympathomimetics

(a) Different agents may act more or less selectively on different receptors.
(b) Type of response varies accordingly.
(c) Injection of inotropic sympathomimetics (dobutamine, dopamine, dopexamine) requires care, as the response may vary markedly with an increase in dose.
(d) Vasoconstrictor sympathomimetics now used less frequently in shock.

SYMPATHOMIMETIC DRUGS WITH A MAINLY PRESSOR ACTION

Adrenaline § (dose: 200–500 micrograms by subcutaneous or intramuscular injection).

Adrenaline (epinephrine) is the natural hormone, formerly obtained from the suprarenal gland, but now made synthetically. It acts on both adrenoceptors, but is now used less frequently as more selective drugs are available. It has a powerful bronchodilator action, but in severe status asthmaticus salbutamol is now preferred as it has fewer cardiac side-effects. In anaphylactic shock, which is characterized by cardiovascular collapse and a sudden fall in blood pressure, with bronchospasm and pulmonary oedema, adrenaline remains the keystone of treatment.

Anaphylactic shock, although uncommon, may occur in a patient who has become sensitized in some way, possibly to a drug, a food or an insect sting or even to an allergen desensitizing injection. It is an emergency requiring prompt treatment to restore the blood pressure, and adrenaline should be given by intramuscular or subcutaneous injection as soon as possible as a 0.5 ml dose of adrenaline solution (1–1000), repeated every 10 minutes as required. (The value of subcutaneous injections has been questioned, but in the early stages of anaphylaxis vasodilatation is marked, and subcutaneous absorption of adrenaline may be rapid, as shown by the response to self-treatment in emergency by pre-filled automatic injection devices. If treatment is delayed and shock occurs, the intravenous injection of adrenaline may be required.)

An antihistamine such as chlorpheniramine should also be given by slow intravenous injection to maintain the response, and continued for 24 hours or more to prevent a relapse. Hydrocortisone may also be given intravenously in a dose of 100 mg, as further supportive therapy, although the action is slow and may not be apparent for some hours.

For individuals known to be at risk from insect stings, syringes pre-filled with adrenaline solution for injection, and an adrenaline aerosol inhalation product (Medihaler-epi §) are now available for emergency use. Adrenaline is occasionally used in the treatment of cardiac arrest by the direct intracardiac injection of 10 ml of a 1–10 000 solution.

Adrenaline is also used for its vasoconstrictor action by its inclusion as an additive in some local anaesthetic solutions to delay absorption and prolong the action, but care is necessary that such adrenaline-containing solutions are not injected into tissues where they could cause ischaemic necrosis.

For the use of adrenaline in the treatment of glaucoma see p. 250.

Noradrenaline § (dose: 8–12 micrograms per minute by intravenous infusion)

Brand name: Levophed §
Noradrenaline (norepinephrine) differs from adrenaline chiefly by exerting its action mainly on the alpha-receptors. It raises the blood pressure by a more general vasoconstriction, although it also has some minor cardiac stimulant action. It has been used in the treatment of shock in doses of 8 micrograms or more per minute by slow intravenous infusion of a well diluted solution, but the dose and rate of administration require considerable care, as the response may fluctuate. Great care must be taken to avoid extravasation, as the intense local vasoconstriction so caused may result in necrosis and gangrene.

Noradrenaline is also used occasionally as a special solution of 200 micrograms for intracardiac injection in cases of cardiac arrest. Like adrenaline, noradrenaline is also added to some local anaesthetic solutions (1 in 80 000 or less) to prolong the anaesthetic action.

The use of noradrenaline and other vasoconstrictor drugs in the treatment of shock is declining, as it is now considered that the general vasoconstriction and rise in blood pressure that it causes may reduce the blood supply to essential organs such as the kidney to a dangerous extent. In any case, vasoconstrictors in shock are of little value if much blood loss has occurred, and reliance is now placed on the restoration of blood volume by expanders, and the use of more selectively acting cardiac drugs such as dopamine and dobutamine, often in association with high doses of hydrocortisone or other corticosteroid.

Dobutamine § (dose: 2.5–10 micrograms/kg per minute by intravenous infusion)

Brand name: Dobutrex §
Dobutamine is a sympathomimetic agent that acts mainly on the β_1-receptors and has a more selective cardiac action than some related drugs. It is used in the treatment of cardiogenic shock associated with myocardial infarction and cardiac surgery, and in heart failure due to organic heart disease.

Dobutamine is given by the slow intravenous drip infusion of a dilute solution in doses of 2.5–10 micrograms/kg per minute according to need and response, followed by slow withdrawal after the condition has been controlled. Its administration requires constant supervision as higher doses may exacerbate heart failure.

Side-effects include nausea and headache, but the onset of tachycardia is indicative of overdose.

Dopamine § (dose: 2–5 micrograms/kg per minute by intravenous infusion)

Dopamine is a natural substance from which noradrenaline is formed, and both compounds have some properties in common. Like dobutamine, dopamine acts on the β_1-receptors, but it has a more potent inotropic action, i.e. it increases the force more than the rate of the heart beat. It increases the cardiac output and tends to correct any haemodynamic imbalance without causing excessive tachycardia. It also appears to act on some 'dopaminergic receptors' in the kidney, so that with small doses renal vasodilatation occurs, renal blood flow increases, and renal efficiency is maintained.

Dopamine is used in the treatment of cardiogenic shock, and of shock unresponsive to the replacement of fluid loss, but its use requires considerable care. It is given in initial doses of 2–5 micrograms/kg per minute by intravenous infusion in 5% glucose injection, preferably into a large vein to avoid tissue necrosis, but the action of the drug is very brief, and continuous control of administration is essential. The dose may be increased according to response, and in exceptional cases a dose as high as 50 micrograms/kg per minute has been given, although large doses may cause vasoconstriction and tend to exacerbate heart failure. A reduction in urine flow is an indication that the dose of dopamine should be reduced. Once the condition is under control, the drug should be slowly withdrawn over some hours as hypotension and anuria may follow sudden withdrawal. As with related drugs, preliminary restoration of a depleted blood volume is necessary.

Dopexamine § (dose: 500 nanograms/kg/minute by intravenous infusion)

Brand name: Dopacard §
Dopexamine is a synthetic catecholamine, related to dopamine, but with a much more powerful action

on the β_2-adrenoceptors. It is indicated in the short-term treatment of acute exacerbations of heart failure, and for support after cardiac surgery. The mode of action is basically that of producing systemic and pulmonary vasodilatation, which results in a reduction in the ventricular afterload, but at the same time it has some inotropic activity that maintains the blood pressure. It also brings about an increase in the renal blood flow. Dopexamine is given by intravenous infusion under careful control in doses of 500 nanograms/kg/minute initially, increased at intervals of 10–15 minutes by increments of 1 microgram/kg/minute up to a maximum of 6 micrograms/kg/minute, adjusted to need and response, including measurement of cardiac output. The half-life of dopexamine is 6–7 minutes, so any excessive response is likely to be short-lived if treatment is withdrawn.

Side-effects include tachycardia, nausea and anginal pain.

Isoprenaline § (dose: 15–10 micrograms)

Brand name: Saventrine §

Isoprenaline is closely related chemically to adrenaline and noradrenaline, but differs in acting almost exclusively on the beta-adrenoceptors. It is used in the emergency treatment of severe bradycardia and heart block and is given by slow intravenous injection in doses of 5–10 micrograms/min under ECG control.

Side-effects include palpitation, nausea, tremor and tachycardia. The drug is now less widely used.

Metaraminol § (dose: 2–10 mg by subcutaneous or intramuscular injection; 15–100 mg by intravenous infusion)

Brand name: Aramine §

Metaraminol has the general vasoconstrictor properties of noradrenaline but it has a longer action. It is used in the severe hypotension of shock, including myocardial infarction, haemorrhage, trauma and surgery. It is given in doses of 15–100 mg by intravenous infusion, after dilution with 500 ml of normal saline or 5% glucose solution. By its extended action it sometimes causes a prolonged rise in blood pressure.

Side-effects include cardiac irregularities.

Methoxamine § (dose: 5–20 mg by injection)

Brand name: Vasoxine §

Methoxamine is a sympathomimetic agent that has a direct stimulating action on the alpha-adrenoceptors. It brings about a prolonged constriction of the peripheral blood vessels with a consequent rise in

the arterial pressure, but it may also markedly reduce renal blood flow. It has little direct action on the heart, although a reflex bradycardia may occur.

Methoxamine is used for its pressor action to maintain blood pressure during spinal anaesthesia, and during and after anaesthesia with halothane or cyclopropane. It is given by intramuscular injection in doses of 10–15 mg or more, repeated if necessary after about 15 minutes. In emergencies, methoxamine may be given by slow intravenous injection in doses of 3–5 mg; intravenous doses up to 10 mg are given to control paroxysmal tachycardia.

Side-effects include nausea, vomiting, headache and bradycardia. Care is necessary in cardiovascular disease. Ephedrine (p. 239) is also given by intravenous injection to reverse hypotension in spinal anaesthesia in doses of 3–6 mg.

Phenylephrine (dose: 2–5 mg by injection)

Phenylephrine is chemically related to adrenaline, but it has a more specific action on the alpha-adrenoceptors, and has a pressor action similar to that of methoxamine. It is used in acute hypotensive states such as circulatory failure, spinal anaesthesia and drug-induced hypotension, and is given in doses of 2–5 mg by subcutaneous or intramuscular injection, or in doses of 100–500 micrograms by slow intravenous injection. Alternatively, phenylephrine may be given in doses of 5–20 mg by intravenous infusion at a rate not greater than 180 micrograms/minute. Phenylephrine has also been used to control paroxysmal supraventricular tachycardia in doses up to 500 micrograms by slow intravenous injection.

Side-effects of phenylephrine include nausea, vomiting, headache and hypertension; care is necessary in cardiovascular disease.

Phenylephrine is also used in ophthalmology as a mydriatic, and to lower intraocular pressure in open angle glaucoma (p. 249).

Xamoterol § (dose: 400 mg daily)

Brand name: Corwin §

Xamoterol is a sympathomimetic agent used only in the treatment of *mild* chronic heart failure. See p. 105.

PARASYMPATHOMIMETIC OR CHOLINERGIC DRUGS

The cholinergic drugs mimic the effects of the parasympathetic nervous system and act on two main acetylcholine-receptor subtypes, namely nicotinic and muscarinic. The names indicate that the natural plant substances nicotine (from the tobacco plant) and muscarine (from the fly agaric mushroom) can compete with acetylcholine for binding sites on their respective receptors where they act as agonists. Nicotinic receptors are found at neuromuscular junctions (see Chapter 19) and autonomic ganglia. The muscarinic receptors mediate acetylcholine effects at postganglionic parasympathetic synapses, mainly heart, smooth muscle and glands (Fig. 6.1). Muscarinic receptors are further subdivided into three main types, namely M_1-receptors found in the CNS, enteric and autonomic ganglia, and on the parietal cells of the stomach, M_2-receptors found on the heart, and M_3-receptors found on exocrine glands, smooth muscle and vascular endothelium.

Parasympathomimetic drugs can be divided into two groups:

1. those that act directly on receptors, i.e. nicotinic and muscarinic agonists
2. anticholinesterases which inhibit the enzyme cholinesterase which normally breaks down acetylcholine. This group thus act indirectly by allowing acetylcholine to accumulate in the synapse and exert its action.

The **side-effects** of cholinergic drugs and anticholinesterases are associated with their general effects of augmenting the action of released acetylcholine or preventing its breakdown. The main side-effects of the anticholinesterases are generally due to their muscarinic properties and include increased salivary and bronchial secretions, increased gastrointestinal activity with nausea, vomiting, colic and diarrhoea, and bradycardia. As atropine is a antagonist muscarinic it antagonizes all the effects of cholinergic drugs, with the exception of the effects on autonomic ganglia and neuromuscular junctions, which are nicotinic. In cases of overdose with cholinergic drugs, atropine is given in doses of up to 1–2 mg by intravenous injection, repeated according to need. It should be noted that certain organophosphorus insecticides are extremely powerful anticholinesterases with a long action, and can cause severe poisoning and death from respiratory failure. Prompt treatment with atropine is essential, and very large doses of up to 50 mg over 24 hours may be required (p. 313).

GROUP 1

Acetylcholine is a transmitter substance found throughout the nervous system, but is broken down so rapidly by cholinesterase that it is of no value therapeutically. In practice, reliance is placed largely on group 2 drugs, but a few choline derivatives and certain plant alkaloids with selective group 1 activity remain in limited use.

Carbachol § (dose: 6 mg daily; 250 micrograms by subcutaneous injection)

Carbachol, or carbamylcholine, has some of the properties of acetylcholine, and has been used in the treatment of acute and chronic retention of urine, as it increases bladder tone by stimulating detrusor muscle contraction.

Carbachol is given orally in doses of 2 mg three times a day before food in chronic retention, but in acute conditions it is given by subcutaneous injection in doses of 250 micrograms, repeated after 30 minutes, and again after a similar interval if required. It is now used less frequently as catheterization is preferred.

Side-effects of carbachol are those of general parasympathetic stimulation, and include nausea, vomiting, blurred vision, sweating and involuntary defaecation. Bradycardia and peripheral vasodilatation leading to hypotension may also occur and for that reason carbachol should not be given by intramuscular or intravenous injection. Carbachol has also been used as a miotic in the treatment of glaucoma as 3% eye-drops (p. 250).

Bethanechol § (dose: 30–120 mg daily; 5 mg by subcutaneous injection)

Brand name: Myotonine §

Bethanechol has the actions, uses and side-effects of carbachol, but cardiovascular disturbances are less likely to occur. It is given in doses of 10–30 mg three or four times a day before food in urinary retention, or in a dose of 5 mg by subcutaneous injection, repeated after 30 minutes, in acute conditions. It is sometimes given by injection in the treatment of postoperative paralytic ileus. Like carbachol, it should not be given by intramuscular or intravenous injection.

GROUP 2

The anticholinesterases permit the accumulation of acetylcholine at nerve endings and so have a wide range of activity as well as side-effects. They have relatively little effect at ganglia, and are used mainly for their nicotinic effects on the neuromuscular junction. Thus, they are of some value in urinary disorders, while others are used in myasthenia gravis, an autoimmune disease associated with dysfunction or loss of the acetylcholine receptors, causing severe skeletal muscle fatigue. It should be noted that atropine, a potent anticholinergic drug, can oppose some but not all of the actions of anticholinesterases.

Neostigmine § (dose: 75–300 mg daily; 1–2.5 mg by injection)

Brand name: Prostigmin §
Neostigmine is a synthetic anticholinesterase that mainly increases the action of released acetylcholine on skeletal muscle, with less action on smooth muscle. It is used mainly in the treatment of myasthenia gravis, a condition characterized by a variably progressive muscular weakness. It may be due to an immunologically induced receptor site abnormality that interferes with normal acetylcholine-mediated muscle contraction, or to a reduction in the number of active receptors. The condition may be alleviated by neostigmine in doses of 75–300 mg daily, given as divided doses modified according to individual need and response, and given at 4-hourly intervals. In more severe conditions, neostigmine may be given by subcutaneous or intramuscular injection in doses of 1–2.5 mg at intervals according to need, up to 2-hourly and a maximum of 20 mg daily.

It should be noted that overdose of neostigmine may have the reverse effects of reducing neurotransmission and increasing the muscle weakness, an effect that must be distinguished from a deterioration of the myasthenic condition.

Neostigmine is also given by injection in doses of 0.5–1 mg in the treatment of paralytic ileus and postoperative urinary retention. It is also used in anaesthesia to cut short the action of muscle relaxants (p. 244).

Side-effects of neostigmine are linked with its cholinergic activity and include nausea, vomiting, salivation, colic and diarrhoea. Bradycardia and hypotension may be indicative of excessive dosage. Neostigmine is contra-indicated in the mechanical obstruction of the intestinal or urinary tract.

Distigmine § (dose: 5–20 mg daily; 500 micrograms by intramuscular injection)

Brand name: Ubretid §
Distigmine has the actions and uses of neostigmine, with the advantage of a longer duration of action that may extend over 24 hours. In myasthenia gravis it is given in an oral dose of 5 mg initially on an empty stomach (to promote absorption) half an hour before breakfast, and increased at intervals of 3 days or so according to response up to a maximum of 20 mg daily.

Distigmine is also useful in the treatment of urinary retention in patients with neurogenic bladder associated with upper motor neurone lesions, and is given in doses of 5 mg daily or on alternate days, preferably half an hour before breakfast. It is sometimes given by injection in doses of 500 micrograms for the prevention and treatment of postoperative urinary retention and intestinal atony.

Side-effects of distigmine are similar to those of prostigmine, but although usually milder, may be more prolonged. If side-effects are severe, treatment with 500 micrograms or more of atropine by injection may be required.

Pyridostigmine § (dose: 300–720 mg daily)

Brand name: Mestinon §
Pyridostigmine has the uses and side-effects of neostigmine, and although less potent, it has a slow and prolonged action. It is useful in those myasthenic states where a less intense action is required, and for night-time use when early morning muscle weakness is a problem. It is given orally in doses of 30–120 mg, taken at intervals during the day linked with need and response, up to a total of 300–720 mg or occasionally more daily.

It does not relieve the symptoms of myasthenia gravis so completely as neostigmine, but its reduced gastro-intestinal side-effects may be an advantage. Like related drugs, pyridostigmine is sometimes used in postoperative paralytic ileus and urinary retention in doses of 60–240 mg as required.

Edrophonium § (dose: 10 mg by intravenous injection)

Edrophonium has the basic properties of neostigmine, but differs markedly in having a very brief action. It is correspondingly valuable in the diagnosis of myasthenia gravis, as in patients with that disease, a dose of 2 mg intravenously, followed, if there is no adverse reaction after 30 seconds, by a further dose of 8 mg, brings about an immediate, definite but transient increase in muscle power. The effect lasts for about 5 minutes, after which the muscle weakness returns.

Edrophonium is also of value in distinguishing between overdose and underdose of an anticholinesterase or cholinergic drug such as neostigmine.

If dosage is inadequate, an intravenous injection of the test dose of 10 mg intravenously will result in an immediate but temporary improvement of the myasthenia, whereas in cases of excessive therapy, the symptoms will be equally rapid but briefly intensified.

Edrophonium has few **side-effects**, but it may cause some respiratory muscle weakness, and care is necessary with asthmatic patients.

ANTICHOLINERGIC OR PARASYMPATHOLYTIC AGENTS

Drugs that inhibit the action of acetylcholine by occupying receptor sites at various points of the parasympathetic nervous system, as well as those of certain sites in the sympathetic system (Fig. 6.1), are antagonists, and are referred to as anticholinergic drugs. The oldest is the alkaloid atropine which is a muscarinic antagonist, but synthetic anticholinergic drugs with greater specificity than atropine are in use.

Attempts have been made to classify the anticholinergic drugs into three groups:

1. those used mainly for their smooth muscle relaxant, antispasmodic and antisecretory properties,
2. those used for their effects on the central nervous system in the treatment of parkinsonism,
3. those used in ophthalmology.

In this chapter they will be divided into natural drugs, synthetic drugs, and those used almost exclusively in the treatment of Parkinson's disease. Those used in ophthalmology are discussed in Chapter 20.

Atropine § (dose: 250 micrograms–1 mg daily orally; 500 micrograms intravenously)

Atropine is the alkaloid originally obtained from belladonna, although it is also prepared synthetically. It brings about a reduction in smooth muscle tone and gastro-intestinal activity, and is given orally in doses of 500 micrograms three times a day, increased if required up to 2 mg daily, for the relief of gastro-intestinal spasm, and in biliary and renal colic.

Atropine is used pre-operatively by injection in doses of 300–600 micrograms to decrease bronchial and salivary secretions. It increases the heart rate by its action on the vagus, and so prevents the bradycardia induced by some inhalation anaesthetics. It is also used in the treatment of bradycardia in myocar-dial infarction by intravenous doses of 300 micrograms–1 mg, up to a maximum of 3 mg over 24 hours. Atropine is also given postoperatively by intravenous injection in doses of 600 micrograms–1.2 mg in association with neostigmine to reverse the action of muscle relaxants (p. 244). Its use in ophthalmology is referred to in Chapter 20.

Side-effects of atropine include dryness of the mouth, dilatation of the pupils, dry skin and bradycardia. It is contra-indicated in prostatic hypertrophy and glaucoma, and should be used with care in the elderly and in cardiac insufficiency. (Note: Belladonna extract, a survivor of older therapy, is still used in some mixed products for the treatment of gastro-intestinal disorders associated with smooth muscle spasm.)

Hyoscine § (dose: 200–600 micrograms orally or by subcutaneous injection)

Hyoscine, also known as scopolamine, is an alkaloid closely related to atropine and has some similar properties. It differs in having a depressant effect on the cerebral cortex, and so it has some hypnotic properties, although sometimes the hyoscine-induced drowsiness may be preceded by a brief period of excitement. Hyoscine is mainly used for premedication in doses of 200–600 micrograms by subcutaneous injection, together with 20 mg of papaveretum or 10 mg of morphine to reduce secretions and facilitate induction. Such combined treatment has also been used in obstetrics to produce analgesia and amnesia.

Hyoscine has a depressant action on the vomiting centre, and it is widely used in the treatment of travel sickness and vertigo. It is given in oral doses of 600 micrograms (150–300 micrograms for children of 6–12 years) about 20 minutes before starting a journey, with subsequent doses three or four times a day as required. Scopoderm TTS § is a patch dressing containing 500 micrograms of hyoscine, for the prevention of travel sickness. It should be applied to a hairless area of the skin about 5 hours before the start of the journey. The slow absorption of the drug from the patch is said to provide an action extending over 72 hours, with the advantage of reduced side-effects. Only one patch should be used at a time, and care should be taken to wash the hands after the application and removal of the patch. The use of hyoscine in ophthalmology is referred to in Chapter 20.

Side-effects of hyoscine are anticholinergic, and include dryness of the mouth, blurred vision and urinary difficulties. It should be used with caution in the elderly, and is contra-indicated in glaucoma.

Hyoscine butylbromide (Buscopan) is a derivative of hyoscine used in the treatment of acute gastro-intestinal spasm. It is given by intramuscular or intravenous injection in doses of 20 mg. Tablets are also available, but response is variable as the absorption is poor.

SYNTHETIC ANTICHOLINERGIC AGENTS

The synthetic anticholinergics or antimuscarinic drugs have reduced side-effects compared to atropine. They do not cross the blood–brain barrier easily, and so are less likely to cause central effects such as confusion or visual disturbances. On the other hand, they are less lipid-soluble and so absorption after oral administration may be poor, and marked differences may exist between oral doses and those given by injection.

These anticholinergic agents are used mainly in the treatment of gastro-intestinal disorders associated with smooth muscle spasm, and by delaying gastric movement they also help to prolong the action of antacids. They are used in urinary frequency and enuresis, as they increase bladder capacity by having a stabilizing action on the detrusor muscle. Anticholinergic drugs may cause confusion in the elderly as well as urinary hesitancy, and care is necessary in glaucoma.

Propantheline is a representative of this group of drugs. Those anticholinergic agents used mainly in the treatment of Parkinson's disease are referred to on p. 98.

Propantheline § (dose: 45–90 mg daily)

Brand name: Pro-Banthine §

Propantheline has the peripheral action of atropine on the response to released acetycholine, and it is used in the treatment of gastro-intestinal disturbances associated with smooth muscle spasm, and in biliary and urinary tract spasm. It is also used in urinary frequency and enuresis, as it reduces the contractions of an unstable detrusor muscle.

Propantheline is given in doses of 15 mg three time a day before meals, with a 30 mg dose at night, subsequently adjusted as required with a maximum dose of 120 mg daily. In the treatment of enuresis, a bedtime dose of 15–45 mg has been used.

Side-effects of propantheline are similar to those of atropine, but in general are less severe.

Other antispasmodics used mainly in gastro-intestinal disturbances are referred to in Chapter 10.

Glycopyrronium § (dose 200–400 mg by injection)

Brand name: Robinul §

Glycopyrronium is a synthetic antimuscarinic agent used like atropine in premedication to reduce salivary secretions. It is given by intramuscular or intravenous injection in doses of 200–400 micrograms. It is also used together with neostigmine as Robinul–Neostigmine to reverse the effects of the non-depolarizing muscle relaxants such as atracurium (p. 244).

PARKINSON'S DISEASE

Originally described in 1817 as the 'shaking palsy', Parkinson's disease, or primary parkinsonism, is a progressive neurodegenerative disease affecting approximately 1% of the population over 50 years of age. It is characterized by the cardinal signs of tremor at rest, bradykinesia, muscle rigidity and postural instability, which ultimately lead to functional disability. The underlying cause is unknown, but the symptoms result from degeneration of the dopaminergic cells within the substantia nigra, leading to deficiency of dopamine in the brain. Secondary parkinsonism may result from injury to the basal ganglia by cerebrovascular disease or infection, or it may be drug-induced as some drugs have an adverse effect on dopamine levels by blocking dopamine receptors or reducing dopamine stores.

The mainstay of pharmacological management of Parkinson's disease is dopamine replacement, with anticholinergic drugs as secondary treatment. Dopamine itself does not cross the blood–brain barrier, but the precursor levodopa enters the CNS and undergoes enzymatic conversion by dopa decarboxylase, to dopamine. However, that enzyme is also present in the periphery and almost 99% of the dose of levodopa is metabolized before it can reach the brain. It is therefore necessary to give larger doses of levodopa to achieve an effective CNS level, with a subsequent increase in side-effects. Carbidopa (a decarboxylase inhibitor) is used to inhibit the enzyme in the peripheral tissues, which in part overcomes the problem.

Treatment with levodopa is palliative, not curative, and does not prevent the slow degenerative nature of the disease, and patients should be warned accordingly. More than 10% of patients fail to respond to treatment with levodopa and with long-term use another 25% experience secondary failure. Dyskinesias, wearing off of dose, abrupt changes in response – the so-called 'on–off' phenomenon – and loss of efficacy has fuelled the search for alternative treatment.

Anticholinergic drugs ameliorate the symptoms of Parkinson's disease by rectifying the imbalance between dopamine and acetylcholine in the striatum, and were the first drugs used to treat the condition. They relieve tremor and salivation, but have little effect on more disabling symptoms such as rigidity or bradykinesia. (They are preferred for drug-induced and postencephalitic parkinsonism.) Treatment should be commenced with, and increased by, small doses as they may cause confusion, particularly in elderly patients, and may precipitate glaucoma and urinary retention.

Other drugs used in Parkinson's disease are dopamine agonists; amantadine is a less potent drug with fewer side-effects.

DOPAMINERGIC AND OTHER DRUGS USED IN PARKINSONISM

Levodopa § (dose: 125–250 mg daily)

In primary parkinsonism levodopa is given by initial doses of 125–250 mg daily in divided doses after food, followed by increasing doses at intervals of 2–4 days according to the response. It is usually given with a dopa-decarboxylase inhibitor such as benserazide or carbidopa, as combined treatment reduces the peripheral and hepatic metabolism of levodopa, so a larger part of a dose reaches the brain for local conversion to dopamine. It also promotes a smoother response with fewer side-effects. Long-term treatment is necessary with doses that provide an adequate response with an acceptable incidence of side-effects.

Some patients do not respond to levodopa therapy, and with those that respond there may be sudden variations in response as treatment is continued, the so-called 'on–off' response, with a reduction in mobility which may last from 2–4 hours. The mechanism of these variations is not clear, and although it may be related to blood levels of levodopa, adjustment of dose frequency has little effect. With extended treatment over some years, the response to levodopa may become less satisfactory, and may be linked with an altered receptor sensitivity as well as with the progressive nature of the disease.

Side-effects of levodopa are numerous. Nausea and anorexia are common, and cardiovascular responses such as postural hypotension, faintness and dizziness may occur, as may flushing, palpitations and sweating.

With longer treatment, agitation, aggression, hallucinations and other psychiatric disturbances may occur. Involuntary movements are common at the optimum dose levels. The urine and other body fluids may be discoloured during levodopa therapy but such changes are of no significance.

Levodopa is contra-indicated in severe psychiatric disturbances, and in closed-angle glaucoma.

Combined products already referred to are Sinemet and Sinemet Plus, containing levodopa 100 mg with carbidopa 10 and 25 mg, respectively (co-careldopa). Madopar 62.5 contains levodopa 50 mg with benserazide 12.5 mg; Madopar 125 and Madopar 250 contain 100 and 200 mg of levodopa with benserazide 25 mg and 50 mg, respectively (co-beneldopa).

Amantadine § (dose: 100–200 mg daily)

Brand name: Symmetrel §
Amantadine is used in less severe parkinsonism, as it improves the hypokinesia and rigidity of parkinsonism, and also the tremor to some extent, but tolerance may occur and not all patients respond well to amantadine. It is given in doses of 100 mg daily, later increased to 100 mg twice a day (the second dose not later than 4 p.m.), often in association with anticholinergic therapy. Larger doses may cause confusion. Amantadine is not suitable for the treatment of drug-induced parkinsonism.

Side-effects include insomnia, nausea, skin discolouration and occasional oedema. Treatment should not be stopped abruptly.

Bromocriptine § (dose: 10–80 mg daily)

Brand name: Parlodel §
Bromocriptine is a dopamine receptor agonist, and acts by stimulating the surviving dopamine receptors. It is mainly used for patients who cannot tolerate adequate doses of levodopa, and is given in initial doses of 1–1.25 mg with food at night for 3–7 days, slowly increased at weekly intervals up to 40 mg or more daily, as three divided doses, with food. Combined therapy with levodopa is sometimes used, but careful balancing of doses is required, as confusion and abnormal movements may occur with such treatment.

Side-effects of bromocriptine are numerous, and include nausea, headache, postural hypotension, drowsiness and confusion. Tolerance may be reduced by alcohol. With higher doses, hallucinations and other psychiatric disturbances may occur, and pleural effusions have been reported.

Lysuride § (dose: 200 micrograms–5 mg daily)

Brand name: Revanil §

Lysuride, like bromocriptine, is a dopamine agonist and has a similar stimulating effect on dopamine receptors. In Parkinson's disease it is given initially in doses of 200 micrograms, with food, at night, followed by weekly increments of 200 micrograms according to response up to a maximum dose of 5 mg. Lysuride may also be given in association with levodopa.

Side-effects include initial hypotension, of which patients should be warned, dizziness, drowsiness, nausea, malaise and psychotic disturbances.

Pergolide § (dose: 50 micrograms–3 mg daily)

Brand name: Celance §

Pergolide resembles both bromocriptine and lysuride in being a dopamine agonist, but differs in having a longer action. It is used mainly as a supplement to levodopa therapy and is given in doses of 50 micrograms daily initially, increased at intervals of 3 days by increments of 250 micrograms up to a maintenance divided dose of 3 mg daily.

Side-effects are similar to those of bromocriptine, and patients should be warned that hypotensive side-effects may be disturbing during the initial days of treatment. Abrupt withdrawal may precipitate hallucinations.

Ropinirole § (dose; 1.5–9 mg daily)

Brand name: Requip §

Ropinirole has a more selective action than related drugs as it is a dopamine D_2-receptor agonist. It is used alone in primary parkinsonism, or as adjunctive therapy to control 'on–off' symptoms, when it may permit up to a 20% reduction in the dose of levodopa. It is given initially in doses of 750 micrograms three times a day, slowly increased over four weeks to maintenance doses of 3–9 mg daily. The **side-effects** are similar to those of bromocriptine.

Selegiline § (dose: 5–10 mg daily)

Brand name: Eldepryl §

Selegiline is an inhibitor of monoamine oxidase-B, and has a selective action in preventing the enzymatic breakdown of levodopa. It is used mainly in association with levodopa in the more severe forms of parkinsonism, as combined therapy may permit a reduction of dose and a smoother response.

Selegiline is given in morning doses of 5 mg, increased if necessary to 10 mg, but a reduction in the associated dose of levodopa by up to 50% may be necessary to prevent an increase in levodopa-linked side-effects. In the elderly, initial doses of 2.5 mg daily should be given. The normal first-pass loss of selegiline given orally can be reduced by the use of freeze-dried tablets (Zelepar §), containing 1.25 mg of selegiline, to be placed on the tongue for rapid absorption.

Unlike conventional monoamine oxidases used in the treatment of depression, selegiline does not cause the so-called 'cheese reaction' or episodes of hypertension.

Side-effects include nausea, hypotension, confusion and agitation.

Apomorphine § (dose: 3–30 mg daily by injection)

Brand name: Britaject §

Apomorphine has a wider range of action than ropinirole, as it stimulates both dopamine D_1 and D_2-receptors, but its emetic properties limit its use in parkinsonism. That disadvantage can be reduced by premedication with domperidone (p. 154), and apomorphine is sometimes used to treat symptoms not controlled by other drugs. It is given by subcutaneous injection or continuous subcutaneous infusion in doses of 3–30 mg daily under close hospital control. It requires well-motivated patients to cooperate with such treatment.

ANTIMUSCARINIC (ANTICHOLINERGIC) DRUGS USED IN PARKINSONISM

In parkinsonism these drugs differ from dopamine-replacement drugs by reducing the central cholinergic activity, and so restore in part the loss of balance between the cholinergic and dopaminergic systems.

Benzhexol § (dose: 2–15 mg daily)

Brand names: Artane §, Broflex §

Benzhexol relieves the muscular rigidity more than the tremor of parkinsonism, but it has little influence on dyskinesia. It is given in doses of 1–2 mg daily initially, slowly increased by incremental doses of 2 mg until 6–15 mg are given daily in divided doses. Patients with postencephalitic parkinsonism tend to require and tolerate larger doses, whereas reduced doses should be given to elderly patients. Combined therapy with levodopa may evoke a better response, and in some cases permit a reduction in the dose of benzhexol, but any change of dose should be carried out slowly. Benzhexol is also used in the treatment of drug-induced parkinsonism, but it should not be used for the tardive dyskinesia associated with long-term antipsychotic therapy, as it may exacerbate the symptoms.

Side-effects of benzhexol are those common to the anticholinergic drugs, and include dryness of the mouth, visual disturbances, occasional tachycardia and confusion. Benzhexol may sometimes cause severe mental disturbances, requiring withdrawal of the drug if adjustment of dose is ineffective.

Benztropine § (dose: 500 micrograms–6 mg daily)

Brand name: Cogentin §

Benztropine is mainly effective in controlling the tremor and rigidity of parkinsonism, and the muscle relaxation thus obtained reduces the discomfort and restlessness at night. It differs from benzhexol in having a sedative action in normal doses, and may be more suitable for elderly patients. Benztropine is also useful in controlling the symptoms of drug-induced parkinsonism. The initial dose is 500 micrograms–1 mg daily, increased very slowly to a maximum of 6 mg daily according to response. In conditions where a prompt action is required, benztropine may be given by intramuscular or intravenous injection in doses of 1–2 mg, repeated according to need. The **side-effects** are similar to those of benzhexol.

Related drugs used in parkinsonism are listed in Table 6.3.

Table 6.3 Anticholinergic drugs for parkinsonism

Approved name	Brand name	Daily dose range
benzhexol	Artane, Broflex	2–15 mg
benztropine	Cogentin	0.5–6 mg
biperiden	Akineton	2–6 mg
orphenadrine	Biorphen, Disipal	150–400 mg
procyclidine	Arpicolin, Kemadrin	7.5–30 mg

Nursing points about drugs used in parkinsonism

(a) Two main types – dopaminergics and antimuscarinics/anticholinergics.
(b) Antimuscarinics are useful initially in patients with mild symptoms; they relieve tremor more than rigidity.
(c) Dopaminergics are basically replacement therapy: value in later stages limited by fluctuations in response – the 'on – off' effect.
(d) Some other drugs act by stimulating surviving dopamine receptors.

DRUG-INDUCED PARKINSONISM

It should be noted that some powerful neuroleptics such as chlorpromazine and related drugs, that function as dopamine-antagonists, may cause extrapyramidal side-effects resembling the symptoms of parkinsonism. Such symptoms may also occur with metoclopramide, particularly in children and young adults. Such **side-effects** can be reduced by the use of one of the antimuscarinic agents used in the treatment of parkinsonism, such as procyclidine, but they should not be used prophylactically as they may cause tardive dyskinesia.

FURTHER READING

Cutson T, Laub K C, Schenkman M 1995 Pharmacological and nonpharmacological interventions in the treatment of Parkinson's disease. Physical Therapy 75:363–373

Fisher M 1995 Treatment of acute anaphylaxis. British Medical Journal 311:731–733

Hodges L C, Rapp C G 1990 New drugs for Parkinson's disease. Journal of Neuroscience Nursing 22(4):254–257

Lusis S A 1997 Pathophysiology and management of idiopathic Parkinson's disease. Journal of Neuroscience Nursing 29(1):24–31

Vernon G M 1989 Parkinson's disease. Journal of Neuroscience Nursing 21(5):273–284

7

Cardiovascular drugs and blood-lipid lowering agents

CARDIOVASCULAR THERAPEUTICS

For people in the industrial world, dysfunction of the cardiovascular system is a major cause of morbidity and so is an important target for drug therapy. The cardiovascular system is a closed circuit, in which blood is supplied to the body tissues, providing oxygen and nutrients and removing waste products. The driving force of the system is the heart, which is a double-sided four-chambered pump with one-way valves. The right side of the heart supplies the pulmonary circulation and the left side the systemic circulation. The heart is a remarkably efficient organ, as during a normal lifetime it may beat over 2500 million times, and in health it can cope with any physiological demands that may be made on it. Its efficiency depends on several factors, including the oxygen supply, the rate and strength of the cardiac muscle contractions, as well as on the speed of conduction of the contractile impulses. In addition cardiac efficiency is also linked with the pressure of the blood entering the heart (pre-load) as well as on that leaving it (after-load).

Heart failure occurs when the cardiac output fails to cope with the physiological demands of the tissues and may be due to:

- coronary artery narrowing so that the heart muscle does not get sufficient oxygen to function fully, usually as a result of atherosclerosis.
- valvular disease, either mitral stenosis when the mitral (bicuspid) valves do not open fully, and so obstruct the flow of blood to the left ventricle, or aortic incompetence when the valves do not close properly, and so allow the blood to leak back into the left ventricle. Both conditions lead to a decrease in cardiac output.
- hypertension, which is usually the result of atherosclerosis or to an excess production of

renin in renal disease. Both cause narrowing of the blood vessels, so the heart has to work harder to pump the blood through the constricted vessels.

- chronic obstructive airways disease, which reduces the ability of the heart to maintain the pulmonary circulation.

In the early stages of heart failure, natural compensatory mechanisms come into play that increase the heart rate and maintain the blood pressure, and the decreasing efficiency of the heart may only manifest itself during exercise and stress. If the heart continues to fail, blood begins to accumulate in the vessels, thus increasing the cardiac pre-load. The increased pressure in the venous circulation affects the capillaries, so more fluid leaks into the tissues than is reabsorbed, and so causes oedema. The oedema may be made worse because kidney efficiency also declines and sodium ions may not be secreted at a rate high enough to maintain an adequate fluid excretion. Eventually the classic symptoms of heart failure, oedema, congestion and cyanosis, develop.

Treatment is aimed at breaking at some point the vicious circle of cardiac weakness – oedema – congestion – reduced renal efficiency – further cardiac weakness, mainly by drugs that stimulate the heart to contract more powerfully, and by diuretics that promote the excretion of fluid and so relieve the oedema, congestion and pre-load. Further support can be provided by drugs that lower the blood pressure, reducing the pre- and after-load on the weakening heart, and when necessary by oxygen to relieve the cyanosis (Fig. 7.1). The use of diuretics in the treatment of heart failure is referred to on p. 161.

CARDIOACTIVE DRUGS

The oldest cardiac stimulant is digitalis, obtained from the leaf of the common foxglove. It was first introduced for the treatment of congestive heart failure by William Withering in 1785, and is still in use as digoxin, the active glycoside, but obtained in greater quantity from the Austrian foxglove. The mode of action of digoxin is a complex one, but it owes its positive inotropic effects to the inhibition of the enzyme-mediated sarcolemmal sodium pump system, also referred to as Na^+/K^+-ATPase. That membrane-bound enzyme converts adenosine triphosphate (ATP) to adenosine diphosphate (ADP) and uses the released energy to move sodium and potassium ions against their concentration gradients through their respective channels in the cardiac cell membrane. The result is that sodium ions are pumped out of the cardiac cells in exchange for potassium ions. When the pump system is inhibited by digoxin, there is a consequent increase in the concentration

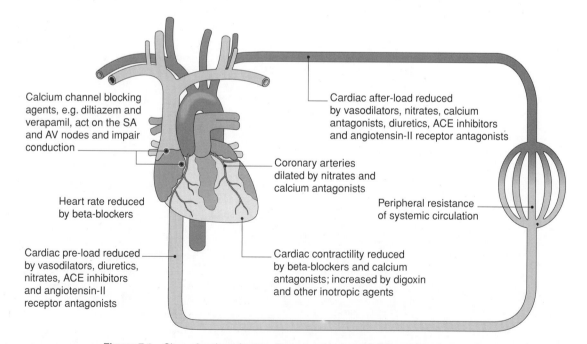

Calcium channel blocking agents, e.g. diltiazem and verapamil, act on the SA and AV nodes and impair conduction

Heart rate reduced by beta-blockers

Cardiac pre-load reduced by vasodilators, diuretics, nitrates, ACE inhibitors and angiotensin-II receptor antagonists

Coronary arteries dilated by nitrates and calcium antagonists

Cardiac contractility reduced by beta-blockers and calcium antagonists; increased by digoxin and other inotropic agents

Cardiac after-load reduced by vasodilators, nitrates, calcium antagonists, diuretics, ACE inhibitors and angiotensin-II receptor antagonists

Peripheral resistance of systemic circulation

Figure 7.1 Sites of action of some drugs used in heart failure and angina.

of intracellular sodium ions, which in turn inhibits the extrusion of calcium ions by the Na^+/Ca^{2+} ion exchanger. The resulting increase in the intracellular calcium ions affects the myocardial contractile fibres and increases their contractile force (Fig. 7.2).

Digoxin §

Digoxin is used in the treatment of congestive heart failure, especially in patients with atrial fibrillation and a high ventricular rate. It improves cardiac efficiency and brings about a general improvement in the circulation. With that improvement, blood flow through the kidneys is increased, and so digoxin has an indirect diuretic action that also helps to relieve oedema and congestion.

Digoxin is well absorbed when given orally, although excretion is slow, and the dose varies according to the severity of the heart failure, and whether rapid digitalization is required. In mild conditions, digoxin is given in doses of 125–250 micrograms twice a day initially, the lower dose being preferred for elderly patients. After about 7 days, the dose should be adjusted to need and response, as the maintenance dose, which may be as low as 62.5 micrograms twice daily, is largely dependent on the rate of elimination of the drug in the urine. For more serious conditions, or when rapid digitalization is desired, a loading dose of 1–1.5 mg may be given as divided doses over 24 hours. When a particularly rapid response is required, digoxin may be given by slow intravenous injection as a single dose of 0.5–1 mg, which produces an effect on the heart rate within 10 minutes. A second injection of 0.5 mg may be given later if required, and then followed by standard oral maintenance doses.

Elderly patients require smaller doses of digoxin, partly because of the increased sensitivity of the myocardium to digoxin in such patients, and partly because of a decrease in the renal elimination of the drug. Children, on the other hand, tolerate relatively large doses of digoxin, and to permit easy adjustment of dose for these two groups of patients, tablets containing 62.5 micrograms of digoxin are available as Lanoxin PG § (paediatric–geriatric). These tablets must be distinguished from the standard tablets which contain 250 micrograms of digoxin and are also available under the brand name Lanoxin §.

Side-effects The margin between the therapeutic and toxic doses of digoxin is small, and side-effects are relatively common; as a precaution, the heart rate should not be allowed to fall below 60 beats/minute. Nausea, vomiting and anorexia are early symptoms of digoxin overdose, as are abdominal pain and diar-

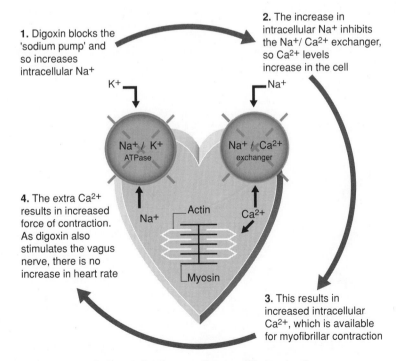

1. Digoxin blocks the 'sodium pump' and so increases intracellular Na^+

2. The increase in intracellular Na^+ inhibits the Na^+/Ca^{2+} exchanger, so Ca^{2+} levels increase in the cell

K^+

Na^+

Na^+/K^+ ATPase

Na^+/Ca^{2+} exchanger

4. The extra Ca^{2+} results in increased force of contraction. As digoxin also stimulates the vagus nerve, there is no increase in heart rate

Na^+

Actin

Ca^{2+}

Myosin

3. This results in increased intracellular Ca^{2+}, which is available for myofibrillar contraction

Figure 7.2 Action of digoxin on a diagrammatic heart cell.

rhoea. Central toxic effects include headache, drowsiness, confusion, hallucinations and visual disturbances such as blurred and coloured vision.

More serious side-effects include disturbances of cardiac rhythm such as bradycardia, atrioventricular block and ventricular extrasystoles which are similar to the symptoms of the cardiac disease under treatment. It can be difficult at times to tell whether a patient is being overdosed or under-dosed with digoxin, so determinations of the plasma level of digoxin should be carried out if overdose is suspected. Toxicity is likely with plasma concentrations greater than 2 nanograms/ml, but marked individual variations may occur.

Hypokalaemia, which may follow the prolonged use of certain diuretics, is also associated with chronic digoxin toxicity, whereas hyperkalaemia occurs in acute overdose. Treatment is the immediate withdrawal of the drug and correction of the potassium imbalance, but in very serious overdose, with life-threatening disturbances of cardiac rhythm and conduction, the toxicity can be rapidly reversed by the use of a specific digoxin antidote (Digibind).

Digibind § is a sheep-derived, digoxin-specific antibody preparation suitable for intravenous injection, and it acts by attracting digoxin away from its receptor sites in the myocardium and binding it as an inert digoxin–antibody complex in the extracellular fluid. The complex is rapidly excreted in the urine, and the symptoms of digoxin toxicity begin to subside within an hour or even less. The dose of Digibind depends on the body load of digoxin, and it is considered that 40 mg of the antidote can detoxify about 600 micrograms of digoxin. Close cardiac control is essential during the use of Digibind, together with monitoring of the serum potassium levels, as symptoms of the original cardiac disease may return as the excess digoxin is mobilized and excreted.

Nursing points about digoxin

(a) Starting dose in mild heart failure 125–250 micrograms twice a day (loading dose not required).
(b) Maintenance dose often once a day.
(c) For rapid digitalization in severe heart failure 0.75–1 mg by intravenous infusion over 2 hours.
(d) Intramuscular injection is painful and not recommended.
(e) Nausea, vomiting and visual disturbances indicate reduction of dose.
(f) Specific antidote is Digibind.
(g) Do not give digoxin if the pulse rate is below 60.

Certain other digitalis glycosides, including *digitoxin*, are occasionally useful as alternatives to digoxin. Digitoxin is extensively bound to plasma proteins, and as enterohepatic reabsorption occurs, it has a long action. The maintenance dose varies from 50 to 200 micrograms daily.

Sympathomimetic drugs which have an inotropic action and increase the force of the heart beat are referred to on p. 90. See also angiotensin-converting enzyme inhibitors (p. 115) and angiotensin-II receptor antagonists (p. 118).

Enoximone § (dose: up to 24 mg/kg daily)

Brand name: Perfan §

Enoximone differs from the cardiac glycosides as it is a synthetic inhibitor of phosphodiesterase, an enzyme that plays an important part in the metabolism of the messenger substance, cyclic AMP. It has a selective action on phosphodiesterase in the myocardium, which leads to a reduced breakdown of cyclic AMP and a rise in intracellular calcium.

Enoximone is used under close control in the treatment of congestive heart failure not responding to other therapy, as it has an inotropic action on the heart, and its vasodilator action also reduces the cardiac workload. It is given by intravenous infusion in doses of 90 micrograms/kg/minute initially, with subsequent supportive doses of 5–20 micrograms/kg/minute up to a total dose if required of 24 mg/kg over 24 hours. It is also given by slow intravenous injection as an initial dose of 0.5–1 mg/kg, followed by 0.5 mg/kg every 30 minutes according to response, up to a maximum of 3 mg/kg.

Side-effects are hypotension, anginal pain, headache and occasional arrhythmias.

Milrinone § (dose: up to 1.13 mg/kg daily)

Brand name: Primacor §

Milrinone resembles enoximone and has similar actions, uses and side-effects. It is used for the short-term treatment of severe congestive heart failure that does not respond to standard therapy. It is given initially by slow intravenous injection over 10 minutes in doses of 50 micrograms/kg, followed by doses of 375–750 nanograms/kg/minute by intravenous infusion, up to a maximum daily dose of 1.13 mg/kg. Treatment may be required for 48–72 hours. It should not be used immediately after myocardial infarction.

Xamoterol § (dose: 400 mg daily)

Brand name: Corwin §

Xamoterol is referred to here as it is used in the treatment of *mild* chronic heart failure in which breathlessness and fatigue are induced by exercise. It is a partial β_1-adrenoceptor agonist that improves myocardial contractility, and reduces the cardiac workload by lowering left ventricular pressure. Xamoterol is given in doses of 200 mg twice daily, and symptoms are said to improve steadily over some weeks. Half-doses should be given in renal impairment. Xamoterol should be withdrawn if the heart failure worsens.

Side-effects include gastro-intestinal disturbances, dizziness and headache. It is contra-indicated in severe heart failure, and caution is necessary in arrhythmias and obstructive airways disease.

DISTURBANCES OF CARDIAC RHYTHM

Cardiac arrhythmias are linked with abnormalities in the conducting system of the heart. The rhythm of the heart is controlled by the sino-atrial node (SA) or pacemaker, which is situated at the junction of the right atrium with the superior vena cava. From the SA node a wave of excitation is conducted across the walls of the atria that causes them to contract. The atrioventricular node (AV) relays the wave of excitation to the Bundle of His and the Purkinje fibres and then to the walls of the ventricles, which in turn contract and pump blood into the aorta and pulmonary artery. After contraction, the heart relaxes and refills with blood for the next contraction.

This cardiac cycle is dependent on the movement of sodium, potassium and calcium ions in and out of cardiac muscle cells. At rest these cells are negatively charged, and the contractile impulse brings about a rapid depolarization (loss of charge) as positively charged sodium ions enter the cell (Phase 0). A refractory period follows during which calcium ions move into the cell, and at that stage the muscle cells will not respond to further stimulation (Phases 1–2). A period of rapid initial repolarization sets in, during which potassium ions flow out of the cell (Phase 3), which goes on to the final stage of repolarization (Phase 4). Sodium ions pass out and potassium ions pass into the cell, which then becomes able to respond to a contractile impulse.

Any disturbance of the cardiac cycle may give rise to arrhythmias, and some precipitating factors are ischaemia with resulting electrolyte and pH abnormalities, excessive myocardial-cell stretch, and exposure to toxins. Disorders of impulse conduction result when the sinus node fails to activate the atria (sino-atrial block), or when there is some defect in conduction of the impulses from the atria to the ventricles (atrioventricular heart block) or to the right or left branches of the Bundle of His (bundle branch block).

In atrial fibrillation and flutter, digoxin is often used to control the heart rate, but in other disturbances of cardiac rhythm a variety of drugs is used, some of which differ widely in their mode of action. They can be classified as in Table 7.1.

Table 7.1 Drugs used to control disturbances of cardiac rhythm

Class	Action	Examples
Class I	These have a cell membrane stabilizing action which may be mediated either by blocking the fast inward current of sodium ions and so reducing the rate of rapid depolarization (phase 0), or by reducing the conduction rate in cardiac cells	quinidine, procainamide, local anaesthetics of the lignocaine type, disopyramide, phenytoin
Class II	These indirectly reduce the activity of the central nervous system on the myocardium by beta-receptor blockade	propranolol
Class III	These act by extending the refractory period of phase 2 and extend the action potential	amiodarone
Class IV	These have a selective action in blocking the movement of calcium ions in the SA and AV nodes	verapamil

Adenosine § (dose: 3–12 mg by intravenous injection)

Brand name: Adenocor §

Adenosine is a natural nucleotide that takes part in many biological processes. It is used therapeutically for the control of paroxysmal supraventricular tachycardia, as it restores sinus rhythm by slowing down conduction through the atrioventricular node, but its use requires careful monitoring. Adenosine is given initially as a dose of 3 mg by rapid intravenous injection, followed if necessary after 1–2 minutes by a further dose of 6 mg. An additional dose of 12 mg may be required.

Side-effects include bronchospasm, severe bradycardia and flushing, but they are usually transient, as adenosine has a very short plasma half-life. It is contra-indicated in second–third degree heart block.

Amiodarone § (dose: 600 mg daily)

Brand name: Cordarone X §

Amiodarone is a class III anti-arrhythmic drug that acts mainly by extending the refractory period of the contractile fibres of both atria and ventricles. It is used only in arrhythmias that are resistant to other drugs. It is of particular value in the Wolff–Parkinson–White (WPW) syndrome, a resistant re-entry supraventricular tachycardia arising from a secondary AV pathway, as the extension of the refractory period may prevent the re-entry of such secondary impulses.

The oral dose of amiodarone is 200 mg three times a day for at least 1 week, as the initial response is slow, followed by maintenance doses of 200 mg daily or on alternate days. In severe conditions, amiodarone may be given by intravenous infusion over 30–120 minutes in doses of 5 mg/kg up to a maximum dose of 1.2 g in 24 hours under ECG control. It increases the response to digoxin and warfarin, and the doses of those drugs should be adjusted accordingly.

Side-effects are numerous and include photosensitivity with occasional skin discolouration (the use of a sunscreen product is recommended); benign corneal microdeposits, and pulmonary alveolitis. Nausea, vomiting and vertigo occur less frequently. Amiodarone is an iodine-containing drug, and it is contra-indicated in thyroid dysfunction, iodine sensitivity, sinus bradycardia and AV block.

Disopyramide § (dose: 300–800 mg daily)

Brand names: Dirythmin §, Rythmodan §

Disopyramide has the membrane-stabilizing action of quinidine (class I) but it also extends the refractory period (class III), and has some of the calcium-blocking activity of verapamil (class IV). It is used in ventricular arrhythmia and tachycardia, especially after myocardial infarction, and in the Wolff–Parkinson–White syndrome. It is also of value in paroxysmal atrial tachycardia, and in the maintenance of rhythm after electroconversion. A standard dose of disopyramide is 100–300 mg twice a day. When a rapid action is necessary, a dose of 2 mg/kg up to 150 mg may be given by *slow* intravenous injection under ECG control, followed by doses of 400 micrograms/kg/hour up to a maximum of 800 mg daily, before transfer to oral therapy.

Side-effects of disopyramide include hypotension, AV block and myocardial depression. It has some anticholinergic properties, and may cause dryness of the mouth. Care is necessary in glaucoma and disturbances of the urinary tract. It is contra-indicated in complete heart block and severe heart failure.

Flecainide § (dose: 200–400 mg daily)

Brand name: Tambocor §

Flecainide is a class I anti-arrhythmic agent of the lignocaine type, and is used mainly in the treatment of severe ventricular and supraventricular tachyarrhythmias and related conditions.

Flecainide is given orally in doses of 100–200 mg twice a day, reduced later according to response, with lower doses in elderly patients where the elimination rate is reduced. In acute conditions, flecainide is given by slow intravenous injection in doses of 2 mg/kg up to a maximum dose of 150 mg, followed by oral therapy as the condition improves. Reduced doses are necessary in cases of renal impairment.

Side-effects of flecainide include dizziness and blurring of vision, which are often transient, and nausea, although uncommon, may occasionally occur. Heart failure and AV block are contra-indications.

Lignocaine §

Brand name: Xylocard §

Lignocaine has a membrane-stabilizing action, and is a class I drug for the rapid control of ventricular tachycardia after an acute myocardial infarction. Treatment is commenced with a bolus dose of 50–100 mg by *slow* intravenous injection, repeated if necessary after 5 minutes, followed by decreasing doses of 4 mg–1 mg per minute as required. Response to lignocaine is linked with a drug plasma level of

1.5–5 micrograms/ml. Reduced doses should be given in hepatic disease and cardiac failure. Adequate plasma levels cannot be obtained by oral therapy as there is a high loss by first-pass liver metabolism.

Side-effects include nausea, vomiting, confusion and epileptiform convulsions. Lignocaine is contra-indicated in AV block and severe myocardial depression.

Mexiletine § (dose: 400 mg–1 g daily orally; 100–250 mg initially by injection)

Brand name: Mexitil §

Mexiletine is a class I drug with the actions of lignocaine, with the advantage of being active orally. It is used mainly to control ventricular arrhythmias following myocardial infarction, and is given by an initial dose of 400 mg, followed by doses of 200–250 mg three to four times a day. In acute conditions, mexiletine is given as a bolus dose of 100–250 mg by intravenous injection over 10 minutes, with ECG monitoring, followed by supportive doses of 500 micrograms/minute according to need. Effective plasma levels are in the range of 0.75–2 micrograms/ml.

Side-effects include hypotension, bradycardia, tremor, dizziness, diplopia, dysarthria and confusion. It is contra-indicated in heart block.

Moracizine § ▼

Brand name: Ethmozine § ▼

Moracizine has a class I-like type of membrane-stabilizing anti-arrhythmic activity and is used in the control of ventricular fibrillation/tachycardia. It is given in doses of 200–300 mg 8-hourly, subsequently adjusted at intervals of 3 days with additional doses of 50 mg 8-hourly for maintenance. In severe conditions, an initial dose of 400–500 mg may be given. In common with related drugs, with moracizine there is a risk of a drug-induced worsening of the arrhythmia.

Side-effects include headache, dizziness, palpitations and dyspnoea.

Phenytoin sodium §

Brand name: Epanutin §

Phenytoin is a class I drug, and has been used to control ventricular arrhythmias associated with digitalis toxicity. It is of little value in cardiac arrhythmias caused by acute or chronic heart disease. Dose by *slow* intravenous injection is 3.5–5 mg/kg, repeated

once if necessary after about 10 minutes. Phenytoin is now largely replaced by other drugs.

Side-effects are bradycardia, hypotension and confusion.

Procainamide § (dose: 1–1.5 g orally; up to 1 g by intravenous injection)

Brand name: Pronestyl §

Procainamide has the membrane-stabilizing (class I) action of quinidine, and also has some class III properties of extending the refractory period, with the advantage of being effective both orally and by injection in the control of ventricular arrhythmias. Procainamide is given orally in initial doses of 1 g, followed by doses of 250 mg 4–6-hourly for prophylaxis and maintenance, but for the control of acute arrhythmias it is given by slow intravenous injection under ECG monitoring in doses of 25–50 mg/minute up to a maximum of 1 g, although a dose over 500 mg is seldom required. A therapeutic response is correlated with a plasma level of 4–8 micrograms/ml. A sustained release preparation containing 500 mg of procainamide is Procainamide Durules.

Side-effects Procainamide may cause nausea, anorexia and diarrhoea, and other side-effects include fever, rash, pruritus and hypersensitivity reactions, as well as cardiac weakness. Prolonged treatment has led to the development of agranulocytosis and a syndrome resembling lupus erythematosus, requiring withdrawal of treatment.

Propafenone § (dose: 450–900 mg daily)

Brand name: Arythmol §

Propafenone is a class I anti-arrhythmic agent of the lignocaine type used in the prophylaxis and treatment of ventricular arrhythmias not responding to other drugs. It is extensively metabolized in the liver, response may be variable, and treatment should be initiated in hospital under ECG control. Propafenone is given orally in doses of 150 mg three times a day, increased at intervals of 3 days as required, up to a maximum of 900 mg daily. The tablets should be taken after food, with a drink, and swallowed whole.

Side-effects include nausea, vomiting, dizziness, blurred vision, bradycardia and other cardiac disturbances. Postural hypotension may occur in the elderly, who should be given smaller doses. It is contra-indicated in heart block and uncontrolled congestive heart failure, and should be avoided in patients with obstructive airways disease as it has some beta-blocking activity.

Nursing points about some anti-arrhythmic drugs

(a) Determine type of arrhythmia by ECG before treatment.
(b) Adenosine in paroxysmal supraventricular tachycardia.
(c) Verapamil is used in supraventricular arrhythmias (not in patients recently treated with beta-blockers).
(d) Propafenone and quinidine may be effective in both supraventricular and ventricular arrhythmias.
(e) Lignocaine and similar drugs in ventricular arrhythmias.
(f) Bretylium is used only in resuscitation.

Quinidine § (dose: 600 mg–1.6 g daily)

Quinidine is the old, original class I or membrane-stabilizing anti-arrhythmic agent. Although its use has declined as more potent drugs have been introduced, quinidine still has a limited place in the prevention of ventricular tachycardias not responding to other therapy. It is given in doses of 200–400 mg three or four times a day, after a test dose of 200 mg to detect any quinidine hypersensitivity. Quinidine may also be given in doses of 500 mg twice a day as a sustained release product (Kinidin §).

Side-effects include nausea and a dose-limiting diarrhoea. Sensitivity reactions, sometimes referred to as cinchonism, are tinnitus, visual disturbances, fever, vertigo and confusion, and may occur in hypersensitive patients after even small doses. It is contra-indicated in heart block.

Cumulative toxic effects of quinidine are ventricular tachycardia and fibrillation.

Quinidine brings about a marked increase in the plasma concentration of digoxin if both drugs are given together, requiring a reduction of digoxin dosage to avoid toxicity. Care is also necessary if combined treatment with amiodarone is given.

Tocainide § (dose: 600–2400 mg daily)

Brand name: Tonocard §
Tocainide is a class I drug chemically related to lignocaine, and with similar anti-arrhythmic properties. It has been used in the treatment of severe or life-threatening ventricular arrhythmias,

particularly those not responding to other therapy. In such acute conditions tocainide is given in doses of 400 mg three times a day or more, up to a maximum of 2.4 g daily, for a plasma level of 6–12 micrograms/ml.

Side-effects of tocainide are numerous and include gastrointestinal disturbances, tremor, dizziness, confusion, fibrosing alveolitis and agranulocytosis. Like procainamide, tocainide may cause a lupus-like syndrome.

Blood counts are essential during treatment. Care is necessary in renal and hepatic impairment.

Verapamil § (dose: 120–360 mg daily)

Brand names: Cordilox §, Securon §, Univer §
Verapamil is a class IV drug and influences the movement of calcium ions in myocardial cells and depresses conduction in the atrioventricular node. It is well absorbed orally, but considerable first-pass liver metabolism occurs. Verapamil is used mainly in the treatment of supraventricular arrhythmias and is given in doses of 40–120 mg, three times a day, but in paroxysmal tachycardias it may be given by slow intravenous injection in a dose of 5–10 mg, repeated if necessary after 5–10 minutes, and followed by oral therapy.

Side-effects are nausea, vomiting and constipation, but after intravenous injection myocardial depression, bradycardia and heart block may occur. Verapamil *should not* be given intravenously (and preferably not orally) to a patient receiving or recently treated with a beta-adrenoceptor blocking agent, as hypotension and asystole may result. Verapamil is contra-indicated in AV node disease, bradycardia and heart block. The use of verapamil as a calcium antagonist in angina is referred to on p. 120.

Bretylium tosylate § (dose: 5 mg/kg, by intramuscular injection)

Brand name: Bretylate §
Bretylium is a class II anti-arrhythmic drug that acts by displacing noradrenaline from storage sites. It is occasionally of value for resuscitation in resistant ventricular arrhythmias, and is given in doses of 5 mg/kg by intramuscular injection, repeated at intervals of 8 hours. Exceptionally, bretylium may be given by *slow* intravenous injection in doses of 5–10 mg/kg, repeated at intervals of 1–2 hours up to a total dose of 30 mg/kg, followed by intramuscular therapy.

Side-effects   include nausea, vomiting and severe hypotension, but noradrenaline and related pressor amines should not be used to restore the blood pressure.

DRUGS USED IN HYPERTENSION AND ANGINA

Blood pressure is the force per unit area exerted on the wall of a blood vessel by the blood it contains. It is affected by three main factors, namely cardiac output (equal to the product of heart rate and stroke volume), peripheral resistance (which is dependent on blood viscosity, vessel length and vessel diameter) and total blood volume. A change in any of these can result in a change of blood pressure.

Blood pressure is regulated in the short-term via the autonomic nervous system. Baroreceptors in the aortic arch and carotid vessels monitor the amount of 'stretch' of the vessel walls, and efferent nerves convey this information to the vasomotor and cardiac centres in the medulla. If the blood pressure falls the sympathetic nerves release noradrenaline which stimulates the alpha-receptors in the arterioles, leading to vasoconstriction. The beta-receptors in the heart are also activated, resulting in increased heart rate and contractile force of the myocardium. Conversely, if blood pressure rises the activity of the sympathetic nervous system decreases and parasympathetic activity increases, so that heart rate slows down, the blood vessels relax and the pressure falls. Other and more long-term factors involved in the regulation of the blood pressure include the renin–angiotensin system (p. 115) and the antidiuretic hormone.

In health, the cardiovascular system responds immediately to any physiological demands and the consequent changes in blood pressure are merely transient. In later life, however, peripheral resistance increases, due to pathological changes such as the narrowing of the diameter of the blood vessels by the formation of atheromatous plaques, and a gradual reduction in the elasticity of the blood vessel walls, all of which lead to a rise in blood pressure.

When the blood pressure is permanently raised, the condition is referred to as 'hypertension'. Sustained hypertension, which may be asymptomatic, causes cardiovascular disease, renal damage, myocardial infarction and stroke, and because of the close control over blood volume by the kidneys, renal damage may increase the hypertension. An elevated blood pressure can be lowered by decreasing peripheral resistance or reducing the cardiac output, and a wide range of drugs is now used in the treatment of hypertension. The aim of treatment, which is indicated in patients with an average diastolic pressure over 100 mmHg, is to reduce the blood pressure to a level consistent with the age and general condition of the patient, although benefit in patients over 80 years of age is unlikely.

The ideal drug would lower the elevated blood pressure slowly and evenly, without any disturbance of the electrolyte balance. In addition, it should not affect the controls that govern normal blood pressure changes, as too great or too sudden a reduction, especially in the elderly, could cause hypotension and an impairment of renal efficiency that might have serious consequences. Such an ideal drug still awaits discovery, and in practice reliance is placed on a range of drugs that act by different mechanisms. They include alpha- and beta-receptor blocking agents, sympathetic neurone blocking agents, centrally acting antihypertensive drugs, angiotensin-converting-enzyme inhibitors, angiotensin-II receptor antagonists, calcium channel blocking agents and diuretics (Chapter 11). Ganglion blocking agents are obsolete, but one survives as trimetaphan, which is used to obtain hypotension during surgery.

An associated condition is angina pectoris, the paroxysmal chest pain that occurs when the supply of oxygenated blood reaching the heart is insufficient to meet physiological requirements. The most common cause is atheromatous narrowing of the coronary arteries, although some forms of angina may be due to coronary spasm (Fig. 7.3). Angina is in effect a stress response to factors that increase cardiac output, such as exercise and emotion, and treatment is with drugs which reduce cardiac drive and oxygen demand. They have little or no effect on the coronary obstruction that is the basic cause of angina. Drugs in use include the nitrates, represented by glyceryl trinitrate, beta-blocking agents and calcium channel blocking agents.

BETA-ADRENOCEPTOR BLOCKING AGENTS

These drugs, often referred to simply as beta-blockers, prevent the access of catecholamines to the beta-adrenergic receptor sites in the heart, bronchi and other organs, and so indirectly inhibit the response to sympathetic stimulation. They protect the heart against excessive stimulation, whether induced by physical or emotional stress, and so

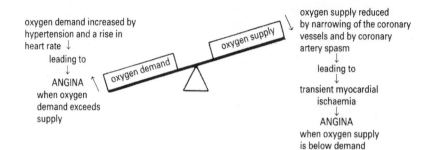

oxygen demand increased by
hypertension and a rise in
heart rate ↓

leading to
↓
ANGINA ↑
when oxygen
demand exceeds
supply

oxygen supply reduced
by narrowing of the coronary
vessels and by coronary
artery spasm
↓
leading to
↓
transient myocardial
ischaemia
↓
ANGINA
when oxygen supply
is below demand

Figure 7.3   Diagram of oxygen balance in angina.

reduce the oxygen requirements of the myocardium. They are widely used in the treatment of hypertension and angina, and are also useful in cardiac arrhythmias, myocardial infarction and thyrotoxicosis. They are also used occasionally in migraine, to allay anxiety, and locally in glaucoma (p. 250).

As a group, the beta-blockers have the same basic action, but they can be divided into two main groups, those that have a general action on the β_1 and β_2-receptors (Group 1) and those that have a more selective action on the β_2 receptors in the heart (Group 2). Some also have a membrane-stabilizing action (p. 105). Others, such as acebutolol, carteolol, oxprenolol and pindolol, have a degree of 'intrinsic

sympathomimetic activity' (ISA), which means that paradoxically they can to some extent stimulate as well as block some beta-receptors, and so function as partial agonists. In practice, beta-blockers with some ISA activity tend to cause less bradycardia. Table 7.2 indicates the range of currently available beta-blockers, of which a few are referred to individually.

In hypertension, combined treatment with a beta-blocker and a thiazide diuretic may increase the response and tend to reduce the hypokalaemia associated with such diuretics. Many combined products are now available, designed mainly to simplify therapy and improve patient compliance. They are useful once control of the hypertension has been achieved, but are not suitable for initial therapy.

Table 7.2   Beta-adrenoceptor blocking agents, some of which are available in slow-release form

Approved name	Brand name	Daily dose range	Type
propranolol	Inderal; Apsolol; Berkolol	40–320 mg	**Group I** $\beta_1 + \beta_2$ or non-cardioselective
betaxolol	Kerlone	20–40 mg	
carvedilol	Eucardic	12.5–50 mg	
nadolol	Corgard	40–240 mg	
oxprenolol	Trasicor; Apsolox	120–480 mg	
pindolol	Visken	7.5–45 mg	
sotalol	Beta-Cardone; Sotacor	160–480 mg	
timolol	Betim; Blocadren	15–60 mg	
acebutolol	Sectral	400–800 mg	**Group II** β_1 or cardioselective
atenolol	Tenormin	50–100 mg	
bisoprolol	Emcor; Monocor	10–20 mg	
celiprolol	Celectol	200–400 mg	
esmolol	Brevibloc	i.v. only	
metoprolol	Betaloc; Lopresor	100–200 mg	
labetalol	Trandate	200 mg–2.4 g	$\beta_1 + \beta_2$ and alpha-receptors

Nursing points about beta-blockers

(a) They all have same basic action, but some (atenolol, nadolol and sotalol) are not lipid-soluble and so are less likely to cause sleep disturbances.

(b) They all cause bradycardia and could precipitate incipient heart failure.

(c) They may bring about histamine release and cause bronchoconstriction.

(d) Patients should be warned about postural hypotension, particularly after sleep.

(e) Coldness in the extremities may occur as the result of the reduced peripheral blood flow.

(f) Treatment should not be stopped abruptly – advise patients not to run out of supplies.

(g) No beta-blocker should be given to a patient recently treated with verapamil.

Some **side-effects**, such as bradycardia, sleep disturbances, bronchoconstriction and reduced peripheral blood flow, are common to all beta-blockers in varying degrees. Sleep disturbances are less likely with atenolol, celiprolol, nadolol and solatol, as they are water-soluble and so do not enter the brain as readily as the lipid-soluble blockers. Bronchoconstriction, which can be severe, is more likely to occur when Group I drugs are used and great care is necessary in initial treatment of patients with a history of asthma. Care is also necessary in patients with cardiac failure and heart block, and the reduced blood flow associated with beta blockade may also influence renal and hepatic efficiency. By the nature of their action, the beta-blockers interact with a wide range of other drugs, which may increase the bradycardia, myocardial depression and other side-effects.

It is of interest that some beta-blockers such as atenolol, metoprolol, propranolol and timolol are used in the long-term secondary treatment of myocardial infarction, as early and prolonged treatment reduces the risk of reinfarction, and increases survival time.

The beta-blockers are also useful in preparing patients for thyroidectomy. If given for 4 days before operation, the clinical aspects of thyrotoxicosis can be temporarily reversed, and the gland becomes less vascular, thus facilitating surgery.

Propranolol § (dose: 40–320 mg daily)

Brand names: Inderal §, Apsolol §, Berkolol §
Propranolol was one of the first of the beta-adrenoceptor blocking agents. It inhibits the normal response to cardiac stimulation, and reduces the contractile force of the heart muscle. It is used in the control of angina, hypertension, thyrotoxicosis, cardiac arrhythmias of varied origin, and the prophylaxis of myocardial infarction and migraine.

Propranolol is given in angina in doses of 40 mg up to three times a day, increasing according to need up to 240 mg daily. In hypertension, it is given in initial doses of 80 mg twice a day, increased at weekly intervals according to response, with maintenance doses varying from 160 to 320 mg daily, often in association with a thiazide diuretic.

For prophylaxis after acute myocardial infarction, treatment is commenced within 1–3 weeks with doses of 40 mg four times a day for a few days, after which the drug is given in doses of 80 mg twice a day.

In arrhythmic emergencies, propranolol may be given by slow intravenous injection, in doses of 1 mg per minute, up to a maximum of 10 mg, preceded by an injection of atropine 1–2 mg to reduce the brady-cardial side-effects.

For migraine prophylaxis, propranolol may be given in doses of 40 mg or more three times a day, and in similar doses for the relief of tremor and palpitation associated with apprehension, stress and anxiety.

Side effects Although propranolol is generally well tolerated, side-effects include bronchospasm in susceptible patients, reduced peripheral blood flow and gastro-intestinal disturbances. In overdose, the bronchospasm may be severe, with bradycardia and hypotension. Propranolol is contra-indicated in asthma, heart failure and heart block, and is not suitable for the treatment of hypertensive emergencies. It should not be given to patients receiving verapamil.

Acebutolol § (dose: 400–800 mg daily)

Brand name: Sectral §
Acebutolol has the actions and uses of propranolol, but is more cardioselective. It also has some intrinsic sympathomimetic activity, and so is less likely to cause bradycardia. In angina and hypertension, acebutolol is given in initial doses of 200 mg twice daily, gradually increased according to need, but doses of more than 1 g daily are seldom necessary. The response to treatment is usually prompt.

Acebutolol has the **side-effects** and contra-indications of propranolol, and although it has less effect on the bronchial adrenoreceptors, it should be used with care in patients with obstructive airway disease. In common with related drugs, acebutolol should not be given to patients receiving intravenous verapamil, as asystole with hypotension may occur.

Atenolol § (dose: 50–100 mg daily)

Brand name: Tenormin §

Atenolol is a cardioselective beta-adrenoceptor blocking agent with an extended action. It is given in hypertension in single doses of 50–100 mg daily, but the full response may not occur until after 1 or 2 weeks. It is often given with a thiazide diuretic to increase the effect. In angina, 100 mg daily as a single or divided dose is adequate, as larger doses are seldom more effective.

Atenolol is also of value in cardiac arrhythmias, and is then given in oral doses of 50–100 mg daily, but in acute conditions it is given by slow intravenous injection in doses of 2.5 mg, repeated at intervals of 5 minutes up to four doses. It may also be given by intravenous infusion in doses of 150 micrograms/kg. Marked bradycardia may follow intravenous use, which can be relieved by the injection of atropine (600 micrograms) as required. Atenolol is also used in the initial acute stage of myocardial infarction as a dose of 5–10 mg by intravenous infusion, followed by supportive oral doses of 50 mg twice daily.

Like acebutolol, it is less likely to provoke bronchospasm, but it should be used with care in asthma and related conditions. It is contra-indicated in untreated heart failure and heart block.

Carvedilol § ▼ (dose: 12.5–50 mg daily)

Brand name: Eucardic § ▼

Carvedilol is a non-cardioselective beta-blocker that also has a vasodilator action mediated by a blockade of alpha-receptors. That dual action reduces peripheral resistance and also the heart-block induced by some beta-blockers. In the treatment of hypertension the initial dose is 12.5 mg daily, doubled after 2–3 days as a single daily dose. Further increases may be made at intervals of not less than 2 weeks up to 50 mg daily. The **side-effects** of carvedilol are those of the beta-blockers generally.

Esmolol § (dose: 50–200 micrograms/kg intravenously)

Brand name: Brevibloc §

Esmolol differs from other beta-blockers in having a very brief action. It has cardioselective properties, and is used in the short-term treatment of supraventricular arrhythmias and tachycardia, and in postoperative hypertension. It is given by intravenous infusion in doses of 50–200 micrograms/kg per minute, but the dosage must be carefully titrated according to individual need.

Labetalol § (dose: 200 mg–2.4 g daily)

Brand name: Trandate §

Labetalol differs from related drugs as it has the double action of blocking both alpha- and beta-adrenoceptors. Blockade of the alpha-adrenoceptors brings about a peripheral vasodilatation, with a fall in blood pressure and a reduction in peripheral resistance. The beta-blockers have little action on the peripheral circulation, as compensatory mechanisms come into play to offset any vasodilator response. With labetalol, the balance of alpha- and beta-blocking activity results in a smoother hypotensive response with fewer side-effects.

Labetalol is useful in hypertensive states generally, in the hypertension of pregnancy, after acute myocardial infarction and in hypertensive crisis. It is sometimes used for controlled hypotension in surgery. In labile hypertension it is given in initial doses of 100–200 mg twice daily with food, increased according to need. High doses are required only in severe conditions. It is not usually necessary to give combined treatment with diuretics. In acute conditions, labetalol can be given by slow intravenous injection in doses of 50 mg, repeated after 5 minutes up to a total dose of 200 mg, or by intravenous infusion in doses of 2 mg/minute up to a similar maximum. The bradycardia that may follow intravenous labetolol may be controlled by atropine in doses of 600 micrograms.

In the acute hypertension of pregnancy and after acute myocardial infarction, doses of 15–20 mg/hour by intravenous infusion may be given, increased according to need up to 120 mg/hour. In hypotensive surgery, doses of 10–20 mg are given by intravenous injection, with a second dose of 5–10 mg after 5 minutes if necessary.

Side-effects include dizziness and lethargy, and postural hypotension may occur after high initial doses. Care is necessary in heart block and asthmatic patients. Severe hepatocellular damage has occurred after labetolol treatment.

Oxprenolol § (dose: 120–480 mg daily)

Brand name: Trasicor §

Oxprenolol is a beta-adrenoceptor blocker of the propranolol type with similar actions and uses. It is given orally in doses of 40–160 mg or more three times a day, according to the condition, adjusted to individual needs and response. Oxprenolol may occasionally cause bronchospasm, and is contra-indicated in heart block.

ALPHA-ADRENOCEPTOR BLOCKING AGENTS

Noradrenaline raises the blood pressure by acting on the postsynaptic alpha-receptors on arterial smooth muscle. Some drugs act as antagonists at those sites, and so bring about a reduction in vascular smooth muscle tone, a lowering of the peripheral resistance and a reduction in blood pressure. They have little effect on skeletal muscles where the blood flow is controlled by beta-receptors. Alpha-adrenoceptor antagonists are of value in hypertensive crisis, and are also used with beta-blockers and diuretics to obtain a smoother response in hypertension. Some newer agents have a more selective action on prostatic and bladder smooth muscle and are used in the symptomatic treatment of benign prostatic hyperplasia (p. 167).

Nursing points about alpha-adrenoceptor blocking agents
(a) Warn patients about hypotension, particularly first-dose hypotension.
(b) Subsequent postural hypotension may be increased by hot baths, long standing and large meals.
(c) Advise patients to rest at any feeling or onset of faintness.

Doxazosin § (dose: 1–16 mg daily)

Brand name: Cardura §
Doxazosin has a more selective and longer action than prazosin (p. 113), and in hypertension it is given in doses of 1 mg initially, slowly increased after 1–2 weeks to 2 mg daily, and subsequently further increased according to need up to a maxi-mum of 16 mg daily. Combined treatment with a beta-blocker and a diuretic is common. Doxazosin may be given in standard doses to the elderly, and to patients with renal insufficiency.

Side-effects are headache, dizziness and postural hypotension.

Indoramin § (dose: 50–200 mg daily)

Brand name: Baratol §
Indoramin also has a more selective and extended

action on the α_1-adrenoreceptors, and lowers the blood pressure by reducing peripheral resistance. In mild hypertension indoramin may be given alone in doses of 25 mg twice a day initially, slowly increased at intervals of 2 weeks up to a maximum of 200 mg daily, usually in association with a beta-blocker and/or a diuretic. Any incipient heart failure should be controlled by digoxin and diuretics before indo-ramin treatment is commenced.

Side-effects include drowsiness, dizziness and dryness of the mouth. Care is necessary in epilepsy, parkinsonism, and hepatic and renal impairment.

Prazosin § (dose: 500 micrograms–20 mg daily)

Brand name: Hypovase §
Prazosin lowers peripheral resistance by dilatation of the arterioles, brought about by a blockade of the post-synaptic alpha-adrenoceptors. Unlike some other drugs, prazosin does not induce a reflex tachycardia and is unlikely to cause or exacerbate bronchospasm. It is used in the treatment of all types of hyper-tension, and is given in doses of 500 micrograms two or three times a day initially, slowly increased according to need up to 20 mg daily. The initial dose of prazosin may cause marked hypotension with loss of consciousness, so the first dose should be taken in the evening, and in bed.

Prazosin is also used in congestive heart failure in maintenance doses of 4–20 mg daily, and in Raynaud's disease lower maintenance doses of 1–2 mg twice a day may be effective. In severe conditions, it may be given in association with a beta-blocker or a diuretic, but dosage requires careful adjustment, and that of prazosin should be reduced by half to avoid an excessive response. It may be used in patients with impaired renal function, as prazosin has little effect on renal blood flow or glomerular filtration rate, even during long-term administration. The use of prazosin in prostatic hypertrophy is referred to on p. 167.

Side-effects are sedation, dizziness, hypotension and weakness. Nasal congestion, depression and palpitations have also been reported.

Terazocin § (dose: 1–10 mg daily)

Brand name: Hytrin §
Terazocin is an antihypertensive agent that produces peripheral vasodilatation by a selective blockade of postsynaptic α_1-adrenoceptors. It is used in mild to moderate hypertension, and is given initially as a

1 mg dose *at night*. That precaution is essential, as an acute hypotensive episode may follow the initial dose within 30–90 minutes, but recurrence is uncommon provided dose increases are kept low.

Subsequent doses may be slowly increased at weekly intervals up to 10 mg or more daily, but doses over 20 mg daily are unlikely to evoke an improved response. No adjustment in dose is necessary in the elderly or in renal impairment. Lower doses of terazocin may be given with a thiazide diuretic.

Side-effects are dizziness, light-headedness, peripheral oedema and postural hypotension.

ALPHA-ADRENOCEPTOR BLOCKING AGENTS AND PHAEOCHROMOCYTOMA

Phaeochromocytoma is a catechol-secreting tumour, usually found in the adrenal medulla, and causes marked hypertension and hypertensive crises. Treatment is with certain alpha-adrenoceptor blocking agents and metirosine.

Phenoxybenzamine § (dose: 10–20 mg initially)

Brand name: Dibenylene §
Phenoxybenzamine is an alpha-adrenoceptor blocking agent with an extended action that is used like phentolamine in the control of hypertensive episodes associated with phaeochromocytoma. It is given in doses of 10 mg initially, increased by 10 mg daily according to need, up to a total daily dose of 1–2 mg/kg (divided into two doses).

Side-effects include postural hypotension and dizziness. In some cases, the tumour may liberate both adrenaline and noradrenaline, and cause marked tachycardia and other arrhythmias, and combined treatment with a beta-adrenoceptor blocking agent such as propranolol may then be necessary to control such side-effects. There is some risk of contact sensitization with phenoxybenzamine, and care should be taken to avoid skin contact with the drug.

Phentolamine § (dose: 5–10 mg by intravenous injection)

Brand name: Rogitine §
Phentolamine is a short-acting alpha-receptor blocking agent used in the diagnosis of phaeochromocytoma and in the control of the associated hyper-

tensive crises. Such tumours release pressor amines such as adrenaline into the circulation, and bring about a rise in blood pressure that can be distinguished from essential hypertension by the intravenous injection of phentolamine. Phentolamine temporarily neutralizes the vasoconstrictor action of pressor amines, with a consequent fall in blood pressure which returns to the previous level within minutes, but in essential hypertension phentolamine causes no significant changes in the blood pressure.

Phentolamine is given in doses of 5–10 mg by intravenous injection, repeated as required, or by intravenous infusion of doses of 5–60 mg over 15–30 minutes according to need and response.

Side-effects include nausea, diarrhoea, tachycardia, hypotension and dizziness. Combined treatment with a beta-blocking agent may be necessary during surgical removal of the tumour.

Metirosine § (dose: 1–4 g daily)

Brand name: Demser §
Metirosine is not an alpha-receptor blocking agent, but is referred to here as it has an action similar to that of phenoxybenzamine. It acts indirectly by blocking the formation of noradrenaline and other catecholamines from tyrosine by inhibiting the enzyme tyrosine hydroxylase.

It is used in the treatment of phaeochromocytoma, as well as in the preoperative preparation of patients with that catecholamine-secreting tumour, but it is not suitable for the treatment of essential hypertension.

Metirosine is given in doses of 250 mg four times a day initially, increased if necessary up to 4 g daily according to laboratory reports of urinary catecholamine levels, which should fall by 50%. If required, combined treatment with phenoxybenzamine may be given.

Side-effects include sedation, diarrhoea and extrapyramidal symptoms. A fluid intake of at least 2 litres daily should be taken to avoid crystalluria.

ANGIOTENSIN-CONVERTING ENZYME INHIBITORS

The renin–angiotensin system is a highly important mechanism concerned with the maintenance of the arterial pressure and the salt and water balance. The kidneys monitor both the pressure in the afferent arterioles supplying the glomeruli and the osmolarity in the distant convoluted tubule of the nephrons. A fall in either the pressure or the osmolarity stimulates the juxtaglomerular cells to release the enzyme renin. Renin splits the plasma protein angiotensinogen and releases angiotensin I.

The next stage is the conversion of inactive angiotensin I to active angiotensin II by the angiotensin-converting enzyme (ACE). Angiotensin II is a powerful pressor agent and has a direct vasoconstrictor action on the smooth muscles of the arterioles and larger arteries, but has much less effect on the venous system. Angiotensin II also stimulates the adrenal cortex to release the hormone aldosterone, which in turn increases the reabsorption of sodium ions by the renal tubules. That reabsorption is accompanied by an increase in water reabsorption, which results in an increase in both blood volume and blood pressure. Hypertension is often associated with high renin plasma levels and consequently with high levels of angiotensin II, and the resulting salt and water retention by the kidneys and the increased peripheral resistance add to the cardiac load. The ideal drug would be a renin inhibitor, but until such a drug is discovered, reliance has to be placed on drugs that act at a later stage and inhibit the conversion of angiotensin I to angiotensin II, e.g. the ACE-inhibitors. More recently, some angiotensin-II receptor antagonists have been introduced, which have certain advantages over the ACE-inhibitors (Fig. 7.4).

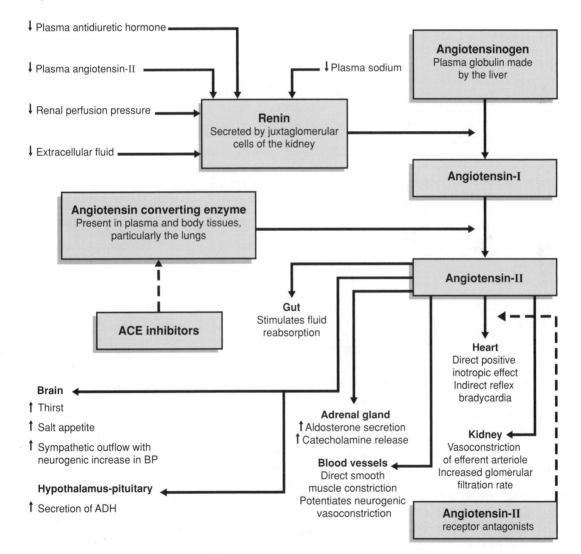

Figure 7.4 The renin–angiotensin system.

The ACE-inhibitors bring about arterial, and to a lesser degree venous, dilatation, reduce arterial tone and venous return, increase cardiac efficiency and improve the circulation. They are used in the early as well as the late and severe stages of heart failure, particularly when beta-blockers or diuretics are insufficient. They are also of value in hypertension and in myocardial infarction. Different ACE-inhibitors differ to some extent in their duration of action, and with some a single daily dose may evoke an adequate response.

The initial use of these drugs requires care, as with some patients there may be a rapid and marked first-dose fall in blood pressure. The risk can be reduced by a low initial dose of the ACE-inhibitor, and the previous withdrawal of any diuretic therapy for a few days. Patients should therefore be kept supine for an hour or two after the first dose, with frequent measurement of the blood pressure. Some ACE-inhibitors may cause renal impairment, so renal efficiency should be checked during treatment, as ACE-inhibitor-induced renal damage may become progressive. Combined use with a NSAID may increase that risk.

The ACE-inhibitors have **side-effects** that are common to some extent to all members of the group, and include headache, dizziness, oedema, fatigue, hypotension and occasional rash and pruritus. A delayed side-effect, often associated with extended treatment, is a persistent and non-productive cough, which may sometimes be severe enough to require withdrawal of the drug. (See angiotensin-II receptor antagonists, p. 118.) A symptom complex has been reported to occur with ACE-inhibitors, which may include fever, myalgia, raised ESR and skin reactions.

Nursing points about ACE-inhibitors

(a) Check renal function and electrolytes before starting and during treatment.
(b) First-dose hypotension may be marked.
(c) Reduce risk by withdrawing diuretic therapy for a few days, and giving a low first-dose at night with the patient in bed.
(d) Discontinue potassium-sparing diuretics or potassium supplements to avoid risk of hyperkalaemia.

Captopril § (dose: 25–150 mg daily)

Brand names: Acepril §, Capoten §
Captopril is used in the treatment of severe hypertension resistant to other therapy, in mild to moderate hypertension, often in association with thiazide diuretics and beta-blockers, and in congestive heart failure. In severe hypertension it is given in initial doses of 12.5 mg twice a day, 1 hour before food, together with a thiazide diuretic. Subsequent doses are slowly increased up to a maximum of 50 mg three times a day. In milder cases, a maintenance dose of 25 mg twice a day, supported by other therapy, is often sufficient. In severe heart failure, initial doses of 6.25–12.5 mg twice a day are given, increased if necessary up to 50 mg three times a day under close supervision. Lower doses are used in renal impairment, and for the elderly. (Capozide § contains captopril 25 mg and hydrochlorothiazide 12.5 mg.)

In all cases initial therapy requires care, as a marked hypotension may occur within an hour or two of the first dose, for which treatment should be immediately available. As a precaution, diuretic therapy should be withdrawn for a few days.

Side-effects include a pruritic rash which tends to disappear with continued treatment, loss of taste, cough and paraesthesia, but more serious side-effects are proteinuria, neutropenia and agranulocytosis. Urinary and blood tests are necessary during captopril treatment.

As captopril decreases aldosterone release, a rise in serum potassium may occur and potassium-sparing diuretics should be avoided (risk of hyperkalaemia), as is combined therapy with allopurinol and procainamide.

Cilazapril § (dose: 1–5 mg daily)

Brand name: Vascace §
Cilazapril has the actions and general uses of the ACE-inhibitors but differs by having a half-life that extends over 9 hours, so that single daily doses may be given. Diuretics should be withdrawn for 2–3 days before starting cilazapril. Initial doses of 0.5–1 mg daily are slowly increased to 2.5–5 mg daily according to response, and diuretic therapy can be reintroduced later if required. The **side-effects** are similar to those of other ACE-inhibitors, and care is necessary in congestive heart failure, ascites and aortic stenosis.

Enalapril § (dose: 5–40 mg daily)

Brand name: Innovace §
Enalapril is a pro-drug, and is slowly hydrolysed following oral administration to enalaprilat, which is the active metabolite. It has the angiotensin-converting-enzyme inhibitory action of captopril, but the effect is more powerful and prolonged. Enalapril is used in all types of essential hypertension, including

that not responding to other drugs, and in the supplementary treatment of congestive heart failure.

In hypertension, it is given in initial doses of 5 mg daily, increased up to a maximum of 40 mg daily. In the elderly, or when renal impairment is present, initial doses of 2.5 mg are used, and in such cases maintenance doses of 1–2 mg daily may be adequate. In congestive heart failure, initial doses of 2.5–5 mg are given in conjunction with digoxin and diuretics. (Innozide § contains enalapril 20 mg with hydrochlorothiazide 12.5 mg.)

Side-effects include hypotension, headache, dizziness, rash, nausea, diarrhoea and persistent cough. Renal function should be checked before and during treatment.

Fosinopril § (dose: 10–40 mg daily)

Brand name: Staril §
Fosinopril is an ACE-inhibitor used mainly in essential hypertension when other drugs are either ineffective or unsuitable. It is given in doses of 10 mg daily initially, rising to 20 mg daily or more to a maximum dose of 40 mg daily. Any diuretic treatment should be withdrawn some days before fosinopril is given and resumed only with care after 4 weeks if the blood pressure is not fully controlled.

Lisinopril § (dose: 2.5–40 mg daily)

Brand names: Carace §, Zestril §
Lisinopril is an analogue of enalapril, with similar actions, uses and side-effects. It has the advantage of a longer action that permits control of blood pressure by a single daily dose. Lisinopril is indicated in essential hypertension of varying severity, and as adjunctive treatment in congestive heart failure. It is given in initial doses of 2.5 mg daily, increased according to need to 10–20 mg daily, up to a maximum of 40 mg daily if required. In diuretic-treated patients, such therapy should be withdrawn for 2–3 days before commencing lisinopril dosage. As with all ACE-inhibitors, care is necessary in renal insufficiency and potassium-sparing diuretics should be avoided. (Carace 20 Plus § and Zestoretic 20 § contain lisinopril 20 mg with hydrochlorothiazide 12.5 mg.)

Moexipril ▼ (dose: 7.5–30 mg daily)

Brand name: Perdix § ▼
Moexepril is a long-acting ACE-inhibitor that is effective in single daily doses. The initial dose is 7.5 mg,

slowly rising to 15–30 mg once daily. If given with a calcium channel blocking agent, and in the elderly, it is given initially in a dose of 3.75 mg under supervision until the blood pressure is stabilized.

Perindopril § (dose: 2–8 mg daily)

Brand name: Coversyl §
Perindopril, like moexipril, is a long-acting ACE-inhibitor that is used for the control of essential hypertension not responding to other drugs. Current treatment with diuretics should be withdrawn 3 days before commencing with perindopril in doses of 2 mg daily before food. Subsequent doses can be increased according to response up to a maximum of 8 mg daily.

Side-effects include cough, headache and malaise.

Quinapril § (dose: 5–40 mg daily)

Brand name: Accupro §
Quinapril, like enalapril, is a pro-drug, and the active metabolite is quinaprilat. It has the actions of the ACE-inhibitors and is useful in all grades of hypertension when other therapy is ineffective or unsuitable because of side-effects. It is also used in congestive heart failure. In hypertension, quinapril is given as an initial dose 5–10 mg daily followed by maintenance doses of 20–40 mg daily. In congestive heart failure, an initial dose of 2.5 mg is given, with subsequent maintenance doses of 10–20 mg daily. (Accuretic § is a mixed product containing quinapril 10 mg with hydrochlorothiazide 12.5 mg.)

Side-effects of quinapril are similar to those of the ACE-inhibitors generally.

Ramipril § (Tritace §) is an ACE-inhibitor with similar actions and uses, given in doses of 1.25–5 mg once daily.

Trandolapril § (dose: 0.5–4 mg daily)

Brand names: Gopten §, Odrik §
Trandolapril is a pro-ACE-inhibitor, as it is hydrolysed in the body to a long-acting metabolite. It is used like other ACE-inhibitors in the treatment of mild to moderate hypertension. Treatment is commenced with doses of 500 micrograms daily, doubled at intervals of 2–4 weeks according to response up to 2–4 mg as a single daily dose for maintenance. Any diuretic therapy should be withdrawn initially to reduce the incidence of hypotensive side-effects. Reduced doses, under supervision, are given in renal or hepatic deficiency and in congestive heart failure.

After myocardial infarction, trandolapril is given in doses of 500 micrograms daily, rising slowly to a maximum of 4 mg daily.

   Side-effects   include cough, headache, dizziness, hypotension and palpitations.

ANGIOTENSIN-II INHIBITORS

Although these drugs act at a later stage than the ACE-inhibitors, they have a basically similar anti-hypertensive action. They are useful for patients who cannot tolerate the ACE-inhibitors, as they do not cause the persistent dry cough which is an undesirable side-effect of those drugs. The cough is thought to be due to the breakdown of bradykinin and other kinins induced by ACE-inhibitors. Care is necessary when angiotensin-II inhibitors are given to patients with renal artery stenosis, and in those taking high-dose diuretics, as the diuresis may bring about a reduction in blood volume and cause hypotension.

Candesartan § (dose: 4–16 mg daily)

Brand name: Amias §
The initial dose of candesartan in essential hyper-tension is 4 mg daily, but half-doses are given in the elderly and in renal impairment. Maintenance dose is 8 mg daily, maximum 16 mg daily. **Side-effects** are mild and transient.

Irbisartan § ▼ (dose: 150 mg daily)

Brand name: Aprovel § ▼
Irbisartan is a long-acting angiotensin-II receptor antagonist for the treatment of hypertension. The initial and maintenance dose is 150 mg daily, rising if necessary to 300 mg daily, but half-doses should be given to elderly patients. **Side-effects** are usually mild and transient.

Losartan § ▼ (dose: 25–100 mg daily)

Brand name: Cozaar § ▼
The initial dose of losartan is 50 mg daily, later increased if necessary up to 100 mg daily. In the elderly and those receiving high-dose diuretic treatment, 25 mg daily should be given, together with monitoring of the plasma potassium levels. The **side-effects** are similar to those of the ACE-inhibitors, but are usually mild.

Valsartan § ▼ (dose: 80–160 mg daily)

Brand name: Diovan § ▼
Valsartan resembles losartan in its actions and uses and is given in doses of 80 mg once daily, increased if necessary after some weeks up to 160 mg daily. Reduced doses in renal impairment.

CALCIUM CHANNEL BLOCKING AGENTS (CCBAs)

Muscle contraction is linked with an influx of calcium ions into the muscle cells via calcium channels in the cell membrane. The channels are normally occupied by calcium ions bound to high-affinity sites, and act as voltage-dependent ionic gates. When stimulated, calcium ions are released, the ionic gate opens, and calcium ions flow through the channels into the cell and stimulate muscle contraction.

   Certain differences in these channels have been recognized, as some are designated receptor-operated channels (ROC) which are activated by acetylcholine and other agents, and others as voltage-operated channels (VOC), which are activated by depolarization of the cell membrane. The VOCs have been differen-tiated as long-lasting (L) channels and transient (T) channels, but the L channels appear to be the main sites of action of calcium channel-blocking agents, as the ROC and T channels are largely insensitive to such blockade.

   When cardiac muscle is stimulated by the flow of calcium ions, the heart rate and myocardial oxygen demand increase, and when that response is exces-sive, cardiac irregularities, coronary artery spasm and angina may occur. Drugs that could block the flow of calcium ions would have wide applications in cardiovascular disease, and drugs of that type are now in use and referred to as calcium channel blocking agents (CCBAs). They act by restricting the movement of calcium ions and so lower the amount of intracellular calcium available to activate contrac-tile proteins. They also reduce the blood pressure and lower the peripheral resistance by a relaxant effect on vascular smooth muscle. They should not be used in heart failure as they may further depress an already reduced cardiac efficiency.

   The CCBAs in current use differ chemically and pharmacologically, as some are more effective in angina than hypertension, so their clinical applications may differ. They can be divided into three groups; one with a dihydropyridine structure, represented by nifedipine, is mainly used in hypertension, stable angina and vasospastic (Prinzmetal's) angina; another group includes diltiazem and consists of benzothiazapine derivatives. The third group is represented by verapamil, a phenylalkylamine derivative. Verapamil has a wider range of activity that includes hypertension, angina, hypertrophic cardiomyopathy, atrial fibrillation and supraventricular tachycardia.

The various CCBAs should not be regarded as interchangeable, and the position is complicated as some have been formulated to provide an extended action. So no alteration from one product to another should be made without good cause and a careful assessment of the risks involved.

Nursing points about calcium channel blockers

(a) Some are used in angina, others in hypertension, as they differ in their pattern of activity.
(b) Not indicated in heart failure (may cause further deterioration).
(c) Nimodipine is exceptional in its use in subarachnoid haemorrhage.
(d) Long-acting products must not be regarded as interchangeable.

Amlodipine § (dose: 5–10 mg daily)

Brand name: Istin §
Amlodipine has the general properties of the CCBAs, although it has less effect on myocardial contractility. It is eliminated more slowly and so has a longer action that permits once daily dosing. It is used in the treatment of angina and hypertension in doses of 5 mg daily, increased if required to 10 mg daily. It can be used as the sole agent in the control of hypertension, or in combination with other antihypertensive agents such as diuretics and beta-blockers, usually without adjustment of dose.

Side-effects include flushing, headache, fatigue and dizziness. The hypotensive episodes and reflex tachycardia that sometimes occur with CCBAs are less likely with amlodipine by virtue of its slower action.

Diltiazem § (dose: 120–360 mg daily)

Brand names: Adizem §, Dilzem §, Slozem §, Tildiem §
Diltiazem is a benzothiazepine calcium channel blocking agent that differs from others by having little inotropic action on the heart. It is used in the treatment of angina and hypertension in doses of 60 mg three times a day, or twice a day for elderly patients, but the individual response may vary and require doses up to 360 mg daily. Diltiazem may be

effective in angina resistant to beta-blocker treatment. It is also used as a slow-release product for the treatment of hypertension in doses of 120 mg twice a day. Diltiazem should be used with care in patients with poor cardiac reserves, as its depressant action on cardiac conduction may precipitate heart failure.

Side-effects include bradycardia, hypotension, ankle oedema, headache and rash. Adizem-SR, Adizem XL, Dilzem SR, Tildiem Retard and Tildiem LA are some sustained action products.

Felodipine § (dose: 5–20 mg daily)

Brand name: Plendil §
Felodipine is a CCBA with a pattern of activity similar to that of amlodipine. It is used in all degrees of hypertension, and is given in initial doses of 5 mg once daily, with subsequent adjustment according to response, up to a maximum of 20 mg daily. It can be given with beta-blockers and diuretics, but the effects may be additive and require adjustment of dose. It is also used in angina in doses of 5–10 mg once daily in the morning.

The **side-effects** of felodipine are similar to those of most other CCBAs, but rash and mild gingival hyperplasia may occur. Felodipine and chemically related CCBAs should be taken with adequate fluid, but not with grapefruit juice, as the flavenoids in the juice may cause a rise in the plasma level of the drug.

Isradipine § (dose: 5–20 mg daily)

Brand name: Prescal §
Isradipine has a higher affinity for calcium channels in arterial smooth muscle than for those in the myocardium and so is largely free from cardiodepressant side-effects. In hypertension isradipine is given in doses of 2.5 mg twice daily initially, increased after 3–4 weeks if the response is inadequate to 5 mg twice a day, or very occasionally up to 20 mg daily. Combined treatment with a beta-blocker/diuretic may permit the use of lower doses. Isradipine undergoes extensive first-pass liver metabolism, and reduced doses should be given to the elderly and in renal impairment. It is not used for angina.

Side-effects include dizziness, headache, tachycardia, rash, weight gain and hypotension.

Lacidipine §

Brand name: Motens §
Lacidipine is chemically related to nifedipine and has similar properties, differing mainly in having a

smoother and more prolonged action. In the treatment of hypertension it may be given alone, or together with other antihypertensive agents such as diuretics and beta-blockers. The standard dose is 2 mg, taken in the morning with food, but half-doses are indicated in the elderly. The development of full response is slow, and 3–4 weeks should elapse before an increase in dose to 4–6 mg daily is considered. Lacidipine is not excreted in the urine, so no modification of dose is required for patients with renal disease.

Side-effects are those of calcium channel antagonists generally. They are usually transient but chest pain may indicate myocardial ischaemia and requires withdrawal of treatment.

Mibefradil § (dose: 50–100 mg daily)

Brand name: Posicor §

Mibefradil is a calcium channel blocking agent that differs from others by acting selectively on the T-channels, whereas most act on the L-channels. In angina and hypertension it is given initially in doses of 50 mg once daily, later slowly increased to 100 mg daily. Care is necessary with combined treatment, as mibefradil may interfere with the plasma levels of drugs metabolized by cytochrome P450 and other enzyme systems. See Manufacturer's Data sheet.

Nicardipine § (dose: 60–120 mg daily)

Brand name: Cardene §

Nicardipine has the general properties of the calcium channel blocking agents. It is used mainly for the prophylaxis and treatment of angina and hypertension as it brings about a direct fall in blood pressure by lowering arteriolar resistance. Nicardipine is given in doses of 20 mg three times a day initially, increased at intervals of not less than 3 days up to a maximum of 120 mg daily.

Side-effects include dizziness, headache, flushing, palpitations, nausea and lower limb oedema. If any ischaemic pain occurs, or is worsened within 30 minutes of the first dose, treatment should be discontinued.

Nifedipine § (dose: 30–60 mg daily)

Brand names: Adalat §, Calcilat §, Coracten §, Nifensar §

Nifedipine is a typical member of the calcium channel blocking agents derived from dihydropyridine. These drugs have a mainly vasodilator action with little influence on cardiac conduction. Nifedipine is used both for the prophylaxis and treatment of angina and in the treatment of hypertension, and is given in doses of 10 mg three times a day initially, slowly increased if required up to 60 mg daily. A liquid-filled capsule of 5 mg is available, and if a rapid effect is required the patient should bite into the capsule and retain the liquid in the mouth. Like chemically related CCBAs, nifedipine has little if any antiarrhythmic activity or depressant action on the myocardium and it may be given together with a beta-blocker. The antihypertensive effects may be additive, and care is necessary to control any marked hypotension that may follow combined therapy.

Adalat Retard and Nifensar XL are sustained action products.

Side-effects are basically similar to those of the CCBAs generally, and are usually transient, but lethargy and hyperplasia of the gums may sometimes occur. Nifedipine may cause or increase ischaemic pain in a few patients within minutes of initiating treatment, and in such cases the drug should be withdrawn.

Nimodipine § (dose: 360 mg daily)

Brand name: Nimotop §

Nimodipine is a calcium antagonist that crosses the blood–brain barrier and has a preferential action on the calcium channels in the cerebral vessels. It is used orally in subarachnoid haemorrhage following rupture of intracranial aneurysm to prevent the development of ischaemic neurological sequelae. Treatment should be commenced within 4 days of the onset of the haemorrhage with nimodipine in doses of 60 mg every 4 hours, and continued for 21 days. If cerebral oedema or ischaemia occurs, oral therapy should be replaced by the intravenous infusion of the drug in doses of 1 mg hourly initially, increased later to 2 mg hourly, and continued for 5 days. Care is necessary in cerebral oedema or increased intracranial pressure.

Side-effects are hypotension and gastro-intestinal disorders.

Nisoldipine § ▼ (Sycor MR §) is a newer CCBA for the prophylaxis of angina and the treatment of hypertension. Dose: 10–40 mg daily before breakfast.

Verapamil § (dose: 240–360 mg daily)

Brand names: Cordilox §, Securon §

Verapamil is the oldest of the calcium channel blocking agents and was used therapeutically before the nature of its function as a CCBA was understood. It has a depressant effect on cardiac conduction mediated by the atrioventricular node, and so is of value in supraventricular arrhythmias and by injection in paroxysmal tachycardia (p. 108). It is also used in the control of angina and hypertension. In angina it is given in doses of 80–120 mg three times a day, and in hypertension up to 480 mg daily. Care is necessary in patients with poor cardiac reserves, as it may precipitate heart failure. For the same reason, combined treatment with a beta-blocker may be hazardous and is contra-indicated.

Securon SR § and Univer § are sustained action products.

Side-effects are nausea, headache and constipation. Verapamil is contra-indicated in bradycardia, heart block and acute myocardial infarction.

POTASSIUM CHANNEL ACTIVATORS

Some drugs are known to cause smooth muscle relaxation by opening up potassium channels in the tissues and so increasing the movement of potassium ions. Such activation in the vascular system leads to vasodilatation, and it is thought that the anti-hypertensive action of diazoxide and minoxidil are mediated in part by potassium channel activation. A new drug with a similar but more selective action is nicorandil, and in view of the therapeutic potential of such activators, others may soon be introduced.

Nicorandil § ▼ (dose: 20–60 mg daily)

Brand name: Ikorel § ▼

Nicorandil is used for the prophylaxis and treatment of angina, and is given initially in doses of 10–20 mg twice a day, later up to 30 mg twice a day if required.

Side-effects include headache, usually transient, nausea, flushing and dizziness.

ADRENERGIC NEURONE-BLOCKING AGENTS

These agents inhibit the release of noradrenaline from postganglionic adrenergic neurones, and may reduce stores of noradrenaline at nerve endings. Drugs of this type, represented by guanethidine, bring about a reduction in peripheral resistance and heart rate, and lower an elevated blood pressure. Careful adjustment of dose or combined treatment with other drugs may be necessary to obtain a smooth and consistent response, as too rapid an action may cause postural hypotension. They are now used mainly in resistant hypertension not fully controlled by other drugs.

Bethanidine § (dose: 10–200 mg daily)

Brand name: Bendogen §

Bethanidine is chemically related to guanethidine and has similar adrenergic neurone blocking properties, but of shorter duration. The initial dose in hypertension is 10 mg three times a day, increased by 5 mg every 2 days up to a maximum daily dose of 200 mg, often with a diuretic and a beta-blocker.

Side-effects such as diarrhoea are less common.

Debrisoquine § (dose: 20–60 mg daily)

Debrisoquine has an antihypertensive action mediated by blocking the transmission of sympathetic nerve impulses at nerve endings. It interferes with the release of noradrenaline, and by lowering sympathetic tone it brings about a reduction in peripheral blood flow and a lowering of the blood pressure. It has little effect on catecholamine stores in the cardiovascular system, and does not affect the cardiac contractile mechanism. Debrisoquine is given in mild hypertension in doses of 10–20 mg once or twice a day, increased according to need and response up to 60 mg daily, although occasionally doses up to 120 mg daily may be needed.

Side-effects include postural hypotension, of which the patient should be warned, but which may be reduced by giving divided doses, with the higher dose at night. Diarrhoea may also occur.

Guanethidine § (dose: 10–20 mg by injection)

Brand name: Ismelin §

Guanethidine is a peripheral sympathomimeic blocking agent that is of value in the control of hypertensive crisis and the toxaemia of pregnancy. It is given in doses of 10–20 mg by intramuscular injection, and a fall in blood pressure may occur within 30 minutes, and reach a maximum in 1 hour. The response may last 4–6 hours, when a further dose may be given. The dose interval should be extended in renal impairment to avoid drug accumulation. Similar doses are given in the toxaemia of pregnancy, but as a drug of last resort when other treatment has failed.

Side-effects include bradycardia, gastro-intestinal disturbance and postural hypotension. The use of guanethidine in glaucoma is referred to on page 251.

CENTRALLY ACTING ANTIHYPERTENSIVE AGENTS

Cardiovascular control centres exist in the brain stem, and by modulating vascular resistance they affect the blood pressure. Some drugs, such as clonidine, reduce the flow of central impulses to the sympathetic nerves as well as reducing the release of noradrenaline at adrenergic nerve endings. The recently introduced moxonidine has a similar but more selective action. It binds with a sub-type of imidazoline receptors (I_1) which modify sympathetic activity, lower sympathetic tone and peripheral resistance, and so induce a fall in blood pressure.

Nursing points about centrally-acting antihypertensives

(a) Now used less frequently.
(b) Clonidine may cause hypertensive crisis if treatment is stopped suddenly.
(c) Methyldopa may be given during pregnancy, and in asthma and heart failure.

Clonidine § (dose: 150 micrograms– 1.2 mg daily)

Brand name: Catapres §
Clonidine is occasionally useful in patients resistant to or unable to tolerate guanethidine or related drugs. It is given in initial doses of 50–100 micrograms three times a day, slowly increasing according to response, although doses of more than 1 mg daily are seldom necessary. Clonidine is also useful in the control of hypertensive crisis, and is given by slow intravenous injection in doses of 150–300 micrograms, repeated if required up to a maximum of 750 micrograms over 24 hours.

Clonidine reduces both the supine and standing blood pressure, and postural hypotension is not uncommon.

In all cases, treatment with clonidine should be withdrawn slowly, as sudden withdrawal may cause a rebound hypertension or precipitate a hypertensive crisis.

Side-effects are sedation, bradycardia, fluid retention and dry mouth. The use of clonidine in the prophylactic treatment of migraine is referred to on p. 56.

Methyldopa § (dose: 0.75–3 g daily)

Brand names: Aldomet §
Methyldopa has a complex action. It has some central effects, and also interferes with an enzyme system concerned with the production of noradrenaline. Instead of noradrenaline, the related methyl-noradrenaline is produced which acts as a 'false

transmitter' of nerve impulses, so the result of treatment is an indirect reduction of peripheral resistance and a lowering of blood pressure.

Possibly as a result of this indirect action, postural hypotension or that induced by exercise is less with methyldopa than with some more directly acting drugs. It also has the advantage of being less likely to cause bronchospasm, and is more suitable for asthmatic patients.

Methyldopa is given orally in all types of hypertension in doses of 250 mg three times a day, together with a thiazide diuretic, increased if necessary up to 3 g daily. In elderly patients, the maximum daily dose should not exceed 2 g. It is sometimes given intravenously in hypertensive crisis in doses of 250–500 mg repeated as required.

Side-effects include drowsiness, diarrhoea, fluid retention, a systemic lupus erythematosus-like syndrome and haemolytic anaemia. Blood and liver function tests are advisable during treatment. Methyldopa may interfere with certain laboratory urine tests and give a false-positive diagnosis of phaeochromocytoma.

Moxonidine § ▼ (dose: 200 micrograms daily)

Brand name: Physiotens § ▼
Moxonidine has a more selective central action than older drugs and is effective in the control of mild to moderate hypertension. It is given in morning doses of 200 micrograms daily, rising after three weeks to 200 micrograms twice a day. It has little affinity for α_2-receptors, so **side-effects** such as dry mouth and sedation are less common than with related drugs.

ANTIHYPERTENSIVE AGENTS WITH A MAINLY VASODILATORY ACTION

A few powerful drugs are available that reduce arteriolar resistance (as distinct from peripheral vasodilators, p. 125). They are used mainly in hypertensive crisis, but are sometimes of value in severe hypertension when given with a beta-blocker and a diuretic.

Diazoxide § (dose: 150 mg–1.2 g over 24 hours)

Brand name: Eudemine §
Diazoxide has a powerful antihypertensive action thought to be mediated by potassium channel activation (see p. 121), resulting in a selective vasodilator effect on the arterioles and a reduction in peripheral resistance. It is used mainly in hypertensive crisis, or

when a very rapid control of severe hypertension is required.

It is given by rapid intravenous injection in doses of 1–3 mg/kg up to 150 mg. A maximum response occurs within about 5 minutes and lasts about 4 hours. Further doses may be given as required up to a maximum of 1.2 g over 24 hours.

Side-effects include marked ECG changes, bradycardia and cerebral ischaemia. The solution is strongly alkaline, so injection requires care.

Diazoxide may cause a sudden hyperglycaemia, which can be controlled by insulin, or if less severe, by a sulphonylurea such as tolbutamide. Because of the powerful action and side-effects of diazoxide, close control is necessary throughout treatment.

The use of diazoxide in the treatment of hypoglycaemia is discussed on p. 202.

Hydralazine § (dose: 50–100 mg daily)

Brand name: Apresoline §
Hydralazine has a direct relaxant action on the arterioles, and is used mainly in the supplementary treatment of the long-term control of moderate to severe hypertension. It is given in doses of 25 mg twice a day, increased according to need up to 100 mg daily, but care is necessary, as a too-rapid reduction in blood pressure may occur even with small doses. It is occasionally given by slow intravenous injection or infusion in doses of 5–10 mg in the control of hypertensive crisis.

Side-effects include nausea, tachycardia, fluid retention and postural hypotension. A syndrome similar to lupus erythematosus, with weight loss and arthritis, has occurred after high-dose therapy.

Minoxidil § (dose: 5–50 mg daily)

Brand name: Loniten §
Minoxidil has a powerful vasodilator action possibly mediated by the opening up of potassium channels (see p. 121). It is used only for the treatment of severe hypertension resistant to other drugs. It is given in doses of 5 mg daily initially, slowly increased at intervals of 3 or more days up to a maximum of 50 mg daily. It must never be used alone, as it causes fluid retention and tachycardia, and combined administration with a diuretic of the frusemide type and a beta-blocker is essential.

Side-effects include nausea, weight gain and hirsutism. As with related drugs, it is contra-indicated in phaeochromocytoma. (It is of interest that minoxidil is used locally for the treatment of alopecia areata, p. 262.)

Sodium nitroprusside § (dose: 0.5–1.5 micrograms/kg per minute by intravenous infusion)

Sodium nitroprusside is a very powerful, short-acting antihypertensive agent that induces vasodilatation by a direct action on the arterioles and blood vessels. It is used in hypertensive crisis, to obtain controlled hypotension during surgery, and in heart failure.

Sodium nitroprusside is given in hypertensive crisis by intravenous infusion in initial doses of 0.5–1.5 micrograms/kg per minute, and in similar doses for controlled hypotension in surgery. In heart failure doses of 10–15 micrograms/minute are given initially, increased every 5–10 minutes as required up to a maximum of 200 micrograms/minute. Constant monitoring of the blood pressure is essential, and sodium nitroprusside should be used only when such monitoring can be carried out, as tachycardia and hyperventilation may occur.

As one of the products of prusside metabolism is cyanide, the plasma concentration of cyanide should be measured if treatment is prolonged.

Trimetaphan § (dose: 3–4 mg/minute by intravenous infusion)

Trimetaphan is a short-acting ganglion blocking agent, and is the surviving representative of a now obsolete group of antihypertensive drugs. It is used solely to obtain controlled hypotension during surgery, and is given by intravenous infusion in doses of 3–4 mg/minute initially, with subsequent doses according to need. Tachycardia and respiratory depression may occur, particularly when muscle relaxants are also used.

Trimetaphan brings about some histamine release, so care is necessary in asthmatics or allergic subjects. It is contra-indicated in severe cardiac disease or atherosclerosis.

NITRATES USED AS VASODILATORS

Although some nitrates have been in use for a long time, it is only in recent years that it has been realized that they act as a source of nitric oxide (NO). It is now known that nitric oxide is a biological mediator with a wide range of activity, exerted mainly by an increased formation of cycloguanosine monophosphate (cGMP), which bring about changes in the intracellular calcium levels. Nitric oxide is released continuously from the vascular endothelium; it maintains the vasodilatation of the cardiovascular system and has a synergistic action with prostacyclin in inhibiting platelet aggregation. The nitrates represent a source of NO, but they have a selective action on the venous system, because the veins produce relatively little endogenous NO and so respond more to the exogenous NO provided by the nitrates. The venodilatation they cause leads to a pooling of the blood in the peripheral veins, so the venous return to the heart is reduced, with a consequent reduction in the cardiac load and oxygen demand. The nitrates are widely used in the prophylaxis and treatment of angina, but tolerance and a reduction in response may occur with their extended use. The risks can be limited by adjustment of dose, so that low blood nitrate levels occur at intervals during the day, or in the case of skin patches, by reducing the time during which they are applied.

Glyceryl trinitrate (dose: 300 micrograms–1 mg)

Glyceryl trinitrate (GTN) was introduced for the treatment of angina pectoris over 100 years ago, but its use is increasing as new methods of presentation are now available, such as long-acting tablets, skin patches and ointment. GTN is used mainly in acute angina, but as it is almost completely inactivated in the liver when given orally, it is often taken as sublingual tablets of 300 or 500 micrograms, which are best taken sitting down to avoid any initial hypotension. The relief is prompt, as the vasodilator action begins in 2 minutes, and lasts up to 20–30 minutes. When used prophylactically, GTN should be taken shortly *before* any exertion likely to cause an attack of angina. Many patients require some nurse-guidance in the use of GTN preparations.

Side-effects include headache (which may subside as tolerance develops), dizziness, flushing and postural hypotension.

In refractory angina associated with severe ischaemia, glyceryl trinitrate is sometimes given by intravenous infusion in doses of 10 micrograms/minute, increased at intervals of 30 minutes up to a dose of 200 micrograms/minute. Nitrocine § and Nitronal § are brand products for such intravenous use after suitable dilution.

Glyceryl trinitrate tablets must be kept in airtight glass containers, and unused tablets should be discarded about 8 weeks after supply to the patient. Many cases of poor response to oral glyceryl trinitrate are due to the use of deteriorated tablets.

Sustac is a long-acting product for prophylactic use. Tablets are available in strengths of 2.6, 6.4 and 10 mg, and should be swallowed whole. Suscard is a buccal tablet presentation of GTN.

Coro-Nitro, Glytrin and Nitrolingual are rapidly acting oral spray products useful as alternatives to sublingual tablets. Percutol is an ointment containing glyceryl trinitrate. Deponit, Minitran, Nitro-Dur and Transiderm-Nitro are self-adhesive patches. They are intended for once daily application to the skin for the extended control of angina. They are also of value for patients who experience attacks at night. The patches should be changed every 24 hours, using a different skin area. (A very different use of GTN ointment is the treatment of anal fissure.)

Isosorbide dinitrate § (dose: 30–120 mg daily)

Brand names: Cedocard §, Isordil §, Sorbitrate §, Isoket §

Isosorbide dinitrate is a longer acting vasodilator given sublingually in doses of 5–10 mg when a prompt action is required, and orally for prophylactic treatment in doses of 5–20 mg three or four times a day. Alternatively, it may be given for the prevention and treatment of acute angina as a sublingual spray (Imtack) in doses of 1.25–3.75 mg.

Some sustained-release oral products are available when an extended action is required. Isosorbide dinitrate is also used in the treatment of left ventricular heart failure, and is then given in larger doses up to a maximum of 240 mg daily. In severe conditions, it may be given by intravenous infusion in doses of 2–10 mg hourly.

Side-effects, including tolerance, are similar to those of glyceryl trinitrate.

Isosorbide mononitrate § (dose: 30–120 mg daily)

Brand names: Elantan §, Ismo §, Monit §, Mono-Cedocard §

The mononitrate is the metabolic derivative of the dinitrate, to which the action of the dinitrate is mainly due. It is well absorbed orally, and largely escapes first-pass metabolism in the liver. In angina it is given in doses of 10–20 mg three times a day; in congestive heart failure the dose is slowly increased according to individual need up to a maximum of 120 mg daily.

Side-effects include headache, dizziness, flushing and palpitations, which are usually transient, but may be relieved by a temporary reduction of dose. Pentaerythritol tetranitrate § (Mycardol §) is also used in the prophylaxis of angina.

Nursing points about nitrate vasodilators

(a) Glyceryl trinitrate tablets (not the long-acting forms) must be given sublingually as the drug is inactivated if swallowed. Tablets must be kept in glass air-tight containers and rejected if more than 2 months old.
(b) Postural hypotension may sometimes limit treatment.
(c) Patches to be applied to a hairless skin area where little movement occurs, and replaced daily at a slightly different site.
(d) Isorbide mono/dinitrate more stable, and can be used for prophylaxis.
(e) Tolerance may occur; risk may be reduced by giving low doses, or by the temporary removal of a skin patch.

PERIPHERAL VASODILATORS

Although peripheral vasodilators are relatively ineffective in the treatment of hypertension, they are considered here as they have some applications in the treatment of peripheral vascular disorders associated with vascular spasm or occlusion, particularly Raynaud's disease. Their value is limited as the vasodilator effect may be more marked in the healthy peripheral vessels, and the blood flow through damaged vessels may be improved to a lesser extent.

Cinnarizine (dose: 225 mg daily)

Brand name: Stugeron Forte
Cinnarizine is an antihistamine with some peripheral vasodilatory activity, and is given in doses of 75 mg two or three times a day in the treatment of peripheral vascular disorders and Raynaud's disease.

It has the **side-effects** of the antihistamines, and care is necessary if hypotension is present. The use of cinnarizine as an anti-emetic is referred to on p. 154.

Nicotinyl alcohol (dose: 100–200 mg daily)

Brand name: Ronicol
Nicotinyl alcohol is partly metabolized to nicotinic acid (page 129) and has a similar but much milder vasodilator action. It is used in peripheral vascular disorders, and given in doses of 25–50 mg four times

a day. It may cause some flushing and dizziness, but symptoms of hypotension are usually mild.

Inositol nicotinate (dose: 3–4 g daily)

Brand name: Hexopal
Inositol nicotinate has vasodilator properties as it is partly metabolized to nicotinic acid. It is sometimes used in cerebral vascular disease as well as disorders of the peripheral circulation in doses of 0.5–1 g three or four times a day.

Oxpentifylline § (dose: 800 mg–1.2 g daily)

Brand name: Trental §
Oxpentifylline is chemically related to theophylline, but it is used only as a vasodilator in peripheral vascular diseases. It is given in doses of 400 mg two or three times a day, and following response, doses of 200 mg three times a day may be given for maintenance.

Side-effects include nausea, dizziness and flushing.

Oxpentifylline may potentiate the action of some antihypertensive agents, and an adjustment of dose of such drugs may be required.

Thymoxamine § (dose: 160–320 mg daily)

Brand name: Opilon §
Thymoxamine (moxisylate) is a selectively acting alpha-adrenergic blocking agent used in the short-term management of Raynaud's disease. It is given in doses of 40 mg four times a day, but if the response is poor after doses of up to 320 mg daily, treatment should be discontinued. A recent development is the use of the drug as Erecnos § by intra-cavernous injection for the pharmacological induction of erection.

Co-dergocrine § (Hydergine §) is a cerebral vasodilator used only for senile dementia in doses of 4.5 mg daily. The response is seldom impressive.

BLOOD-LIPID LOWERING AGENTS

Hyperlipidaemia is a broad term referring to a general rise in the level of blood lipids which is also a broad term that includes cholesterol, triglycerides and phospholipids. Cholesterol, derived from dietary fats, is the substance from which steroids are formed by biosynthesis; triglycerides are present in many animal and vegetable fats and are derivatives of glycerin and fatty acids that function as an energy source; phospholipids are components of cells of the nervous system. Blood lipids are present in the plasma as protein complex particles (lipoproteins) and have a core of cholesterol and triglycerides and an outer shell of phospholipids and protein. They are classified according to the varying amounts of their constituents. (See Table 7.3.)

The chylomicrons transport dietary fat to the liver where the VLDLs are formed, and when these VLDLs enter the circulation much of their triglyceride content is removed by the action of lipoprotein lipase, an enzyme present on the surface of capillary endothelial cells, and they become low density lipoproteins. These LDLs are involved in the transport of cholesterol to the peripheral tissues. The HDLs are formed in the liver and small intestines and function as cholesterol scavengers, as they pick up any free cholesterol in the circulation and return it to the liver for excretion or conversion to bile acids. Attempts have been made to classify the hyperlipidaemias according to variations in the different lipoprotein levels, and the Fredrickson/WHO classification is outlined in Table 7.4.

The most common form of hyperlipidaemia is a rise in the blood level of cholesterol (hypercholesterolaemia) and although diet and smoking play an important role in its development, genetic factors may also have an influence. It leads to the formation of lipid deposits (atheromas) in the arterial linings, particularly the coronary arteries, resulting in atherosclerosis and ischaemic heart disease. As the blood supply to the heart is restricted, and becomes insufficient to meet the oxygen demands of the body, the ischaemia may be manifested by angina and myocardial infarction. Ischaemic heart disease is the main cause of death in industrial countries. A

Table 7.4 Fredrickson/WHO classification of hyperlipidaemias

Type	Frequency	Notes
I	Rare	High triglyceride levels; symptoms may occur in childhood with symptoms of acute pancreatitis
IIa	Common	High cholesterol levels, high risk of CHD
IIb	Common	High cholesterol and triglyceride levels, high risk of CHD
III	Uncommon	High cholesterol and triglyceride levels, with risk of diabetes, high risk of CHD and peripheral vascular disease
IV	Common	High risk of peripheral vascular disease
V	Uncommon	High triglyceride and chylomicron levels with risk of diabetes

CHD = coronary heart disease

lowering of the cholesterol levels in hypercholesterolaemia, particularly when the level rises above 6.5 mmol/l, reduces the risks of ischaemic heart disease, and may also reduce the rate of the progressive atherosclerosis. A rise in the HDL may also have a protective effect by reducing tissue stores of cholesterol.

The main treatment of hyperlipidaemia is a strict low-fat diet, weight reduction and cessation of smoking. Drug treatment should be regarded as adjunctive, and is mainly indicated for patients unable to tolerate, or who do not respond to, such dietary restrictions. The range of drugs used includes bile acid binding agents, lipase-stimulating drugs derived from fibrinic acid, enzyme inhibitors and nicotinic acid derivatives. The varying sites of action are indicated in Fig 7.5.

Table 7.3 Classification of lipoproteins

Name	Main constituents	Function
Chylomicrons	Almost entirely triglycerides	Transport dietary fat to the liver.
Very-low-density lipoproteins (VLDLs)	Mainly triglycerides	Transport hepatic synthesized triglycerides to the tissues
Intermediate density lipoproteins (IDLs)	Fairly equal mixture of triglycerides, cholesterol and protein	Breakdown product of VLDL; precursor of LDL by uptake of triglyceride and cholesterol from HDL
Low-density lipoproteins (LDLs)	Mainly cholesterol, with some phospholipids and protein	Transport cholesterol to the peripheral tissues
High-density lipoproteins (HDLs)	Mainly protein with small amounts of triglycerides and cholesterol	Transport cholesterol from peripheral cells back to the liver

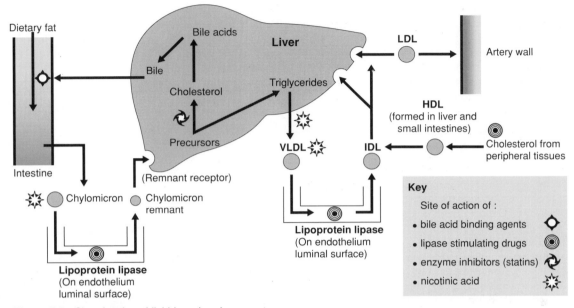

Figure 7.5 Site of action of lipid lowering drugs.

Nursing points about blood-lipid lowering agents

(a) Exchange resins bind intestinal bile acids and so act indirectly on lipid formation.
(b) The fibrate group of drugs reduce blood levels of lipids partly by enzyme activity.
(c) The statins inhibit the synthesis of cholesterol in the liver.
(d) They can all cause a myositis-like syndrome.
(e) The nicotinic acid derivatives are also peripheral vasodilators and may cause undesirable flushing.

BILE ACID BINDING AGENTS

Bile acid binding agents act by binding to and preventing the reabsorption of bile acids from the small intestine, and so interrupt the normal enterohepatic recirculation of those acids. The insoluble bile acid–binding agent complex is excreted in the faeces. The bile acids that the body requires are then derived from stores of cholesterol in the liver, and those stores are replaced in turn from cholesterol-containing low-density lipoproteins (LDL). With the extended use of such binding agents, which are exchange resins, the

Table 7.5 Table of blood-lipid lowering agents

Type of drug	Approved name	Brand name	Daily dose	Main lowering effect on
Bile acid binding resins	cholestyramine colestipol	Questran Colestid	12–24 g 10–30 g	Cholesterol
Fibric acid derivatives	bezafibrate ciprofibrate clofibrate fenofibrate gemfibrozil	Bezalip Modalim Atromid-S Lipantil Lopid	400–600 mg 100–200 mg 2 g 300–400 mg 1–5 g	Cholesterol and triglycerides
HMG CoA reductase inhibitors (the statins)	fluvastatin cerivastatin pravastatin simvastatin	Lescol Lipostat Zocor	20–40 mg 10–80 mg 10–40 mg 10–40 mg	Cholesterol
Nicotinic acid derivatives	acipimox	Olbetam	500–1200 mg	Cholesterol and triglycerides
Unclassified	omega-triglycerides	Maxepa	10 g	Triglycerides

plasma levels of cholesterol and LDL are slowly reduced. They are used mainly in the treatment of the more common hyperlipidaemias (IIa and IIb), particularly in patients who have not responded to other therapy, but prolonged treatment is necessary. They are also used in the prophylactic treatment of middle-aged men with resistant hyperlipidaemia.

Cholestyramine § (dose: 12–24 g daily)

Brand name: Questran §
Cholestyramine is a bile acid binding exchange resin used in hyperlipidaemias, particularly Type IIa, that have not responded to diet, and in the early prevention of coronary heart disease. It is given orally as a powder, often sprinkled on food, in doses of 8 g initially, slowly increased over 3–4 weeks up to 24 g or more, in single or divided doses. Some patients may find treatment more acceptable if the drug is taken as a drink with fruit juice or soup. Nausea, flatulence and abdominal disturbances are the main **side-effects**. It is of no value in biliary obstruction, as in that state no bile acids reach the intestinal tract.

Cholestyramine may reduce the absorption of certain other drugs such as digoxin and warfarin and thiazide diuretics, and any combined therapy should be given at least 1 hour before cholestyramine, or 4 hours afterward to prevent any interference with absorption. With prolonged treatment, the absorption of fat-soluble vitamins may be reduced, and supplementary treatment may be required.

Cholestyramine is also used in doses of 4–8 g daily in the treatment of pruritus associated with partial biliary obstruction, and in standard doses in the treatment of diarrhoea caused by Crohn's disease, ileac resection and radiotherapy.

Colestipol § (Colestid §) is another bile acid binding anion exchange resin used in hyperlipidaemia, and is given in doses of 10 g initially, slowly increased up to 30 g daily.

THE FIBRATE GROUP OF LIPID LOWERING AGENTS (LIPASE-STIMULATING DRUGS)

The fibrates, of which clofibrate was the first to be introduced, reduce the plasma levels of both cholesterol and triglycerides. The mode of action is not yet clear, but they appear to increase the activity of lipoprotein lipase, augment the removal of triglycerides from chylomicrons, and promote the uptake of cholesterol by high density lipoproteins. They are used in the treatment of most forms of hyperlipid-aemia in patients who have not responded to other therapy, but reduced doses should be given in renal insufficiency and they are contra-indicated in severe renal and hepatic impairment and gall bladder disease, and in pregnancy.

Gemfibrozil differs chemically from other fibrates, and is used mainly when response to other drugs is inadequate. The **side-effects** of the fibrates include abdominal discomfort, flatulence and nausea. An uncommon reaction that may occur with any member of the group is a myositis-like syndrome, particularly in patients with renal impairment.

Bezafibrate § (dose: 600 mg daily)

Brand names: Bezalip §; Bezalip-Mono §
Bezafibrate is a typical member of the fibrate group, and is used in the treatment of most types of hyper-lipidaemia with the exception of Type I. It is given in doses of 200 mg three times a day, preferably after food, although doses of 200 mg twice daily may be adequate in hypertriglyceridaemia. Bezalip-Mono is a delayed release product containing 400 mg of bezafibrate, for administration at night. The **side-effects** are those of the fibrates generally. Bezafibrate is contra-indicated in severe renal and hepatic disease, biliary cirrhosis and gall bladder dysfunction.

Clofibrate § (dose: 1–1.5 g daily)

Brand name: Atromid-S §
Clofibrate is used in the treatment of most types of hyperlipidaemia with the exception of Type I. It is given in doses of 500 mg three times a day after food. It has the disadvantage of increasing the biliary excretion of cholesterol, and may promote gallstone formation, and is now used mainly in patients who have undergone cholecystectomy.

Side-effects are abdominal discomfort, nausea and flatulence.

Gemfibrozil § (dose: 0.9–1.5 g daily)

Brand name: Lopid §
Gemfibrozil is usually given in doses of 600 mg twice a day and is effective in most types of hyperlipidaemia (except Type I) that have not responded to other treatment. It is also used for the prevention of coronary heart disease in men in the 40–55 year age group with hyperlipidaemia unresponsive to diet or drug therapy. It differs structurally from other fibrates, and blood counts and liver function tests are necessary before long-term treatment with gemfibrozil is considered.

Side-effects are those of the fibrates generally and include dizziness, blurred vision and painful extremities. Other fibrates are listed in Table 7.5.

THE STATINS (ENZYME INHIBITORS)

This group of drugs offers a different approach to the treatment of hyperlipidaemia, as they have a direct action on the biosynthesis of cholesterol in the liver. The rate-limiting enzyme in the cascade of reactions involved in cholesterol synthesis is hydroxy-methylglutaryl co-enzyme A reductase (HMG-CoA-reductase). Inhibition of that enzyme would interrupt the hepatic synthesis of cholesterol at an early stage. Such an interruption would in turn lead to a compensatory increase in the number of active LDL receptors in the liver, and so further increase the take-up and removal of cholesterol from the circulation. Currently available inhibitors of HMG-CoA-reductase are listed in Table 7.5.

They are given in doses of 10–40 mg daily in the treatment of primary hypercholesterolaemia (Type IIa). They tend to have more effect than the exchange resins in lowering LDL levels, but are less active than the fibrates in lowering triglyceride levels.

Side-effects include gastro-intestinal disturbances, headache and rash. Myositis is an uncommon side-effect, but it and other reactions may occur more frequently during combined therapy with fibrates and nicotinic acid and patients should be advised to report any muscle pain or tenderness without delay. Liver function tests should be performed before such combined therapy is considered. Multiple treatment with an exchange resin, on the other hand, may have an additive effect, but when so given the resin should be given some hours before the statin to avoid loss of the drug by resin-binding.

NICOTINIC ACID AND DERIVATIVES

Nicotinic acid is a member of the vitamin B group, and has been found to lower the plasma levels of cholesterol and triglycerides. It reduces the biosynthesis of VLDLs and increases the clearance of chylomicrons and VLDLs from the plasma. It also inhibits the release of free fatty acids from fat stores in the tissues, so reducing the amount of those acids available for take-up by the liver for cholesterol synthesis and LDL production.

Acipimox § (dose: 500–750 mg daily)

Brand name: Olbetam §

Acipimox is effective in most types of hyperlipidaemia and acts mainly by inhibiting the release of fatty acids from stores in adipose tissues, so causing a gradual lowering of blood lipids. It is given in divided doses of 500–750 mg daily with the main meals, adjusted individually according to the plasma lipid levels. Reduced doses should be given in renal impairment.

Side-effects are peripheral vasodilatation with flushing and itching, which tend to subside as treatment is continued.

Nicotinic acid (dose: 3–6 g daily)

Nicotinic acid is given in doses of 1–2 g three times a day, but its therapeutic value is limited by the intense flushing caused by such high doses. Treatment is best commenced with small initial doses of 100–200 mg three times a day for 2–4 weeks before increasing the dose slowly to a therapeutic level. The flushing, which appears to be mediated by prostaglandins, may also be relieved in some cases by the administration of a low dose of aspirin about half an hour before the dose of nicotinic acid.

Other **side-effects** include dizziness, nausea, abdominal discomfort, pruritus and urticaria.

Fish oil concentrate

Brand name: Maxepa

The low incidence of coronary heart disease in Greenland Eskimos has been linked with their dietary intake of polyunsaturated fish oils. These oils contain eicosapentaenoic acid (EPA) and decosahexanoic acid (DHA), sometimes referred to as the omega-3-fatty acids, and differ from the 6-fatty acids in western diets.

A fish oil concentrate containing EPA 18% and DHA 10% (and merely negligible amounts of vitamins A and D) is used in some hyperlipidaemias as it brings about a sustained fall in plasma triglyceride levels. It is given in doses of 5 ml twice daily with food in severe triglyceridaemia, and in patients at risk of ischaemic heart disease. It also inhibits platelet aggregation, so care is necessary in patients already receiving anticoagulants.

FURTHER READING

Berkin K E, Ball S G 1988 Cough and angiotensin converting enzyme inhibition. British Medical Journal 296:1279–1280

Breckenridge A 1988 Angiotensin converting enzyme inhibitors. British Medical Journal 296:618–620

Garratt C J et al 1992 Adenosine and cardiac arrhythmias. British Medical Journal 305:3

Heber M E 1990 Effectiveness of the once-daily antagonist lacidipine in controlling 24-hour ambulatory blood pressure. American Journal of Cardiology 66:1228–1232

Horowitz L N 1990 Role of moracizine in the management of ventricular arrhythmias. American Journal of Cardiology 65:41D–46D

Jordan S 1992 Reducing hypertension. Nursing Times 88(21):44–47

Keen P J 1993 Channel modulators – new therapeutic opportunities. Pharmaceutical Medicine 7:175–182

Kenny J 1985 Calcium channel blocking agents and the heart. British Medical Journal 291:1150–1152

Laniado M E, Lalani E N 1997 Ion channels: new explanations for old diseases. British Medical Journal 315:1171–1172

O'Connor P et al 1990 Lipid lowering drugs. British Medical Journal 300:667–672

Poole-Wilson P A, Lindsay D 1992 Advances in the treatment of chronic heart failure. British Medical Journal 304:1067–1070

Pritchett E L C 1992 Management of atrial fibrillation. New England Journal of Medicine 326:1264–1271

Purcell H, Fox K 1993 Potassium channel activators in ischaemic heart disease. British Journal of Clinical Practice 47(3):150–154

Simpson J, Smith R 1997 Treating anal fissure. British Medical Journal 314:1638–1639

Smith G D, Pekkanen J 1992 Should there be a moratorium on the use of cholesterol lowering drugs? British Medical Journal 304:431–434

Smith S 1987 Drugs and the heart. Nursing Times 83(21):24–26

Vallance P, Collier J 1994 Biology and clinical relevance of nitric oxide. British Medical Journal 309:453–457

Wright J M 1995 Pharmacological management of congestive heart failure. Critical Care Nursing 18(1):32–44

8

Anticoagulants and haemostatics

Blood is the transport fluid of the body and contains plasma, red and white blood cells and platelets. The distributive functions include the delivery of oxygen, nutrients and hormones to the body cells, and the removal of metabolic waste products. The protective functions are maintenance of the blood pH and volume, the prevention of infection and the control of haemostasis. Haemostasis is the complex process by which blood loss from damaged vessels is limited and repair initiated.

ANTICOAGULANTS

Vascular damage results in a cascade of reactions involving a variety of blood factors concerned with the formation of a blood clot. The initial stage is vasoconstriction, which reduces the immediate blood loss, and is followed by the aggregation of blood platelets at the damaged site under the influence of thromboxane A_2. The platelets adhere to each other and to the damaged vessel and form a temporary plug that further reduces blood loss. More platelets are attracted to the area, where they degranulate and release thromboplastin. At the same time the initial damage causes a release of tissue thromboplastin which forms a complex with calcium. Further inter-active stages include the activation of Factor X, which converts plasma prothrombin to thrombin, which in turn converts soluble fibrinogen to insoluble fibrin. The fibrin mesh so formed entraps further blood cells, and the process ends with the formation of a stable clot. (See Fig. 8.1.) Subsidiary factors include Factor VIII, a deficiency of which causes haemophilia A, Factor IX, also known as the Christmas factor, which if lacking results in haemophilia B, prostacyclin (p. 135), nitric oxide (p. 123) and vitamin K (p. 288).

131

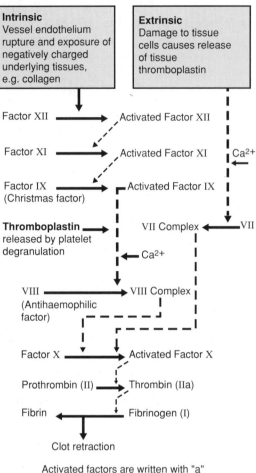

| **Intrinsic**
Vessel endothelium rupture and exposure of negatively charged underlying tissues, e.g. collagen | **Extrinsic**
Damage to tissue cells causes release of tissue thromboplastin |

Factor XII ⟶ Activated Factor XII

Factor XI ⟶ Activated Factor XI Ca^{2+}

Factor IX (Christmas factor) ⟶ Activated Factor IX

Thromboplastin released by platelet degranulation ⟶ VII Complex ⟵ VII

⟵ Ca^{2+}

VIII (Antihaemophilic factor) ⟶ VIII Complex

Factor X ⟶ Activated Factor X

Prothrombin (II) ⟶ Thrombin (IIa)

Fibrin ⟵ Fibrinogen (I)

Clot retraction

Activated factors are written with "a" after the number, e.g. XIIa

Figure 8.1 Simplified fibrin clot formation pathway.

In health the whole system is so well balanced that although minor clotting occurs as part of the normal repair process of the vascular system, intravascular clotting does not occur. However, that delicate balance may be disturbed by damage to the vascular epithelium and cause some intravascular clotting, and if that takes place in one of the coronary arteries, the consequent restriction in the blood flow to the heart may result in coronary thrombosis. Thrombosis may also occur in the deep veins of the legs, where the clot may have a long tail that waves in the direction of the blood flow. This is particularly likely during prolonged bed rest, with the added danger that part of the tail may become detached and cause pulmonary embolism. A longer-term effect of deep vein thrombosis is damage to the valves, which gives rise to venous hypertension and leg ulceration.

The treatment of thrombosis is accordingly based on drugs that interfere at various points in the blood-clotting cascade system and those that act at a later stage and degrade already formed fibrin clots. They include antithrombin agents, antiplatelet drugs and fibrinolytic agents, and are used in the prophylaxis and treatment of deep vein thrombosis and pulmonary embolism where the clots consist mainly of platelets and dead cells. They are less effective in arterial thrombosis, as in the faster-flowing arterial circulation the clots consist largely of aggregated platelets with little fibrin. The major anticoagulants are heparin, given by injection, and warfarin, given orally. It is of interest that leech bites continue to bleed because in biting an anticoagulant, huridin, is transferred to the bite. Huridin can now be extracted in a pure form, and may become therapeutically available as a useful anticoagulant.

HEPARINS

Nursing points about heparin
(a) Standard heparin is given by intravenous or subcutaneous injection under laboratory control. (b) Fractionated or low molecular weight heparins are for subcutaneous injection only; they have a longer action that permits single daily doses. With such products laboratory control is not necessary. (c) Effects of heparin can be neutralized rapidly by an injection of protamine.

Heparin § (dose: 5000–10 000 units intravenously or subcutaneously).

Brand names: Calciparine (s.c.) §, Minihep (s.c.) §, Monoparin (i.v.) §, Multiparin (i.v.) §, Pump-Hep (i.v.) §, Unihep (i.v.) §, and Uniparin (s.c.) §

Heparin is a complex mucopolysaccharide present in mast cells, the endothelial cells of the blood vessels and in the plasma. For therapeutic use it is obtained from animal lung and intestinal mucosa, and as the batch potency varies, the dose of heparin is measured in units. It acts by inhibiting the action of thrombin as well as some of the co-factors of coagulation, and in deep vein thrombosis and pulmonary embolism it is given in a preliminary dose of 5000–10 000 units hourly by intravenous injection, followed by maintenance doses of 1000–2000 units, by continuous infusion under daily laboratory control. Alternatively, maintenance doses of 15 000 units may be given 12-hourly by subcutaneous injection. In prophylaxis, heparin is given 2 hours before surgery in subcutaneous doses of 5000 units, followed by similar doses 8–12-hourly for 7 days. During such maintenance treatment laboratory control is not required.

Similar doses are given for prophylaxis against thrombosis in general surgery.

Heparin is also used (50–200 units) to flush out and maintain the patency of catheters when they are in place for more than 48 hours (Canusal, Hep-Flush, Heplok, Hepsal). For short-term use, saline solution may be equally effective.

Low molecular weight heparins

The heparin molecule has a complicated structure, but fragments of that large molecule can be split off, some of which have modified anticoagulant properties, and these low molecular weight heparin fractions are in use for the prophylaxis and treatment of venous thromboembolism. They have a longer action than standard heparin, and are given by once daily subcutaneous injection. With such doses laboratory control is not necessary (Table 8.1). Such heparins are also used to prevent clotting in extracorporeal circuits.

Side-effects of heparin include bruising, haemorrhage, transient alopecia and hypersensitivity reactions. Osteoporosis has occurred after prolonged use. It is contra-indicated in peptic ulcer, severe hypertension, severe liver and renal disease, thrombocytopenia, and any haemorrhagic disorder.

Heparin overdose

Platelet counts should be measured in patients receiving heparin for more than 5 days, and treatment withdrawn if thrombocytopenia develops. Haemorrhage due to slight overdose can be controlled by withdrawal of the drug, but if severe, a rapid reversal of the anticoagulant action can be obtained by the intravenous injection of protamine sulphate, which is a specific antidote.

Protamine is a simple protein obtained from salmon sperm and is given as a 1% solution in doses depending on the degree of heparin overdose (as 1 mg will neutralize 80–100 units of heparin), up to a total dose of 50 mg, if given within 15 minutes of overdose. Lower doses are adequate after a longer interval, as heparin is rapidly excreted and, paradoxically, an overdose of protamine has an anticoagulant effect.

ORAL ANTICOAGULANTS

Oral anticoagulants are synthetic substances that differ from heparin in both nature and mode of action, as they function as vitamin K antagonists. That vitamin is essential for the formation in the liver of prothrombin (Factor II) as well as Factors VII, IX and X. The oral anticoagulants act by interfering with the biosynthesis of those factors and they may also inhibit the further synthesis of vitamin K. They therefore have an indirect anticoagulant action that is slow in onset (36–48 hours), as the plasma level of circulating clotting factors has to fall by normal metabolism before the inhibition of prothrombin synthesis can exert its effects.

Oral anticoagulants are used in the prophylaxis and treatment of deep vein thrombosis. Although they have no effect on established clots, they prevent extension of such preformed thromboses, and so reduce the possibility of secondary thromboembolic complications.

Table 8.1 Low molecular weight heparins

Approved name	Brand name	Dose by subcutaneous injection
certoparin	Alphaparin	3000 units 1–2 hours before surgery, then 3000 units daily 7–10 days
dalteparin	Fragmin	2500 units before surgery, then 2500 units daily 5–7 days
enoxaparin	Clexane	2000 units before surgery, then 2000 units daily 7–10 days
tinzaparin[1]	Innohep	3500 units before surgery, then 3500 units 7–10 days

[1]This product contains sulphites; in asthmatic and hypersensitive patients it may precipitate bronchospasm and shock.
Danaparin (Orgaron) is a heparinoid with similar actions and uses. It is given in doses of 750 units subcutaneously 1–4 hours before surgery; later twice daily for 7–10 days.

In practice, when an immediate anticoagulant action is required, therapy is commenced with both heparin and an orally active drug and the former continued for 48 hours, after which heparin may be discontinued, as by that time the oral anticoagulant drug should have become effective. In all cases, laboratory control of dose in relation to the prothrombin time in terms of the International Normalized Ratio (INR) is essential throughout treatment. Omission of dose requires reassessment of the prothrombin time. All patients receiving anticoagulant therapy should have an official treatment booklet.

Warfarin § (dose: 3–10 mg daily)

Brand name: Marevan §

Warfarin is a coumarin derivative that is widely used as an orally active anticoagulant in the treatment and prevention of venous thrombosis and pulmonary embolism, in the treatment of transient cerebral ischaemia, and to prevent the formation of clots on prosthetic heart valves. It is also used prophylactically against deep-vein thrombosis in high-risk surgery.

Warfarin is usually given as an initial dose of 10 mg daily for 2 days, and subsequent doses are designed to maintain the INR between 2 and 3 for prophylaxis, with a higher ratio in deep vein thrombosis and pulmonary embolism. Maintenance doses range from 3 to 9 mg daily, best taken at the same time every day. Warfarin is usually well tolerated, and is regarded as a first-choice drug, but it should be used with care in hepatic and renal disease and after surgery. It is contra-indicated in pregnancy, severe hypertension, or any potentially haemorrhagic condition.

Side-effects include nausea, alopecia and skin reactions, but the most serious side-effect is haemorrhage from almost any organ of the body. Early signs of overdose are bleeding from the gums and the presence of erythrocytes in the urine, but severe haemorrhage requires withdrawal of the drug, and the administration by slow intravenous injection of phytomenadione (vitamin K_1) in a dose of 5 mg, together with a blood factor product (see p. 288) or up to 1 litre of fresh frozen plasma. In less severe overdose, phytomenadione may be given orally in doses of 2–20 mg. Phytomenadione has a slow action that may take up to 12 hours to develop and may persist for as long as 2 weeks or more.

The action of warfarin may be modified by many other drugs, including aspirin and anti-inflammatory drugs such as the NSAIDs. The anticoagulant action is reduced by rifampicin and griseofulvin, and poten-

tiated by clofibrate and related drugs, by sulphonamides and some antibiotics, and combined treatment requires care.

Nicoumalone § (dose: 1–12 mg daily)

Brand name: Sinthrome §

Nicoumalone has the actions, uses and side-effects of warfarin but is used much less frequently. A standard scheme of dosage is a single dose of 8–12 mg on the first day of treatment, 4–8 mg on the second day, followed by maintenance doses of 1–8 mg or more daily, under laboratory control.

Phenindione § (dose: 50–200 mg daily)

Brand name: Dindevan §

Phenindione was once the most widely used of the oral anticoagulants, but it has now been largely replaced and is mainly used for patients who cannot tolerate warfarin. Treatment is commenced with a dose of 200 mg, followed by 100 mg on the second day, with maintenance doses of 50–150 mg according to laboratory reports of the prothrombin time.

Side-effects It may colour the urine pink. Phenindione may cause hypersensitivity reactions, ulcerative colitis, renal and hepatic damage and agranulocytosis.

Nursing points about oral anticoagulants

(a) The dose should be taken about the same time every day to avoid changes in the blood level of the anticoagulant.
(b) Clotting times must be closely monitored.
(c) Observe any unusual bruising or bleeding such as bleeding from nose or gums; tarry stools; excessive menstrual flow.
(d) Patients should be advised not to make any substantial alterations in their diet.
(e) Alcoholic beverages are best avoided; they may reduce the absorption of vitamin K.
(f) Patients should be advised to avoid aspirin, and not to take any other non-prescribed product without informing their doctor.
(g) Patients must always carry some indication that they are taking an anticoagulant, and inform a dentist before treatment.

PLATELET AGGREGATION INHIBITORS

Conventional anticoagulants are of value in the prophylaxis and treatment of venous thrombosis, but have little influence on thrombus formation on the arterial side of the circulation. Increasing attention has been turned towards the development of drugs that inhibit platelet aggregation and adhesion, and thus prevent clot formation in the arterial circulation.

Platelet aggregation is normally controlled by a balance between thromboxane A_2 (TXA_2) which is present in the platelets and induces aggregation, and prostacyclin, found mainly in the vascular endothelium, which has the opposite effect. Platelets stick to each other and to areas of vascular epithelium damaged by hypertension or disease by linkage with adhesive glycoproteins. Such glycoproteins are normally contained within the intact lining of the epithelium, but are released by damage, and the platelets thus activated also release TXA_2, and so start the chain reaction that leads to the development of a thrombus (Fig. 8.1).

Aspirin (dose: 75–300 mg daily)

Aspirin has an antiplatelet action mediated by binding with cyclo-oxygenase (see p. 206) and so preventing the formation of TXA_2. The binding is irreversible, as the platelets are unable to synthesize new cyclo-oxygenase, and new platelets must be formed before aggregation ability is restored, a process that takes 7–10 days. By the same binding action aspirin inhibits the formation of prostacyclin, but the effect is reversible and so less prolonged, as the vascular epithelium has the ability to re-synthesize cyclo-oxygenase. However, the amount of aspirin required to inhibit platelet activity is less than that needed to inhibit prostacyclin synthesis, which may explain why low doses of aspirin are sometimes given in antiplatelet therapy.

Aspirin is used for the secondary prophylaxis of myocardial infarction and cerebrovascular disease, although the optimum dose is open to question as it is given in doses of 75–300 mg daily. It is also used for the prevention of occlusion after by-pass surgery, and may be of value in the management of venous leg ulcer. The **side-effects** of aspirin are referred to on p. 54. Products containing 75 mg of aspirin are Angettes and Caprin.

Dipyridamole § (dose: 300–600 mg daily)

Brand name: Persantin §
Dipyridamole is given in doses of 100–200 mg three times a day, and its antithrombotic action is mediated by enhancing the action of prostacyclin and by inhibiting the enzyme phosphodiesterase (see enoximone, p. 104). It is used, together with anti-

coagulants, for the prevention of thrombosis in prosthetic heart valves. It has also been given in doses of 50 mg three times a day for the treatment of chronic angina.

Side-effects are nausea, diarrhoea, headache and rash.

Epoprostenol §

Brand name: Flolan §
Epoprostenol, also known as prostacyclin, is a prostaglandin produced in the intima of blood vessels and it is the most potent inhibitor of platelet aggregation yet known. It has a very short half-life (2–3 minutes), and must be given by continuous intravenous infusion. It is used mainly to inhibit platelet aggregation during renal dialysis. Specialist literature should be consulted for details of dose and preparation of the injection solution.

Abciximab §

Brand name: ReoPro §
Abciximab is a monoclonal antibody that selectively binds with glycoproteins on the surface of platelets, and so prevents platelets aggregating together to form a thrombus. It is used as an adjunct to heparin and aspirin for the prevention of cardiac ischaemic complications in patients undergoing percutaneous transluminal coronary angioplasty (PTCA), where there is a risk of the abrupt closure of the treated vessel. It is given initially as a bolus intravenous dose of 0.25 mg/kg, followed by doses of 10 micrograms per minute by continuous infusion for 12 hours, together with heparin therapy. See specialist literature.

FIBRINOLYTIC AGENTS

In health, the small blood clots that are formed as part of the natural repair process of the vascular system are broken down by plasmin, a fibrinolytic agent derived from plasminogen by an activator present in the vascular endothelium. If clotting activity is excessive, deep vein thrombosis and pulmonary embolism may occur. In such conditions, normal fibrinolysis can be increased by treatment with plasminogen activators, which by an enzymatic action break down the fibrin into small soluble peptides which are swept away in the blood stream (Fig. 8.2).

Early use is essential, and in acute myocardial infarction the anticipated response should be balanced against the risks of treatment.

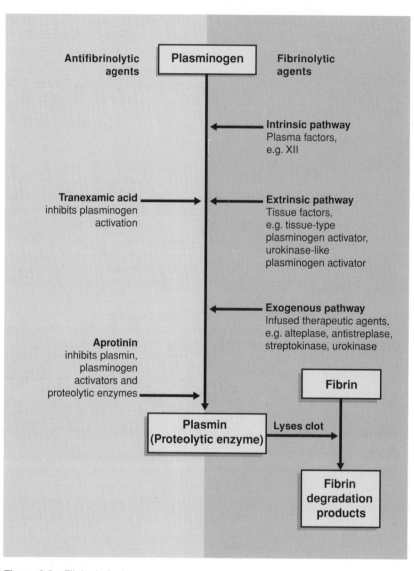

Figure 8.2   Fibrinolysis.

Alteplase § (dose: 10–15 mg initially)

Brand name: Actilyse §

Alteplase is a recombinant form of human plasminogen activator, and so has the advantage of being non-antigenic. It is given intravenously and is virtually inactive until it reaches and binds to fibrin, for which it has an increased affinity. Such binding activates the digestive properties of plasmin and causes a breakdown of the occlusive clot. In myocardial infarction it is given within 6–10 hours as an initial intravenous dose of 10–15 mg, followed by a dose of 50 mg by intravenous infusion over one hour, then four doses of 10 mg at 30 minute intervals up to a total dose of 100 mg over three hours. In pulmonary embolism the initial dose of 10 mg is followed by the infusion of 90 mg over 2 hours. Delayed treatment is less effective.

Side-effects   include nausea, vomiting and bleeding. Bleeding can be severe and include cerebral haemorrhage requiring withdrawal of the drug and anticoagulant/antifibrinolytic therapy. Contraindications are cardiovascular disease, severe hypertension and surgery.

Anistreplase § (dose: 30 units)

Brand name: Eminase §

Anistreplase is an inactive complex of plasminogen and streptokinase, used in myocardial infarction as a fibrinolytic agent. Following intravenous injection it binds firmly to the fibrin clot, and is then activated at a steady state within the occlusion to release free and active plasmin, leading to the breakdown and dissolution of the clot. Anistreplase is given as a single dose of 30 units by intravenous injection over 4–5 minutes as soon as possible after the infarction, and not more than six hours after.

Side-effects are similar to those of other plasminogen activators. The development of antistreptokinase antibodies limits repeated treatment for at least six months.

Stanozolol § (dose: 10 mg)

Brand name Stromba §

Stanolzolol is a steroid with some fibrinolytic properties. It is used in the treatment of the vasculitis of Behçet's disease. Dose 10 mg daily.

Streptokinase § (dose: 100 000–1 500 000 units)

Brand names: Kabikinase §; Streptase §

Streptokinase is a protein obtained from cultures of beta-haemolytic streptococci. It combines with plasminogen and activates the fibrinolytic system, and so promotes the dissolution of intravascular thrombi and pulmonary emboli. It is used mainly in the treatment of deep vein thrombosis, acute arterial thromboembolism and severe pulmonary embolism. Streptokinase is given by intravenous infusion as a loading dose of 250 000 units over 30–60 minutes, followed by maintenance doses of 100 000 units hourly for 24–72 hours. Further treatment, if required, should be continued for not more than three more days. In myocardial infarction doses of 150 000 units are given with aspirin 150 mg daily as supportive therapy, continued for at least four weeks. Occasionally streptokinase has been given by direct intracoronary injection.

Streptokinase should not be used after recent surgery, nor in early pregnancy as it may cause placental separation. Its use should be avoided after any streptococcal infection as the blood may then contain streptokinase-neutralizing antibodies; for the same reason a second course of streptokinase therapy should not be given for at least six months.

Side-effects include anaphylactic reactions, fever, rash and haemorrhage. The latter, if severe, can be controlled by tranexamic acid (see p. 138).

Urokinase § (dose: 4400 units/kg; 5000 units)

Urokinase is an enzyme obtained from male urine that has fibrinolytic properties mediated by the activation of plasminogen to plasmin. It is given in deep vein thrombosis and pulmonary embolism in doses of 4400 units/kg hourly by intravenous infusion, but it is mainly of value in the dispersal of blood clots in the eye, particularly when the anterior chamber is filled and there is a rise in the intraocular pressure. A solution containing 5000 units of urokinase is injected into the clot, and following disintegration of the clot the cavity is washed out with saline. Urokinase is also used to clear arteriovenous shunts by the instillation of 5000–25 000 units in 2–3 ml of saline solution.

As urokinase is of human origin, it is non-antigenic.

HAEMOSTATICS AND ANTIFIBRINOLYTIC AGENTS

Bleeding from wound surfaces can be reduced by direct application of adrenaline solution to the wound, or by the use of calcium-sodium-alginate dressings (p. 300). In surgery, menorrhagia and other haemorrhagic conditions, local treatment is not possible and reliance is placed on drugs that have an inhibitory action on fibrinolysis.

Aprotinin § (dose: 500 000–1 000 000 units)

Brand name: Trasylol §

Aprotinin is a polypeptide obtained from bovine lung tissue. It inhibits the action of various proteolytic enzymes such as trypsin, plasmin and plasmin activators, and so has haemostatic properties. It is used to prevent excessive blood loss during open heart surgery with extracorporeal circulation, in haemophiliacs, in Jehovah's Witnesses, in patients with blood dyscrasias, and in life-threatening haemorrhage due to hyperplasminaemia. It is also used to reduce an excessive response to streptokinase.

In surgery aprotinin is given by slow intravenous infusion as a dose of 2 million units, of which 50 000 units should be given initially to reveal any hypersensitivity to the drug. Maintenance doses of 500 000 units are given hourly during the operation. In hyperplasminaemia an initial dose of 500 000 units is given, followed by doses of 200 000 units until the bleeding is controlled. At any sign of a hypersensitivity reaction, treatment must be stopped and anti-allergic drugs given immediately. Local thrombophlebitis may occur at the injection site.

Ethamsylate § (dose: 2 g daily)

Brand name: Dicynene §
Ethamsylate is a synthetic agent that does not influence normal clotting mechanisms, but appears to act by maintaining the stability of the vascular walls, increasing the degree of platelet adhesion and by inhibiting the action of those prostaglandins that reduce platelet aggregation. It is used to control bleeding due to damage of small blood vessels during surgery, and in menorrhagia and haematuria. In menorrhagia treatment should be given as soon as the bleeding starts, as premenstrual use is not recommended. Ethamsylate is given orally in doses of 500 mg four times a day, or in severe conditions by intramuscular/intravenous injection in doses of 500 mg every 4–6 hours. Doses of 12.5 mg/kg are given by injection 6-hourly to low birth weight infants for the prophylaxis and treatment of periventricular haemorrhage. Occasional **side-effects** include nausea, headache and rash.

Tranexamic acid § (dose: 2–6 g daily)

Brand name: Cyklokapron §
Tranexamic acid acts as an antifibrinolytic agent by inhibiting the conversion of plasminogen to plasmin. It is used to control the haemorrhage due to local fibrinolysis associated with prostatectomy, menorrhagia, epistaxis and in the dental treatment of haemophiliacs. The standard dose of tranexamic acid is 1–1.5 g two or three times a day; in severe conditions it is given in doses of 0.5–1 g three times a day by intravenous injection, followed by oral therapy. **Side-effects** are gastrointestinal disturbances, which subside with a reduction in dose.

SOME BLOOD PRODUCTS USED AS HAEMOSTATICS

Some of the factors concerned with the formation of a blood clot are shown in Fig. 8.1, and certain products containing one or more of those factors have a limited use as haemostatics. They are mainly used in haemophilia and other factor-deficiency conditions.

Human fibrin and thrombin

Human fibrin formed by mixing fibrinogen and thrombin can be prepared as a dry, spongy product. It is used occasionally as a haemostatic in surgery, where bleeding cannot be controlled by other methods. Fibrin glue is a mixture of fibrinogen, thrombin, other blood factors and aprotinin that is applied as a spray to bleeding surfaces.

Factor VIII

A deficiency of Factor VIII is the cause of haemophilia A. Concentrated preparations of that factor obtained from plasma have been used as replacement therapy, but have caused allergic reactions due to the presence of fibrinogen. More highly purified products are now available, such as Monoclate-P § and Replenate §. Recently, recombinant forms of Factor VIII have been introduced, with which the risks of allergy and the transmission of blood-borne viruses are avoided (Kogenate § ▼, Recombinate § ▼).

The dose of Factor VIII products is based on the degree of deficiency, the weight of the patient and the severity of the bleeding.

Factor IX

A deficiency of Factor IX is the cause of haemophilia B (Christmas disease). Alphanine §, Mononine § and Replenine § are highly purified preparations of that factor, and although they may contain other clotting factors, they are less likely to cause allergic reactions than the older, less purified products. The dose is based on the degree of Factor VIII deficiency.

Factor VIIa

Factors VIII and IX are converted to activated forms in the circulation, and haemophiliac patients may develop neutralizing antibodies that inhibit activation and and so affect the response to treatment. Factor VIIa bypasses that neutralizing action, as it acts at a later stage in the conversion of fibrinogen to fibrin, functions independently of Factors VIII and IX, and does not induce antibody formation. It has a local action, and forms a haemostatic plug at the haemorrhagic site. It is used to control serious bleeding in haemophiliac patients, and during surgery, but requires specialist supervision (Novoseven § ▼).

FURTHER READING

Apple S 1996 New trends in thrombolytic therapy. Registered Nurse 59(1):30–35

Auer I K 1996 The role of pharmacologic agents in blood conservation. AACN Clinical Issues 7(2):260–276

Bonnar J, Sheppard B L 1996 Treatment of menorrhagia during menstruation: randomised controlled trial of ethamsylate, mefenamic acid and tranexamic acid. British Medical Journal 313:579–582

Brigden M L 1992 Oral anticoagulant therapy. Postgraduate Medicine 91(2):285–296

Butler M 1995 Use of anticoagulants in hospital and community. Nursing Times 91(13):36–37

Hirsh J 1991 Heparin. New England Journal of Medicine 324:1565–1574

Kessler C M 1991 The pharmacology of aspirin, heparin, coumarin and thrombolytic agents. Chest (Suppl) 99(4):97S–112S

Layton A, Ibbotson S, Davies J A, Goodfield M 1994 Randomised trial of oral aspirin for chronic venous leg ulcers. Lancet 344:164–165

Prandoni P et al 1992 Subcutaneous low-molecular-weight heparin compared with intravenous standard heparin in the treatment of proximal vein thrombosis. Lancet 339:441–445

Sandercock P A G et al 1997 The international stroke trial (IST): a randomised trial of aspirin, subcutaneous heparin, both, or neither among 19 435 patients with acute ischaemic stroke. Lancet 349:1569–1581

Scott A K 1989 Prescribing anticoagulants. Prescribers' Journal 29:24–30

Tuten S H, Gueldner S H 1991 Efficacy of sodium chloride versus dilute heparin for maintenance of peripheral intermittent intravenous devices. Applied Nursing Research 4(2):63–71

Workman M L 1994 Anticoagulants and thrombolytics: what's the difference? AACN Clinical Issues 5(1):26–35

9

Anti-anaemic and haematopoietic agents and drugs used in neutropenia

Anaemia can be broadly defined as an insufficiency of mature red cells in the blood. The most frequent and important cause is impaired blood formation, but excessive blood loss or destruction of red cells may also lead to anaemia. Red blood cells develop in the bone marrow from megaloblastic stem cells which form pro-erythroblasts, which later diminish in size, acquire haemoglobin and form normoblasts. Later still the normoblasts lose the nucleus and form reticulocytes, which mature into erythrocytes (Fig. 9.1). The main function of the erythrocytes is to transport oxygen from the lungs to the tissues, and convey carbon dioxide away from the tissues. The oxygen transport molecule is haemoglobin, an iron-containing protein enclosed in a lipid membrane within the erythrocytes. Many factors are concerned with formation of haemoglobin-carrying red blood cells, including thyroxine, adrenocorticotrophic hormone, erythropoietin, vitamins, iron and other minerals, and the absence of any of those factors may result in some degree of anaemia.

IRON-DEFICIENCY ANAEMIA

Iron-deficiency anaemia is the most common type of anaemia and results from reduced dietary intake, impaired absorption, excessive blood loss, or pregnancy. The dietary intake of iron should be about 10–15 mg daily to replace the 1–2 mg lost daily in the urine and faeces, and in women the 30 mg lost monthly in menstruation. The intake of iron must be greater than the loss because much dietary iron is in the ferric non-absorbable state, and is excreted bound to phosphates and phytates in the faeces. Only a small amount of ferric iron is reduced to the ferrous state by gastric acid and made available for absorp-

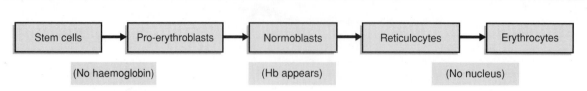

Figure 9.1   Red blood cell development.

tion, and even that small amount may be reduced if antacids are taken. The absorption of iron is a function of the intestinal mucosa, and is a complex process. When the iron stores of the body are low, iron is absorbed and transported by a plasma protein as transferrin, or is combined with a protein (apoferritin) to form ferritin, in which form iron is stored in the body within a protein shell (Fig. 9.2). When the body stores of iron are adequate, there is little apoferritin available for iron uptake, a condition referred to as the mucosal block, and the surplus dietary iron is excreted in the faeces. When the iron stores are low, ferritin is released and enters the circulation as the iron–protein complex transferrin, and is converted to haemoglobin in the bone marrow, and to myoglobin and iron-containing enzymes in the tissues. Ferritin also functions as a recycling agent, as it is concerned with the re-use of iron made available by the breakdown of dead red cells. Apart from the normal loss of iron already referred to, the body has no mechanism for the excretion of excess iron, so iron overload may occur as the result of repeated blood transfusion.

The treatment of iron deficiency is basically replacement therapy, and the following products are in use.

Ferrous sulphate (prophylactic dose: 200 mg daily; therapeutic dose: 600–900 mg daily)

Ferrous sulphate is one of the most widely used therapeutic forms of iron, as it is soluble, effective and inexpensive. It is usually given as tablets containing 200 mg, equivalent to 60 mg of elemental iron. The drug is astringent and may cause occasional gastric disturbance, which can be reduced by taking the tablets after food. Ferrous sulphate may also be given in solution as Ferrous Sulphate Oral Solution (Paediatric Ferrous Sulphate Mixture) which is a very suitable product for the administration of iron to small children. Iron salts should not be given with the tetracycline group of antibiotics, as the absorption of both drugs may be mutually reduced.

Many alternatives have been introduced with the aim of reducing the side-effects associated with ferrous sulphate, although some better tolerated products merely contain smaller doses of iron. A few, such as Feospan, Ferrograd and Slow-Fe contain ferrous sulphate in a slow-release form.

Tablets of ferrous sulphate are usually coated to prevent oxidation, and have been taken by children in mistake for sweets. Such an overdose may cause severe gastrointestinal damage, leading to haematemesis, shock and hypotension. Severe liver damage and coma may occur later. Many deaths have occurred in small children from this cause. Immediate treatment includes gastric lavage and intravenous desferrioxamine (Desferal). See p. 312. Desferrioxamine is a chelating agent that binds iron as a water-soluble non-toxic complex which is excreted in the urine. Iron overload may also occur after repeated blood transfusions, and desferrioxamine has been given in doses up to 2 g with each transfusion. It is also given by subcutaneous infusion in doses of 20–40 mg/kg daily for 5–7 days. The effects in iron overload can be increased by the oral use of ascorbic acid (vitamin C) in doses of 200 mg daily between meals. Desferrioxamine is also useful in the treatment of aluminium overload in patients on maintenance haemodialysis.

Ferrous gluconate (prophylactic dose: 600 mg daily; therapeutic dose: 1.2–1.8 g daily)

Ferrous gluconate has the same action as ferrous sulphate, but is less irritant and is often acceptable when ferrous sulphate is not tolerated. Weight for weight it contains less iron than the sulphate, so that larger doses are required (300 mg is equivalent to 35 mg of iron).

Ferrous gluconate is present in a number of proprietary iron preparations, many of which contain vitamins. Such vitamin supplements, with the exception of vitamin C, do not increase the absorption of iron and are of little therapeutic value.

Other iron salts

Ferrous fumarate and ferrous succinate are other iron salts with reduced side-effects, and are present in a number of proprietary anti-anaemic preparations. They are useful for patients who cannot tolerate other forms of iron, but have few other advantages.

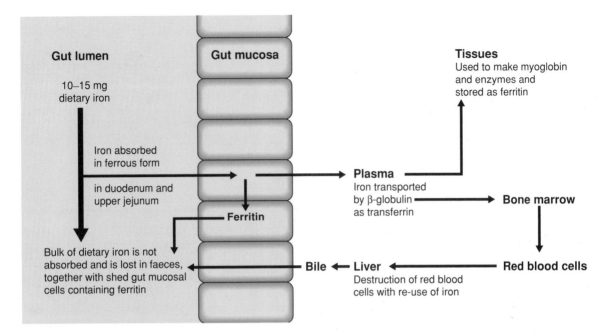

Figure 9.2 Transportation and utilization of iron.

Sodium iron-edetate (Sytron) is a liquid preparation in which the iron is combined as an organic complex. It breaks down in the body and releases the iron in an absorbable form. It is useful when gastric intolerance to other oral iron preparations is severe. Niferex is a similar product in which iron is bound as a polysaccharide complex.

Some iron deficiency is common in pregnancy, and if associated with a folic acid deficiency, it may manifest itself in late pregnancy as a folate-deficiency-megaloblastic anaemia. Several preparations of iron and folic acid are now available for prophylactic use throughout pregnancy, and are often used routinely. A representative product is Pregaday, but the use of such a preparation in older patients is not advised, as in undiagnosed pernicious anaemia, neurological symptoms could be precipitated.

Iron-sorbitol injection § (1 ml = 50 mg iron)

Brand name: Jectofer §

Iron-sorbitol injection is a stabilized complex of iron, sorbitol and citric acid. It is given in severe iron deficiency, or when oral iron is not tolerated or when the patient fails to cooperate with standard treatment. It is given under haematological control in doses equivalent to 1.5 mg/kg of iron daily by deep intramuscular injection, the total dose being based on the degree of iron deficiency. Oral iron should be discontinued before injection therapy is commenced.

Deep intramuscular injection is necessary to reduce the risk of subcutaneous staining, and should be made only into the muscle mass of the upper and outer quadrant of the buttock, employing a Z-track injection technique. That involves a lateral displacement of the skin before the needle is inserted, and after injection of the drug, pausing for a few seconds before withdrawing the needle. That will allow the muscle mass to accommodate the volume of the injection, and so minimize the risk of leakage up the injection track. To further minimize the risk, the patient should be warned not to rub the injection site.

PERNICIOUS ANAEMIA

A progressive, megaloblastic and macrocytic anaemia, resistant to iron therapy, may occur even when an adequate diet is taken, and its failure to respond to treatment led to the disease being described as 'pernicious anaemia'. In 1926 it was discovered that raw liver could relieve some of the symptoms, and later it was found that the anti-anaemic factor present in liver was vitamin B_{12} (cyanocobalamin). Dietary vitamin B_{12}, sometimes termed the extrinsic factor, is absorbed from the terminal ileum after combination with the intrinsic factor secreted by the parietal cells of the stomach. After absorption, the B_{12}-intrinsic factor complex is stored in the liver and released as required for red cell formation in the bone marrow (Fig. 9.3).

Pernicious anaemia is basically a deficiency disease caused by an inability to absorb vitamin B_{12}, and the most common cause is a lack of production of the intrinsic factor, which may be due to atrophic gastritis, autoimmune disease, or as a consequence of gastric or intestinal surgery. The deficiency of vitamin B_{12} not only causes pernicious anaemia, but may also result in neurological damage, such as degeneration of the spinal cord. Treatment is replacement therapy by injections of vitamin B_{12}, usually as hydroxocobalamin.

Hydroxocobalamin § (dose: 1 mg by injection)

Brand names: Neo-Cytamen §, Cobalin-H §
Hydroxocobalamin is the preferred form of vitamin B_{12} as it has a longer action than cyanocobalamin. It binds more firmly with specific plasma proteins, and is excreted more slowly. In vitamin B_{12} deficiency states it is given in initial doses of 1 mg by intramuscular injection, repeated at intervals of 2–3 days until a total dose of 5 mg has been given. Subsequent maintenance doses of 1 mg are then given at 3-monthly intervals, usually for life. It is also given prophylactically after gastrectomy. Hydroxocobalamin is also used in the megaloblastosis that occurs after prolonged inhalation of nitrous oxide, as the gas inactivates vitamin B_{12}.

Cyanocobalamin § (dose: 250 micrograms–1 mg by injection)

Brand names: Cytamen §, Cytacon §
Cyanocobalamin, originally extracted from liver, is obtained as a by-product of the growth of various microorganisms. It has been given in doses of 1 mg monthly by intramuscular injection. It is of no value orally.

Folic acid § (dose: 200 micrograms–5 mg)

Folic acid is a member of the vitamin B complex, and is one of the many factors concerned in blood formation, particularly the maturation of red blood cells. Deficiency of folic acid may lead to a megaloblastic anaemia, and the administration of folic acid is of value in dietary deficiency anaemias, and in some disturbances of fat metabolism such as tropical sprue. Folic acid is also used prophylactically during pregnancy, and is given in doses of 200–500 micrograms daily, usually with iron (p. 143). When given to prevent neural tube defect, doses of 5 mg daily should be taken and continued until the twelfth week of pregnancy. Folic acid was used at one time in the treatment of pernicious anaemia, but such use may precipitate degeneration of the spinal cord and has been abandoned.

HAEMATOPOIETIC AND ANABOLIC AGENTS

Erythropoietin §

Brand names: Eprex §, Recormon §
Erythropoietin is a glycoprotein hormone synthesized in the renal cortical cells, and is the main regulator of red blood cell production. The kidneys are sensitive to the amount of oxygen in the circulation, and hypoxia of kidney tissue leads to the release of erythropoietin which reaches the bone marrow and stimulates the pro-erythroblasts to mature more quickly into reticulocytes. The process is controlled by a feedback mechanism (see Fig. 9.4).

The main clinical use of erythropoietin is the treatment of patients with end-stage renal failure, where normal production of the hormone has broken down as the kidney cells are largely destroyed, resulting in severe chronic anaemia. The condition may deteriorate still further, as such patients are often maintained by haemodialysis which is associated with further blood loss, and so erythropoietin must be provided exogenously. The natural hormone is not readily available, but large amounts are now obtained by recombinant DNA technology and referred to as epoietin.

Two forms of epoietin are available, epoietin alpha and epoietin beta, and the dose varies to some extent according to the product used; although they are clinically interchangeable, the prescriber must specify the type required. Close haematological control is necessary during erythropoietin therapy, and specialist literature should be consulted for dosage details. Any deficiency

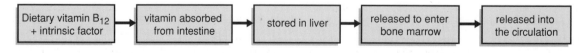

Figure 9.3   Outline of vitamin B_{12} absorption and release.

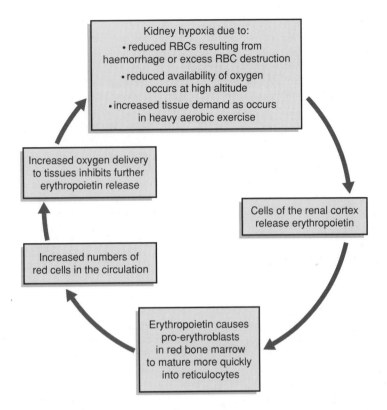

Figure 9.4 Negative feedback regulation of erythropoiesis.

of iron or folate should be dealt with before treatment with epoetin therapy is commenced.

Other therapeutic applications of epoietin include the anaemia of cancer chemotherapy, and the anaemia of premature babies of low birth-weight. Such infants lack both epoietin and adequate red blood cells. Epoietin may also have applications in the treatment of the anaemia associated with chronic inflammatory conditions such as rheumatoid arthritis.

Side-effects include headache, a dose-dependent increase in blood pressure and influenza-like symptoms. A sudden migraine-like pain may be a warning of an incipient hypertensive crisis. Seizures have occurred in patients with poor renal function.

DRUGS USED IN NEUTROPENIA

Neutropenia is an abnormal reduction in the number of circulating neutrophils, one of the forms of leuco-cytes concerned with phagocytosis and the removal of invading bacteria. In neutropenia, which is often caused by depression of bone-marrow activity by cytotoxic drugs, the risks of infection are correspond-

ingly increased. The production of neutrophils and other blood cells is regulated in part by the granulocyte-macrophage-colony-stimulating factor (GM-CSF), which stimulates the development of blood cell progenitors, and more selectively by the granulocyte-colony-stimulating factor (G-CSF), which promotes neutrophil development only. Recombinant forms of those factors are now used to stimulate neutrophil production, and to reduce the risks of infection associated with the neutropenia caused by cancer chemotherapy, bone marrow transplantation and advanced HIV infection. They are used only under expert supervision.

Filgrastim § ▼ (dose: 500 000 units/kg)

Brand name: Neupogen § ▼
Filgrastim is a recombinant form of G-CSF, and is given in doses of 500 000 units/kg daily by subcutaneous injection or intravenous infusion beginning not less than 24 hours after the end of chemotherapy. The injections should be continued until the normal neutrophil count has been restored, which may take up to 2 weeks.

Side-effects are muscle pain and dysuria.

Lenograstim § ▼ (dose: 150 micrograms (19.2 million units)/m² daily)

Brand name: Granocyte § ▼

Lenograstim is another recombinant form of G-CSF with the actions and uses of filgrastim. In the treatment of drug-associated neutropenia in malignancy it is given in daily doses of 150 micrograms/m² of body area by subcutaneous injection, commenced the day after the end of the course of chemotherapy. Treatment should be continued until the neutrophil count has reached a satisfactory level for up to a maximum of 28 days. A similar course is given by slow intravenous injection after bone marrow transplantation.

Molgramostim § ▼ (dose: 60 000–110 000 units/kg)

Brand name: Leucomax § ▼

Molgramostim is a recombinant form of GM-CSF, and is similar in actions and uses to filgrastim and lenograstim. In cytotoxic chemotherapy it is given subcutaneously in doses of 60 000–110 000 units/kg daily, starting 24 hours after the end of such treatment, and continued for 7–10 days. Similar doses are given as an adjunct to treatment with ganciclovir. In bone marrow transplantation a dose of 110 000 units/kg is given daily by intravenous infusion after transplantation for up to 30 days. Blood counts are necessary during lenograstim treatment.

Side-effects are numerous – see specialist literature.

Amifostine § ▼ (dose: 910 mg/m²)

Brand name: Ethylol § ▼

Amifostine is a different type of antineutropenic agent, as it is an organic thiophosphate with a cytoprotective action. It can prevent or minimize the myelosuppressive and nephrotoxic effects of cancer chemotherapy, as it protects normal cells from exposure to such therapy, without affecting the susceptibility of cancer cells to such attack. It is used mainly in advanced ovarian cancer treated with cyclophosphamide or cisplatin to reduce the risks of neutropenia-related infection. Amifostine is given by intravenous infusion as a once daily dose of 910 mg/m², given 30 minutes before chemotherapy. The infusion should be stopped if any significant fall in blood pressure occurs, but it can be restarted if the blood pressure returns to normal within five minutes. Any anti-emetic therapy should be given previously. See specialist literature.

Nandrolone § (dose: 50–100 mg weekly)

Brand name: Deca-Durabolin §

Anabolic steroids such as nandrolone have been used in high doses for the treatment of aplastic and haemolytic anaemias, but the mode of action is not clear and the response is variable. It is given in doses of 50–100 mg weekly by deep intramuscular injection. Treatment for 3–6 months is necessary, and with such long therapy, virilizing **side-effects** are likely to occur.

GLUCOSE 6-PHOSPHATE DEHYDROGENASE DEFICIENCY

One form of haemolytic anaemia, found in some African and Asian populations and also known to occur in the Mediterranean area, is due to a deficiency of the enzyme glucose 6-phosphate dehydrogenase (G6PD). That enzyme plays a key role in red blood cell (RBC) activity and integrity, and a deficiency of G6PD, which occurs mainly but not exclusively in males, leads to an increased sensitivity of the RBCs to oxidative breakdown by certain drugs, resulting in a haemolytic anaemia. The degree of susceptibility is subject to individual variation, and may be dose-related to some extent, but care is necessary in treating any patient known to be G6PD deficient with sulphonamides, nalidixic acid and other quinolones, dapsone, nitrofurantoin, primaquine, pamaquin and methylene blue. Some patients may also be susceptible to aspirin, chloroquine, menadione, quinine and quinidine.

FURTHER READING

Bergstrom J 1993 New aspects of erythropoietin treatment. Journal of International Medicine 223:445–462

Fried W 1995 Erythropoietin. Annual Review of Nutrition 15:353–377

Temple R M 1994 Uses of epoetin in the management of renal anaemia. Hospital Update 20(3):165–171

Wald N J, Bower C 1995 Folic acid and the prevention of neural tube defects. British Medical Journal 310:1019–1020

Watson N J, Hutchinson C H, Atta H R 1995 Vitamin A deficiency and xerophthalmia in the United Kingdom. British Medical Journal 310:1050–1051

Wimberley T H, Parks B 1991 Iron preparations: it's elementary my dear. Pediatric Nursing 17(3):274–275

Winearls C G et al 1986 Effects of human erythropoietin derived from recombinant DNA on the anaemia of patients maintained by chronic haemodialysis. Lancet ii:1175–1178

10

Drugs acting on the gastrointestinal tract

Gastrointestinal disturbance is a common affliction, and its frequency is matched by the variety of preparations available to treat it. These preparations vary widely in nature and pharmacological properties, and will be considered under the headings antacids, carminatives and bitters, peptic ulcer healing agents, anti-emetics, intestinal sedatives, adsorbents and laxatives.

ANTACIDS

Antacids are used to reduce gastric acidity and provide symptomatic relief in gastritis, heartburn and other forms of hyperacidity. The ideal antacid would reduce gastric acidity but not neutralize it, as otherwise a compensatory over-secretion of acid might occur. It should also have a long action without side-effects. In practice, however, mixtures of antacids are often used to obtain the best response, and many proprietary antacids are available. In some the action is augmented by the inclusion of auxilliary drugs such as atropine to reduce gastric spasm, or by dimethicone to reduce foaming and flatulence by causing gas bubbles to collapse. Gastric reflux can be reduced by products containing alginic acid such as Gaviscon, which reacts with gastric acid to form a gel that protects the stomach and oesophagus from acid attack. In the past, antacids were widely used for the treatment of peptic ulcer, but they have been superseded for that purpose by the histamine H_2-receptor antagonists (p. 148). Recently, some of these antagonists have become over-the-counter products and are now promoted as 'antacids'.

Aluminium hydroxide

Brand names: Aludrox, Alu-cap
Aluminium hydroxide, usually used as aluminium

hydroxide gel or mixture (dose: 5–10 ml) but also available as capsules and tablets, has antacid properties that are useful in the treatment of dyspepsia. It has a slow and extended action with few side-effects, but unlike magnesium-based antacids it may cause constipation. Magaldrate (Dynese) is a complex of aluminium and magnesium hydroxides and sulphates available as a suspension containing 800 mg per 5 ml. It is given in dyspepsia in doses of 5–10 ml after food, and at night.

Nursing points about antacids

(a) Used for the symptomatic relief of ulcer and non-ulcer dyspepsia and similar conditions.
(b) Often best taken between meals.
(c) Should not be taken with other drugs as they may reduce absorption or form insoluble complexes.
(d) May affect the special coating of some slow-absorption products.

Calcium carbonate (dose: 1–5 g)

Chalk is natural calcium carbonate and has a useful and extended antacid action. It is often used in association with magnesium carbonate as Calcium Carbonate Compound Powder.

Magnesium carbonate (dose: 250–500 mg)

Magnesium carbonate is a slow-acting antacid and is a constituent of a wide range of proprietary products sold for dyspepsia and mild acidity. It is also used as Aromatic Magnesium Carbonate Mixture. Magnesium hydroxide (cream of magnesia) also has mild antacid action, but is used mainly as a laxative (p. 157).

Magnesium trisilicate (dose: 0.5–2 g)

Magnesium trisilicate has a slow and prolonged antacid action, as in the stomach it forms a gel which has a local protective action. It is usually given in association with magnesium carbonate and sodium bicarbonate as Compound Magnesium Trisilicate Mixture (BP) (dose: 10 ml) or Compound Magnesium Trisilicate Oral Powder (dose: 1–5 g).

Sodium bicarbonate (dose: 1–4 g)

Sodium bicarbonate is soluble in water and neutralizes gastric acid very quickly, with the evolution of carbon dioxide. Continued use may lead to alkalosis and rebound acid formation, and it is therefore seldom given alone except for the immediate relief of gastric pain. The carbon dioxide liberated in the stomach by the reaction of gastric acid with the sodium bicarbonate may also relieve distension as the gas is eructed, and such eructation is useful as a proof to the patient of the efficacy of the antacid.

CARMINATIVES AND BITTERS

These are survivors of traditional medicine. Carminatives produce a feeling of warmth in the stomach, and tend to relieve gastric distension by belching. They are represented by tincture of ginger and oil of peppermint, and are regaining some favour. Peppermint oil has a useful role in the treatment of dyspepsia and abdominal colic, and is being promoted for use in irritable bowel syndrome and as a colonic antispasmodic during endoscopy. It is available as Colpermin and Mintec capsules. Ginger root has been shown recently to have some anti-emetic properties, and has been given to reduce the incidence of nausea and vomiting after major gynaecological surgery. Bitters are vegetable products that promote a reflex secretion of gastric juice and so stimulate the appetite. Gentian is a traditional bitter, and is still in use as Alkaline Gentian Mixture and Acid Gentian Mixture.

PEPTIC ULCER-HEALING DRUGS

The term peptic ulcer refers to the mucosal erosion caused by the digestive action of gastric acid and pepsin, and includes stomach, duodenal and oesophageal ulcers. They are caused by an excessive production of hydrochloric acid or by an insufficient supply of mucus, as often happens in old age. Almost without exception, peptic ulcers do not develop in the absence of acid and the 'No-acid-no-ulcer' theory is the basis of anti-ulcer treatment; in the past, reliance was placed on the regular use of antacids.

However, a completely new approach to the control of acid secretion stemmed from the finding that the acid-producing parietal cells are stimulated by histamine. Yet conventional antihistamines used in the treatment of allergy have no influence on gastric acid production. The anomaly was solved when it was found that two types of histamine receptors exist, the H_1-receptors associated with allergy and the H_2-receptors concerned with the production of gastric acid. A search for selective H_2-receptor antagonists led to the introduction of cimetidine, which revolutionized the treatment of peptic ulcer. Such antagonists are now widely used in the control of benign gastric and duodenal ulcer and related disorders, as well as the Zollinger–Ellison syndrome, a rare condition caused by a gastrin-secreting tumour of the pancreas. They are also useful in the prophylaxis and treatment of gastric ulcers induced by non-steroidal anti-inflammatory drugs (NSAIDs).

The final stage in the formation of gastric acid is the movement of hydrogen ions into the gastric lumen in exchange for potassium ions, followed by combination with chloride ions to form hydrochloric acid. That exchange is mediated by the enzyme H^+K^+-ATPase, and the system is referred to as the proton pump. A selective inhibitor of that pump system would be free from some of the disadvantages of the H_2-receptor antagonists, and the first drug of that type was omeprazole. It is highly active and is particularly useful in patients with severe gastric hypersecretion, and in reflux oesophagitis with severe ulceration, a condition usually resistant to other drugs. Figure 10.1 indicates the sites of action of some ulcer-healing drugs.

An interesting twist in the treatment of peptic ulcer is the finding that a subsidiary problem is often an infection with *Helicobacter pylori*. It was once believed that no bacteria could survive in the acid conditions of the stomach, but *H. pylori* has a protective envelope. The eradication of *H. pylori* from the stomach requires intensive therapy with omeprazole, amoxycillin and/or metronidazole or clarithromycin. Eradication, once achieved, usually results in long-term remission, although reinfection remains a possibility.

In all cases, and especially in the elderly, the possibility of malignancy should be excluded before peptic ulcer therapy is commenced.

Cimetidine § (dose: 800 mg to 1.6 g daily)

Brand names: Galenamet §, Tagamet §, Zita § †
Cimetidine was the first of the H_2-receptor antagonists to be introduced and has the general properties of that group of drugs. In benign peptic ulcer it is given in doses of 200 mg morning and evening, or alternatively in some cases as a single dose of 800 mg at night.

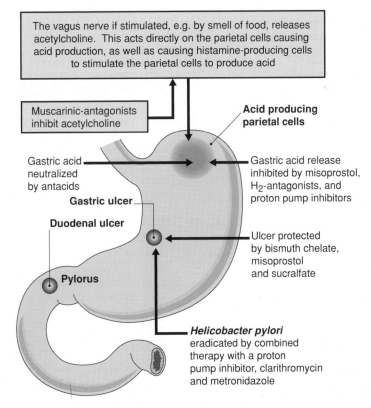

The vagus nerve if stimulated, e.g. by smell of food, releases acetylcholine. This acts directly on the parietal cells causing acid production, as well as causing histamine-producing cells to stimulate the parietal cells to produce acid

Muscarinic-antagonists inhibit acetylcholine

Acid producing parietal cells

Gastric acid neutralized by antacids

Gastric acid release inhibited by misoprostol, H_2-antagonists, and proton pump inhibitors

Gastric ulcer

Duodenal ulcer

Ulcer protected by bismuth chelate, misoprostol and sucralfate

Pylorus

Helicobacter pylori eradicated by combined therapy with a proton pump inhibitor, clarithromycin and metronidazole

Figure 10.1 Sites of action of ulcer-healing drugs.

Those doses should be taken for at least 4 weeks, or longer in ulcers linked with NSAID therapy. In the latter, increased doses of 400 mg four times a day may be required. Subsequent maintenance doses vary from 400 mg once or twice a day. Cimetidine is given in similar doses for reflux oesophagitis, but doses up to 1.6 g daily or more may be required in the Zollinger–Ellison syndrome. In severe cases, cimetidine may be given by intramuscular or slow intravenous injection or intravenous infusion in doses of 200 mg at intervals of 4–6 hours. It is also used preoperatively when a reduction in gastric acid secretion is required. Cimetidine is also used in standard doses to reduce the breakdown of pancreatin in the treatment of pancreatitis and cystic fibrosis (p. 159).

Side-effects   Cimetidine is usually well tolerated, but diarrhoea, dizziness and rash may occur. It may cause confusion in the elderly and severely ill patients, which rapidly subsides if the drug is withdrawn.

Cimetidine binds to androgen receptors, and may sometimes cause gynaecomastia. It can modify the action of many other drugs, and care is necessary in hepatic and renal impairment. (Algitec § is a mixed product containing cimetidine with alginic acid as a mucosal protectant.)

Nursing points about ulcer-healing drugs.

(a) Malignancy should be excluded before starting treatment in elderly patients.
(b) Treatment with H_2-receptor antagonists is basically symptomatic, not curative.
(c) Extended maintenance treatment necessary.
(d) Cimetidine, more than other antagonists, increases plasma levels of warfarin, phenytoin, theophylline and other drugs by inhibiting their metabolism.
(e) Proton pump inhibitors have a similar influence.
(f) Prostaglandin derivatives have a protective action by promoting mucus production.

Famotidine § (dose: 20–40 mg daily)

Brand name: Pepcid §
Famotidine has the actions, uses and side-effects of cimetidine, but it is effective in smaller doses and has a more prolonged action. In peptic ulcer it is given as a nightly dose of 40 mg for 4–8 weeks, followed by maintenance doses of 20 mg, also at night. In the Zollinger–Ellison syndrome, larger doses of 20 mg

---

†Small packs of cimetidine and some related drugs are available without prescription solely for the short-term treatment of heartburn, dyspepsia and hyperacidity.

every 6 hours are necessary. Unlike cimetidine, famotidine does not affect drug metabolism mediated by hepatic microsomal enzymes.

Nizatidine § (dose: 150–300 mg daily)

Brand name: Axid §
Nizatidine has the general properties and uses of the H_2-receptor antagonists, but has a more prolonged action. In the treatment of duodenal and benign gastric ulcer, it is given in doses of 300 mg at night, or 150 mg twice a day for at least 4 weeks. For the prevention of recurrence after ulcer healing, evening doses of 150 mg are given, and prolonged treatment for some months may be required. In short-term hospital treatment, nizatidine is given by continuous intravenous infusion in doses of 10 mg/hour.

Nizatidine is excreted mainly in the urine, and in renal impairment a reduction in dose to 150 mg daily or on alternate days may be necessary. Part of a dose is also excreted in breast milk, and its use during lactation should be avoided.

Reported **side-effects** include myalgia, chest pain, abnormal dreams and pruritus.

Ranitidine § (dose: 150–300 mg daily)

Brand name: Zantac §
Rantidine resembles cimetidine in its general pattern of activity, and in peptic ulcer it is given in doses of 150 mg twice a day or as a 300 mg dose at night for 4–8 weeks, with maintenance doses of 150 mg at night. In severe conditions, ranitidine may be given by intramuscular or slow intravenous injection in doses of 50 mg at intervals of 6–8 hours. It is also given by injection before surgery to prevent acid aspiration. Large doses up to 6 g daily may be necessary to reduce the gastric acid secretion in the Zollinger–Ellison syndrome. Ranitidine bismuth citrate (Pylorid) has similar properties and uses, and is sometimes given for the elimination of *Helicobacter pylori* (p. 149).

Ranitidine is well tolerated and has few **side-effects**, although it may cause confusion in some elderly patients and care is necessary in renal impairment. It is less likely to interfere with the metabolism of other drugs such as the oral anticoagulants.

Omeprazole § (dose: 20–40 mg daily)

Brand name: Losec §
Omeprazole is proton pump inhibitor (p. 149). It is taken up selectively by the parietal cells, as only traces remain in the circulation after 24 hours, and

brings about a more rapid rate of ulcer healing than the H_2-receptor antagonists. It is the preferred drug in the treatment of the Zollinger–Ellison syndrome. Omeprazole is used in the treatment of gastric and duodenal ulcers that have not responded to other drugs, including ulcers associated with NSAID therapy, and is given in doses of 20 mg daily for 4 weeks initially (8 weeks in gastric ulcer) with daily doses of 20 mg for maintenance treatment. Initial doses can be increased to 40 mg daily in severe conditions. Similar doses are given in erosive reflux oesophagitis. In the Zollinger–Ellison syndrome, initial doses of 60 mg daily are required, with subsequent maintenance doses varying from 20 to 120 mg daily according to need and response. The capsules should be swallowed whole, but if preferred, they may be cut open and the contents mixed with fruit juice. Omeprazole is also used in the triple therapy scheme for the eradication of *Helicobacter pylori* (p. 149).

Side-effects Omeprazole is well tolerated, and side-effects of headache and gastrointestinal disturbances are usually mild and transient. Adjustment of dose may be necessary in patients receiving warfarin, diazepam and phenytoin, as omeprazole also inhibits the action of the liver enzyme cytochrome P450, which is concerned with drug elimination.

Lansoprazole § (dose: 30 mg daily)

Brand name: Zoton §
Lansoprazole is a proton pump inhibitor of the omeprazole type. In duodenal ulcer it is given in morning doses of 30 mg daily for 4 weeks, but for 8 weeks in gastric ulcer. Similar doses are given in reflex oesophagitis. **Side-effects** are similar to those of omeprazole.

Pantoprazole § ▼ (dose: 40 mg daily)

Brand name: Protium § ▼
Pantoprazole is a proton pump inhibitor with the actions and uses of omeprazole. Dose 40 mg daily in the morning for 2–4 weeks, according to the response. Alternate day treatment is advisable in hepatic impairment.

Misoprostol § (dose: 400–800 micrograms daily)

Brand name: Cytotec §
Prostaglandins (p. 204) are mediators in the maintenance of the mucosal lining of the alimentary tract, and the biosynthesis of endogenous prostaglandins may be impaired in patients with peptic ulcer, and inhibited by non-steroidal anti-inflammatory agents (NSAIDs). Misoprostol is a synthetic prostaglandin analogue that inhibits gastric acid secretion and promotes mucus production, and is used in the treatment of established peptic ulcer as well as in the prophylaxis of NSAID-induced ulceration, particularly in the elderly (see p. 204). It is given in doses of 800 micrograms daily in two or four divided doses, taken with meals, and a last dose at night. Although early symptomatic relief may be obtained, treatment should be continued for at least 4 weeks or longer, up to 8 weeks if necessary. Doses of 200 micrograms two to four times a day are given for the prophylaxis of NSAID-induced peptic ulcers. Misoprostol is not indicated in simple dyspepsia.

Side-effects include diarrhoea (requiring a reduction in dose), nausea, abdominal pain and occasional abnormal vaginal bleeding. Care is necessary in cardiovascular disease, as misoprostol may cause hypotension. Misoprostol should not be given to women of child-bearing age unless such treatment is essential.

Arthrotec § and Napratec § are mixed products containing misoprostol 200 micrograms with a NSAID.

Bismuth chelate (dose: 480 mg daily)
(tripotassium dicitro-bismuthate)

Brand name: DeNol; De-Noltab
Bismuth chelate is a bismuth–potassium–citrate complex that appears to promote peptic ulcer healing by forming an insoluble protective coating over the ulcerated area. In addition, it has some toxic action on *Helicobacter pylori*, and the healing response may be longer than with other drugs, but the risk of relapse remains a possibility. It is given in doses of 120 mg four times a day, increased to 240 mg six times a day if necessary. As the complex may coat food as well as an ulcer, it should be taken with plenty of water half an hour before meals. Milk, except in nominal amounts, should be avoided.

Side-effects are a darkening of the tongue and blackening of the faeces.

Sucralphate § (Antepsin §) is a complex of aluminium hydroxide with sulphated sucrose, and has a similar ulcer-protective action but little antacid activity. Dose 1–2 g four times a day before meals and at night. If antacids are also used, they should be given well before or after sucralphate dosing.

Carbenoxolone §

Brand names: Bioplex §, Bioval §
Carbenoxolone is a derivative of an acid present in liquorice root. It has some anti-inflammatory properties

and is used locally for mouth ulcers. It is also used in association with antacids as Pyrogastrone § for the control of oesophageal ulceration. Extended treatment for 6–12 weeks may be required. It is contra-indicated in cardiac failure, hepatic or renal impairment, and in patients over 75 years of age.

Cisapride § (dose: 30–40 mg daily)

Brand name: Prepulsid §
Cisapride is used in the treatment of gastro-oesophageal reflux. At one time antacids were widely used, but the reflux may be due more to a delay in gastric emptying than to acidity and treatment is now directed towards stimulating gastric transit. Cisapride has some of the required properties and its gastric stimulation action appears to be linked with a local release of acetylcholine. It is given for the relief of the symptoms of reflux and non-ulcer dyspepsia in doses of 10 mg three or four times a day, continued for some weeks. It should be taken about 15–30 minutes before meals to obtain the optimum benefit, with a dose at night to prevent nocturnal reflux.

Combined administration with drugs that prolong the QT interval should be avoided, as should the antibiotics clarithromycin and erythromycin, and the antifungal agents fluconazole, itraconazole, ketoconazole and miconazole.

Some **side-effects** such as abdominal pain and diarrhoea are associated with the gastric stimulant action of the drug, but occasional headache, light-headedness and convulsions have occurred.

Spasmolytics

Spasmolytics are used as supplementary treatment in a variety of disturbances of the gastro-intestinal tract, including non-ulcer dyspepsia and the irritable bowel syndrome. They are mainly antimuscarinic (anticholinergic) in action, and so have a relaxing effect on smooth muscle. Atropine is one of the oldest spasmolytics (p. 95) but its **side-effects** such as dryness of the mouth limit its value.

Table 10.1 indicates some available products, but others, not listed, may contain auxilliary substances such as antacids.

ULCERATIVE COLITIS

Ulcerative colitis and Crohn's disease are inflammatory bowel disorders. The former affects the mucosa

Table 10.1 Intestinal antispasmodics

Approved name	Brand name	Daily dose
alverine	Spasmonal	180–360 mg
dicyclomine	Merbentyl	30–60 mg
hyoscine butylbromide	Buscopan	40–80 mg
mebeverine	Colofac	405 mg
peppermint oil	Colpermin, Mintec	0.2 ml
poldine	Nacton	8–16 mg
propantheline	Pro-Banthine	75 mg

and occasionally the submucosa of the colon and rectum, whilst the latter may affect the entire alimentary tract. The symptoms include attacks of bloody diarrhoea, colic, weight loss and anaemia, with apparently capricious periods of remission and exacerbation. Drug treatment is based on corticosteroids and the aminosalicylates such as sulphasalazine, although in some resistant conditions azathioprene (p. 278) in doses of 2 mg/kg daily may be effective. Budesonide § (Entocort CR §) is a glucocorticoid used to induce remission in Crohn's disease in doses of 9 mg once daily after breakfast.

Sulphasalazine § (dose: 2–8 g daily)

Brand name: Salazopyrin §
Sulphasalazine is a sulphonamide derivative. It appears to be taken up selectively by the connective tissues of the intestinal tract with the release of 5-aminosalicylic acid (mesalazine), the active part of the molecule. It is used in the treatment of ulcerative colitis and regional enteritis (Crohn's disease), often in association with a corticosteroid, but the response is variable.

Sulphasalazine is given initially in doses of 1–2 g four times a day together with adequate fluids for 2–3 weeks for the control of acute attacks, reduced to maintenance doses of 500 mg four times a day when remission occurs. For children initial doses of 40–60 mg/kg daily are used, with maintenance doses of 20–30 mg/kg daily. Oral therapy can be supplemented by daily retention enemas of 3 g, or suppositories of 500 mg twice a day. Extended maintenance treatment should be given to avoid relapse.

Side-effects include nausea, headache, fever, rash, pruritus and neurotoxicity. Patients should be warned to report immediately if soreness of the throat, fever or malaise occurs, as blood disorders require prompt withdrawal of treatment. It is contra-indicated in patients known to react to sulphonamides or salicylates.

Mesalazine § (dose: 1.2–2.4 g daily)

Brand names: Asacol §, Pentasa §, Salofalk §
Mesalazine is the active metabolite of sulphasalazine, but it is absorbed too rapidly to be suitable for the treatment of ulcerative colitis. Absorption can be delayed by using the drug as slow-acting products from which the active constituent is released in the lower intestinal tract. It is given in doses of 400–800 mg three times a day when the side-effects of the parent drug are unacceptable.

Side-effects Mesalazine may cause nausea, diarrhoea and abdominal pain. Salicylate sensitivity is a contra-indication. Suppositories of mesalazine (250 and 500 mg) and retention enemas (1 and 2 g) are also available, and may be useful in patients with the distal form of the disease.

Osalazine § (dose: 1.5–3 g daily)

Brand name: Dipentum §
Osalazine represents an attempt to avoid the side-effects of sulphasalazine, which are mainly due to the splitting of the molecule, the release of the sulphonamide fragment, and the over-rapid absorption of the active derivative mesalazine. In osalazine, the sulphonamide has been eliminated, as the compound is a combination of two molecules of mesalazine. The major part of a dose reaches the colon unchanged, where the compound is broken down by intestinal bacteria to release the active substance. In the treatment of ulcerative colitis, osalazine is given in doses of 500 mg–1 g three times a day, increased in severe conditions to 3 g daily. For maintenance, doses of 500 mg twice a day are given for long periods.

The main **side-effect** is a watery diarrhoea. Osalazine is contra-indicated in patients sensitive to salicylates. Balsalazide § (Colazide §) is a related drug. Dose: 6.75g daily

ANTI-EMETICS

Vomiting is a complex reflex and protective mechanism that promotes the rejection of ingested toxins, but it may be stimulated by a variety of other factors, including fear, pain, movement and drugs, and may then not serve any useful purpose. The stimulating factors reach the vomiting centre in the medulla oblongata by several pathways, including the vagus nerve and the chemoreceptor trigger zone (CTZ), Fig. 10.2. That zone is found in the floor of the fourth ventricle of the brain, and can be reached by substances not capable of penetrating the blood–brain barrier. Once the vomiting centre is stimulated, it co-ordinates the motor responses that result in vomiting, namely the muscles of the diaphragm, the abdominal wall and pyloric end of the stomach, together with relaxation of the oesophagus and body of the stomach, and closing off of the airway.

The receptors of four neurotransmitter systems have been identified as being involved in mediating the emetic response, namely the dopamine (D_2), the

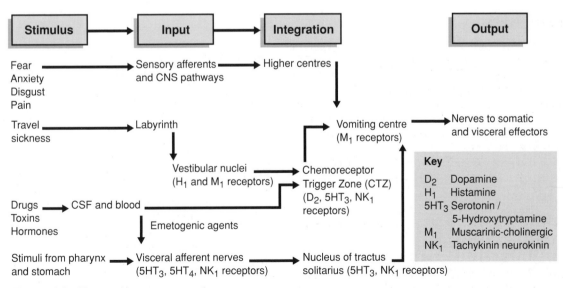

Figure 10.2   The vomiting response pathways

histamine (H_1), the serotonin ($5HT_3$) and the acetylcholine (M_1) receptors. The anti-emetic drugs available may act on different receptors, and the most effective one in any individual may have links with the underlying cause of the nausea or vomiting. The main aim of treatment is to promote patient comfort, as well as to prevent complications such as dehydration and electrolyte imbalance. The introduction of highly emetogenic anticancer drugs such as cisplatin highlighted the importance of anti-emetics, as the intense nausea induced by such agents has caused some patients to refuse further treatment. The vomiting of pregnancy is another special case, and during the first trimester anti-emetics should not normally be used because of the risks of drug-associated fetal damage. If treatment is essential, short-term therapy with an antihistamine or promethazine could be tried.

In view of the complexity of the vomiting process, it is not surprising that anti-emetic activity is found in a wide range of drugs, some of which have some degree of central depressant activity. Hyoscine is present in many travel sickness remedies, and certain antihistamines such as cyclizine (Valoid), dimenhydrinate (Dramamine) and promethazine theoclate (Avomine) are other useful anti-emetics. Betahistine § (Serc §), dose 8–16 mg, and cinnarizine (Stugeron), dose 15–30 mg, represent drugs of value in Meniere's disease, vertigo and other labyrinthine disturbances. Many of the phenothiazine-derived antipsychotic drugs also have antiemetic properties (Table 10.2) and prochlorperazine § (Stemetil §) and trifluoroperazine are representative compounds. The newer and much more powerful anti-emetics used in cancer therapy are serotonin inhibitors (see p. 156).

Nursing points about antiemetics

(a) Hyoscine and antihistamines are useful in motion sickness.
(b) Some phenothiazines, but not thioridazine, are effective in more severe vomiting.
(c) In severe nausea and vomiting secondary to disease and cytotoxic therapy, domperidone and nabilone are effective.
(d) The selective serotonin antagonists are valuable in severe cytotoxic drug-induced vomiting not controlled by other antiemetics.

Domperidone § (dose: 30–120 mg daily)

Brand name: Motilium §

Domperidone is a potent dopamine antagonist, and by preventing the access of dopamine to receptors in the chemoreceptor trigger zone (CTZ), the activation of that zone by emesis-provoking stimuli is inhibited. It also binds selectively with dopamine D_2-receptors in the stomach, and so inhibits the

---

Table 10.2 Anti-emetics

Type of antiemetic	Mode of action	Examples	Antiemetic uses
Anticholinergics (antimuscarinics)	M_1-receptor antagonist	Hyoscine	Travel sickness, postoperation
Antihistamines	H_1-receptor antagonist	Cyclizine, Dimenhydrinate	Travel sickness, postoperation, labyrinthine disorders
Gastrokinetic	D_2-receptor antagonist 5HT-receptor antagonist	Metoclopramide	Post operation, migraine, gastro-duodenal disorders, drug induced (but not cytotoxic drugs)
Butyrophenones	D_2-receptor antagonist	Haloperidol Domperidone	Cancer chemotherapy, very severe nausea and vomiting
Phenothiazines	D_2-receptor antagonist	Prochloperazine	Postoperation, severe vomiting, labyrinthine disorders
Serotonin antagonists	$5HT_3$-receptor antagonist	Granisetron Ondansetron Tropisetron	Cancer chemotherapy, radiotherapy
Miscellaneous • Tricyclic antidepressants	$M_1 + H_1$ receptor antagonists	Amitriptyline Nortriptyline,	Cancer chemotherapy
• Cannabinoids	Opiate receptors	Nabilone	Cancer chemotherapy

dopamine-mediated propulsive waves in the stomach that can result in vomiting. Domperidone does not cross the blood–brain barrier easily, and is less likely to cause sedation, extrapyramidal symptoms and other central side-effects of the anti-emetics of the phenothiazine type. It is given orally in doses of 10–20 mg every 4–8 hours, or by suppositories of 30 mg. Domperidone also increases gastro-intestinal mobility and has been used in functional dyspepsia, and to expedite the transit of barium sulphate in gastro-intestinal radiological investigations.

Metoclopramide § (dose: 15–30 mg daily)

Brand name: Maxolon §
Metoclopramide is a dopamine antagonist and has a central effect by depressing the threshold of activity of the vomiting centre, and by its weak serotonin antagonist properties. It also reduces the sensitivity of nerves linking that centre with the pylorus and duodenum and increases gastric peristalsis.

Metoclopramide is given in doses of 10 mg, orally or by injection, up to three times a day, and is useful in many conditions associated with nausea and vomiting. (Gastrobid Continus §, Gastromax § and Maxolon SR § are slow-release products.) In the control of the nausea due to cytotoxic therapy, meto-clopramide is given in large doses (2–4 mg/kg) by intravenous infusion up to a maximum of 10 mg/kg over 24 hours, the initial dose being given before cytotoxic therapy is commenced.

Side-effects Metoclopramide is usually well tolerated, but it should not be given to patients under 20 years of age unless the vomiting is severe. In young patients it may have extra-pyramidal side-effects and cause involuntary movements.

Nabilone § (dose: 2–6 mg daily)

Brand name: Cesamet §
Nabilone is a synthetic cannabinoid with antiemetic properties of value in the nausea and vomiting associated with cytotoxic therapy. It is not a dopamine antagonist, and appears to act on certain opiate receptors. It is given in oral doses of 1–2 mg twice a day during each period of treatment (commencing before such therapy) and continued for 24 hours after the end of the course.

Side-effects include drowsiness, confusion, hallu-cinations, depression and hypotension. Nabilone should be used with care in patients with a history of psychosis, and if renal impairment is present.

Prochlorperazine § (dose: 10–30 mg daily)

Brand names: Buccastem §, Stemetil §
Prochlorperazine is a chlorpromazine-like drug with similar actions and uses. It is used in the prophyl-axis and treatment of severe nausea and vomiting, as well as in labyrinthine disorders. In prophylaxis, doses of 5–10 mg are given two or three times a day, but for the treatment of nausea and vomiting the initial dose is 20 mg, followed by doses of 10 mg as required. Alternatively, an initial dose of 25 mg may be given by suppository. In severe conditions, prochlorperazine can be given in doses of 12.5 mg by deep intramuscular injection, followed by oral therapy. Buccastem is a product designed for buccal administration to provide a longer action from a 3 mg dose of prochlorperazine. In labyrinthine disorders, initial doses of 5 mg three times a day may be increased slowly up to 30 mg daily; extended treat-ment may be required.

Side-effects such as sedation, dryness of the mouth and drowsiness are usually mild but extrapyramidal reactions may occur with high doses, especially in children and the elderly.

SEROTONIN (5HT$_3$)-RECEPTOR ANTAGONISTS

Cytotoxic chemotherapeutic agents and radiotherapy can cause very severe nausea and vomiting, con-sidered to be due to the release of serotonin (5HT) from the enterochromaffin cells in the intestinal mucosa, which contain most of the body stores of serotonin. Such released serotonin acts on a specific subgroup of receptors in the gut, identified as the 5HT$_3$-receptors, which in turn leads to stimulation of the vagus nerve and activation of central 5HT$_3$-receptors in the chemoreceptor trigger zone (CTZ), and subsequent initiation of the vomiting reflex.

When the anti-emetic properties of metoclo-pramide were found to be linked with its weak serotonin antagonist action, attention was turned to the development of more selective and powerful 5HT$_3$-receptor antagonists, represented by granisetron, ondansetron and tropisetron. These drugs act on the 5HT$_3$-receptors in the gut and CTZ, and have no action on other types of serotonin receptors. They have no dopamine antagonist properties, and so are unlikely to cause the extrapyramidal side-effect of metoclopramide. To obtain the best anti-emetic response, these 5HT$_3$-receptor antagonists should be given before chemotherapy or radiotherapy is commenced.

Granisetron § (dose: 2 mg daily)

Brand name: Kytril §

Granisetron is a $5HT_3$-receptor antagonist with the general properties of that group of drugs. It is given for the prophylaxis and treatment of nausea and vomiting induced by cytotoxic therapy in doses of 1 mg orally, preferably an hour before treatment, followed by doses of 1–2 mg daily during treatment. Alternatively, granisetron may be given as a 3 mg dose by intravenous infusion, repeated at intervals if necessary up to a total dose of 9 mg in 24 hours. **Side-effects** include headache and constipation.

Ondansetron § (dose: 24 mg daily)

Brand name: Zofran §

Ondansetron is another $5HT_3$-receptor antagonist used like granisetron and tropisetron for drug-induced nausea and vomiting. When severe vomiting is anticipated it is given before chemotherapy in a dose of 8 mg by intravenous injection, followed by doses of 8 mg at intervals of 2–4 hours. Alternatively, an intravenous dose of 1 mg hourly for up to 24 hours may be given. A dose of 20 mg of dexamethasone, given intravenously before chemotherapy may enhance the anti-emetic response. In less severe vomiting, the initial intravenous dose of 8 mg can be followed by oral therapy in doses of 8 mg 8-hourly. Maintenance treatment is with doses of 8 mg 8-hourly for up to 5 days. Ondansetron is well tolerated, but **side-effects** include constipation, headache and a sensation of flushing or warmth.

Tropisetron § (dose: 5 mg daily)

Brand name: Navoban §

Tropisetron is a $5HT_3$-receptor antagonist that differs from others by its extended action which permits single daily dosage. It is used as a 6-day treatment for the prevention of cancer chemotherapy-induced nausea and vomiting, and is given initially as a single dose of 5 mg by intravenous infusion. Over the next 5 days it is given orally as a single morning dose of 5 mg, to be taken well before food. Tropisetron is generally well tolerated, but **side-effects** such as headache, constipation, dizziness and gastro-intestinal disturbances may occur.

ADSORBENTS

Adsorbents are solids that have the ability to bind with gases and other substances, including bacterial toxins, and so prevent their absorption. They are used mainly in the treatment of mild diarrhoea. Activated charcoal is also used in the treatment of poisoning by some toxic drugs (p. 310).

Kaolin (dose: 15–60 g)

Kaolin, or china clay, is a purified silicate of aluminium. It is used in the treatment of food poisoning, enteritis, dysentery and diarrhoea. Mixture of Kaolin and Morphine BP, BNF is widely employed in the treatment of mild gastro-intestinal disturbances, as the kaolin adsorbs any toxins and the morphine constituent reduces gastro-intestinal motility.

Charcoal (dose: 4–8 g)

Activated charcoal has adsorbent properties similar to those of kaolin, and is sometimes used in the treatment of flatulence and distension, and in poisoning by alkaloids and related drugs. It is also used by the charcoal perfusion technique in cases of poisoning by methyl alcohol, lithium salts and salicylates.

ANTIDIARRHOEAL DRUGS

Diarrhoea is the result of alterations in intestinal mobility, impaired absorption and an increased secretion of fluid into the intestinal lumen. Treatment includes Kaolin and Morphine Mixture for mild diarrhoea and antimotility drugs for acute diarrhoea. The latter include codeine phosphate, dose 15–30 mg, which is also present in some proprietary products (Diarrest §; Kaodene) and co-phenotrope. Co-phenotrope (Diaphen §; Lomotil §; Tropergen §) contains diphenoxylate 2.5 mg, which binds with opioid receptors in the gut, and the anticholinergic agent atropine 25 micrograms. Loperamide (Arret; Diasorb; Imodium) has similar properties. Both co-phenotrope and loperamide are useful in acute and chronic diarrhoea.

In simple acute diarrhoea, particularly in children and the elderly, it is essential to replace fluid and electrolyte loss as soon as possible, and this should precede drug therapy. Compound Sodium Chloride and Glucose Powder, or Oral Rehydration Salts (ORS) are suitable products for that purpose, or alternatively, for short periods, a solution of glucose or sugar with a small amount of salt may be used. Proprietary products for oral rehydration therapy include Diocalm, Diorylate, Electrolade, Gluco-lyte, Rapolyte and Rehidrat. Infective diarrhoeas are usually caused by viruses and are self-limiting; antibacterial drugs are seldom required.

In more 'severe and extended diarrhoeas, the cause, such as ulcerative colitis, should be sought, as more specific drugs may be required (p. 152).

LAXATIVES

Sometimes termed aperients, laxatives are substances which stimulate peristalsis, promote evacuation and relieve constipation. At one time they were used extensively regardless of need, but their routine use has declined. Their use is primarily indicated for the treatment of constipation in (1) illness and pregnancy, (2) elderly patients with inadequate diets and poor abdominal muscle tone, (3) when intestinal activity has been reduced by medication, and (4) preparation for surgery or diagnosis. They can be classified as osmotic, stimulant, bulk and lubricant laxatives (faecal softeners).

OSMOTIC LAXATIVES

Osmotic laxatives are those that when taken orally are not absorbed, and the osmotic pressure they set up reduces the absorption of fluid from both the small and large bowel. They include magnesium sulphate and magnesium hydroxide; the latter is converted by gastric acid to magnesium chloride, and so has the same action as magnesium sulphate (Epsom salts). When given in doses of 5–15 g, well diluted, in the morning on an empty stomach, their laxative action is rapid and effective.

Bowel cleansing solutions such as Citromag are used to evacuate the bowel before colonoscopy, radiology and surgery. Citromag is an effervescent preparation of magnesium citrate; Klean-Prep contains sodium sulphate and other electrolytes. In use, such products are taken well diluted on the morning before the examination.

STIMULANT LAXATIVES

Stimulant laxatives include the old anthraquinone-containing vegetable products and the few synthetic laxatives. They are all thought to stimulate Auerbach's plexus in the large intestine and increase the rate of peristaltic movement. The vegetable laxatives are slow in action and are best taken at night. They may cause abdominal cramp, and are now used much less extensively than in the past. Their chronic use should be discouraged as they may then exacerbate the problem of constipation by inducing an atonic colon, as well as causing electrolyte loss, particularly potassium. Some are excreted to a limited extent in breast milk and can affect the infant.

Vegetable laxatives

The powerful vegetable purgatives such as aloes are now rarely used.

Cascara

Cascara bark has a mild slow action that results in the passage of a soft stool. Used mainly as standardized tablets, dose 1 or 2 at night.

Senna (dose: 0.5–2 g)

Both the leaves and the seed pods of senna have laxative properties, and have long been used domestically as 'senna tea'. Senna is very effective but may cause some griping. Senokot is a proprietary product containing a standardized extract of senna, which is more consistent in action and better tolerated.

Castor oil (dose: 5–20 ml)

Castor oil was formerly given as a purgative in diarrhoea and food poisoning, but is now rarely used. It survives as an emollient in Zinc and Castor Oil Cream.

Synthetic laxatives

Bisacodyl (dose: 5–10 mg)

Brand name: Dulcolax
Bisacodyl is not absorbed when given orally but has a stimulant action on the walls of the colon. It is sometimes described as a contact laxative, and is useful not only as a general laxative, but also to secure evacuation of the colon before X-ray examination. Tablets containing 5 mg and suppositories of 10 mg are available. Danthron has similar properties, but it is used only for constipation in the aged and terminally ill, as the drug may have some carcinogenic potential.

Docusate sodium (dose: 50–500 mg)

Brand name: Dioctyl
Docusate sodium, also known as dioctyl sodium sulphosuccinate, is a surface-active agent, and acts as a faecal softener by increasing the amount of water that remains in or penetrates into the faeces. It is also present with danthron in the mixed product co-danthramer, which is used mainly for constipation in the elderly and terminally ill patients.

Lactulose (dose: 50% solution, 15–50 ml)

Brand names: Duphalac, Lactugal, Osmolax, Regulose
Lactulose is an artificial sugar that escapes digestion and reaches the colon unchanged, and so functions as a slow-acting osmotic laxative. It is later broken down by bacteria to form lactic and other acids, and promotes the formation of softer faeces of low pH.

Lactulose solution is given in doses of 15 ml twice a day. It is also of value in doses of 30–50 ml three times a day in hepatic encephalopathy, as it limits the formation and absorption of nitrogenous breakdown products in the intestinal tract. Such breakdown products are normally converted in the liver to urea, and could accumulate when liver damage has occurred. The **side-effects** of lactulose are flatulence, abdominal cramp and intestinal discomfort.

Lactitol is a semisynthetic sugar similar in actions and uses to lactulose. For constipation it is given as a single daily dose of 10–20 g, mixed with food and taken with adequate fluid. In hepatic encephalopathy, it is given in doses of 500–700 mg/kg three times a day.

Phenolphthalein (dose: 50–300 mg)

Phenolphthalein has a mild irritant action on the intestines, and is used in habitual constipation. It is absorbed in part by the enterohepatic circulation and excreted later in the bile, so that the action may extend over several days. It may cause rash and albuminuria, and its use has now declined. It is present in some proprietary laxative products and patients should be warned that it may colour the urine pink.

Sodium picosulphate (dose: 5–15 mg)

Brand names: Laxoberal, Picolax
Sodium picosulphate is a synthetic laxative of the bisacodyl type, and is used for similar purposes. It is slow acting (10–12 hours), and is useful for bowel evacuation before surgery. Sodium Picolate Elixir is the official product (dose 5–15 ml) at night). Products of this type are not suitable for prolonged use.

BULK LAXATIVES

Bulk laxatives are vegetable substances of a mucilaginous nature and are hydrophilic. They are not digested, but absorb water, swell and so increase the bulk of the faeces. That increase stimulates peristalsis as well as the rectal reflexes that promote defaecation. They are therefore useful in the treatment of constipation where the faeces are dry and hard, but they may not be suitable when the intake of fluid is inadequate or in cases of faecal impaction.

Typical products are bran, ispaghula and psyllium seeds which form the basis of proprietary bulk laxatives such as Fybogel, Isogel, Metamucil, Normacol, Proctifibe, Regulan and Trifyba. Celevac contains methylcellulose. All these bulk laxatives should be taken with an adequate amount of water to reduce the risk of intestinal obstruction.

LUBRICANT LAXATIVES AND FAECAL SOFTENERS

Liquid paraffin (dose: 8–30 ml)

Liquid paraffin is a mineral oil that passes through the alimentary tract unchanged and acts as a simple lubricant laxative. It is particularly valuable in producing a soft stool after intestinal and rectal operations or in cases of haemorrhoids. It is now used mainly as Liquid Paraffin Oral Emulsion.

Although liquid paraffin has been in use for many years, the Committee on Safety of Medicines has recommended that its use should be restricted, as prolonged use may cause malabsorption of fat-soluble vitamins, foreign body reactions in the small intestine (paraffinoma) and anal leak.

LAXATIVE ENEMAS

Locally acting laxatives are sometimes useful in softening impacted faeces and facilitating evacuation. Those used as enemas may contain oils, osmotic laxatives or surface-active faecal-softening agents, and the following are some representative products: arachis oil retention enema, magnesium sulphate enema, phosphates enema, Micralax, Relaxit and Veripaque.

MISCELLANEOUS DRUGS

This section refers to a few drugs that are not easily classified but have exceptional value in some less common metabolic disorders.

Alglucerase § ▼ (dose: 60 units/kg every 14 days)

Brand name: Ceredase § ▼

Gaucher's disease is an uncommon recessive disorder of lipid metabolism due to the deficiency of a specific enzyme. Treatment is replacement therapy with alglucerase intravenously in doses of 60 units/kg every 14 days according to need and response. Prolonged treatment is required.

Carnitine § (dose: 200–400 mg/kg daily)

Brand name: Carnitor §

Carnitine is present in skeletal and cardiac muscle and is concerned with the transport of long-chain fatty acids. A deficiency may be due to an inborn error of metabolism, or it may be the result of reduced carnitine production in severe liver failure or excessive loss during renal dialysis. Treatment is with carnitine in doses of 200–400 mg/kg daily, or by intravenous injection in doses of 100 mg/kg daily.

Side-effects are dose-related and include nausea and vomiting.

Penicillamine § (dose: 1.5 g daily)

Brand names: Distamine §, Pendramine §

Penicillamine, also referred to on p. 207, is used in the treatment of Wilson's disease, a hepatolenticular degeneration brought about by the excessive retention of copper in the body. Penicillamine binds with and mobilizes the excess copper as a soluble chelate, which is excreted in the urine. It is given in doses of 500 mg three times a day before food, but treatment must be continued indefinitely with maintenance doses of 750 mg daily once a negative copper balance has been achieved. Hypersensitivity reactions may limit prolonged treatment.

It is also used in the treatment of cystinuria, as it combines with cystine to form a more soluble complex. It is given initially in divided doses of 1–3 g daily before food, aimed at reducing urinary cystine excretion to 200 mg/litre. Subsequent maintenance doses are 0.5–1 g, together with a fluid intake of at least three litres daily.

Penicillamine is also used in the treatment of poisoning by lead, mercury, copper and gold.

Trientine § ▼ (dose: 1.2–2.4 g daily)

Trientine is also a copper chelating agent used in the treatment of Wilson's disease, but it is usually reserved for patients unable to tolerate penicillamine. It is given in doses of 300–600 mg four times a day before food. Trientine may cause nausea and interfere with the absorption of iron.

Cholelitholytic drugs

Cholelitholytic drugs are those that are used orally for the dissolution of cholesterol-containing gallstones present in a functioning gall bladder. They appear to act by inhibiting the hepatic synthesis of cholesterol, and as the bile becomes less saturated with cholesterol, so steroid-containing gallstones tend to dissolve, but stones larger than 15 mm are less likely to dissolve completely. They are suitable for the treatment of radiolucent stones only, as calcium-containing or bile-pigment stones are unlikely to dissolve.

Chenodeoxycholic acid (Chendecon §, Chenofalk §) is given in doses of 750–1250 mg daily; ursodeoxycholic acid (Destolit §, Ursofalk §) is given in doses of 450–600 mg daily. Combidol § and Lithofalk § contain both acids, and are given in doses of 500–750 mg daily. They are used only when surgery or other biliary techniques are inadvisable, as very prolonged treatment is required and recurrence is common within a year after treatment is discontinued. Oestrogen-containing oral contraceptives and drugs of the clofibrate type, which increase bile cholesterol, should be avoided.

Pancreatin

Pancreatin is obtained from mammalian pancreas and contains a mixture of the enzymes protease, amylase and lipase necessary for the digestion of proteins, carbohydrates and fats. It is given orally in the treatment of cystic fibrosis and other conditions of pancreatic deficiency.

It is used as a powder or granules, and may be taken mixed with food or fluids, which should not be too hot, and not allowed to stand before being taken, otherwise enzyme inactivation may occur.

Inactivation by gastric acid may also occur, but the risk can be reduced by taking pancreatin with an antacid or an acid-inhibiting agent of the cimetidine type. Some preparations of pancreatin are supplied as enteric-coated granules, by which means larger amounts of lipase and other enzymes escape inactivation and reach the duodenum unchanged. Nurses should advise patients that these enteric-coated granules should be swallowed whole, and not chewed, otherwise the benefits of the enteric coating will be lost. The standard dose of pancreatin is up to 8 g daily, but requires individual adjustment according to need and the nature and frequency of the stools.

Side-effects include nausea, vomiting and abdominal discomfort; anal irritation may also occur. Some very high strength pancreatin preparations have been used in cystic fibrosis, but recent reports indicate that with these high potency products, there is a risk that fibrotic strictures of the colon may develop with extended treatment and require major surgery. Until the extent of the risk becomes known,

the Committee on Safety of Medicines has recommended that high potency pancreatin products should not be given to patients aged 15 or less; the total daily dose should not exceed 10 000 units of lipase per kg. If symptoms indicative of gastrointestinal obstruction occur with any pancreatin preparation, the possibility of bowel stricture should be reported without delay.

Pancreatin preparations

Creon; Nutrizym GR; Nutrizym 10; Pancrease; Pancrex; Pancrex V.

High potency pancreatin products*

Creon 25000; Nutrizym 22; Pancrease HL, (A different product for the treatment of cystic fibrosis is dornase alfa, p. 241).

FURTHER READING

Andrews C 1994 Ulcer-healing drugs, their actions and side-effects. Nursing Times 90(33):38–40

Axon A T R et al 1997 Randomised double blind controlled study of recurrence of gastric ulcer after treatment for eradication of *Helicobacter pylori* infection. British Medical Journal 314:565–568

Bone M E, Wilkinson D J, Young J R et al 1990 Ginger root – a new antiemetic. The effect of ginger root on postoperative nausea and vomiting after major gynaecological surgery. Anaesthesia 45:669–671

Booth S, Booth B 1986 Aperients can be deceptive. Nursing Times 82(39):38–39

Bountra C, Gale J D, Gardner C J et al 1996 Towards understanding the aetiology and pathophysiology of the emetic reflex. Oncology 53 (suppl 1):102–109

Cook D J, Reeve B K, Scholes L C 1994 Histamine-2-receptor antagonists and antacids in the critically ill population: stress ulceration versus nosocomial pneumonia. Infection Control and Hospital Epidemiology 15(7):437–442

Hills M J, Aaronson P I 1991 The mechanism of action of peppermint oil on gastrointestinal smooth muscle. Gastroenterology 101:55–65

Kelly J 1994 Drug therapy and peptic ulceration. British Journal of Nursing 3(21):1129–1134

Maton P M 1991 Omeprazole. New England Journal of Medicine 324:965–975

Pervan V 1993 Understanding anti-emetics. Nursing Times 89(10):36–38

Tate S, Cook H 1996 Postoperative nausea and vomiting 2: management and treatment. British Journal of Nursing 5(17):1032–1039

11

Drugs acting on the urinary system

DIURETICS

Diuretics act on the kidney and increase water and electrolyte excretion, and are used to treat the oedema and congestion of heart failure, renal disease and liver cirrhosis. They are also useful in hypertension, and in lowering an elevated intracranial or intraocular pressure. In congestive heart failure they are first-line drugs, as by increasing the urinary output they reduce the plasma volume, lower the venous return and so reduce the cardiac preload.

The site of action of the diuretics is the nephron, of which there are about a million in each kidney. Each nephron consists of a Bowman's capsule containing a knot of fine blood vessels that form the glomerulus, and two tubules connected by the loop of Henle (Fig. 11.1). In health about 1500 ml of blood passes through the kidneys every minute, and the glomerulus acts as a size-selective filter, as the blood cells, plasma proteins and lipids are retained in the circulation, and the filtrate contains the electrolyte and other water-soluble constituents of the plasma. As the filtrate passes through the tubules, much of the water and the solutes, glucose, sodium chloride, sodium bicarbonate and potassium chloride are reabsorbed and pass back into the circulation by active and passive transport systems. Re-absorption occurs mainly in the proximal tubule where most of the water, 70% of the sodium, all the potassium and varying amounts of the other solutes are taken up. Another 20% of sodium is reabsorbed in the loop of Henle, and about 20 ml of the original filtrate reaches the distal tubule, where the filtrate is further concentrated and, depending on the electrolyte concentration, more sodium is absorbed in exchange for potassium. The remaining filtrate passes on to the

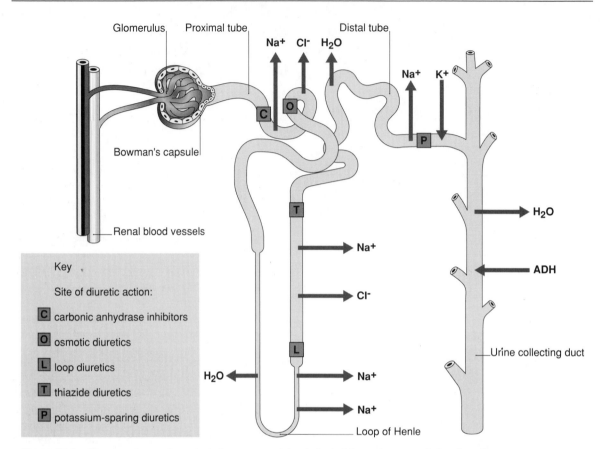

Figure 11.1 Diagram of a nephron, including some points of electrolyte exchange and diuretic action.

collecting duct, where under the influence of the antidiuretic hormone more water may be absorbed and pass back into the circulation.

Diuretics and electrolyte balance

In health, the kidneys are capable of maintaining the electrolyte balance of the blood within narrow limits in spite of varying intake of fluid or extremes of climatic conditions. However, if the blood supply to the kidneys is reduced by heart failure, liver disease or drug-induced hypotension, the glomerular filtration rate slows down. Yet tubular re-absorption continues unaltered, so excess water and electrolytes that are normally excreted begin to accumulate in the tissues, causing congestion and oedema. Diuretics act by inhibiting tubular re-absorption, and so increase the elimination of water and electrolytes. That re-absorption process is mediated by pump or carrier systems which transfer ions into and out of the nephron in the process of concentrating the

glomerular filtrate, and different diuretics act at different points.

The most powerful diuretics are the 'loop diuretics' which act on the thick segment of the loop of Henle and prevent the transport of sodium chloride out of the distal tubule into the interstitial tissues, and so back into the circulation, by inhibiting the Na^+/K^+2Cl^- carrier system in the loop membrane. In consequence, a sodium-rich filtrate passes on to the distal tubules, but their ability to take up electrolytes and water is soon overwhelmed, so larger amounts pass on to the collecting ducts to be excreted.

An equally important group of diuretics, the thiazides, also act on the distal tubules where they decrease the active reabsorption of sodium and chloride by binding to Na^+/Cl^- co-transport system and inhibiting its action. Unlike the loop diuretics, the thiazides have no action on the thick segment of the loop of Henle.

The diuretics that act on the distal tubule tend to alter the sodium/potassium balance, so less potassium is reabsorbed and more passes on to be excreted. Occasionally that imbalance may cause some hypokalaemia, and the oral administration of potassium supplements may be necessary, either as effervescent potassium tablets (Kloref; Sando-K), or as a slow release product (Slow-K). Such products should always be taken with plenty of water and with the patient in a sitting or standing position to avoid the risk of oesophageal damage.

Although the loop and thiazide diuretics have a similar action, the latter are used mainly in mild to moderate heart failure where pulmonary oedema is not present. In smaller doses they are widely used in the treatment of hypertension, often in association with other antihypertensive drugs. The loop diuretics are used mainly in the relief of pulmonary oedema associated with left ventricular failure, and in those patients with chronic heart failure who no longer respond to a thiazide diuretic.

These potent diuretics are in general well tolerated, but the reported **side-effects** are numerous and include gastro-intestinal disturbances, hyperglycaemia, hypokalaemia, hyperuricaemia, metabolic acidosis, gout, rash and thrombocytopenia. The loop diuretics may cause tinnitus and deafness. Care is necessary in renal and hepatic impairment. Small initial doses should be given to the elderly, who are often particularly susceptible to the side-effects of potent diuretics. Aldosterone antagonists are referred to on p. 165.

Table 11.1 indicates the range of diuretics now in use. They are best taken in the morning, a time when the subsequent diuresis is less likely to interfere with sleep.

Nursing points about diuretics

(a) Thiazides are used mainly to reduce oedema due to heart failure, and in hypertension.
(b) Loop diuretics are of value in pulmonary oedema caused by left ventricular failure, and when response to thiazides is inadequate.
(c) Hypokalaemia is potentially dangerous in patients with coronary heart disease receiving digoxin or anti-arrhythmic drugs.
(d) Best taken in the morning to reduce nocturia.
(e) May cause postural hypotension, especially after sleep.
(f) Note any signs of electrolyte disturbances such as tachyarrhythmias; muscle weakness (hypokalaemia); lethargy (hyponatria); tingling and numbness (hypocalcaemia); bone pain, nausea and confusion (hypercalcaemia).

THIAZIDE DIURETICS

Chlorothiazide § (Saluric §, dose: 0.5–2 g) was the first thiazide diuretic, but it has been largely replaced by more potent drugs.

Bendrofluazide § (dose: 2.5–10 mg daily)

Brand names: Aprinox §, Neo-NaClex §
Bendrofluazide is representative of the thiazide diuretics generally, and is in wide use for congestive heart failure and hypertension, and occasionally in premenstrual tension. In heart failure it is given in morning doses of 5–10 mg; similar doses may be given for maintenance once to three times a week. In hypertension a dose of 2.5 mg daily is usually adequate, as larger doses have less influence on the blood pressure and may cause electrolyte disturbances.

LOOP DIURETICS
Frusemide § (dose: 40 mg–2 g daily)

Brand names: Lasix §, Dryptal §, Diuresal §
Frusemide is a powerful loop diuretic and is frequently effective in oedema and the oliguria of renal failure when other diuretics fail to evoke an adequate response. Frusemide is given in doses of 40 mg or more daily, and the onset of diuresis is rapid and may extend over 6 hours. Maintenance doses may vary from 20 to 80 mg daily according to need and response.

If a very rapid diuresis is required, as in pulmonary oedema, frusemide may be given by intramuscular or slow intravenous injection in doses of 20–50 mg, and the response may be dramatic both in its rapidity and in the magnitude of the diuresis. Nausea and weakness may follow the copious diuresis, and some hypotension may occur. In severe oliguria associated with renal failure, much larger doses are given, ranging from 250 mg 4–6-hourly up to a maximum single dose of 2 g, although such a high dose is seldom required. Alternatively, treatment may be commenced with a dose of 250 mg by intravenous infusion, increased if necessary to 500 mg–1 g spread over four hours. Further doses can be repeated every 24 hours.

Side-effects are many and include rash, tinnitus, deafness and hypokalaemia. Care is necessary in diabetes and gout. It is contra-indicated in cirrhosis of the liver and renal failure with anuria.

Bumetanide § (dose: 1–5 mg daily)

Brand name: Burinex §
Bumetanide is a loop diuretic with a rapid but brief

Table 11.1 Diuretics

Approved name	Brand name	Products
Thiazide and thiazide-type diuretics		
bendrofluazide	Aprinox	Tablets 2.5 & 5 mg
	Neo-Naclex	
chlorothiazide	Saluric	Tablets 500 mg
chlorthalidone	Hygroton	Tablets 50 mg
cyclopenthiazide	Navidrex	Tablets 500 micrograms
hydrochlorothiazide	HydroSaluric	Tablets 25 & 50 mg
hydroflumethiazide	Hydrenox	Tablets 50 mg
indapamide	Natrilix	Tablets 2.5 mg
mefruside	Baycaron	Tablets 25 mg
metolazone	Metenix	Tablets 5 mg
polythiazide	Nephril	Tablets 1 mg
xipamide	Diurexan	Tablets 20 mg
Loop diuretics		
bumetanide	Burinex	Tablets 1 mg
		Ampoules 1–2 mg
ethacrynic acid	Edecrin	Vials 50 mg
frusemide	Lasix	Tables 20 & 40 mg
torasemide	Torem	Tablets 2.5; 5; 10 mg
Potassium-sparing diuretics		
amiloride	Amilospare	Tablets 5 mg
triamterene	Dytac	Capsules 50 mg
Aldosterone antagonists		
spironolactone	Aldactone	Tablets 25; 50; 100 mg
	Spiroctan	
potassium canrenoate	Spiroctan-M	Ampoules 200 mg

Note: Several mixed diuretic products are available. Others contain added potassium, usually indicated by the suffix 'K'. It should not be assumed that these mixed potassium products contain the same amount of diuretic as the plain tablet. In some such products the potassium chloride is contained in an enteric-coated core of the tablet, and the release of the potassium chloride in the small intestine may occasionally cause bowel ulceration and obstruction. Patients taking such tablets should be advised to report any gastrointestinal disturbances.

action and is effective in a dose as low as 1 mg daily, but a second dose may be given after 6–8 hours if required. Larger doses of 5 mg or more daily have been given in oliguria. In pulmonary oedema, bumetanide may be given by intravenous or intramuscular injection in doses of 1 or 2 mg, repeated if required after 20 minutes or later, or doses of 2–5 mg may be given by slow intravenous infusion. Much larger doses may be required in patients whose renal function is impaired, but may cause deafness and myalgia. The action of bumetanide is similar to that of frusemide, and electrolyte disturbances and loss of potassium may occur as with other diuretics. In the elderly, the rapid relief of oedema may cause sudden disturbances of the circulation with hypotension and collapse.

Ethacrynic acid § (dose: 50–400 mg daily)

Brand name: Edecrin §

Ethacrynic acid is a 'loop' diuretic with an action similar to that of frusemide and may evoke a prompt and copious diuresis in patients who are resistant to other diuretics. It has been given orally in doses of 50–250 mg in refractory oedema, but is now used only by slow intravenous injection or infusion in cases where urgent diuresis is essential, as in acute pulmonary oedema. A single dose of 50 mg is usually adequate, but a second dose, if required, should be given at a different site to avoid thrombophlebitis. The possibility of a marked response causing an acute hypotensive episode with electrolyte disturbance should be borne in mind.

Side-effects include gastro-intestinal disturbances, occasionally with a watery diarrhoea. Deafness has been reported as a side-effect after intravenous use, especially with high doses and in reduced renal efficiency. Potassium supplements may be required with continued therapy, as potassium loss, although less with ethacrynic acid than with some diuretics, may still occur.

Torasemide § (dose: 5–40 mg daily)

Brand name: Torem §

Torasemide is a loop diuretic with the actions and uses of related drugs. In oedema it is given in morning doses of 5 mg initially, slowly increased as required up to 20 mg as a single daily dose, and less frequently up to 40 mg daily. In severe congestive heart failure and pulmonary oedema it can be given by slow intravenous infusion in doses of 10–20 mg daily, increased up to 40 mg daily according to need and response. Exceptionally, doses up to 200 mg have been given in the oedema of renal disease. Torasemide is also used in hypertension, and is given in doses of 2.5–5 mg daily. The **side-effects** and contra-indications are those of the loop diuretics generally.

POTASSIUM-SPARING DIURETICS

These drugs have a relatively weak diuretic action as they have a selective effect by reducing the normal loss of potassium by the distal tubules. For that reason they are often given together with a thiazide or loop diuretic.

Amiloride § (dose: 5–20 mg daily)

Brand name: Midamor §

Amiloride may be given alone in congestive heart failure and hypertension as a daily dose of 10 mg, or in doses of 5 mg when given together with more potent diuretics.

The **side-effects** are mainly those of related drugs.

Co-amilozide is a mixed product containing amiloride 2.5 mg and hydrochlorothiazide 25 mg. Co-amilofruse contains amiloride 2.5 mg and frusemide 20 mg. Navispare is a mixed product containing amiloride 2.5 mg and cyclopenthiazide 25 mg. Co-amilofruse (Burinex A) contains amiloride 2.5 mg and frusemide 20 mg.

Triamterene § (dose: 150–250 mg daily)

Brand name: Dytac §

Triamterene is a potassium-sparing diuretic similar to amiloride, and is given in initial doses of 50 mg three to five times a day, adjusted after 1 week according to need, and given on alternate days. If given with a thiazide diuretic, the overall diuretic effect is increased, and such combined treatment may be useful in resistant oedema.

Co-triamterzide § (Dyazide §) is a mixed product containing triamterine 50 mg and hydrochlorothiazide 25 mg. Dytide § contains triamterine 50 mg and benzthiazide 25 mg.

Side-effects are nausea, dry mouth and rash. Patients should be advised that, in some lights, the urine may appear bluish. Potassium supplements should not be given with triamterene, or with any other potassium-sparing diuretic.

ALDOSTERONE ANTAGONISTS

Spironolactone § (dose: 100–400 mg daily)

Brand names: Aldactone §, Spiroctan §

Spironolactone is a synthetic steroid that has a limited diuretic action mediated by blocking the aldosterone receptors in the distal tubule. Aldosterone is one of the steroid hormones of the adrenal cortex, and is concerned with the re-absorption of sodium and the excretion of potassium. Spironolactone inhibits that action, and so indirectly inhibits the potassium loss and has a potassium-sparing effect. Some patients with cirrhosis or ascites secrete excessive amounts of aldosterone which in turn limits the response to diuretics. In such resistant conditions spironolactone promotes diuresis by its aldosterone-blocking action, and increases the effects of other diuretics.

In congestive heart failure, ascites and oedema, spironolactone is given in doses of 25–50 mg four times a day, together with other diuretic therapy. The initial response may be slow, and after five days the dose may need to be increased up to 400 mg daily.

Side-effects are headache, drowsiness and disturbances of the electrolyte balance, and treatment should be discontinued if hyperkalaemia develops. Care is necessary in renal and hepatic impairment.

Potassium canrenoate § (Spiroctan-M §) is similar, and is given by slow intravenous infusion/injection in doses of 200–400 mg.

OSMOTIC DIURETICS

Osmotic diuretics are pharmacologically inert substances that pass through the glomerulus, and increase the osmotic pressure of the filtrate. In consequence they reduce the amount of water normally re-absorbed by the tubules and Henle's loop, and so increase the urinary volume. However, they have little effect on sodium re-absorption, so in heart failure associated with sodium retention they are of little value, and may have the adverse effect of increasing blood volume. On the other hand, they have a use independent of their diuretic action in the treatment of acute cerebral oedema due to a high intercranial pressure, by withdrawing water from the tissues. By the same action they are also used in glaucoma in acute ocular hypertension. The only representative of the group at present is mannitol.

Mannitol § (dose: 50–200 g)

Mannitol is a carbohydrate used to reduce the intracranial pressure in cerebral oedema. It is given by intravenous infusion of a 10–20% solution in doses of 50–100 g over 24 hours, after an intravenous sensitivity test dose of 200 mg/kg. Careful control of the fluid balance and plasma electrolytes is necessary to prevent circulatory overload.

Side-effects of mannitol are chills, fever, nausea and tachycardia. Care is necessary to avoid extravasation, as necrosis may occur.

DRUGS USED IN SOME URINARY TRACT DISORDERS AND IN BENIGN PROSTATIC HYPERPLASIA

Urinary frequency and bladder spasm

Many of the anticholinergic drugs of the propantheline type are useful in the treatment of urinary frequency and incontinence, and other drugs with anticholinergic (antimuscarinic) **side-effects**, such as amitriptyline and other tricyclic antidepressants, are also given in enuresis and similar conditions. They act mainly by reducing the contractile activity of the detrusor muscle, but they have the disadvantages of most anticholinergic agents of causing dryness of the mouth and blurred vision. Care is also necessary in the elderly, as they may precipitate glaucoma, and in males may add to the problems of prostatic hyperplasia. Some other drugs used in the treatment of urinary frequency and other bladder disorders are represented by the following.

Desmopressin § (dose: 10–40 micrograms intranasally; 200–400 micrograms orally)

Brand names: DDAVP §, Desmospray §, Desmotabs §
Desmopressin is an analogue of vasopressin (p. 176) and is used in the control of primary nocturnal enuresis in children and adults. It is given by nasal spray at bedtime in doses of 10–20 micrograms, increased to a maximum of 40 micrograms if necessary. Alternatively, it may be given orally in doses of 200 micrograms at night, increased to 400 micrograms only if the response to the lower dose is inadequate. It is not recommended for children under 5 years of age. The response should be checked at 3-monthly intervals by suspending treatment for a week. Although desmopressin has little pressor activity, care should be taken in hypertension, cardiovascular disorders and in renal impairment. Its use in diabetes insipidus is referred to on p. 177.

Ephedrine § (dose: 30–60 mg daily)

Ephedrine is a sympathomimetic amine (p. 90) that has been used in nocturnal enuresis. Dose 30–60 mg at night according to age.

Flavoxate § (dose: 600 mg daily)

Brand name: Urispas §
Flavoxate has some smooth muscle relaxant properties, and is indicated in the control of spasm of the urinary tract and in the symptomatic relief of dysuria, urgency and cystitis. It is given in doses of 200 mg three times a day.

Side-effects may include headache, nausea and blurred vision. Like related drugs, it should be used with care if glaucoma is present.

Oxybutynin § (dose: 10–20 mg daily)

Brand names: Cystrin §, Ditropan §
Oxybutynin resembles flavoxate in having antispasmodic properties, and is useful in relieving the symptoms of neurogenic bladder instability, such as frequency and urgency. It is given in doses of 5 mg two to four times a day according to need. Children and the elderly may be more susceptible to the atropine-like **side-effects** of oxybutynin, and should be given half-doses.

BENIGN PROSTATIC HYPERPLASIA

Benign prostatic hyperplasia (BPH) is common in men over 50 years of age, and causes urinary frequency and urgency, nocturia and decreased urinary flow. The associated incomplete emptying of the bladder may promote infection and secondary inflammation of the bladder which may also involve the upper urinary tract. Surgery is the radical treatment, but when that is contra-indicated or has to be postponed, treatment with alpha-adrenoceptor blocking agents or an anti-androgen may give symptomatic relief. Testosterone has a considerable influence on prostatic growth, mediated by its conversion to the more potent metabolite dyhydrotestosterone by the enzyme 5-alpha-reductase. In prostatic hyperplasia an inhibitor of that enzyme could lead to a reduction in prostatic size, an improvement in the urinary flow and a reduction in the volume of residual urine. An enzyme inhibitor of the required type is finasteride, which in effect functions as an anti-androgen.

The alternative treatment of BPH with alpha-adrenoceptor blocking agents is based on the finding that prostatic smooth muscle contraction is a response to sympathetic nerve stimulation, mediated specifically by the α_{1A}-adrenoceptors. In BPH a blockade of those receptors could lead to prostatic muscle relaxation, with consequent relief of the typical symptoms of benign prostatic hyperplasia. Several drugs with α_{1A}-adrenoceptor blocking action are now available, and are listed in Table 11.2.

They have a number of **side-effects** in common, particularly first-dose postural hypotension. The first dose should always be taken at night with the patient in bed, with a warning to lie down at once if giddiness or sweating develops with subsequent doses.* The elderly should commence treatment with half-doses.

By the nature of their action these drugs have some antihypertensive properties, and patients already receiving blood-pressure lowering drugs should be given reduced doses under supervision.

Finasteride § (dose: 5 mg daily)

Brand name: Proscar §

Finasteride is given as a single daily dose of 5 mg, but prolonged administration is necessary to bring about an adequate shrinkage in size of the prostate gland, and the response should be reviewed after six months' treatment.

Side-effects are linked with the anti-androgen nature of finasteride, and include impotence, breast tenderness and hypersensitivity reactions such as rash and lip-swelling. Finasteride has a highly selective action, and has no affinity for androgen receptors in other tissues.

Table 11.2 Drugs used in benign prostatic hyperplasia

Approved name	Brand name	Daily dose range
Alpha$_{1A}$-adrenoceptor blocking agents		
alfuzosin	Xatral	5–10 mg
doxazosin	Cardura	1–8 mg
indoramin	Doralese	40–100 mg
prazosin	Hypovase	1–4 mg
tamsulosin	Flomax	400 micrograms
terazosin	Hytrin BPH	1–10 mg
5-alpha-reductase inhibitor		
finasteride	Proscar	5 mg

*Tamsulosin is the exception. It has little action on the cardiovascular system and the daily dose should be taken with water after breakfast.

FURTHER READING

Gormley G J et al 1982 The effect of finasteride in men with benign prostatic hyperplasia. New England Journal of Medicine 327:1185–1191

Jardin A et al 1981 Alfuzosin for the treatment of benign prostatic hypertrophy. Lancet 337:1457–1461

12

Drugs acting on the uterus and vagina

The oestrogenic and other hormones play an important part in the development and continuing function of the uterus, but there are also a few unrelated compounds that have a powerful action on the pregnant uterus. Of chief value are those that increase uterine contractions once labour has commenced (the oxytocics), and those that inhibit premature labour. Of the former group, sometimes referred to as myometrial stimulants, ergot is one of the most effective drugs.

OXYTOCICS

Ergot is a fungus that develops in the ear of rye and some other cereals, when instead of the normal grains, dark-coloured, long and tapering 'grains' are produced. These fungal bodies contain the alkaloids ergometrine and ergotamine. The former is widely used in the later stages of labour and in the control of post-partum haemorrhage; ergotamine is used in migraine (p. 56).

Flour made from infected rye can cause severe ergot poisoning, and epidemics due to such poisoning have often occurred in the past, and are not unknown today. This poisoning, once known as 'Saint Anthony's Fire' is characterized by extreme pain in the limbs, which is eventually followed by gangrene, and also by epileptiform convulsions.

Ergometrine maleate § (dose: 0.5–1 mg orally; 0.2–1 mg by injection)

Ergometrine is the principal alkaloid of ergot, and is used mainly during the third stage of labour. Following oral doses of 0.5–1 mg, uterine contractions commence within a few minutes and persist for about an hour. When there is a high risk of post-partum haemorrhage, or in emergency, ergometrine may be given intravenously in doses of 125–250 micrograms. Oral ergometrine is also of value in the control of minor post-partum haemorrhage in doses of 500 micrograms three times a day for up to 3 days.

Oxytocin §

Brand name: Syntocinon §
Oxytocin has a selective stimulating action on uterine muscle, but it has no pressor or antidiuretic properties. The degree of activity is related to the physiological state of the uterus, and is greatest during the late stages of pregnancy. In practice oxytocin is used mainly in uterine inertia and for the induction of labour. It is given by intravenous drip infusion in dextrose solution, in small doses of 1–3 milliunits per minute, as the rapid response requires careful control of the dose with monitoring of the fetal heart rate.

Oxytocin is also used to control post-partum haemorrhage, and is given in doses of 5–10 units by slow intravenous infusion. Doses of 2–5 units may also be given by intramuscular injection, often together with 500 micrograms of the longer-acting ergometrine, as Syntometrine. Oxytocin is also used by intravenous infusion in the management of missed abortion.

PROSTAGLANDINS

The prostaglandins have a wide range of activity (see p. 206), but prostaglandins E and F are of value in midwifery and obstetrics as they cause contractions of both the non-pregnant and pregnant uterus. Prostaglandin analogues are now used in the induction of labour and to induce abortion, as they cause softening of the tissues and reduce the resistance of cervical tissues. They are also used for the termination of early pregnancy as the uterine muscle is relatively insensitive to oxytocin.

Two of the main disorders of menstruation, dysmenorrhoea (painful periods) and menorrhagia (excessive blood loss) are associated with abnormal prostaglandin production. In the latter there is an increased production of PGE_2 and PGI_2, which causes an increased vasodilatation of the endometrial blood vessels, together with an increased production of prostacyclin resulting in a reduction in haemostasis. In spasmodic dysmenorrhoea there is an increase in the availability of the spasmogenic prostaglandins PGE_{2a} and PGF_{2a}. It is on that basis that NSAIDs (p. 203) are used for treatment.

Carboprost §

Brand name Hemebate §
Carboprost has an action on the uterus similar to that of ergometrine and oxytocin, and is used in the control of post-partum haemorrhage not responding to those drugs. It is given by deep intramuscular injection in doses of 250 micrograms at intervals of 90 minutes, or less according to need, but a total dose of 2 mg should not be exceeded, i.e. 8 doses. Nausea, diarrhoea and flushing are among the many **side-effects** of carboprost.

Dinoprost §

Brand name: Prostin F2 alpha §
Dinoprost is a prostaglandin used for the induction of labour as well as for the therapeutic termination of pregnancy and abortion. It is given by intra-amniotic injection as well as intravenously, but intravenous injection is associated with an increased risk of **side-effects** such as shivering, pyrexia, dizziness and diarrhoea. See Manufacturer's Data Sheet for dose.

Dinoprostone §

Brand names: Prepidil §, Prostin E2 §
Dinoprostone is a prostaglandin used for the induction of labour as well as for the termination of pregnancy and for abortion. It is given orally in doses of 500 micrograms at hourly intervals up to a total of 1.5 mg, and as a vaginal gel containing 400 micrograms/ml, and as vaginal tablets containing 3 mg. For abortion it is given by intravenous infusion or slow extra-amniotic injection, under close hospital supervision.

Note. Prepidil cervical gel is used for cervical softening and dilation before induction; Prostin E2 vaginal gel is for the induction of labour. Prostin E2 vaginal tablets are used for the same purpose, but contain different doses of dinoprostone, and must not be regarded as equivalent products. Specialist literature should be consulted.

Gemeprost §

Brand name: Cervagem §
Gemeprost is a prostaglandin used to dilate the cervix uteri and facilitate operation in first trimester

abortion, and is given as a 1 mg pessary 3 hours before surgery. For details of dose and risks, specialist literature should be consulted.

Mifepristone §

Brand name: Mifegyne §
Mifepristone is not a prostaglandin but an antiprogestogen, and is considered here as it is used in the termination of pregnancy (up to 63 days duration). It appears to sensitize the uterus to local prostaglandins, and is given under close control as a single oral dose of 600 mg. If abortion is not complete after 36–48 hours, a pessary of gemoprost (1 mg) should be used, but careful observation of the patient is necessary for 6 hours, as gemoprost may cause marked hypotension. Both smoking and alcohol should be avoided by patients likely to need gemoprost, and the drug is contra-indicated in patients over 35 years who smoke.

Side-effects include nausea, diarrhoea, shivering and pyrexia. Severe uterine pain and bleeding may also occur. Mifepristone is under investigation for use in metastatic breast cancer, and as a postcoital contraceptive.

Alprostadil §

Brand name: Prostin VR §
Alprostadil or prostaglandin E_1 is used only to maintain the patency of the ductus arteriosus in neonates with ductus dependent heart defects, who are awaiting corrective surgery. It is given by intravenous infusion in doses of 50–100 nanograms/kg/minute, reduced according to need.

Alprostadil has many **side-effects**, and intensive care facilities must be available.

Indomethacin has the opposite action, and is used under specialist supervision when closure of the ductus arteriosus is required. The dosage scheme is complex and depends on age; consult specialist literature.

PREMATURE LABOUR

To prevent premature labour a drug is required that has a powerful and selective relaxant action on the uterus, and is free from toxic side-effects. Suitable myometrial relaxants are few, but some of the required uterine muscle-relaxant properties are found in some sympathomimetic drugs with a selective stimulant action on the β_2 adrenoceptors

(p. 238). They are indicated in the control of uncomplicated premature labour between the 24th and 33rd weeks, but the use of these drugs requires care, and the dose must be adjusted to need and response; attention should be paid to the fetal as well as the maternal heart rate. Tachycardia is a common **side-effect**, and may increase to a serious extent if atropine has already been given during premedication. These drugs are contra-indicated in haemorrhagic conditions.

Ritodrine §

Brand name: Yutopar §
Ritodrine has a relaxant action on uterine muscle, and is given by intravenous infusion as soon as possible after the onset of premature labour in doses of 50 micrograms/minute, increased as required up to 150–350 micrograms/minute. The optimum dose should be continued for 12–48 hours after the contractions have been brought under control, and the response maintained by intramuscular doses of 10 mg 4-hourly before transfer to oral therapy with doses of 10 mg as required, and continued as long as necessary. Intravenous doses of 50 micrograms/minute are also given in cases of fetal asphyxia due to uterine hypertonicity while preparing for delivery.

Side-effects are those of the sympathomimetic agents and include tachycardia, nausea, hypotension and flushing. Ritodrine is contra-indicated in eclampsia, cardiac disorders and antepartum haemorrhage. Pulmonary oedema has occurred with ritodrine therapy, but is possibly linked with fluid overload.

Salbutamol §

Brand name: Ventolin §
Salbutamol is a β_2-adrenoceptor stimulant (p. 238) used in the control of uncomplicated premature labour. It is given by intravenous infusion in doses of 10 micrograms/minute initially, gradually increased to 45 micrograms/minute until contractions have ceased. Dosage can then be slowly reduced according to response, followed by intramuscular injections in doses of 100–250 micrograms before changing to oral therapy in doses of 4 mg 6–8-hourly.

Terbutaline §

Brand name: Bricanyl §
Terbutaline resembles salbutamol in its action and is given by intravenous infusion in doses of

5 micrograms/minute for 20 minutes, and gradually increased to 10 micrograms/minute until contractions have ceased. Later treatment is the subcutaneous injection of the drug in doses of 250 micrograms 6-hourly for 3 days, when oral therapy with 5 mg doses 8-hourly may be given for maintenance therapy as required.

Side-effects of terbutaline are similar to those of other myometrial relaxants used in the treatment of premature labour.

Eclampsia

Eclampsia is a severe form of toxaemia of pregnancy, characterized by convulsions, hypertension and oedema. The cause is unknown, but the primary treatment is the intravenous infusion of 4 g of magnesium sulfate. Diazepam is sometimes preferred for the immediate control of the convulsions.

ENDOMETRIOSIS

Endometriosis affects 1–2% of the female population, and is due to the presence of functional endometrial tissue in parts of the body other than the uterus. Such tissue is mainly found in the pelvis but may be present elsewhere. The symptoms that arise from such ectopic endometrium include dysmenorrhoea, menorrhagia, dyspareunia and infertility. The aims of treatment are pain relief, resolution of the ectopic tissues, and when wanted, restoration of fertility. The dependence of endometrial tissue on ovarian hormones, particularly oestrogen, has led to the use of therapy aimed at ovarian suppression and the inhibition of cyclic menstruation with progestogens, androgens and gonadotrophin-releasing agonists such as buserelin, and the gonadotrophin inhibitor danazol.

Buserelin § (dose: 900 micrograms daily)

Brand name: Suprecur §
Buserelin is a synthetic analogue of gonadotrophin that indirectly suppresses ovarian steroid production and is used as a nasal spray for the symptomatic relief of endometriosis. A dose of 150 micrograms is sprayed into each nostril three times a day, starting on the first day of the menstrual cycle. Prolonged treatment for up to 6 months may be required. A second course is inadvisable, as buserelin may bring about a reduction in bone density. From the nature of its action buserelin has many **side-effects**,

including menstrual and menopause-like symptoms, breast tenderness, nervousness and mood changes.

Danazol § (dose: 200–800 mg daily)

Brand name: Danol §
Danazol is a steroid with androgenic properties that has a suppressive action on gonadotrophin secretion. It is used mainly in endometriosis; other therapeutic applications are menorrhagia, gynaecomastia and hereditary angio-oedema. In endometriosis it is given in doses of 100–200 mg four times a day, starting on the first day of the cycle, and continued for some months. Doses of 200–400 mg daily are given in gynaecomastia. It is given occasionally in mastalgia when gamolenic acid is ineffective (p. 173).

Side-effects are linked with its androgenic action, and include weight gain, oedema, acne and voice changes.

Gestrinone § (dose: 5 mg weekly)

Brand name: Dimetriose §
Gestrinone is an antiprogestogen that appears to have a multiple action in endometriosis. It is believed to reduce gonadotrophin activity and subsequent ovarian steroid production, to increase androgen levels and to have a direct effect on endometrial tissues. It is given in doses of 2.5 mg twice a week, starting on the first day of the cycle, with the second dose 3 days later. As with other drugs used in endometriosis, treatment for 6 months may be required. Care is necessary in patients with cardiac or renal disease as gestrinone may cause some fluid retention. Diabetic patients and those with hyperlipidaemia require increased monitoring during gestrinone treatment.

Side-effects are similar to those of danazol.

Goserelin §

Brand name: Zoladex §
Goserelin has the actions, uses and side-effects of buserelin, but differs in being given as a *single* course of treatment by subcutaneous injection into the anterior abdominal wall in doses of 3.6 mg every 28 days, starting on the 1st–5th day of the cycle. Like buserelin, treatment for up to 6 months may be required. It may cause local irritation at the injection site, and the use of a local anaesthetic may be necessary. Leuprorelin § (Prostap SR §) has a similar action and is given by subcutaneous or intramuscular injection in doses of 3.75 mg every 28 days. Goserelin is also used in the treatment of advanced premenopausal breast cancer (p. 223).

Nafarelin §

Brand name: Synarel §
Nafarelin, like buserelin, is given in endometriosis as a spray of 200 micrograms in one nostril each morning, and a similar dose in the other nostril in the evenings for a maximum period of 6 months. A repeat dose may be given if sneezing occurs during or immediately after use; nasal decongestants should be avoided before and after treatment.

Side-effects are similar to those of buserelin.

Gamolenic acid §

Brand name: Efamast §
Gamolenic acid is not a hormone, but is referred to here as it is used for the relief of mastalgia or breast pain, and is better tolerated than danazol. It is given in doses of 120–160 mg (as evening primrose oil) twice daily for 8–12 weeks, or longer with lower maintenance doses.

VAGINAL THERAPY

Most of the drugs referred to in this section are those used locally for vaginal candidiasis or mixed infections. Those agents that are given orally and have a systemic action are dealt with in more detail in Chapter 5.

Clotrimazole

Brand name: Canestan
Clotrimazole is one of the imidazole group of antifungal agents used topically in various dermatomycoses, but it is also useful in candidal or mixed candidal–trichomonal vaginal infections. It is used as a vaginal tablet containing 100 mg of the drug, for insertion high in the vagina at night for at least 6 nights. A cream is available for more frequent use.

Metronidazole §

Brand names: Flagyl §
Metronidazole is an antimicrobial agent that is also used in the treatment of infections caused by the flagellate protozoan *Trichomonas vaginalis*. That organism causes a low-grade vaginitis, which may be treated with metronidazole in oral doses of 200–400 mg three times a day for 7–10 days, or 800 mg in the morning and 1200 mg at night for 2 nights.

For vaginitis of combined trichomonal and candidal origin, a mixed product of metronidazole and nystatin is available as Flagyl Compak §. The use of metronidazole in systemic anaerobic infections is referred to on p. 72.

Miconazole §

Brand names: Femeron §, Gyno-Daktarin §, Monistat §
Miconazole is another imidazole antifungal agent that is mainly used systemically (p. 84), but it is also effective when used locally in the treatment of vulvovaginal candidiasis. It is used both as a pessary (100 mg) and as a vaginal cream (2%) and two pessaries or two applications of the cream should be used nightly for 7 nights, and subsequently repeated if necessary. Fenticonazole § (Lomexin §) has similar actions and uses.

Nystatin §

Brand name: Nystan §
Nystatin is an antifungal antibiotic used orally in intestinal candidiasis (p. 83) but it is also effective in vaginal candidiasis. It is used mainly as pessaries containing 100 000 units, two of which should be inserted high in the vagina nightly for 14 nights. Cream, gel and ointment are available for intravaginal or local use. Econazole (Ecostatin; Pevaryl §), isoconazole (Travogyn §), ketoconazole (Nizoral §) and amphotericin (Fungilin §) are other products used locally for vaginal infections. Clindamycin (Dalacin cream 2% §) is used in bacterial vaginosis.

FURTHER READING

Buckman R 1994 Endometriosis: pharmacologic alternatives to surgery. Journal of Practical Nursing 44(3):47–58
Donaldson K et al 1994 RU 486: An alternative to surgical abortion. Journal of Obstetric, Gynecologic and Neonatal Nursing 23(7):555–557
Fox R, Draycott T 1996 Diazepam is more useful than magnesium sulphate for immediate control of eclampsia. British Medical Journal 312:1669–1670
Garner C 1994 Uses of GnRH agonists. Journal of Obstetric, Gynecologic and Neonatal Nursing 23(7):563–570
Glasier A et al 1992 Mifepristone (RU 486) compared with high-dose estrogen and progestogen for emergency postcoital contraception. New England Journal of Medicine 327(15):1041–1044

Guillebaud J 1990 Medical termination of pregnancy. British Medical Journal 301:352–354

Mackenzie S, Yeo S 1997 Pregnancy interruption using mifepristone (RU-486). Journal of Nurse-Midwifery 42(2):86–90

Narrigan D 1994 Postcoital contraception. Journal of Nurse-Midwifery 39(6):363–369

Nielson J P 1995 Magnesium sulphate: the drug of choice in eclampsia. British Medical Journal 311:702–703

Peyron R et al 1993 Early termination of pregnancy with mifepristone (RU 486) and the orally active prostaglandin misoprotol. New England Journal of Medicine 328(21):1509–1513

Rennie J M, Cooke R W I 1991 Prolonged low-dose indomethacin for ductus arteriosus of prematurity. Archives of Diseases in Childhood 66:55–58

Report of working group on the management of genital candidiasis 1995 British Medical Journal 310:241–244

Shaw R W 1992 Treatment for endometriosis. Lancet 340 (8830):1267–1270

Summers L 1997 Methods of cervical ripening and labor induction. Journal of Nurse-Midwifery 42(2):71–85

Wright S 1991 Abortifacient drugs: ethico-legal issues. Nursing Standard 5(24):36–37

13

Hormones and the endocrine system

THE ENDOCRINE SYSTEM

The endocrine system is part of the chemical communication system of the body and complements the nervous system. The latter evokes rapid but short-term responses whereas the former causes slower and more sustained effects. The endocrine system consists of small ductless glands spread throughout the body which secrete hormonal messenger substances into the circulation. These hormones interact with receptors on certain cell surfaces, or in the case of the steroid hormones, with receptors within the cells, and bring about a physiological response. The hormone-regulated processes include the stress response, the maintenance of the salt, water and nutrient balance of the body and the regulation of cell metabolism.

The endocrine glands are stimulated to release their hormones by other hormones (termed trophic hormones), by humoral stimuli such as the blood levels of calcium or sugar or by neural stimuli. The hormone levels in the blood are controlled by negative feedback mechanisms, but in certain circumstances the nervous system can over-ride or modulate hormonal activity via hypothalamic control.

Many of the natural hormones have now been synthesized, and in addition some synthetic analogues are available that are more potent than the natural products. More recently, genetic engineering has allowed the production in quantity of chemically identical hormones. A number of hormones and hormone antagonists are now used therapeutically in the management of a variety of illnesses.

THE PITUITARY GLAND

The pituitary gland or hypophysis is situated in the sella turcica of the spheroid bone at the base of the skull, and is attached to the hypothalamus by a stalk. It has two lobes, the anterior lobe or adrenohypophysis, and the posterior lobe or neurohypophysis. The anterior lobe produces and secretes a number of hormones, whereas the posterior lobe stores hormones produced by the hypothalamus.

The relationship between the pituitary gland and the many hormones it produces is indicated in Figure 13.1.

POSTERIOR LOBE

This part of the pituitary gland is a store for two hormones, vasopressin and oxytocin, derived from the hypothalamus. Vasopressin is the antidiuretic hormone. It affects the permeability of the collecting duct of the nephron, and so plays an essential part in maintaining the water balance of the body. Oxytocin stimulates contractions of uterine smooth muscle, particularly at the end of pregnancy (see p. 170).

Vasopressin, now obtained by recombinant technology, increases the re-absorption of water by the renal tubules when the fluid intake is low, and so reduces the urinary output, whereas with a high intake of fluid it decreases absorption and preserves

the fluid balance by increasing urinary excretion. Vasopressin is used mainly in the treatment of diabetes insipidus which is caused by pituitary dysfunction. It is a deficiency condition that may occur abruptly at almost any age, or it may follow injury, and is characterized by thirst and a high output of very dilute urine. A correspondingly high fluid intake is required that may amount to several litres a day. Two forms of the disease are recognized, pituitary diabetes insipidus (PDI), and nephrogenic or partial diabetes insipidus (NDI). The former can be treated by vasopressin, but in practice vasopressin is used mainly for the diagnosis of PDI, and its differentiation from NDI. In nephrogenic diabetes insipidus the kidneys are resistant to exogenous ADH and treatment is with chlorpropamide, chlorthalidone and carbamazepine. Those drugs appear to sensitize the renal tubules to respond to any remaining endogenous vasopressin.

Vasopressin § (dose: 5–20 units)

Brand name: Pitressin §

Vasopressin is used in the diagnosis and treatment of pituitary diabetes insipidus and is given in doses

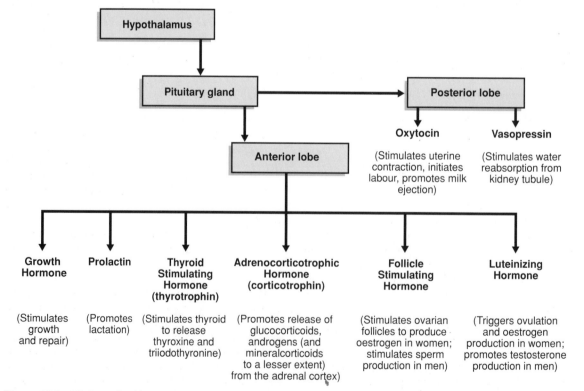

Figure 13.1 Pituitary gland hormones.

of 5–20 units by subcutaneous or intramuscular injection every 4 hours. When the diabetes insipidus is due to injury, only short-term treatment may be necessary. For long-term use treatment with alternative drugs such as desmopressin, lypressin and terlipressin is usually preferred, which in some cases can be given by nasal spray. Vasopressin is also used for the control of variceal bleeding, and is then given in doses of 20 units by intravenous infusion.

Side-effects of vasopressin are nausea and intestinal disturbances, cramp and occasionally angina.

Desmopressin §

Brand names: DDAVP §, Desmospray §, Desmotabs §
Desmopressin is a synthetic analogue of vasopressin with a much longer antidiuretic action and reduced pressor side-effects. It is used in pituitary diabetes insipidus as nasal drops or spray once or twice a day in doses of 10–20 micrograms (one to two puffs), or orally in doses of 100–200 micrograms three times a day. It may also be given by intramuscular or intravenous injection in doses of 1–4 micrograms daily. Liquid intake must be adjusted during desmopressin treatment to avoid fluid retention and hyponatria. **Side-effects** of desmopressin are similar to those of vasopressin. Desmopressin is sometimes useful in nocturnal enuresis when endogenous vasopressin may be deficient. In doses of 20–40 micrograms at night it may control the eneuresis without affecting day-time kidney function. It may also be of value in nocturia associated with multiple sclerosis. Withdrawal of such treatment should be carried out after 3 months to permit an assessment of renal function.

Lypressin § (dose: 2.5–10 units as required)

Brand name: Syntopressin §
Lypressin resembles desmopressin in action, and in pituitary diabetes insipidus it is given as a nasal spray in doses of 2.5–10 units (one to four puffs) 3–4 times a day. Local **side-effects** are nasal congestion and ulceration; it may also cause nausea and abdominal pain.

Terlipressin § (dose: 1–2 mg by injection)

Brand name: Glypressin §
Terlipressin is a vasopressin analogue for the treatment of bleeding from oesophageal varices. It is given by intravenous injection as an initial dose

of 2 mg, followed by doses of 1–2 mg 4- to 6-hourly until bleeding is controlled up to a maximum of 12 doses. The **side-effects** of terlipressin are similar to those of vasopressin, but less marked.

ANTERIOR LOBE

The anterior lobe of the pituitary gland is one of the most important glands of the body. It secretes at least six hormones, four of which are trophic hormones stimulating other endocrine glands (Fig. 13.1). Some are used therapeutically, others in diagnosis, but as they are protein in nature they are not effective orally and must be given by injection.

With a few exceptions their therapeutic use is disappointing. Their action is basically that of stimulating the related endocrine gland, i.e. the thyrotrophic hormone controls the activity of the thyroid gland, and in therapy the use of the hormones of the gland concerned is preferred.

Corticotrophin §

Corticotrophin, the adrenocorticotrophic hormone, sometimes referred to as ACTH has a direct action on the cortex of the adrenal gland, and stimulates the production of hydrocortisone, cortisone and other steroids. The final action of the hormone is basically that of hydrocortisone, and direct treatment with that drug or related steroids is now preferred.

Corticotrophin exerts its effects through the medium of the adrenal gland, and in health there is a balance between the activity of the gland and the level of corticosteroids in circulation. The balance is achieved by a 'feedback' mechanism, as a rise in the blood corticosteroid level causes a fall in corticotrophin secretion. That fall results in a reduction in the release of the steroids from the adrenal cortex, which then stimulates the anterior pituitary gland to produce more corticotrophin, so the level of corticosteroids again rises, and this 'see-saw' rise and fall in hormone production is an essential part of the physiological balance of the body.

When the cortex is damaged, as in Addison's disease, corticotrophin is of no value and corticosteroid replacement therapy is necessary. Corticotrophin has been used in the treatment of chronic asthma and many other disorders but its use has declined as the response is unreliable. It remains in limited use in the tetracosactrin test of the efficiency of adrenocortical function.

ADRENAL CORTEX

When the adrenal cortex is stimulated by adrenocorticotrophic hormone (ACTH) it releases two types of steroidal hormones, both synthesized from cholesterol, namely the corticosteroids and the adrenal androgens. The corticosteroid hormones can be divided into two main groups, the glucocorticoids which are exemplified by hydrocortisone and which control carbohydrate and protein metabolism, and the mineralocorticoids represented by aldosterone which influence salt and water balance. This distinction is useful, but not exact as natural glucocorticoids also influence water and electrolyte balance. Some synthetic derivatives have a more selective action, and fludrocortisone is exceptional in having marked mineralocorticoid potency.

GLUCOCORTICOIDS

The glucocorticoids influence a wide range of physiological activities (Fig. 13.2) and so have extensive therapeutic uses.

Hydrocortisone (cortisol) and cortisone are well known examples of natural glucocorticoid hormones, and are closely related as cortisone is converted in the liver to hydrocortisone, although many synthetic analogues are now in use. They are potent drugs with a wide range of action and uses, and have many side-effects. They are mainly used to suppress inflammation and allergic/ immune responses, and are valuable in rheumatoid arthritis, vasculitis, ulcerative colitis and Crohn's disease. They are also used locally in inflammatory eye disorders, and skin conditions such as psoriasis and eczema. Their basic action is mediated by the stimulation of lipocortin synthesis in the leukocytes. That protein inhibits the enzyme phospholipase A_2, which is concerned with the formation of arachidonic acid, the precursor of prostaglandin and leukotriene inflammatory mediators (p. 204).

Glucocorticoids also reduce the release of histamine from basophils, and so are useful in allergic states. In bronchial asthma and other obstructive diseases of the airways they reduce bronchial inflammation and mucus production and increase airway calibre. They also have a marked immunosuppressive action, and on that account they are used in association with other drugs such as azathioprine to prevent the rejection of transplanted organs. As they also inhibit cell division by interfering with DNA synthesis, glucocorticoids are also used in combination with cytotoxic drugs in the treatment of leukaemia, lymphoma and other cancerous conditions. Dexamethasone in particular is used to reduce cerebral oedema. By their mineralocorticoid activity they are of value in the treatment of shock.

In deficiency states, such as Addison's disease, the secretion of corticosteroids by the adrenal cortex is diminished or absent, and for replacement therapy reliance is largely placed on hydrocortisone supplemented by fludrocortisone. The latter has an increased mineralocorticoid activity that provides the balance for complete replacement therapy.

The potency of the corticosteroids is such that they should be used with great care, and in principle they should be used in the lowest effective dose for the shortest period of time. Patients should carry a card stating that they are receiving the drugs, so that in cases of emergency, treatment can be adapted to the patient concerned, as continuity of treatment is important, and higher doses may be necessary in illness. Table 13.1 shows the anti-inflammatory doses of some corticosteroids, although larger doses may be required in allergic conditions (p. 256).

Nursing points about corticosteroid therapy

(a) They are potent drugs; lowest effective dose should be given and response balanced against the potential dangers.
(b) In long-term treatment, the side-effects may be worse than the disabilities caused by the illness being treated.
(c) In chronic conditions, treatment should be withdrawn very slowly to permit the return of normal adrenocortical function.
(d) Corticosteroids are best taken in the morning to reduce suppressive effects on pituitary–adrenal function.
(e) All patients should carry a steroid warning card.
(f) Great care is necessary in anaesthesia, and measures must be taken to avoid a potentially precipitous fall in blood pressure due to corticosteroid therapy.

Table 13.1 Comparable doses of some corticosteroids

Corticosteroid	Dose
Betamethasone	0.75 mg
Cortisone	25.0 mg
Hydrocortisone	20.0 mg
Deflazacort	6.0 mg
Prednisone	5.0 mg
Methylprednisolone	4.0 mg
Triamcinolone	4.0 mg
Dexamethasone	0.75 mg

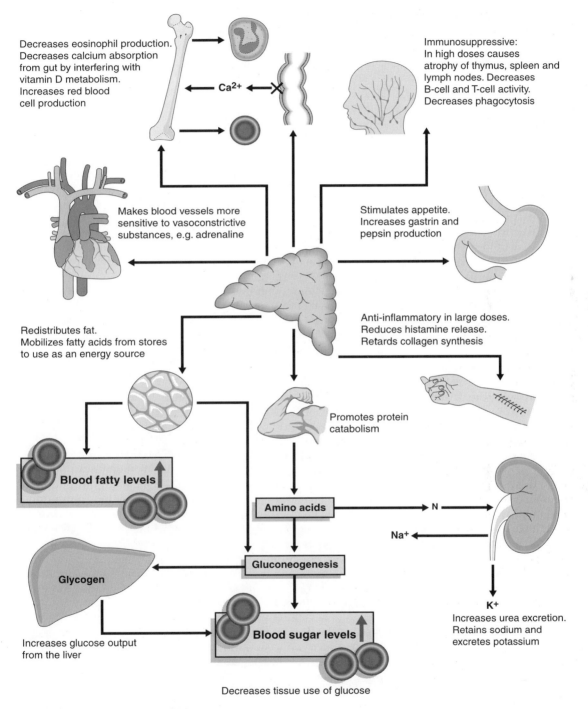

Decreases eosinophil production. Decreases calcium absorption from gut by interfering with vitamin D metabolism. Increases red blood cell production

Ca²⁺

Immunosuppressive: In high doses causes atrophy of thymus, spleen and lymph nodes. Decreases B-cell and T-cell activity. Decreases phagocytosis

Makes blood vessels more sensitive to vasoconstrictive substances, e.g. adrenaline

Stimulates appetite. Increases gastrin and pepsin production

Redistributes fat. Mobilizes fatty acids from stores to use as an energy source

Anti-inflammatory in large doses. Reduces histamine release. Retards collagen synthesis

Promotes protein catabolism

Blood fatty levels ↑

Amino acids → N →

Na⁺ ←

Glycogen

Gluconeogenesis

Blood sugar levels ↑

Increases glucose output from the liver

K⁺
Increases urea excretion. Retains sodium and excretes potassium

Decreases tissue use of glucose

Figure 13.2 Effects of glucocorticoids.

Side-effects The glucocorticoids have many side-effects, and so they must be used with care. Suppression of the pituitary–adrenal axis can occur within 10 days of starting treatment, and thus withdrawal of the drug can lead to hypoadrenalism, which may cause an Addisonian crisis. Therefore, the drug must be withdrawn slowly. Patients should also carry a card stating that they are taking steroids, as suppression of the gland means that it is unable to respond in times of stress, and so patients will need to be given extra glucocorticoids to compensate. Giving twice the dose of glucocorticoid on alternate days can be effective in treating some conditions while minimizing adrenal suppression. The inhibitory effects of corticosteroids on adrenal secretion are greater at night than during the day and so can be minimized by giving the drug early in the day.

Metabolic problems are common. High doses quickly cause a moon-face and fat is redistributed from the extremities to the trunk, which can give rise to a 'buffalo-hump'. Increased appetite can lead to weight gain. Disturbed carbohydrate metabolism can lead to hyperglycaemia and diabetes, while protein loss from skeletal muscles causes wasting, weakness, and a negative nitrogen balance. An increase in bone catabolism may cause osteoporosis, especially in children and postmenopausal women. Purple striae, petechiae, hyperpigmentation and thinning of the skin occur as the protein content of skin and blood vessels are affected.

Fluid retention, hypokalaemia and hypertension may occur with drugs with a significant mineralocorticoid activity. Potassium supplements may be required to reduce muscle weakness and cardiac irregularities that can result from prolonged treatment. There is increased susceptibility to infections which may progress unrecognized because the normal indicators of infection, for example pyrexia, are suppressed. Nascent infections, for example tuberculosis, may be reactivated. Wound healing is also inhibited due to the negative affects on inflammation, wound debridement and proliferation of collagen. In children retardation of growth occurs and epiphyseal closure may be delayed. Administration of corticosteroids during pregnancy may suppress fetal adrenal function and cause cleft palate.

Other **side-effects** include depression, which can be serious in patients with a history of mental disturbances, psychosis, cataracts, reversible glaucoma which is unpredictable and results from a genetic susceptibility, peptic ulceration due to increased gastric acidity, and hirsutism.

Care is also necessary with locally used products; if applied over large areas, especially under occlusive dressings, systemic absorption may occur. Also, as their action is suppressive, the condition may return when treatment is discontinued.

Hydrocortisone §

Brand names: Efcortelan §, Efcortesol §, Hydrocortone §, Solu-Cortef §

Hydrocortisone is the main glucocorticoid hormone of the adrenal cortex. It is used orally for replacement therapy in Addison's disease and other conditions of adrenal cortex deficiency in doses of 20 mg in the morning and 10 mg at night, adjusted to need, and supplemented by fludrocortisone, which has an increased mineralocorticoid activity. In severe deficiency states, and in the crises of Addison's disease, hydrocortisone is given by intravenous injection in doses of 100 mg every 6–8 hours, followed by oral therapy as the condition is controlled.

Large doses of hydrocortisone intravenously are also used in the emergency treatment of severe acute asthma, and to supplement adrenaline injections in acute hypersensitivity reactions. It is also given intravenously for the treatment of septic shock in doses up to 300 mg, although the value of such therapy has been questioned. Large doses have been given orally in conditions such as pemphigus and exfoliative dermatitis. A retention enema containing hydrocortisone 100 mg is sometimes used in ulcerative colitis to supplement other therapy.

Hydrocortisone is also highly effective when applied locally in the treatment of many inflamed and itching skin conditions (see p. 256).

Cortisone §

Brand name: Cortisyl §

Cortisone is a glucocorticoid with the actions and side-effects of hydrocortisone, to which it is converted in the liver. Hydrocortisone is now the preferred drug.

Prednisolone § and prednisone §

Prednisolone brand names: Deltastab §, Precortisyl §, Prednesol §

Prednisolone and prednisone are derivatives of hydrocortisone and cortisone respectively, but are about five times more potent. They have the same general action and uses of the parent drugs, but the increased glucocorticoid action is accompanied by a decrease in mineralocorticoid potency, with a reduction in some **side-effects** Prednisolone is now the preferred drug.

Prednisolone is used in a wide range of conditions requiring systemic corticosteroid therapy, including the suppression of the inflammatory reactions of rheumatoid arthritis, in allergic states, systemic lupus erythematosus and pemphigus, to name but a few. It is given orally in doses that may range from 5–60 mg daily in divided doses, but for the extended treatment of rheumatoid conditions doses above 10 mg daily are seldom required. In such long-term treatment, alternate-day, early-morning dosage may reduce side- effects by causing less depression of the pituitary– adrenal axis. For serious conditions such as acute lymphoblastic leukaemia and pemphigus, large doses are given, as the need to control the condition outweighs the risks of side-effects. In other cases, it may be given by intramuscular injection as prednisolone acetate in doses of 25–100 mg once or twice a week.

One of the chief disadvantages of corticosteroid therapy generally is the disturbance caused in the salt and water balance of the body. Although these disturbances are less with prednisolone and other derivatives, in all cases, and especially with long-term treatment, the maintenance dose should be the lowest dose that evokes a satisfactory response. Intermittent rather than daily doses have been recommended as pituitary–adrenal suppression may occur if treatment is prolonged. When treatment is to be discontinued, slow withdrawal of a corticosteroid over a period of weeks may be required to permit the natural production of corticosteroids to rise to a normal level.

The reduced tendency of some derivatives to cause salt and water retention is of advantage when long-term therapy is needed, but conversely, they are less suitable for the treatment of Addison's disease, and in such cases a salt-retaining corticosteroid such as fludrocortisone is required.

Corticosteroids such as prednisolone are given in high doses of 30–40 mg for the control of acute asthma, but for long-term use their systemic side-effects may cause complications. The difficulty has been solved to some extent by the introduction of some corticosteroids that are effective in asthma when given by oral inhalation. Beclomethasone (Becotide §, Becloforte §) and budesonide (Pulmicort §) are available products, supplied in metered dose aerosols, and given in doses of 50–200 micrograms up to four doses daily. Fluticasone (Flixotide §) is a newer derivative effective in doses of 25–120 micrograms. They are used in conditions of chronic airway obstruction not responding adequately to drugs of the salbutamol type, and regular use is necessary to obtain the maximum response. Patients should be given detailed instructions in the use of these aerosol products to obtain the maximum penetration of the drug (p. 13).

In some cases, the use of corticosteroid inhalations may permit a transfer from oral therapy, with a consequent reduction in side-effects, but such transfer must be made very slowly.

Dexamethasone §

Brand name: Decadron §

Dexamethasone has the general properties and uses of the corticosteroids, but it has little, if any, mineralocorticoid potency. It is given orally in doses of 0.5–9 mg daily, although larger doses up to 15 mg daily in divided doses may be required in severe conditions. Doses by intravenous injection range from 1 to 20 mg, but in the treatment of shock, doses of 2–6 mg/kg by intravenous infusion or injection have been given.

Dexamethasone is also of great value in the treatment of raised intracranial pressure, as in cerebral oedema, which can result from trauma or oxygen deprivation, and is then given intravenously as an initial dose of 10 mg, followed by intramuscular doses of 4 mg 6-hourly, continued if required for some days. The more selective action of dexamethasone on the hypothalamus–pituitary–adrenal axis is made use of in the dexamethasone suppression test for the diagnosis of Cushing's syndrome, in which a single dose of 1 mg is given at night. The degree of suppression of corticotrophin secretion is measured by the urinary excretion of certain hydroxycorticosteroids. Betamethasone (Betnelan §, Betnesol §) is a related compound with similar actions and uses.

MINERALOCORTICOSTEROIDS

Hydrocortisone and analogous compounds are known as glucocorticoids because their main effect is on carbohydrate metabolism. Other hormones of the adrenal cortex, represented by aldosterone, are concerned with the maintenance of the electrolyte balance of the body, and are referred to as mineralocorticoids. One synthetic compound, however, fludrocortisone, has both glucocorticoid and a marked mineralocorticoid activity.

Fludrocortisone acetate § (dose: 50–300 micrograms)

Brand name: Florinef §

Fludrocortisone is a fluorine-containing derivative of hydrocortisone, and is characterized by a marked increase in potency and salt-retaining properties of value in Addison's disease. In that disease the adrenal glands have been damaged or destroyed by tubercular infection, or have atrophied from other causes, and in consequence there is deficiency of adrenal corticosteroids. As a result of the absence of those sodium and water-retaining factors, large amounts of salt and fluid are excreted. Fludrocortisone can restore the electrolyte and fluid balance but doses of fludrocortisone that just maintain the electrolyte balance may not evoke an adequate glucocorticoid response. Therapeutically it is used only for partial replacement treatment of adrenocortical insufficiency in Addison's disease to supplement hydrocortisone therapy. Fludrocortisone is given in doses of 50–300 micrograms daily, together with hydrocortisone 20–30 mg daily, carefully adjusted to individual need and response. Both salt and fluid intake should be controlled to avoid the development of oedema, hypertension and weight gain. Occasionally, potassium supplements may be required.

INHIBITORS OF CORTICOSTEROID SYNTHESIS

These are considered here because of their biochemical association with hydrocortisone.

Metyrapone §

Brand name: Metopirone §
Metyrapone blocks the synthesis of hydrocortisone precursors at a specific point, and is used to test anterior pituitary gland activity. In the diagnosis of ACTH-dependent Cushing's syndrome it is given in doses of 750 mg 4-hourly for six doses, and the consequent reduction in the level of glucocorticoids in the plasma stimulates the anterior pituitary to secrete more corticotrophin. That increase stimulates the production of more precursors, but as further conversion to hydrocortisone is inhibited by metyrapone these precursors are excreted in the urine, and can be measured as an assessment of activity of the gland. Metyrapone has also been used in the treatment of Cushing's syndrome, in doses based on hydrocortisone production, under specialist supervision.

Trilostane § (dose: 120–480 mg daily)

Brand name: Modrenal §
Trilostane is a steroid antagonist that inhibits a particular stage in the biosynthesis of corticosteroids by the adrenal cortex. It is used in the treatment of Cushing's syndrome, primary aldosteronism, and

other conditions of adrenal cortex hyperfunction. The standard dose is 60 mg four times a day for 3 days, afterwards adjusted to need. Much larger doses have been given, and prolonged treatment is usually required, with monitoring of the blood corticosteroid and electrolyte levels. Caution is necessary in liver and kidney dysfunction.

Trilostane has a secondary use in the treatment of breast cancer when oestrogen antagonists such as aminoglutethimide (p. 222) are no longer effective.

GONADOTROPHIC HORMONES

These hormones stimulate the gonads in both sexes. Two separate hormones are known, the follicle-stimulating hormone (FSH) and the luteinizing hormone (LH). They are produced in the anterior lobe of the pituitary gland and released under the influence of gonadorelin, the gonadotrophin releasing hormone (GnRH) of the hypothalamus. Their function is complex, as in the female the follicle-stimulating hormone (FSH) controls the development of the ovarian follicles and the production of oestrogens. The luteinizing hormone (LH) is concerned with the development in the ovary of the corpus luteum and the formation of progesterone, whereas in the male the LH controls the production of androgens.

It has not proved possible to extract these hormones from anterior pituitary glands except in very small amounts, but large quantities of hormones with very similar actions are obtainable from other sources. The urine of pregnant women contains a hormone derived from the placenta and referred to as chorionic gonadotrophin (HCG), which resembles the luteinizing hormone. It is the presence of HCG in urine that forms the basis of some pregnancy tests. Human follicle-stimulating hormone is obtained from the urine of postmenopausal women. Some semi-synthetic hormone products are also available.

Chorionic gonadotrophin §

Brand names: Gonadotrophon LH §, Pregnyl §, Profasi §
Human chorionic gonadotrophin (HCG) is used in infertility caused by inadequate levels of natural gonadotrophins. It is given to induce ovulation after follicle development has been stimulated by injections of follicle-stimulating hormone, in doses based on individual need, and a course of treatment may require a total dose of 5000–10 000 units. The use of

HCG requires care to avoid hyperstimulation and multiple pregnancy. In males, HCG has been given in doses of 500 units or more to stimulate the production of testosterone in delayed puberty.

Side-effects include headache, mood changes and oedema.

Human gonadotrophins §

Humegon § and Normegon § are preparations of human menopausal gonadotrophin (HMG) containing the follicle-stimulating hormone (FSH) and the luteinizing hormone (LH). They are used in the treatment of female fertility disorders associated with hypopituitarism. Dose is based on the individual response. Metrodin § is a preparation of urofollitrophin, the follicle-stimulating hormone.

Intramuscular injections of FSH, followed by injections of HCG are used in anovulatory sterility due to low gonadotrophin secretion, particularly in patients who have not responded to clomiphene.

Gonadorelin § (LH-RH)

Brand names: Fertiral §, Relefact LH-RH §, HRF §
Gonadorelin is a synthetic form of the gonadotrophin-releasing hormone (LH-RH) that controls the formation and release of the follicle-stimulating and luteinizing hormones of the anterior pituitary gland. It is used as a diagnostic agent to assess pituitary function as a single intravenous dose of 100 micrograms, after which the level of circulating luteinizing hormone is assayed.

It is also used in the treatment of amenorrhoea and infertility due to a deficiency of endogenous gonadorelin. In such cases, gonadorelin is given by subcutaneous or intravenous pulsatile pump injections in initial doses of 10–20 micrograms, repeated every 90 minutes under careful control. Treatment is continued for 6 months unless conception occurs earlier.

Analogues of gonadorelin have an initial stimulating action on the production of gonadotrophin, followed by a secondary inhibition of ovarian and testicular activity. They have applications in the treatment of endometriosis and metastatic prostatic cancer (see pp. 172 and 222).

Sermorelin §

Brand name: Geref 50 §
Sermorelin is an analogue of somatorelin, the growth hormone releasing hormone (GHRH). It is given in a dose of 1 microgram/kg by intravenous injection after an overnight fast to determine the release of the growth hormone.

OTHER COMPOUNDS WITH HORMONE-LIKE ACTIVITY

Clomiphene citrate § (dose: 50–200 mg daily)

Brand names: Clomid §, Serophene §
Clomiphene is not a gonadotrophin but an anti-oestrogen, and is considered here because of its selective influence on ovulation. It blocks the actions of oestrogens on receptor sites in the hypothalamus, and by disturbing the normal hormone balance, indirectly increases the release of pituitary gonadotrophins, and stimulates the maturation of the ovarian follicles.

Clomiphene is used in the treatment of infertility provided that the patient is still capable of responding to an ovulatory stimulus. It is given in doses of 50 mg daily for 5 days, commencing about the 5th day of the menstrual cycle, or at any time if amenorrhoea is present, and may induce ovulation and produce an endometrium favourable to the establishment of pregnancy. The dose may be increased, if ovulation does not occur, up to 100 mg daily for 5 days as the cycle of treatment is continued, but if pregnancy is not achieved after three cycles, further treatment is unlikely to be successful. Treatment for more than six cycles may increase the risk of ovarian cancer.

Side-effects include visual disturbances, hot flushes, weight gain, dizziness and occasional hair loss. Care must be taken to avoid hyperstimulation, as multiple births have occurred. Clomiphene is contra-indicated in conditions of abnormal uterine bleeding, or if ovarian cysts are present.

Bromocriptine § (dose: 2.5–7.5 mg daily)

Brand name: Parlodel §
The hypothalamus both stimulates and inhibits the secretion of prolactin by the anterior pituitary gland, and the inhibitory factor is thought to be dopamine. Bromocriptine is a dopamine agonist, and so has the effect of inhibiting prolactin release, and is used for the suppression of lactation and the relief of galactorrhoea. It is given in doses of 2.5 mg initially, followed by doses of 2.5 mg twice a day for 14 days. In galactorrhoea, the initial daily dose is increased to 7.5 mg daily up to a maximum of 30 mg daily. Doses of 2.5 mg twice daily are also used in some types of infertility.

Bromocriptine also inhibits the release of growth hormone; and has been used in the treatment of acromegaly in doses of 20 mg daily.

Side-effects are numerous and include nausea, dizziness, postural hypotension, confusion and dyskinesia. Pleural effusions with high doses may require withdrawal.

The use of bromocriptine in the treatment of parkinsonism is referred to on p. 97.

Cabergoline § ▼ (dose: 1 mg)

Brand name: Dostinex § ▼

Cabergoline, like bromocriptine, is a dopamine agonist and has similar actions and uses, but with the advantages of a longer duration of action and fewer side-effects. For the inhibition of lactation cabergoline is given as a single dose of 1 mg during the first post-partum day. For the suppression of established lactation it is given in doses of 0.25 mg every 12 hours for 2 days. In the treatment of hyperprolactinaemia, cabergoline is given in doses of 0.25 mg twice a week initially, gradually increased by 0.5 mg at monthly intervals. Subsequently doses range from 0.25 to 2 mg weekly. Serum prolactin levels tend to return to normal within 2–4 weeks, and monthly determinations of such levels should be carried out. Slow recurrence of the hyperprolactinaemia usually occurs when treatment is withdrawn. Cabergoline is better tolerated than bromocriptine, but dizziness, vertigo, headache, dyspepsia and hypotension are some of the many **side-effects**. Care is necessary if antihypertensive or antipsychotic therapy is also given. Pregnancy should be excluded before commencing cabergoline therapy. It should not be given with macrolide antibiotics or any dopamine antagonist.

Quinagolide § ▼ (dose: 25–150 micrograms daily)

Brand name: Norprolac § ▼

Quinagolide is a selective dopamine D_2-agonist. Although it has an action similar to that of bromocriptine, it is used mainly in the control of hyperprolactinaemia. It is given in initial doses of 25 micrograms at night for three nights, slowly increased at 3-day intervals to a daily maintenance dose of 75–150 micrograms or more. The **side-effects** are those of bromocriptine, but the initial hypotensive response may be more marked, requiring monitoring of the blood pressure.

Danazol § (dose: 200–800 mg daily)

Brand name: Danol §

Danazol has a wide range of pharmacological activity mediated by its inhibitory action on pituitary gonadotrophins, but is used mainly in endometriosis. It is also used in menorrhagia, gynaecomastia and severe cyclical mastalgia when the response to other therapy is inadequate. Doses vary from 200–800 mg daily, starting on the first day of the menstrual cycle.

Side-effects are those associated with its androgenic activity and include nausea, weight gain, oedema, voice changes and hirsutism.

OESTROGENS

Oestrogens are synthesized mainly by the growing ovarian follicle and the corpus luteum in response to follicle stimulating and luteinizing hormones. They are also produced by the placenta and the adrenal cortex, while some tissues such as the liver can also convert steroid precursors to oestrogen. Oestrogens have many effects, including development of secondary sexual characteristics, cyclical ovulation, repair and proliferation of the endometrium during the menstrual cycle, breast development in preparation for lactation, alteration in haemostatic mechanisms which may limit blood loss during childbirth, inhibition of bone re-absorption, and sodium and water retention.

Oestrogens can be classified into three groups: endogenous oestrogens (estradiol, oestriol, oestrone), esters and conjugates of natural oestrogens (oestropipate, polyoestradiol), and synthetic oestrogens (ethinyloestradiol, stilboestrol, dienestrol). Therapeutically oestrogens have a variety of uses. Alone they are used to treat genital hypoplasia, primary amenorrhoea, delayed puberty, and as a topical formulation to manage senile vaginitis and pruritus vulvae. They are used in the palliative treatment of postmenopausal breast cancer and to relieve the pain associated with bony metastases, as well as being valuable in the treatment of carcinoma of the prostate gland where they may give considerable symptomatic relief, although side-effects can be troublesome. Oestrogens are also used in combination with progestogen as an oral contraceptive (p. 187), as replacement therapy in ovarian insufficiency and for the management of menstrual disturbances such as menorrhagia and dysmenorrhoea. They are used as hormone replacement therapy (HRT) to prevent the symptoms of the menopause caused by a decline in the natural secretion of oestrogen. Their use in breast cancer is referred to on p. 184.

Oestrogens were formerly used for the suppression of lactation, but dopamine agonists such as bromocriptine are now preferred, as they are less likely to cause thromboembolism.

Ethinyloestradiol § (dose: 10–50 micrograms daily)

Ethinyloestradiol has the action of the natural hormone, but is some 20 times more potent and has fewer side-effects. It is active in controlling menopausal symptoms in doses as low as 10 micrograms daily, and it is also used in primary amenorrhoea, functional uterine bleeding, sometimes in association with a progestogen. In general, long-term treatment should be avoided.

Side-effects include nausea, breast enlargement, weight gain and disturbances of liver function. Care is necessary in hypertension and cardiac disease.

Other oestrogens are represented by oestriol (Ovestin), conjugated oestrogens (Premarin), piperazine-oestrone (Harmogen) and polyoestradiol (Estradurin).

Stilboestrol § (dose: 100 micrograms– 20 mg daily)

Stilboestrol, also known as diethylstilboestrol, is a synthetic compound that is unrelated to the natural oestrogens, yet it has powerful oestrogenic properties. It is effective orally and has been used in all conditions requiring oestrogen therapy, but nausea and vomiting are common with stilboestrol and it is now used much less frequently.

HORMONE REPLACEMENT THERAPY (HRT)

The vasomotor disturbances of the menopause are due to the natural decline in oestrogen production, and can be relieved by suitable replacement therapy. The primary use of HRT is the relief of symptoms associated with the menopause, such as hot flushes, palpitations and mood swings. The secondary use is the extended protection of the skeletal and cardiovascular systems, as after the menopause women may experience a rapid decline in bone density that may lead to osteoporosis and the increased risk of fracture. The risks of cardiovascular disease may also increase.

Hormone replacement therapy usually consists of oestrogen and progestogen, with the oestrogen being given continuously and the progestogen being used cyclically, tricyclically or continuously. The oestrogen in HRT is given for its beneficial effects on bone and heart, and its relief of menopausal symptoms. The progestogen is given to prevent endometrial hyperplasia which can occur with unopposed oestrogen therapy, but women who have had a hysterectomy do not require progestogen. The oestrogen can be given orally, by transdermal patch, gel or subcutaneous implant, and progestogens are given orally or combined with oestrogen as a transdermal patch. The advantage of the non-oral routes is that they do not undergo first-pass metabolism, which may be important for women with a history of liver disease, thrombosis, hypertension or diabetes. If patches are used they should be applied to clean, unbroken and dry skin below the waistline and detached after 3–4 days. Fresh patches should be applied to a different area.

Side-effects include breast tenderness, nausea and leg cramps due to the oestrogen, while progestogens can cause bleeding, irritability, premenstrual tension (PMT), headaches and a bloated feeling. The risk of developing breast cancer as a result of HRT is increased, markedly after treatment with hormone replacement therapy for more than five years, and women should be informed about the degree of risk.

HRT is contra-indicated in women with an oestrogen-dependent tumour, active liver disease, undiagnosed bleeding or otosclerosis, while care must be taken if there is a history of thrombosis, untreated hypertension, fibroids, endometriosis, diabetes or previous myocardial infarction.

Alternative drug treatments to HRT include clonidine (Dixarit §) in doses of 50–75 micrograms twice daily (p. 56) to reduce menopausal flushing, and to promote vaginal lubrication to relieve dryness. Research is ongoing to find new and better treatment such as progesterone-releasing intrauterine devices.

The following products are available §:
Oestrogen only:
Climaval, Progynova, Premarin, Harmogen, Hormonin, Zumenon
Oestrogen/progestogen
Climagest, Cyclo-Progynova, Menophase, Nuvelle, Prepak, Trisequens
Patches
Dermestril, Estraderm, Evorel, Estracombi, Estrapak

Tibolone §

Brand name: Livial §

Tibolone is a synthetic steroid with progestogen and oestrogen activity. It is used mainly to control the flushing and other vasomotor disturbances of the menopause, and the daily dose of 2.5 mg should be continued for at least 3 months without interruption. The **side-effects** are those of related compounds. It is contra-indicated in cardiovascular disease and in hormone-dependent neoplasm. Vaginal bleeding is an occasional side-effect of tibolone, and it should not be used within one year of the last natural menstrual period.

PROGESTOGENS AND RELATED SUBSTANCES

Progesterone is the hormone secreted by the corpus luteum in the second half of the menstrual cycle. Its main function is to prepare the uterus for the implantation of a fertilized ovum, but if that does not occur progesterone secretion stops abruptly and that sudden action is the main cause of the onset of menstruation. When implantation occurs, progesterone prevents uterine contraction and maintains the pregnancy, and together with oestrogen prepares the breasts for lactation. Therapeutically, progestogens have been used in threatened abortion, but they are now used mainly in dysfunctional uterine bleeding and other menstrual disorders, and as secondary drugs in the treatment of breast cancer. In menorrhagia, tranexamic acid (p. 138) is usually preferred.

Progesterone §

Brand name: Gestone §

Progesterone is the natural hormone, and is given by deep intramuscular injection as an oily solution. In dysfunctional uterine bleeding doses of 5–10 mg may be given for a week before menstruation is expected. In the premenstrual syndrome it is given as a pessary or suppository (Cyclogest §) of 200–400 mg twice daily.

Proluton Depot § (hydroxyprogesterone hexanoate) is a long-acting derivative. In habitual abortion it is given in doses of 250–500 mg by intramuscular injection at weekly intervals during the first half of pregnancy, but its value has been questioned.

Side-effects of progesterone include acne, urticaria and weight gain. It should be used with care in cardiac and renal disease, epilepsy, asthma, or conditions associated with fluid retention.

Medroxyprogesterone § (dose: 2.5–30 mg daily)

Brand names: Farlutal §, Provera §

Medroxyprogesterone has the general properties of the progestogens, and is given in doses of 2.5–10 mg daily for 5–10 days in dysfunctional uterine bleeding. In endometriosis doses of 10 mg three times a day are given continuously for 3 months, but tranexamic acid may be more effective. See p. 224 for its use as a cytotoxic agent.

Gestronol § (Depostat §), dose 200–400 mg weekly by intramuscular injection, and megestrol (Megace §), dose 40–320 mg daily, are other progestogens used in large doses in the treatment of breast cancer. (See p. 224.)

Norethisterone § (dose: 10–30 mg daily)

Brand names: Menzol §, Primolut N §, Utovlan §

Norethisterone is an orally active progestogen, which is used mainly in the treatment of amenorrhoea, functional uterine bleeding and endometriosis. It has also been used in dysmenorrhoea and the premenstrual syndrome. Doses vary from 5 to 10 mg three times a day, at different stages of the menstrual cycle according to the condition under treatment.

It has been used to postpone menstruation in doses of 5 mg three times a day. It is also used as a second-line drug in the treatment of breast cancer (see p. 224.). It is also a constituent of many oral contraceptive products (see p. 188).

Dydrogesterone § (dose: 5–30 mg daily)

Brand name: Duphaston §

Dydrogesterone is a potent, orally active progestogen, and it is used in the treatment of endogenous progesterone deficiency. It is exceptional as it does not inhibit ovulation, yet it is capable of relieving the pain of dysmenorrhoea. It is given in doses of 10 mg twice daily for 3 weeks, followed by a break of 7 days before treatment is recommenced. It is also useful in some forms of endometriosis, dysfunctional uterine bleeding, infertility and abortion, and in control of the premenstrual syndrome.

FERTILITY CONTROL

The explosive rise in population in recent years, particularly in underdeveloped countries, has led to the development of drugs for controlling fertility and birthrates.

It has long been recognized that the inhibition of ovulation by oestrogens would be effective, and later it was found that lower doses could be used if a progestogen was also given. Following the production of synthetic and highly active progestogens, oestrogen–progestogen preparations that can inhibit ovulation for long periods, apparently without influencing subsequent fertility, are now used as oral contraceptives (see Table 13.2). These products are in general well tolerated, but some nausea, acne, gain in weight, liver damage and thrombosis may occur.

The possible relationship between thromboembolism and the use of oral contraceptives has caused some concern. The magnitude of the risk is difficult to assess, as thrombosis and pulmonary embolism may occur in a woman of child-bearing age who is not taking oral contraceptives. This risk appears to be associated with the oestrogen content, and many products now have a reduced dose of oestrogen. Some progestogen-only oral contraceptives are also available, but menstrual irregularities are more likely with these products.

It has also been suggested that there may be a possible link between breast cancer in women up to the age of 45 years and the prolonged use of oral contraceptives before a first pregnancy. An oral contraceptive containing the lowest suitable doses of both oestrogen and progestogen is recommended. The use of any oral contraceptive product should be discontinued if side-effects such as migraine-like headaches, visual disturbances, or any signs of thromboembolism or jaundice occur.

It should be noted that some drugs that induce hepatic enzyme activity, such as phenytoin, griseofulvin and carbamazepine, and some antibiotics, particularly rifampicin, may reduce the efficacy of oral contraceptives, and others such as ampicillin may hinder their absorption.

ANDROGENS

Testosterone is the main natural androgen, which is synthesized by the interstitial cells of the testis in response to luteinizing hormone. It is also produced by the ovary and the adrenal cortex. It stimulates the development of the secondary sexual characteristics and promotes sperm production, and also has anabolic or powerful tissue-building properties and causes the rapid physical development of the male at puberty.

Therapeutically, the androgens are used mainly in hypogonadism in the male, and in carcinoma of the breast in females. Some modified androgens with a reduced virilizing action are described later under 'Anabolic steroids'.

Testosterone §

Brand names of testosterone esters: Primoteston §, Restandol §, Sustanon §, Virormone §

Testosterone is the natural androgen, now prepared synthetically. In testicular deficiency or hypogonadism it is given as long-acting esters such as testosterone propionate by intramuscular injection in doses varying from 25 to 250 mg at intervals of 2–3 weeks. An alternative method is the subcutaneous implantation of sterile pellets. A pellet dose of 200–600 mg will provide a slow release of testosterone over a period of more than 6 months. Recently, a testosterone skin patch for daily application has been introduced as Andropatch § ▼.

Testosterone undecanoate (Restandol) is given orally in doses of 120–160 mg daily initially, with subsequent maintenance doses varying from 40 to 120 mg daily.

Mesterolone §

Brand name: Pro-Viron §

Mesterolone is an orally active androgen used in the treatment of hypogonadism and male infertility due to oligospermia. It is given in doses of 25 mg three or four times a day, but prolonged treatment for some months is required. Mesterolone is less likely to cause hepatic disturbances and other toxic effects.

ANABOLIC STEROIDS OR NON-VIRILIZING ANDROGENS

Attempts have been made to exploit the protein-building properties of androgens in the treatment of wasting disease, but the results were largely disappointing. Such modified androgens are still used to a limited extent in the treatment of postmenopausal osteoporosis, and also in some aplastic and resistant anaemias, as steroids have some stimulating action on erythropoiesis. The response is highly variable.

Table 13.2 Oral contraceptives

	Brand name	Progestogen dose of product
Mixed products containing 50 micrograms of mestranol	Norinyl-1 Ortho-Novin 1/50	norethisterone 1 mg
Mixed products containing 50 micrograms of ethinyloestradiol	Ovran	levonorgestrel 250 micrograms
Mixed products containing 35 micrograms of ethinyloestradiol	Brevinor Cilest Norimin Ovysmen	norethisterone 500 micrograms norgestimate 250 micrograms norethisterone 1 mg norethisterone 500 micrograms
Mixed products containing 30 micrograms of ethinyloestradiol	Eugynon 30 Femodene Loestrin 30 Marvelon Microgynon 30 Minulet Ovran 30 Ovranette	levonorgestrel 250 micrograms gestodene 75 micrograms norethisterone 1.5 mg desogestrel 10 micrograms levonorgestrel 150 micrograms gestodene 75 micrograms levonorgestrel 250 micrograms levonorgestrel 150 micrograms
Mixed products containing 20 micrograms of ethinyloestradiol	Loestrin 20 Mercilon	norethisterone 1 mg desogestrel 150 micrograms
Progestogen-only products	Femulen Micronor Microval Neogest Norgeston Noriday	ethynodiol 500 micrograms norethisterone 350 micrograms levonorgestrel 30 micrograms norgestrel 75 micrograms levonorgestrel 30 micrograms norethisterone 350 micrograms

Logynon, Logynon ED, BiNovum, Synphase, Tri-Minulet, Triadene, Trinordiol and Trinovum are mixed products containing tablets of different strengths of ethinyloestradiol and norethisterone or levonorgestrel, and are designed to produce a phased hormonal response that mimics the natural hormone cycle more closely than is possible with fixed dose packs.

The progestogen-only products appear to act by increasing the viscosity of cervical mucus, and so reduce sperm penetration. Unlike mixed products, they are given continuously as single daily doses, to be taken at the same time every day. Additional protection is necessary for the first 14 days, or if any dose is omitted. In general, they are considered less reliable than the mixed products. Depo-Provera (medroxyprogesterone) is an injectable contraceptive, and is given as a single dose of 150 mg by deep intramuscular injection between the third and fifth day of the cycle, repeated after 3 months for long-term protection. Similarly, norethisterone enanthate (Noristerat) may be given in a dose of 200 mg by deep intramuscular injection, repeated after 8 weeks.

Post-coital contraception has been obtained by the use of mixed products containing levonorgestrel 250 micrograms and ethinyloestradiol 50 micrograms (Ovran and PC4). Treatment should be commenced within 72 hours of intercourse with a dose of two tablets, followed by a second dose 12 hours later. The risk of drug-induced vomiting can be reduced by an antiemetic such as prochlorperazine.

Levonorgestrel is a progestogen widely used in oral contraceptives, but it is now available as implants (Norplant) claimed to have an action extending over 5 years. The product consists of six capsular implants each containing 38 mg of the drug, for subcutaneous insertion. The drug is slowly released from the capsules, and binds with progesterone receptors, and acts by thickening the cervical mucus so that it is impenetrable by spermatozoa. Suppression of ovulation may also occur. Should it be necessary to remove the implants, levonorgestrel plasma levels become undetectable within a few days.

They should not be given to children to stimulate growth, as premature closing of the epiphyses may occur. Representative compounds include nandrolone (Decadurabolin §), given by deep intramuscular injection in doses of 25–50 mg at intervals varying from 1–3 weeks, and stanozolol (Stromba §), given orally in doses of 5–10 mg.

Cyproterone §

Brand name: Androcur §

Cyproterone is referred to here as it has anti-androgenic properties and is used in the treatment of hypersexuality in the male. It is given in doses of 50 mg twice daily.

On the basis that sebum secretion is linked with androgen activity, cyproterone is used in the treatment of severe acne in women not responding to other treatment, as Dianette § (cyproterone 2 mg with 35 micrograms of ethinyloestradiol), once daily for 21 days a month for several months.

Side-effects of cyproterone in full doses are fatigue and weight gain; care is necessary in hepatic dysfunction, and blood counts should be made at regular intervals. The use of cyproterone in the treatment of prostatic carcinoma is referred to on p. 223.

THYROID HORMONES

The thyroid is one of the largest of the endocrine glands and is located in the neck, overlying the trachea. It consists of two lateral lobes joined by an isthmus and has an extensive blood supply. The thyroid gland extracts iodine from the blood to synthesize thyroxine and tri-iodothyronine, which are stored in the gland as thyroglobulin. Those hormones are released in response to pituitary thyroid stimulating hormone and increase the rate of cellular metabolism. Excess production results in hyperthyroidism or thyrotoxicosis, while reduced production of thyroid hormones results in reduced metabolic rate, and in the adult causes hypothyroidism or myxoedema. As thyroid hormone is required for brain and nervous system development in the fetus and infant, lack of that hormone in the young child results in cretinism.

Calcitonin, another hormone of the thyroid gland, has a different function (see p. 191).

Nursing points about thyroid drugs

(a) Early diagnosis and treatment are essential in cretinism.
(b) In hypothyroidism, maintenance doses should be taken before breakfast.
(c) Liothyronine is used in severe conditions when a rapid action is required, and is given by intravenous injection in hypothyroid coma.

Thyroxine § thyroxine sodium § (dose: 25–200 micrograms daily)

Thyroxine is used mainly in the control of thyroid deficiency states (hypothyroidism or myxoedema), and in neonatal hypothyroidism or cretinism. In myxoedema, treatment is commenced with small doses of 25–50 micrograms daily, slowly increased until a metabolic balance has again been achieved. Maintenance doses are 100–200 micrograms daily. The reason for these small initial doses is that the myocardium is often affected in myxoedema. Large initial doses of thyroxine may increase the heart rate and add to the cardiac burden before the myocardium has had time to recover.

In cretinism early diagnosis and prompt treatment are essential, as if delayed, mental damage may occur which cannot be reversed by subsequent thyroid treatment. The initial dose for a cretinous infant is about 10 micrograms/kg daily, rising to 100 micrograms daily by about 5 years of age, and controlled by laboratory reports on plasma thyroxine levels. Maintenance doses in adults range from 100 to 200 micrograms daily, and treatment must be continued for life.

Side-effects, which may be associated with over-rapid therapy, include tachycardia, diarrhoea, restlessness, anginal pain and weight loss. Many such side-effects disappear with an adjustment of dose.

Liothyronine § (dose: 5–60 micrograms daily)

Brand names: Tertroxin §, Triiodothyronine §

The latent period of 10 days or so that elapses before thyroxine exerts a full effect is due to a slow conversion of the drug into liothyronine, which is the form of the hormone which finally affects the metabolism.

Liothyronine is used when a rapid action is required, as it is effective within a few hours, but the action is correspondingly short and the drug is not suitable for maintenance treatment. It is given in initial doses of 20 micrograms a day, slowly increased to 60 micrograms daily according to need. In severe myxoedema, when coma may be imminent or present, liothyronine may be given by intravenous injection in initial doses of 50 micrograms, gradually reduced to 25 micrograms twice daily. Alternatively, doses of 5–20 micrograms may be given intravenously 12-hourly or more frequently as required.

Side-effects are similar to those of thyroxine, and care is necessary in hypertension and cardiovascular disease.

THYROID INHIBITORS†

Excessive activity of the thyroid gland, referred to as hyperthyroidism or thyrotoxicosis, is characterized

---

†These are not hormones, but are considered here because of their use in thyroid disease.

by rapid pulse, loss of weight, raised metabolic rate and enlargement of the thyroid. At one time surgical removal of much of the gland was the only effective treatment, but since the introduction of certain anti-thyroid substances, oral therapy has become an established method of control.

Nursing points about thyroid inhibitors

(a) Bone marrow suppression may occur.
(b) Withdraw treatment if any evidence of neutropenia.
(c) Advise patients to report sore throat or other indications of possible infection.
(d) White cell counts if any evidence of infection.

Carbimazole § (dose: 5–60 mg daily)

Brand name: Neo-Mercazole §
Carbimazole is the most effective and least toxic of the antithyroid drugs. These compounds reduce the formation of thyroxine and liothyronine in the thyroid gland by combining with the iodine absorbed from the blood. By this means the iodine necessary for the biosynthesis of thyroxine is made unavailable, and carbimazole brings about an indirect lowering of the basal metabolic rate by this interference with hormone synthesis.

Carbimazole is active orally, and the dose depends on the degree of thyrotoxicosis. An average initial dose is 30 mg daily, and the patient may feel better within 10–14 days, but the full response is slow as the thyroxine already formed and stored in the gland must first be metabolized, and the raised basal metabolic rate may not return to normal until after 3–5 weeks. The dose of carbimazole can then be slowly reduced to a maintenance dose of 5–15 mg daily and prolonged treatment for months is usually required. Resistance to carbimazole is uncommon, and a poor response may indicate that the patient is not complying with treatment. Occasionally, carbima-zole and thyroxine are given together in the so-called 'blocking-replacement regimen'.

Side-effects are most common in the early stages of treatment, and include gastro-intestinal dis-turbances, pruritus, nausea and headache. Macropapular rash may also occur, usually controlled by antihistamine therapy. Severe reactions such as agranulocytosis and aplastic anaemia have also been reported. It should be noted that carbimazole and related drugs may appear in breast milk, and may depress the thyroid activity of a breast-fed infant.

Propylthiouracil § (dose: 300–600 mg daily) also has an antithyroid action, but is more liable to cause toxic effects than carbimazole. It is useful occasion-ally when the rash caused by carbimazole is severe and not controlled by antihistamines.

Iodine

Although iodine in very small amounts is necessary for normal thyroid activity, larger doses can depress thyroid function for short periods, and temporarily relieve the symptoms of thyrotoxicosis. The effect of large doses is at a maximum after about 2 weeks, and iodine is often given to reduce the basal metabolic rate during the preparation of patients for thyroid-ectomy. It also reduces the hyperplasia and vascularity of the gland, making it smaller and firmer, and so making subsequent surgery easier. It is usually given as Lugol's Solution (Aqueous Solution of Iodine) in doses of 0.1 to 0.3 ml well diluted, three times a day for 2 weeks before operation. Potassium iodide in doses of 60 mg three times a day is also effective. Lugol's Iodine Solution has been given in doses of 2 ml (after dilution with saline) by slow intravenous injection in thyrotoxic crisis.

Beta-adrenergic blocking agents are also used in thyrotoxicosis as they inhibit the adrenergic-mediated action of thyroxine, and so reduce tachycardia and tremor. They are used for short-term treatment in association with other antithyroid drugs. Propranolol is often used, in doses of 10–50 mg 6-hourly for a few days before thyroidectomy, and nadolol and sotalol are other beta-blockers used for the sympto-matic treatment of thyrotoxicosis.

Propranolol is also used in association with other antithyroid drugs in the emergency treatment of thy-rotoxic crisis, and is given by intravenous injection in doses of 5 mg every 6 hours, together with hydro-cortisone 100 mg 6-hourly. Radioactive iodine (p. 226) is occasionally used in the diagnosis of thyroid dys-function, in the treatment of thyrotoxicosis resistant to other drugs, and in cancer of the thyroid.

OTHER HORMONES

Lactogenic hormone (Prolactin)

Prolactin is concerned with milk formation. During pregnancy, premature lactation is suppressed by the relatively large amounts of oestrogen in the blood, but following delivery there is a sharp fall in the oestrogen level, and release of prolactin. In the breast prepared during pregnancy, prolactin stimulates milk production at term, and sustains subsequent lactation. It should be noted that some drugs, such as methyldopa and the phenothiazines, may cause galactorrhoea as a side-effect via stimulation of prolactin release.

Oestrogens were formerly used to suppress lactation, but dopamine receptor agonists such as bromocriptine (p. 183) are now preferred.

Growth hormone (somatrophin); Somatropin §

Brand names: Genotropin §, Humatrope §, Norditropin §, Saizen §, Zomacton §
Somatropin is the recombinant form of somatotrophin, the human growth hormone, used to stimulate growth in children with a deficiency of somatotrophin. The dose is 0.5–0.7 unit/kg weekly by subcutaneous or intramuscular injection. It is also used in Turner's syndrome (gonadal dysgenesis). Growth hormone is contra-indicated if epiphyseal closure has already taken place.

Octreotide § (dose: 50–600 micrograms daily by injection)

Brand name: Sandostatin §
Octreotide is a synthetic analogue of the natural regulatory hormone somatostatin. That hormone inhibits the release from the anterior pituitary gland of the growth hormone somatotrophin, as well as other pituitary hormones such as the thyroid stimulating hormone, corticotrophin and prolactin. It also acts on the pancreas and inhibits the release of insulin, glucagon, gastrin and the vasodilator intestinal peptide (VIP), and so blocks their action on the target tissues. Somatotrophin has too short a plasma life to be of therapeutic value, but octreotide is a derivative with a much longer action. It is used for the symptomatic relief of the flushing and severe diarrhoea of the carcinoid syndrome, which is associated with tumours that secrete excessive amounts of vasoactive substances such as VIP into the circulation.

Octreotide is given in doses of 50 micrograms by subcutaneous injection twice daily, increasing to 200 micrograms three times a day according to need. In most cases a complete remission of symptoms may be achieved, but the drug should be withdrawn in the absence of a response after 1 week's treatment. It may also be given by intravenous injection under ECG control when a rapid response is required. It should be noted that octreotide has no antitumour action, and has no effect on the underlying cause of the carcinoid syndrome. Similar doses have been given in the treatment of acromegaly. An occasional **side-effect** is a sudden loss of control and a rapid return of symptoms with increased severity.

PARATHYROID GLAND, CALCITONIN AND CALCIUM-REGULATING AGENTS

The skeleton is more than a bony supporting structure, as bone is constantly being broken down and reformed, a process referred to as 'bone turnover', in which the parathyroid gland and the hormone calcitonin have a controlling influence.

The parathyroid glands are situated in the neck, near the thyroid glands, and their function is the control of calcium and phosphate metabolism. A deficiency of parathyroid activity, or an accidental removal of the glands during thyroidectomy results in a lowering of blood calcium and an increase in the phosphate level. The former, if unchecked, leads to severe tetany which can be relieved by the administration of calcium salts. For an acute attack, calcium gluconate solution (10%) can be injected intravenously or intramuscularly in doses of 10–20 ml, and treatment may be maintained by the oral administration of calcium gluconate or calcium lactate (dose: 1–5 g). Vitamin D (calciferol) and related drugs may also be given in the long-term control of calcium deficiency (p. 286).

Calcitonin § Salcatonin §

Brand names: Calcitare § (pork), Calsynar § (salmon)
Calcitonin is a hormone present in the thyroid gland, and together with the parathyroid hormone it controls the calcium balance of the body. It lowers the blood calcium by inhibiting bone turnover, and is used for the treatment of hypercalcaemic conditions, in osteoporosis, and in the severe hypercalcaemia that may occur in neoplastic disease. Calcitonin is also useful in relieving the pain and neurological complications of Paget's disease, including deafness. It is also used in the treatment of postmenopausal osteoporosis.

Calcitonin can be obtained from pig thyroid, but a synthetic form is salcatonin (salmon calcitonin). Salcatonin is more potent than calcitonin, and is suitable for long-term treatment, as it is less likely to produce antibodies.

In Paget's disease, salcatonin is given in doses of 50 units three times a week by subcutaneous or intramuscular injection. In hypercalcaemia, doses up to 10 units/kg are given, based on need and bio-chemical response. In the short-term treatment of the severe bone pain of malignancy, doses by injection of 200 units 6-hourly for 48 hours are given. For longer treatment the bisphosphonates are preferred. In post-menopausal osteoporosis 100 units of salcatonin are injected daily, with vitamin D and calcium supplements orally. If calcitonin is used, the dose should be adjusted on the basis that 80 units are equivalent to 50 units of salcatonin.

Side-effects are nausea, flushing and tingling. Skin tests should be carried out before treatment in patients with a history of allergy.

BISPHOSPHONATES

Bisphosphonates are considered here as, although they are unrelated to calcitonin, they are also used in disturbances of bone metabolism such as Paget's disease and hypercalcaemia. Paget's disease is caused by an over-activity of osteoclasts, and is a chronic skeletal disorder in which localized areas of normal bone are replaced by softened and enlarged osseous cells. The excessive bone turnover results in abnormal formation of new bone. Treatment is with bisphos-phonates which are adsorbed on the hydroxyapatite (calcium-containing) crystals of bone, and reduce their rate of growth as well as their subsequent dissolution. They thus reduce the rapid turnover of bone that occurs in Paget's disease, and reduce the pain as well as the further development of the disease. In hypercalcaemia they act by inhibiting the normal mobilization of skeletal calcium. The bisphosphonates are also useful in osteoporosis.

Alendronate § ▼ (dose: 10 mg daily)

Brand name: Fosamax § ▼
Alendronate is used mainly in postmenopausal osteoporosis, as it inhibits osteoclast activity and strengthens bone. It is given in doses of 10 mg daily in the *morning*, but care is necessary as it may cause oesophageal damage. Patients should be instructed to swallow alendronate tablets whole with a full glass of water at least 30 minutes before breakfast, and should remain sitting or standing until after breakfast has been taken. Medical attention should be sought if symptoms of oesophageal irritation occur. Other **side-effects** include gastro-intestinal disturbances, headache and rash. Care is necessary in renal impairment.

Nursing points about bisphosphonates
(a) Used in Paget's disease of bone, osteoporosis and hypercalcaemia.
(b) When given orally, the dose should be taken 30 minutes to 2 hours before food, according to the preparation used, with ample fluid. The patient should remain sitting or standing until after the food has been taken.
(c) Milk, calcium, iron and other mineral-containing products should be avoided.

Disodium etidronate § (dose: 5–10 mg/kg daily)

Brand names: Didronel §, Dodronel PMO §
In Paget's disease etidronate is given as a single daily dose of 5 mg/kg, but prolonged administration for up to 6 months may be necessary. Doses of 10 mg/kg daily are sometimes given for shorter periods. In vertebral osteoporosis a 90-day cycle of treatment is given, with etidronate 400 mg daily for 14 days, followed by calcium carbonate 1.25 g daily as Didronel PMO. The serum phosphates and phosphatase levels should be measured before and during treatment. Food, antacids, iron, calcium and other mineral-containing products should be avoided for at least 2 hours before and after each dose.

Nausea and diarrhoea are **side-effects**, and an increase in bone pain with risks of fracture may occur with higher doses. Much of the drug is excreted in the urine, and severe renal impairment is a contra-indication.

Disodium pamidronate § (dose: 10–60 mg)

Brand name: Aredia §
Pamidronate is given in Paget's disease in doses of 30 mg by intravenous infusion once a week for 6 weeks, or at longer intervals up to a total dose of 360 mg. In skeletal bone metastases and osteolytic lesions, doses of 90 mg are given every 4 weeks. **Side-effects** are numerous and specialist literature should be consulted.

Sodium clodronate § (dose: 1.6–3.2 g daily)

Brand names: Bonefos §, Loron §
Clodronate has the actions and uses of other bisphosphonates, and is given for the relief of the pain of skeletal metastases and in hypercalcaemia as a single oral dose of 1.6–3.2 g daily, with adequate

fluid. Food and mineral products should be avoided for one hour before and after clodronate therapy. In malignant hypercalcaemia it is given by intravenous infusion in doses of 300 mg daily for 5–7 days.

Side-effects are nausea and diarrhoea; it is contra-indicated in renal impairment.

Tildronate § ▼ (dose: 400 mg daily)

Brand name: Skelid § ▼

Tildronate (tiludronic acid) resembles other bisphosphonates in reducing bone resorption, and in Paget's disease it promotes the normalization of bone turnover. It is given in single daily doses of 400 mg for up to 12 weeks; a second course may be given after 6 months. The food intake precautions, **side-effects** and contra-indications are those of the bisphosphonates generally.

Sodium cellulose phosphate (dose: 15 g daily)

Brand name: Calcisorb

Sodium cellulose phosphate functions in the intestinal tract as an ion-exchange substance, and binds with dietary calcium, thus preventing its absorption. It is used in the treatment of hypercalcaemia, and is given in doses of 5 g three times a day in association with a low-calcium diet.

Diarrhoea is an occasional **side-effect**, and renal impairment and congestive heart failure are considered to be contra-indications.

Trisodium edetate § (Limclair §) has been used in hypercalcaemia in doses up to 70 mg/kg daily by intravenous infusion, but its use is not without risk, and very close control of the plasma calcium level is essential during the administration of the infusion.

REFERENCES

Abernethy K 1997 The menopause and hormone replacement therapy. Nursing Standard 11(31):49–56

Abernethy K 1997 Hormone replacement therapy. Professional Nurse 12(10):717–719

Auer I K 1996 The role of pharmacologic agents in blood conservation. AACN Clinical Issues 7(2):260–276

Baxter J 1992 The effects of glucocorticoid therapy. Hospital Practice 27(9):111–134

Beex L et al 1989 Pamidronate and hypercalcaemia of malignancy. Lancet ii:617

Compton J E 1994 The therapeutic use of bisphosphonates. British Medical Journal 309:711–715

Coleman R E 1994 Therapeutic use of bisphosphonates in oncology. British Medical Journal 309:1233

Council on Scientific Affairs 1990 Medical and nonmedical uses of anabolic-androgenic steroids. Journal of the American Medical Association 264(22):2923–2927

Frazer H M, Waxman J 1989 Gonadotrophin releasing hormone analogues for gynaecological disorders and infertility. British Medical Journal 298:475–476

Kessenich C R 1996 Update on pharmacologic therapies for osteoporosis. Nurse Practitioner 21(8):19–24

Lichtman R 1991 Perimenopausal hormone replacement therapy: review of the literature. Journal of Nurse-Midwifery 36(1):30–48

Mitchell D H, Owens B 1996 Replacement therapy: arginine vasopressin (AVP), growth hormone, cortisol, thyroxine, testosterone and estrogen. Journal of Neuroscience Nursing 28(3):110–153

Price E H, Littel H K 1996 Women need to be fully informed about risks of hormone replacement therapy. British Medical Journal 312:1301

Ralston S H et al 1990 Use of bisphosphonates in hypercalcaemia due to malignancy. Lancet 335:737

Wilson B A, Malseed R T 1993 Understanding corticosteroids: pharmacologic adverse effects. MEDSURG Nursing 2(4):322–324

14

Insulin and other hypoglycaemic agents

Insulin and other hypoglycaemic agents are used in the treatment of diabetes mellitus, an endocrine disorder in which there is a lack of effective insulin. It is characterized by a high level of glucose in the blood (hyperglycaemia), as in health the blood sugar level rarely exceeds 7 mmol/l.

Two types of the illness are known: Type 1, juvenile-onset or insulin-dependent diabetes mellitus (IDDM), and Type 2, non-insulin-dependent diabetes mellitus (NIDDM). Type 1 may occur at any age but is most common in the young, and it may be caused by an altered immune response, possibly triggered off by some environmental factor such as a virus. Such patients produce little or no endogenous insulin, so life-long insulin replacement therapy is required. Patients with NIDDM, sometimes referred to as maturity-onset diabetes, continue to produce some endogenous insulin, but its normal release mechanism is impaired and some insulin-resistance may be present. There is a strong genetic factor in the development of NIDDM, and the condition can be precipitated by obesity. In NIDDM treatment with an oral hypoglycaemic agent coupled with a suitable diet is usually effective in controlling the condition.

Insulin is one of several hormones produced by the pancreas, which also releases digestive enzymes into the duodenum. It is formed and released from the beta-cells (the islets of Langerhans) and is essential for the utilization and storage of food-derived glucose, amino acids and fats. It has a multiple action by:

- stimulating the transport and take-up of glucose by body cells
- stimulating glycogenesis (the conversion of glucose to glycogen for storage in the liver)
- controlling glycogenolysis (breakdown of glycogen)
- controlling glyconeogenesis (production of glucose from fats and proteins)

195

- promoting the uptake of amino acids and protein synthesis
- stimulating lipogenesis (synthesis of fats) and inhibiting lipolysis (fat breakdown).

In insulin deficiency, glucose cannot be metabolized completely as a source of energy, and as a result muscle and fat stores are catabolized, leading to loss of weight, weakness and lethargy. Without glucose, the body is unable to metabolize fats completely to carbon dioxide, so in diabetes the end-products of fat metabolism are intermediate substances known as ketones. Ketones are excreted in part in the urine, but those retained in the circulation cause ketoacidosis. The increasing amounts of under-used glucose in the blood cause hyperglycaemia. Part of the excess glucose is excreted in the urine and functions as an osmotic diuretic, causing thirst and dehydration. If the diabetes is untreated, the ketoacidosis, hyperglycaemia and dehydration lead to coma and death (Fig. 14.1).

The management of diabetes mellitus involves the replacement of the insulin deficiency and balancing the dose required against diet and exercise. Insulin is a polypeptide, so it is ineffective orally and is given by subcutaneous injection. Insulin can be extracted from the pancreas of cattle and pigs, but human-type insulin is now available as enzyme-modified pork insulin (H-emp), or by recombinant DNA technology from *Escherichia coli* (H-prb) or from yeast cells (H-pyr). These human-type insulins differ slightly from animal insulins in the arrangement of certain amino acids, but they are now being used to an increasing extent. Although they are considered to have a potency comparable with that of standard insulins, care must be taken when transferring a patient from animal to human-type insulin. Hypoglycaemia may occur during the change-over period without the patient experiencing the normal warning symptoms of giddiness, tremor and palpitation, although some authorities consider that those risks have been over-exaggerated.

Type 2 diabetes (NIDDM) is usually treated with an oral hypoglycaemic agent such as a sulphonylurea or a biguanide, although in some cases small doses of supplementary insulin may be required. The sulphonylureas act by:

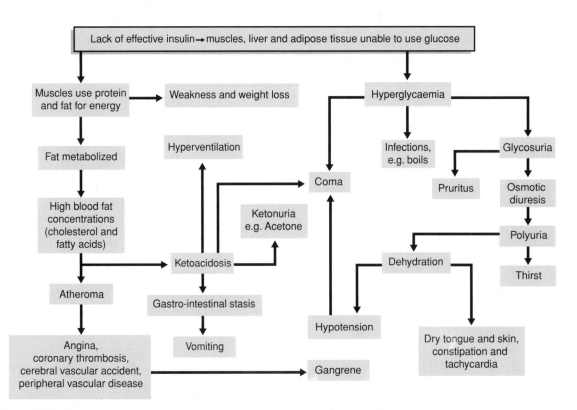

Figure 14.1 Physiology of undersecretion of insulin.

- increasing beta-cell sensitivity to glucose, and so promoting the release of insulin from the pancreas
- increasing the number of insulin receptors on cell surfaces and so improving glucose uptake
- reducing free fatty acids in the plasma by stimulating lipogenesis.

Metformin is the only biguanide in current use. It slows down the absorption of glucose from the gut, increases insulin-mediated glucose uptake by increasing insulin-receptor binding, and inhibits gluconeogenesis and glycogenolysis. The action of metformin results in weight loss, which is an advantage in the treatment of obese NIDDM patients.

The underlying cause of NIDDM is thought to be insulin resistance, and a new approach to the problem is the introduction of troglitazone, an oral insulin enhancer. It brings about a reduction in blood sugar levels similar to that following other oral agents, together with a beneficial effect on the blood lipid profile. It appears to increase sensitivity to endogenous insulin, although part of its action may be mediated by promoting the efficiency of the β-cells of the pancreas. It is possible that long-term therapy may reduce the microvascular complications of NIDDM such as retinopathy, as well as the more serious sequelae.

In all cases, the type and dose of insulin or other hypoglycaemic agent must be adjusted to the needs of the individual patient, together with modifications of diet and lifestyle to achieve the optimum degree of control. Blood or urine tests to determine glucose levels should be carried out regularly and reagent test strips are available for visual or meter measurement. Such tests may show variations throughout the day, and patients should be warned about such fluctuations, but levels between 4 and 10 mmol/l of blood glucose for most of the time should reduce the risks of diabetic complications. Car drivers should be very careful to avoid hypoglycaemia and its consequences, and on long journeys should carry out a blood glucose test every 2 hours.

MAIN TYPES OF INSULIN

Three main types of insulin are in use: the short-acting, the intermediate and the long-acting insulins (Table 14.1). They are usually given by subcutaneous injection, as insulin, being a polypeptide, is inactivated by gastric enzymes. For stable, well motivated diabetic patients some automatic self-injection devices are available, involving the use of insulin cartridges. These devices permit some adjustment of dose and offer advantages over conventional syringe injection, and Autopen, B-D Pen, Diapen, NovoPen and Penject are examples of such self-injection devices. Another method is the administration of soluble insulin by continuous subcutaneous injection via an infusion pump system. Such a device provides a basic insulin level, with pre-meal supplementary doses as required, but it is suitable only for use by competent patients who are aware of the risks as well as the advantages of continuous insulin infusion. For such patients, the method offers a considerable improvement in the quality of life.

Soluble insulin injection (neutral insulin)

Soluble insulin is the standard form of insulin, and is the product to be used when insulin injection or neutral insulin is prescribed. Following subcutaneous injection it is rapidly absorbed, and a peak effect is reached in about 3 hours. With a suitable dose, the high blood-sugar level falls rapidly, the depleted glycogen reserves are restored, ketone bodies are oxidized, and as glucose is no longer excreted in the urine, the characteristic thirst and polyuria of diabetes are relieved.

Soluble insulin is used in the initial treatment of severe diabetes, in doses dependent on the degree of insulin deficiency and the condition of the patient. Soluble insulin is also the product of choice for the treatment of diabetic emergencies, and for increased control during operation. If required, it may be given by intramuscular or intravenous injection when the subcutaneous route is not indicated, but the onset of action is rapid and duration correspondingly brief.

A recently introduced alternative to soluble insulin is insulin lispro (Humalog). It is a human insulin analogue with a shorter duration of action, and may be useful for patients who experience pre-meal hypoglycaemia.

Protamine zinc insulin (PZ insulin)

Protamine zinc insulin is a suspension of insulin combined with protamine, a simple protein obtained from fish sperm, and a trace of zinc chloride. This modified insulin is not soluble in water, and a single daily dose may be sufficient to control the symptoms of diabetes when suitable dietary adjustments are made.

For patients who require a product with a more rapid initial action, yet with a sustained effect, a mixed injection of suitable doses of soluble and PZ insulin, prepared at the time of use, may be given. With such mixtures in the same syringe, part of the soluble insulin becomes bound to the PZ insulin, thus modifying the effect, and the use of PZ insulin has declined.

Isophane (NPH) and biphasic insulins

These are modifications of insulin that have an action midway between those of soluble and PZ insulins. Isophane insulin is a neutral suspension of an insulin–protamine–zinc complex, and when given twice daily evokes a smooth response. Biphasic isophane insulins are mixtures of soluble insulin and isophane insulin, and the rapidity of action depends on the proportion of soluble insulin present in a particular product.

INSULIN ZINC SUSPENSIONS

These preparations are protamine-free suspensions of zinc insulin but the rate of absorption of these modified insulins is markedly influenced by the size of the insulin particles present in the suspension. When the particles are extremely small (amorphous zinc insulin) absorption is rapid; with larger crystalline particles the absorption is slower, but the action more prolonged. For many diabetics, the use of a form of insulin zinc suspension may permit control with a single daily injection. These insulin modifications are basically for the maintenance control of stabilized diabetics. They are not suitable for emergency use, neither should they be mixed with any other form of insulin. Three forms of these insulins are in use:

Insulin zinc suspension (amorphous)

This product has slower but longer action than that of soluble insulin.

Insulin zinc suspension (crystalline)

The form with a duration of action that may extend over 24 hours.

Insulin zinc suspension (mixed)

This preparation contains both the amorphous and crystalline forms of zinc insulin. It has a peak effect about 6 hours after injection with a duration of activity of about 22 hours. It is often given twice a day; although with some patients a single daily dose may be adequate. Human as well as bovine and porcine preparations of insulin zinc suspension are available, but human forms have a shorter duration of activity.

Adverse reactions

Insulin overdose may cause hypoglycaemia, with faintness, giddiness and weakness, and if untreated may lead to coma, convulsions and death. The immediate treatment is sugar or glucose as a highly sweetened cup of tea if the patient is still able to swallow, but in severe hypoglycaemia intravenous glucose will be required.

All diabetic patients should carry some glucose sweets for immediate use should they feel faint, as well as a warning card indicating that they are diabetics. Hypoglycaemic coma must be distinguished from diabetic coma, where the blood sugar is high, with marked acidosis, and treatment is the administration of repeated small doses of soluble insulin, if necessary by careful intravenous injection.

Modified insulins

The frequency with which injections of soluble insulin must be given has led to the development of a number of modified insulins with varying durations of effect to obtain a smoother control of the diabetic state. Some, such as isophane insulin and biphasic insulin can be given twice daily, others such as protamine zinc insulin and insulin zinc suspension permit once-daily administration. Table 14.1 indicates the range of products available and their approximate duration of activity.

Nursing points about insulins

(a) Usually injected subcutaneously.
(b) Soluble insulin has a rapid action and so is given 15–30 minutes before food.
(c) They are injected intravenously in emergencies, but action disappears after about 30 minutes.
(d) Soluble insulin may be mixed in the syringe with most other forms of insulin of the same type (bovine, porcine, human), but the soluble form should be drawn up first.
(e) Vials of insulin suspension should be rotated and inverted to ensure even mixing; shaking will cause froth.
(f) Date vial when first withdrawal is made.
(g) Rotate injection site to reduce risk of local fat hypertrophy.
(h) Where appropriate, confirm by showing the vial to the patient that the prescribed type of insulin has been supplied.

Table 14.1 Insulin products

Product	Brand or other name	Origin	Approximate duration of action in hours
Short-acting insulins			
soluble insulin		Beef	6–8
insulin lispro		Human	2–4
neutral insulin			
	Human Actrapid	H-pyr	6–8
	Human Velosulin	H-emp	6–8
	Humulin S	H-prb	6–12
	Hypurin Neutral	Beef	6–8
	Velosulin	Pork	6–8
Intermediate-acting insulins			
insulin zinc (amorphous)	Semitard MC	Pork	12–16
biphasic insulin			
biphasic isophane insulin	Human Mixtard 10	H-pyr	14–24
(mixtures of isophane and soluble	Human Mixtard 20	H-pyr	14–24
insulin in varying proportions)	Human Mixtard 30	H-pyr	14–24
	Human Mixtard 40	H-pyr	14–24
	Human Mixtard 50	H-pyr	14–24
	Pork Mixtard 30		10–22
	Humulin M1	H-prb	6–20
	Humulin M2	H-prb	6–20
	Humulin M3	H-prb	6–20
	Humulin M4	H-prb	6–20
	Humulin M5	H-prb	6–20
isophane insulins	Human Insulatard	H-pyr	8–20
	Humulin I	H-prb	8–22
	Hypurin Isophane	Beef	8–22
	Insulatard	Pork	8–22
insulin zinc suspension	Human Monotard	H-pyr	8–22
(mixed)	Humulin Lente	H-prb	8–22
	Hypurin Lente	Beef	8–22
	Lentard MC	Beef and pork	8–22
Long-acting insulins			
insulin zinc suspension	Human Ultratard	H-pyr	22–30
(crystalline)	Humulin Zn	H-prb	8–22
protamine zinc insulin	Hypurin Protamine Zinc	Beef	24–30

Minor reactions to insulin include local irritation, and a lipoma may occur at a repeatedly used injection site. Such lipomas are of little importance except from the cosmetic point of view. An insidious long-term complication of diabetes is diabetic nephropathy, with proteinuria, a decline in glomerular filtration and a rise in blood pressure. ACE-inhibitors (p. 115) may reduce the glomerular pressure by dilating the arteries, and may slow down the progression to end-stage renal failure.

Some of the complications of diabetes mellitus appear to be associated in part with the abnormal accumulation of certain glucose metabolites, particularly the sugar sorbitol. The production of sorbitol is mediated by the enzyme aldose reductase, and an inhibitor of that enzyme would have therapeutic value in controlling the incidence and severity of diabetic complications. Some experimental studies have confirmed the potential value of such enzyme inhibitors, and the marketing of a drug of that type can be expected with some confidence.

ORAL HYPOGLYCAEMIC AGENTS

Tolbutamide § (dose: 0.5–2 g daily)

Brand name: Rastinon §

Many attempts have been made to find orally active

hypoglycaemic drugs, and thus avoid the need to inject insulin, but no real success was obtained until tolbutamide was discovered. Tolbutamide is a sulphonylurea, and brings about a lowering of the blood glucose level by stimulating the release of endogenous insulin from the still-functioning beta-cells of the pancreas. It is not an orally active insulin substitute, and is of no value in the absence of functioning beta-cells.

Tolbutamide is most effective in middle-aged and elderly patients who are well stabilized on low doses of insulin or who fail to respond solely to dietary restrictions. Therapy with tolbutamide or related drugs is not suitable for Type 1 (juvenile) diabetes or unstable diabetics.

Transfer from insulin to tolbutamide should be made slowly over a few days, and the initial doses depend to some extent on the dose of insulin being given. With small insulin requirements (less than 20 units daily), the insulin may be withdrawn and the change-over commenced with an initial tolbutamide dose of 1 g twice a day, reduced steadily to a maintenance dose of 1 g daily or less.

Larger doses, or a reversion to insulin, may be necessary during illness and other periods of stress. Tolerance to tolbutamide may occur in a few patients after treatment for some months, necessitating a change of therapy.

Tolbutamide is well tolerated and may be preferred in renal impairment, as it is largely metabolized in the liver.

Occasional **side-effects** are gastrointestinal disturbances, skin rash and weight gain, and it should be used with care in liver disease. Depression of bone marrow activity is uncommon, especially with low doses. Hypoglycaemia is indicative of overdose, requiring prompt adjustment.

Glibenclamide § (dose: 5–15 mg)

Brand names: Daonil §, Euglucon §
Glibenclamide is an example of several oral hypoglyaemic agents introduced after tolbutamide, and effective in lower doses as listed in Table 14.2. They all have an affinity for the sulphonylurea receptors present on B-cells, and the varying doses used reflect differences in the potency of that affinity, and their different abilities to stimulate insulin release. Clinically there is little difference between the sulphonylureas, but gliclazide and tolbutamide are thought to act more rapidly, and may be more suitable for elderly patients who may have some degree of renal impairment.

The initial dose of glibenclamide is 5 mg daily with breakfast, rising as required up to a maximum of 15 mg daily. The **side-effects** are similar to those of tolbutamide.

Metformin § (dose: 1–2 g daily)

Brand name: Glucophage §
Metformin differs both chemically and pharmacologically from the sulphonylureas as it belongs to the biguanide group. It does not influence the islets of Langerhans to produce more insulin, but appears to act by reducing the absorption of glucose from the gut, and increasing its utilization by the tissues.

Type 2 or maturity-onset diabetes may result from a disturbance of the sugar-regulating mechanism, and not a lack of insulin, and metformin may correct this disturbance. Like the sulphonylureas, the biguanides are active only when functioning pancreatic islet cells are present.

Table 14.2 Oral hypoglycaemic drugs (sulphonylureas and biguanides)

Approved name	Brand name	Daily dose range
Sulphonylureas		
glibenclamide	Daonil, Euglucon, Libanil, Malix, Calabren	5–15 mg
gliclazide	Diamicron	40–320 mg
glipizide	Glibenese, Minodiab	2.5–30 mg
gliquidone	Glurenorm	45–180 mg
tolazamide	Tolanase	100 mg–1 g
tolbutamide	Rastinon	500 mg–2 g
Biguanide		
metformin	Glucophage	1.5–3 g
troglitazone	Romozin	200–600 mg

Metformin is given in initial doses of 500 mg two or three times a day, gradually increasing over a period of 10 days according to response to a maximum dose of 3 g daily. Metformin is usually well tolerated, but it may cause some metabolic abnormalities, such as lactic acidosis, especially in patients with renal failure, for whom it should not be prescribed.

The main value of metformin is in the treatment of non-insulin-dependent diabetics who have failed to respond to sulphonylureas and dieting, although it is also useful in overweight diabetics.

Side-effects are nausea, anorexia and diarrhoea. Lactic acidosis requires withdrawal of the drug.

Troglitazone § ▼ (dose: 200–600 mg daily)

Brand name: Romozin § ▼

Troglitazone enhances the action of endogenous insulin and is a new approach to the treatment of NIDDM. It is given as an initial dose of 200 mg daily with breakfast, slowly increased if necessary at intervals of 2–4 weeks up to a single daily dose of 600 mg. It may be given as monotherapy in a patient not fully controlled by diet, or in combination. If a patient is switched from another oral drug, both medications should be continued for two weeks, as the onset of action of troglitazone is slow.

Side-effects include gastro-intestinal disturbances, headache and fatigue. Oral contraceptives should be avoided during troglitazone therapy.

At the time of writing, the prescribing of troglitazone has been suspended while reports of liver damage are being investigated. Even if troglitazone is withdrawn, interest in insulin enhancers is such that another drug of that type will be marketed in time.

Nursing points about oral hypoglycaemic agents

(a) Effective only when some residual beta-cell activity is present.
(b) Insulin therapy may be required during illness, surgery and pregnancy.
(c) Elderly more at risk of hypoglycaemia, particularly with long-acting sulphonylureas.
(d) Alcohol may cause facial flushing if taken with chlorpropamide.

SUPPLEMENTARY HYPOGLYCAEMIC AGENTS

Acarbose § (dose: 100–200 mg daily)

Brand name: Glucobay §

Acarbose, obtained from cultures of actinomycetes, is an inhibitor of alpha-glucosidase. That enzyme is involved in the breakdown of dietary carbohydrates into monosaccharides such as glucose that can be readily absorbed. Acarbose binds with alpha-glucosidase, and so slows down the rate of carbohydrate breakdown, which in turn reduces the amount of glucose available for immediate absorption. The use of acarbose leads to smoother daily blood glucose levels, and reduces the post-food peaks of hyperglycaemia that normally occur. Acarbose is indicated in the long-term treatment of non-insulin-dependent diabetes mellitus (NIDDM) in patients not otherwise adequately controlled, and is given initially in doses of

50 mg three times a day, just before or with food, and with water. The dose is increased after 6–8 weeks up to 300 mg daily according to need and response, as individual intestinal levels of glucosidase activity may vary widely.

Side-effects are flatulence, abdominal discomfort and diarrhoea.

Guar gum (dose: 21 g daily)

Brand name: Guarem

Guar gum has been used for many years as a thickening agent in food preparation, but if taken in large doses it retards the subsequent absorption of glucose. It is used in the treatment of diabetes mellitus, especially in diabetics poorly controlled by standard therapy, as it complements the hypoglycaemic action of insulin, the sulphonylureas and biguanides.

It may also have a supplementary action in promoting the lowering of plasma cholesterol levels, as such levels are often elevated in diabetes mellitus and may be a factor in the development of atherosclerotic disease in diabetics. Guar gum is given as granules in doses of 7 g three times a day, and half a dose should be taken before a meal with at least 100 ml of fluid, with the other half sprinkled over the food. An adequate fluid intake with each dose is essential. Treatment is continued for 6 weeks initially, after which the dose is reduced to 7 g twice a day.

Side-effects are flatulence, which may be marked, abdominal discomfort and intestinal obstruction.

HYPERGLYCAEMIC AGENTS

Glucagon § (dose: 0.5–1 mg by injection)

An overdose of insulin in a diabetic patient causes a lowering of the blood-sugar level. If mild, this hypoglycaemia may be controlled by oral glucose, but if severe, or if a state of insulin coma has occurred, prompt reversal of the hypoglycaemia is essential. As an alternative to intravenous dextrose, glucagon may be given and is often a first-choice drug.

Glucagon is a hormone secreted by the *alpha* islet cells of the pancreas, and increases blood glucose concentrations by a rapid mobilization of liver glycogen and release of glucose. A dose of 0.5–1 mg by injection brings about a rapid rise in the blood-sugar level, which in hypoglycaemia should be supported by the administration of glucose to prevent a relapse. The dose of glucagon, which may be given by subcutaneous, intramuscular or intravenous injection, may be repeated if required after an interval of 20 minutes. It is ineffective in chronic hypoglycaemic states.

Diazoxide § (dose: 5 mg/kg daily)

Brand name: Eudemine §

Diazoxide is a synthetic drug that inhibits the release of insulin, and as a result the blood-sugar level rises. It is of value in restoring a normal blood-sugar level in cases of hypoglycaemia associated with abnormally high insulin secretion due to islet-cell hyperplasia or pancreatic tumours, and also in the severe idiopathic hypoglycaemia of infancy. It is given orally in divided doses of 5 mg/kg daily initially, adjusted as soon as possible according to need and response. Care is necessary in cardiac disease, renal impairment and pregnancy. Diazoxide is of no value in the treatment of acute hypoglycaemia.

Side-effects of diazoxide include nausea, common in the early stages of treatment, oedema, hypotension, which may be severe and require treatment, tachycardia and extrapyramidal symptoms. Blood examinations are necessary during prolonged treatment.

The use of diazoxide in hypertensive crisis is referred to on page 122.

FURTHER READING

Chan A W, MacFarlane I A 1988 The pharmacology of oral agents used to treat diabetes mellitus. Practical Diabetes 5(2):59–64

Clissold S P, Edwards C 1988 Acarbose. Drugs 35:214–243

Jacques A 1993 The use of insulin in diabetes mellitus. Professional Nurse 9(3):190–192

Gallichan M 1995 Treatment options for managing diabetes mellitus. Nursing Times 91(8):40–41

Krentz A J 1996 Insulin resistance. British Medical Journal 313:1385–1389

McLellan A R 1993 Insulins. Medicine International 21(7):250–251

McLellan A R 1993 Oral hypoglycaemic agents. Medicine International 21(7):255–256

McPherson M L 1992 Pharmacotherapy of diabetes mellitus. Journal of Home Health Care 4(3):20–27

Petrie J, Small M, Connell J 1997 'Glitazones' a prospect for non-insulin-dependent diabetes. Lancet 349:70–71

Practical Diabetes 1993 Acarbose – review of new oral anti-diabetic agent. Supplement to Practical Diabetes 10(6):S3–31

Tomlinson D R 1994 Aldose reductase: its importance in diabetes. Practical Diabetes 11(2):51–54

15

Antirheumatic and uricosuric agents

ANTIRHEUMATICS

Rheumatoid arthritis is a common inflammatory disease of the peripheral synovial joints, mainly involving the fingers, wrists and knees. Unlike osteoarthritis, which occurs in weight-bearing joints and is the result of wear and tear, rheumatoid arthritis is a symptom of a systemic disorder characterized by the presence of auto-antibodies. Initially the affected joints become swollen, painful and warm, but the disease is progressive and in time the synovium becomes thickened and inflamed, leading eventually to articular cartilage damage and joint deformity. Inflammation is part of the normal healing process, but in rheumatoid arthritis the immune system of the body has turned against itself and inflammatory mediators such as histamine, serotonin, bradykinin and prostaglandin perpetuate rather than heal damage to the synovial membranes.

NSAIDs AND PROSTAGLANDINS

In severe inflammatory conditions such as rheumatoid arthritis, treatment is largely based on the nonsteroidal anti-inflammatory drugs (NSAIDs), which include aspirin. The corticosteroids (Chapter 13) are now less widely used except for acute conditions, and secondary drugs like penicillamine and gold are potent drugs used when the response to a NSAID is inadequate. The NSAIDs act by interrupting the synthesis of prostaglandins from arachidonic acid by inhibiting the enzyme cyclo-oxygenase (prostaglandin synthetase). The process is a complex one, outlined in Fig. 15.1, and the prostaglandins normally synthesized form a group referred to as the prostanoids.

It should be noted (Fig. 15.1) that leukotrienes are also formed from arachidonic acid. That process is inhibited by the glucocorticoids, which stimulate the production of lipocortin, which in turn inhibits the enzyme phospholipase A_2. That process explains the powerful anti-inflammatory action of the glucocorticoids. (The other uses of the prostaglandins are referred to on p. 170.) The prostanoids, particularly PGE_2, interrupt the inflammatory response to mediators of inflammation such as bradykinin and histamine. They also appear to inhibit inflammatory cell migration, as well as preventing the release of other inflammatory factors, and their value in rheumatoid conditions is increased by their intrinsic analgesic potency. Their action is palliative, as they do not alter the underlying disease process.

Although all NSAIDs appear to have the same basic mechanism of action, individual members of the group vary in activity, and there is also a wide variation in individual response to therapy. Some differences in action may be due to variations in the degree of tissue binding, or the subsidiary mechanisms that may contribute to the overall anti-inflammatory response, and the best drug is the one that gives the individual patient optimum relief of symptoms with minimal side-effects.

The NSAIDs generally have a number of **side-effects**, which may be severe, including gastric irritation with nausea and vomiting which may lead to gastric erosion, and bleeding. Such reactions are linked with the inhibitory effects of NSAIDs on the synthesis of prostaglandins E and F, which normally inhibit gastric acid secretion and control mucosal blood flow. These gastric irritant side-effects can be reduced by administration of the drug with food or milk, and patients should be advised accordingly.

More recently, misoprostol (p. 151) has been used for the prophylaxis of NSAID-induced gastroduodenal ulceration. Other side-effects include headache, vertigo, tinnitus and dizziness that may interfere with driving. Care is also necessary in renal and hepatic impairment. Of particular importance is the risk of hypersensitivity reactions such as bronchospasm, angioneurotic oedema and rash. NSAIDs should be avoided in asthmatic patients, especially if it is known that the asthma is provoked by aspirin. Some NSAIDs may become highly protein bound,

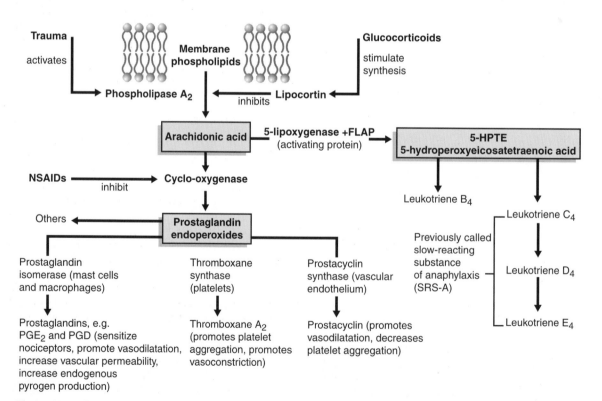

Figure 15.1 Scheme of prostaglandin synthesis.

Table 15.1 Non-steroidal anti-inflammatory drugs (NSAIDs)

Approved name	Brand name	Average daily dose
aceclofenac▼	Preservex▼	100–200 mg
acemetacin	Emflex	120 mg
azapropazone	Rheumox	600 mg–1.2 g
diclofenac[a]	Voltarol	75–150 mg
diflunisal	Dolobid	500 mg–1 g
etodolac	Lodine	400–600 mg
fenbufen	Lederfen	600–900 mg
fenoprofen	Fenopron	900 mg–2.4 g
flurbiprofen	Froben	150–300 mg
ibuprofen	Brufen	600 mg–1.2 g
indomethacin[a]	Imbrilon, Indocid	50–200 mg
ketoprofen[a]	Orudis, Oruvail	100–200 mg
mefenamic acid	Ponstan	1.5 g
meloxicam[a]▼	Mobic▼	7.5–15 mg
nabumetone	Reliflex	1 g
naproxen[a]	Naprosyn, Synflex	500 mg–1 g
phenylbutazone	Butacote	200–600 mg
piroxicam[a]	Feldene	20–40 mg
sulindac	Clinoril	200–400 mg
tenoxicam	Mobiflex	20 mg
tiaprofenic acid	Surgam	600 mg
tolmetin	Tolectin	600 mg–1.8 g

[a]Suppositories available for use at night to reduce morning stiffness.

Nursing points about NSAIDs

(a) Treatment should be initiated at a low dose level.
(b) Patients vary considerably in response, and a change of drug may be necessary to obtain the optimum response.
(c) Should not be given in active peptic ulcer or a history thereof or to the elderly unless other therapy is ineffective.
(d) *All* NSAIDs are contra-indicated in patients hypersensitive to aspirin.
(e) Some NSAIDs can be obtained without prescription; deterioration in the condition of an asthmatic patient may be due to self-medication with a NSAID.
(f) Photosensitivity may occur with azapropazone (Rheumox); patients should be advised accordingly.

---

and the doses of oral anticoagulants and hyperglycaemic agents may require adjustment.

Many NSAIDs are derivatives of phenylpropionic acid. A few examples of representative compounds are discussed here and on page 206, and Table 15.1 indicates the wide range available, but it should be noted that etodolac, although used in the treatment of rheumatoid arthritis, has little analgesic activity.

Some NSAIDs are used locally for the symptomatic relief of mild rheumatoid and muscular pain and soft tissue inflammation. Representative products are Feldene Gel (piroxicam), Proflex Cream (ibuprofen), Traxam (felbinac) and Voltarol Emulgel (diclofenac). Small amounts should be rubbed into the affected areas three or four times a day, but occlusive dressings should not be used.

Aspirin (dose: 2–8 g daily)

The use of aspirin (acetylsalicylic acid) as a mild analgesic as well as its side-effects are referred to on page 54, but its associated anti-inflammatory action is of value in the treatment of the pain and inflammation of rheumatoid disease and musculoskeletal disorders generally. It is given in doses of 0.5–1 g up to 4-hourly, but in acute inflammatory conditions doses up to 8 g daily may be required to obtain an adequate response. Doses of 3 g daily or less have little anti-inflammatory activity.

Aspirin is also given for Still's disease (juvenile rheumatoid arthritis) in doses varying from 80–130 mg/kg daily, but otherwise it is now recommended that aspirin should not be given to children under 12 years of age, as there is a possible link between the use of aspirin and Reye's syndrome (acute encephalopathy with fatty degeneration of the viscera).

Benorylate, in which aspirin is combined with paracetamol, is also used in the treatment of the pain and inflammation of rheumatic disorders.

Naproxen § (dose: 500 mg–1 g daily)

Brand names: Naprosyn §, Nycopren §, Synflex §
Naproxen is one of the most widely used NSAIDs. It has analgesic as well as anti-inflammatory and antipyretic properties, and although rapidly absorbed, much of the drug becomes bound initially to plasma proteins, followed by relatively slow release. In rheumatoid conditions, naproxen is given as an initial dose of 250 mg twice a day, later increased to 500 mg twice daily. When morning stiffness causes difficulties the daily dose can be so divided that a larger dose is taken at night. Alternatively, suppositories of 500 mg can be used at night for a prolonged action and they are also useful when naproxen is not well tolerated orally.

Naproxen is also of value in the symptomatic treatment of acute gout, and is then given in doses of 750 mg initially, followed by 250 mg 8-hourly. It has also been used for the relief of the pain of dysmenorrhoea.

Side-effects of naproxen are those of the NSAIDs generally. As cross-sensitivity to aspirin and other NSAIDs may exist, naproxen should not be given to patients known to be sensitive to such drugs. Some reversible hair loss has occurred in children receiving naproxen.

Napratec § is a combination pack containing misoprostol tablets 200 micrograms together with naprosyn tablets 500 mg for prophylaxis against NSAID-induced peptic ulcer.

Fenbufen § (dose: 600–900 mg daily)

Brand name: Lederfen §
Fenbufen is a pro-drug, as it is not effective until metabolized after absorption into active metabolites. It has the analgesic and anti-inflammatory properties of naproxen, and in rheumatoid disease and musculoskeletal disorders it is given in doses of 450 mg twice daily, or 300 mg and 600 mg morning and evening respectively.

It has the **side-effects** and hypersensitivity risks of the NSAIDs, although rash is more common, in which case the drug should be withdrawn immediately, as an allergic lung reaction may follow. Ibuprofen is a related drug now used more extensively as a mild analgesic (p. 55).

Indomethacin § (dose: 50–200 mg daily)

Brand names: Imbrilon §, Indocid §
Indomethacin is a derivative of indole-acetic acid, and is a potent anti-inflammatory agent with analgesic properties. It is used in the treatment of the inflammation and pain of rheumatoid arthritis and other musculoskeletal disorders, and is effective in doses of 25 mg two to four times a day with food, increased if necessary up to 200 mg daily. For a longer action in the control of night pain and morning stiffness, indomethacin may be used at night as a suppository of 100 mg. It is sometimes used in the treatment of acute gout in doses of 50 mg four times a day. Indomethacin has been used in the relief of the pain of dysmenorrhoea in doses of 25 mg three times a day.

Side-effects of indomethacin are those of related NSAIDs, including hypersensitivity reactions, which are a contra-indication, as is peptic ulcer. Headache is common with initial treatment, but if it persists the drug should be withdrawn. Ocular side-effects and corneal deposits have occasionally been reported.

Piroxicam § (dose: 20–40 mg daily)

Brand name: Feldene §
Piroxicam is an analgesic/anti-inflammatory agent with the advantage of a longer action that permits a single daily dose. In rheumatoid conditions it is given in doses of 20–30 mg daily, but in acute gout piroxicam is given in doses of 40 mg daily for 4–6 days. It is usually well tolerated, but extended treatment with doses of more than 30 mg daily may increase the incidence of gastro-intestinal disturbances. Suppositories containing 20 mg of piroxicam are also available. In acute conditions it is sometimes given by deep intragluteal injection in doses of 20 mg. Feldene Melt § is a tablet product designed to melt and dissolve in the mouth.

Phenylbutazone § (dose: 400–600 mg daily)

Brand name: Butacote §
Phenylbutazone has powerful anti-inflammatory and analgesic properties, but its value is limited by its **side-effects**. These include an acute pulmonary syndrome, fluid retention that can lead to cardiac failure, agranulocytosis and aplastic anaemia. The use of phenylbutazone is now restricted to the hospital treatment of ankylosing spondylitis. It is given in doses of 100 mg two or three times a day, but prolonged treatment may be necessary.

PROSTAGLANDINS

As the prostaglandins are closely concerned with the onset and maintenance of the inflammatory processes, and many anti-inflammatory agents such as the NSAIDs act by inhibiting prostaglandin biosynthesis, it is convenient briefly to review here that interesting group of substances.

The prostaglandins are derivatives of arachidonic acid, a long-chain unsaturated fatty acid, linked with phospholipids, present in many body cells. Their release is mediated by the enzyme phosphatase A_2, and they are then metabolized by prostaglandin synthetase, also known as cyclo-oxygenase, to prostaglandin endoperoxides, which are later differentiated into a number of separate prostaglandins (Fig. 15.1).

As a group, the prostaglandins are concerned in the regulation of almost all biological functions and have widely varying actions, as they are involved in the contraction and relaxation of smooth muscle in the blood vessels, bronchi and uterus, and affect blood platelet aggregation and the inhibition of gastric secretion. Some important members of the group are designated as PGE, PGF, prostacyclin and thromboxane A_2 (TXA_2), and are sometimes referred to collectively as the prostanoids. PGE and PGF have been differentiated into certain sub-groups represented by PGE_1 and PGF_2.

Leukotrienes are associated substances formed from arachidonic acid by lipoxygenase and also have inflammatory and allergic properties. The slow-reacting substance of anaphylaxis (SRS-A) is one of the leukotrienes.

Other prostaglandins of interest include epoprostenol (prostacyclin) and thromboxane A_2 which are concerned with the maintenance of blood flow (p. 135). Prostaglandins with a selective action on the uterus are referred to on page 170.

Prostaglandins are also involved in the patency of the ductus arteriosus, which normally closes soon after birth with the changes in oxygen tension that occur. Babies born with congenital heart defects may still require a patent ductus for adequate oxygenation, and to maintain such patency until corrective surgery can be carried out, alprostadil is used (p. 171). On the other hand, when the ductus fails to close normally after birth, indomethacin has been used to induce closure by its antiprostaglandin activity. Misoprostol is a synthetic analogue of alprostadil that inhibits gastric secretion, and is used to prevent NSAID-induced gastric disturbances (p. 151).

Caverject § is an alprostadil preparation for the treatment of erectile dysfunction. It is given in doses of 2.5 micrograms by direct intracavernous injection.

SPECIFIC SUPPRESSANTS OF INFLAMMATION

A few non-analgesic drugs appear to have an unusual and largely specific action on the local inflammatory processes of rheumatoid disease. They are regarded as second-line drugs for use when response to NSAIDs fails, when treatment with corticosteroids is undesired, or when there is a deterioration of the rheumatoid condition, but they should be used before joint damage has become irreversible. They are powerful drugs with which extended therapy is required, and their use requires care. They are sometimes referred to as disease-modifying antirheumatic drugs (DMARDs) as the onset of their action is slow.

Penicillamine § (dose: 0.25–1 g daily)

Brand names: Distamine §, Pendramine §
Penicillamine, a chelating agent obtained by the acid degradation of penicillin, was introduced to increase the urinary excretion of copper in Wilson's disease

---

Nursing points about gold, penicillamine and related drugs

(a) Used only in active inflammatory joint disease after certain diagnosis, and when NSAID treatment is ineffective or unacceptable.
(b) Treatment should be initiated before joint damage becomes irreversible.
(c) Response is slow and may take 4–6 months to appear with gold therapy, 6–12 weeks with penicillamine.
(d) If no benefit after 6 months with gold, 1 year with penicillamine, discontinue treatment.
(e) Development of a rash requires withdrawal of the drug.
(f) Relapse after gold treatment should be avoided, as response to a second course of gold therapy is usually poor or absent.
(g) Blood counts are necessary at regular intervals.
(h) Long treatment with chloroquine carries risk of retinal damage; regular eye tests necessary.

(p. 159), but it is also useful in some cases of severe active rheumatoid arthritis as an alternative to gold therapy. The adult dose is 250 mg daily before food, increasing at monthly intervals to a maintenance daily dose of 500 mg or more. Treatment may be required for 6–12 weeks before a response is obtained, and not all patients respond. Penicillamine is also used in juvenile chronic arthritis (Still's disease). It is also used in the control of chronic active hepatitis (p. 159).

Side-effects Penicillamine is potentially toxic, and regular blood and urine tests are essential. Blood dyscrasias and kidney damage require cessation of treatment, but therapy can be recommenced after a rest period if renal function and blood counts return to normal. Other side-effects include nausea, rash and proteinuria. Loss of taste may occur in the early weeks of treatment, but usually returns later. Hypersensitivity reactions or a late-occurring rash may require withdrawal of the drug.

Sodium aurothiomalate § (dose: 10–50 mg weekly by injection)

Brand name: Myocrisin §
This gold compound is used for its anti-inflammatory action in rheumatoid arthritis and Still's disease as a second-line drug when NSAIDs are no longer effective. It is indicated in severe conditions when joint inflammation is progressive, but treatment must be commenced before irreversible joint damage has occurred. Sodium aurothiomalate is also useful in patients with severe rheumatoid arthritis requiring large doses of corticosteroids to control the

symptoms, as it may permit a reduction in the dose of such steroids. Gold therapy is ineffective in other forms of arthritis, and is of no value when extensive deformities have developed.

Treatment with sodium aurothiomalate is commenced with a test dose of 10 mg to assess tolerance. It must be given by deep intramuscular injection, and the area should be massaged gently. If the drug is well tolerated, treatment is continued with increasing doses up to 50 mg weekly until remission of symptoms occurs or a total dose of 1 g has been injected. The response to treatment is slow, and may not occur until 500 mg have been given, but when it occurs, the interval between doses may be increased to 2–4 weeks.

A remission, once achieved, should continue to be treated with the effective dose for prolonged periods for 5 years or more. Maintenance of therapy is important, and if a relapse occurs, the dose should be increased at once to 50 mg weekly to regain control, after which the dose may be reduced to the previous maintenance level. The response to a second course of gold therapy after a complete relapse is seldom satisfactory.

Side-effects Blood and urine tests should be carried out before each injection, as the side-effects of sodium aurothiomalate are sometimes severe and include skin reactions, oedema and renal disorders and pruritus. Blood disorders that may occur can require intensive supportive therapy if a fatal outcome is to be avoided. The drug should be withdrawn if a rash develops after prolonged treatment, and it is contra-indicated in renal or hepatic disease, blood disorders, severe anaemia or dermatitis.

Auranofin § (dose: 6–9 mg daily)

Brand name: Ridaura §
Auranofin is a water-soluble gold compound with the actions, uses and side-effects of sodium aurothiomalate, and the advantage of being active orally. It is used in severe and progressive rheumatoid arthritis when other drugs are ineffective. It is given in doses of 3 mg after food twice daily initially, which, if well tolerated, may then be given as a single daily dose of 6 mg.

The response to treatment is slow, and if a 6 mg daily dose of auranofin is ineffective, 3 mg may be given three times a day, withdrawn after 3 months if the response remains unsatisfactory. Blood counts and tests for proteinuria should be performed throughout treatment, and auranofin should be withdrawn if thrombocytopenia occurs or is suspected.

The most common **side-effect** of auranofin is diarrhoea, which may be severe enough in some patients to require withdrawal of the drug. Other side-effects include rash, mouth ulcers, nausea, intestinal pain and pruritus. Blood and urine tests should be carried out monthly, as blood disorders sometimes develop suddenly.

Auranofin should be used with caution in patients with renal or hepatic disease, a history of bone marrow depression or rash. It does not interfere with the action of oral contraceptives.

Ridaura is presented as a tablet of unusual shape that permits easy handling by arthritic patients, as the tablet tilts when placed on a flat surface.

Chloroquine § (dose: 150 mg daily)

Brand names: Avloclor §, Nivaquine §
Some antimalarials such as chloroquine may evoke a response in severe active rheumatoid arthritis similar to that induced by penicillamine, auranofin or sodium aurothiomalate. Chloroquine is given in doses of 150 mg daily after food, but prolonged treatment for up to 2 years may be necessary. On the other hand, some physicians consider that antimalarial agents are of greatest value in early, mild rheumatoid arthritis.

A potential danger with such long treatment is the risk of irreversible retinal damage, although the risk is slight when the dose does not exceed 4 mg/kg daily, or when the total cumulative dose does not exceed 100 g. As a precaution, an 8-week rest period from treatment every year has been recommended. In all cases, a full ocular examination is advisable before treatment, and twice-yearly thereafter.

Other **side-effects** include nausea, diarrhoea, pruritus, skin reactions, tinnitus, photosensitization, corneal opacities and blood disorders. Chloroquine should be used with caution in elderly patients, as it may be difficult to distinguish drug-induced retinopathy from age-related ocular changes.

Hydroxychloroquine (Plaquenil §) is a related drug with similar actions, uses and side-effects, but is less likely to cause retinal problems. Dose 200–400 mg daily, after food.

Sulphasalazine § (dose: 2–3 g daily)

Brand name: Salazopyrin §
Sulphasalazine, used chiefly in ulcerative colitis (p. 152), is sometimes effective in suppressing the inflammatory symptoms of rheumatoid arthritis. It is given in doses of 500 mg initially, increased up to

2–3 g daily over 4 weeks but haematological distur-bances may occur and full blood counts are necessary, particularly during the first 6 months of treatment. Liver function tests should also be carried out. Patients should be warned to report immediately if soreness of the throat, fever or malaise occurs, as blood disorders require prompt withdrawal of treatment.

For other **side-effects** see p. 152.

IMMUNOSUPPRESSANTS

Several immunosuppressants represented by azathio-prine, which is used to prevent rejection in transplant surgery (p. 278), have an action similar to that of gold and chloroquine in rheumatoid arthritis and other conditions thought to be auto-immune in origin, such as the connective tissue disorder lupus erythe-matosus. They are sometimes useful as alternative therapy in patients not responding to other drugs.

Azathioprine § (Imuran §) is given in doses of 1.5–2.5 mg/kg daily, but as the drug causes some bone marrow depression, blood counts should be carried out monthly. Nausea and diarrhoea may occur in the early stages of treatment, and may be severe enough to require withdrawal of the drug.

Chlorambucil § (Leukeran §) is an alkylating agent (p. 216) with an action in rheumatoid arthritis similar to that of azothioprine, and is given in doses of 2.5–7.5 mg daily. Blood counts are necessary during treatment. Cyclophosphamide § (Endoxana §) (p. 216) has a similar action, and is given in doses of 1–5 mg/kg daily.

Methotrexate § (Maxtrex §) is a cytotoxic agent (p. 218) with immunosuppressant properties. In severe active rheumatoid arthritis not responding to other therapy it is given in doses of 7.5 mg once weekly initially, rising according to need and response to a maximum dose of 30 mg weekly. Full blood counts and liver function tests are essential during methotrexate treatment. **Side-effects** include myelo-suppression and mucositis, which can be reduced by folinic acid (p. 219). Methotrexate is contra-indicated in marked renal impairment.

Cyclosporin § (Neoral §; formerly Sandimmun), the immunosuppressive agent referred to on p. 278, is also used in the treatment of severe, active rheumatoid arthritis in adult patients resistant to other therapy. The initial dose is 2.5 mg/kg daily, and after 6 weeks the dose can be increased accord-ing to need and response, but should not exceed 4 mg/kg daily. Cyclosporin may be used with care together with a NSAID, but combined treatment increases the risks of renal and liver damage.

URICOSURIC DRUGS

Uricosuric drugs are used mainly in the treatment of gout, which is a painful metabolic disorder charac-terized by deposits of sodium urate crystals in the joints and tendons. Gout is caused by an excessive production of purines or a reduced renal clearance of uric acid, and an inflammatory response to the deposits of sodium urate causes the typical attack of acute gout, which usually arrives without warning. The long-continued deposit of the crystals results in the tophi of chronic gout as well as erosive damage to and deformity of the joints. Most drugs used in the treatment of gout act by reducing the inflam-matory response, increasing the urinary excretion of uric acid and by decreasing its further production.

Some NSAIDs such as naproxen and indomethacin are used to relieve the inflammatory symptoms of acute gout, as is colchicine, but for chronic gout allo-purinol is preferred. In all treatment with uricosuric agents, a high fluid intake is essential, and the urine should be made alkaline with sodium bicarbonate or potassium citrate to prevent the recrystallization of urates during excretion.

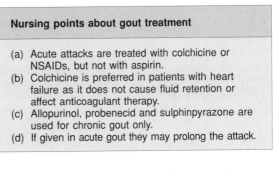

Nursing points about gout treatment

(a) Acute attacks are treated with colchicine or NSAIDs, but not with aspirin.
(b) Colchicine is preferred in patients with heart failure as it does not cause fluid retention or affect anticoagulant therapy.
(c) Allopurinol, probenecid and sulphinpyrazone are used for chronic gout only.
(d) If given in acute gout they may prolong the attack.

Colchicine §

Colchicine is the alkaloid obtained from the autumn crocus, and is an old but specific drug for the treat-ment of acute gout. It acts by binding to microtubules in white blood cells, and prevents their migration to areas of uric acid deposition and so reduces the inflammatory response. Colchicine is given in doses of 1 mg initially, followed by doses of 500 micrograms every 2–3 hours until relief is obtained, or until a total dose of 10 mg has been given. The response is usually dramatic, although sometimes adequate dosing is limited by **side-effects** such as nausea, vomiting, abdominal pain and diarrhoea.

Colchicine is also used in doses of 500 micrograms two or three times a day to prevent the attacks of acute gout that may occur during the initial stages of treatment of chronic gout with allopurinol, or uricosuric drugs. It should be used with care in the elderly, and in cases of renal impairment.

Allopurinol § (dose: 200–600 mg daily)

Brand names: Zyloric §, Caplenal §

Allopurinol has a unique action in the treatment of chronic gout. It inhibits xanthine oxidase, an enzyme linked with the formation of uric acid from purines, and so reduces the plasma concentration of that acid by a different mechanism from that of the uricosuric drugs. Allopurinol is widely used in the prolonged treatment of chronic gout, and may be of particular value in patients with impaired renal function not responding to uricosuric agents as it bypasses such impairment by its different mode of action.

Allopurinol is given in doses of 100 mg daily initially (after any attack of acute gout has subsided), and slowly increased over 3 weeks to a dose of 300 mg or more daily. The dose is later adjusted until the plasma uric acid level falls to 60 micrograms per ml, with maintenance doses of 200–300 mg daily. As allopurinol may precipitate an attack of acute gout during initial therapy, combined treatment with colchicine or a NSAID for at least 4 weeks is recommended. A high fluid intake and alkalization of the urine are necessary during allopurinol therapy. Allopurinol is also used to control the hyperuricaemia that may follow the use of some cytotoxic drugs, and should be commenced before such treatment is given.

Allopurinol is usually well tolerated, but intestinal disturbances may occur and alopecia has been reported. A rash with fever indicates withdrawal of treatment.

Probenecid § (dose: 1–2 g daily)

Brand name: Benemid §

Probenecid influences renal tubular activity, as it increases the rate of excretion of some substances such as uric acid and so is of value in the treatment of chronic gout. It is given in doses of 250 mg twice daily initially, increased as required up to a maximum of 2 g daily. Dosage should be adjusted later according to the plasma uric acid level.

Probenecid is generally well tolerated, but headache, flushing and dizziness may occasionally occur. It should be noted that in the initial stages of treatment, probenecid may precipitate attacks of acute gout as the stores of urate are mobilized and excreted. Such attacks may be controlled by colchicine or naproxen.

Sulphinpyrazone § (dose: 200–800 mg daily)

Brand name: Anturan §

Sulphinpyrazone promotes the renal excretion of urates by inhibiting tubular reabsorption. It brings about a lowering of uric acid level in the blood and the mobilization of urate tophi in the tissues that is of value in the treatment of chronic gout. Unlike the NSAIDs, it has no analgesic properties, and is of no value in acute gout.

Sulphinpyrazone is given in doses of 100–200 mg daily initially, with food, but as it may precipitate attacks of acute gout, colchicine or a NSAID such as naproxen may be given concurrently for a time to reduce the risks of such attacks. Subsequently, increasing doses of sulphinpyrazone up to 600 mg daily may be given, and adjusted later to a maintenance dose of 200 mg or more daily as required. In resistant gout, combined treatment with allopurinol is sometimes effective.

Sulphinpyrazone is usually well tolerated, but it may cause occasional gastro-intestinal disturbances and it should not be used in cases of peptic ulcer. It should be noted that sulphinpyrazone may influence the action of oral anticoagulants and sulphonylureas, and an adjustment of dose of those drugs may be necessary.

FURTHER READING

Agambar L, Flower R 1980 Anti-inflammatory drugs: history and mechanism of action. Physiotherapy 76(4):198–202

Akil M, Amos R S 1995 Rheumatoid arthritis–I; Clinical features and diagnosis. British Medical Journal 310:587–589

Akil M, Amos R S 1995 Rheumatoid arthritis–II; Treatment. British Medical Journal 310:652–655

Bateman D N, Kennedy J J G 1995 Non-steroidal anti-inflammatory drugs and elderly patients. British Medical Journal 310:817–818

Bradlow A, David J 1995 Recent advances in rheumatology. British Medical Journal 310:637–640

Brick J E, DiBartololomeo A G 1992 Rethinking the therapeutic pyramid for rheumatoid arthritis. Post Graduate Medicine 91(2):75–91

Buckley C D 1997 Treatment of rheumatoid arthritis. British Medical Journal 315:236–239

McConkey B, Amos R, Durham S et al 1980 Sulphasalazine in rheumatoid arthritis. British Medical Journal 287:442–444

Spittle M 1995 Misoprostol in patients taking non-steroidal anti-inflammatory drugs. British Medical Journal 311:1518–1519

Veale D, Pullar T 1994 Drug therapy of rheumatic diseases. Hospital Update February:93–100

16

The chemotherapy of malignant disease

Cancer is the second killer of adults after heart disease, and although some risk factors have been identified, the reason why normal body cells begin to differentiate into cancer cells is not yet fully understood. In some cases a genetic abnormality may be the cause, but most cancers are the result of contact in some way with carcinogens. These are often chemical substances, but viruses and radiation may also be involved. Normal body cells divide up to a maximum of about 50 times before they are replaced by new cells, but occasionally a few escape control and continue to divide, and undifferentiated growth takes place. Not all cells that go out of control progress far enough to be harmful, as their abnormality may not permit extended survival, and others may be destroyed by the body's immune system because they are recognized as not being normal body cells. Those abnormal cells that do survive grow haphazardly and may spread throughout the body.

Several theories have been developed to explain carcinogenesis. One suggests that cancer is a multistep process, in which some carcinogens may act as initiators and bring about irreversible changes in cells, while others may act more as promotors and modify the expression of altered genes that leads to tumour development. The viral hypothesis suggests that when a virus infects a cell, some viral genetic material is inserted into that of the host in such a way that the gene controlling normal replication of the host is modified. In consequence, the infected cell starts to reproduce uncontrollably and eventually develops into a cancer.

The 'oncogene' theory is based on the suggestion that normal cells contain genes referred to as oncogenes. Oncogenes are thought to function by maintaining cell division during early development, and by inhibiting it at a later stage. It has been

213

proposed that cancers develop when oncogenes are subsequently re-activated in some way. For example, genes that normally inactivate oncogenes may lose their potency by mutation, oncogenes themselves may resist inactivation by mutation, and infective viruses may introduce uncontrollable oncogenes into normal cells.

Once cells escape from the controls governing normal growth they may change significantly, become undifferentiated and revert to a more primitive type of new growth. These growths are referred to generically as neoplasms, and are of two main types, the benign and the malignant. Benign growths are made up of more or less differentiated cells; they are slow-growing, encapsulated, and do not infiltrate adjacent tissues or spread to distant organs. They are not usually serious, although they may cause pressure symptoms or the overproduction of certain hormones, and can often be treated by surgical removal. Malignant neoplasms or cancers differ sharply in being fast-growing, undifferentiated, unencapsulated and capable of being carried by the blood and lymph to distant organs. These secondary growths are termed metastases. Once a malignant tumour has spread it is difficult to treat by surgery or radiotherapy, and chemotherapy is often the only choice.

CHEMOTHERAPY

The aim of treatment with chemotherapeutic agents is to destroy malignant cells with minimal damage to normal cells, but few drugs are so selective. The majority of anticancer agents (with the exception of hormonal drugs) attack all rapidly dividing cells, which accounts for their severe side-effects. The potency depends on the fact that malignant cells, as compared with normal cells, are more susceptible to drug attack, have a reduced capacity for repair, and are slower in recovering from the effects of cytotoxic drugs, although cells that reach the resting phase of the cycle (Fig. 16.1) may survive attack.

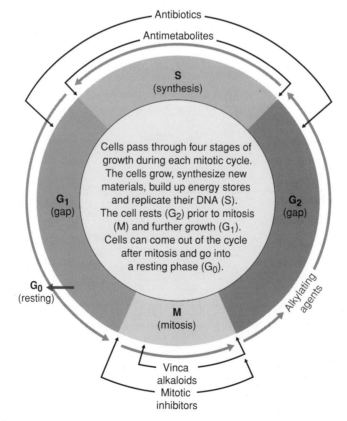

Figure 16.1 Cell cycle and points of cytotoxic drug attack.

The cytotoxic drugs in current use can be divided into five main groups: the alkylating agents, the antimetabolites, the cytotoxic antibiotics, the antimitotics, and an ill-defined group of unrelated substances that have a cytotoxic action, such as carboplatin and some hormone inhibitors. Some act at different stages of the cell cycle, so combined therapy may increase the anti-tumour activity and reduce side-effects, and a number of multi-drug dosage schemes are in use, usually identified by the initial letters of the drugs concerned, as ABVD, CHOP, and CMF.

Combination therapy may also tend to limit the development of drug resistance, which may occur with several cytotoxic agents. The cause is usually a plasma membrane protein identified as phosphoglycoprotein (PGP). It is a cytoprotective agent, and has the ability to extrude foreign substances from the cell by an ATP-activated pumping process, thus preventing the intracellular concentration of a cytotoxic drug from reaching a destructive level. The pump may be inactivated by certain drugs such as nifedipine, tamoxifen and verapamil, and attempts are being made to inhibit PGP activity by combined therapy. Some tumours respond well to chemotherapy, and in the case of childhood leukaemias, tetromas, Burkitt's lymphoma and advanced Hodgkin's disease a curative response may be obtained. In other cases chemotherapy may be adjunctive or palliative treatment. The search for new and more effective cytotoxic agents is continuous, and methods of improving the targeting of drugs more effectively are studied, as by the use of monoclonal antibodies. Low-dose continuous infusion may permit a cytotoxic drug to attack a cancer cell at the most sensitive phase of the cell-growth cycle, so advances in cancer chemotherapy can be expected.

Side-effects Chemotherapy has multiple side-effects, some of which may be severe enough to limit treatment. Depression of bone marrow activity, which may be severe, is a common side-effect of cytotoxic drugs, with the exceptions of bleomycin and the vinca alkaloids. The speed of onset of such depression varies, and may be delayed. It is also linked with an immunosuppressant action involving cell-mediated immunity, thus increasing the risks of infection during cytotoxic therapy, and may be a limiting factor in the chemotherapy of malignant disease. The drug-induced neutropenia can be reduced by injections of the human granulocyte-colony stimulating factor (G-CSF). See filgrastim, lenograstim and molograstim (pp. 145–146).

Other common and often severe side-effects are gastrointestinal toxicity with mouth ulceration, anorexia, nausea and vomiting. The latter, once experienced, may become anticipatory, as the thought of further treatment may provoke vomiting. Fortunately, pre-treatment with the powerful antiemetics now available (p. 156) can prevent such nausea and vomiting. Electrolyte disturbances may also occur, including hypercalcaemia, and hyperuricaemia may follow the breakdown of nuclear proteins (see allopurinol, p. 210). Almost all cytotoxic drugs may cause a loss of hair. Such alopecia is usually reversible when the chemotherapy is withdrawn, but it may have a highly undesirable effect on body image and morale.

Cytotoxic drugs are, by their nature, extremely toxic to embryonic tissues, and should not be used during pregnancy.

Handling cytotoxic drugs

Cytotoxic agents are toxic agents, and so should always be handled with great care. Some, especially the alkylating agents and certain antibiotics, are known to cause contact dermatitis and irritation of the skin and mucous membranes. That should be taken as a general warning, as it is *not repeated* when referring to individual drugs. Commonsense precautions should always be taken during the preparation and administration of cytotoxic drugs, including using protective clothing. Contact or spillage should be dealt with by immediate washing and dilution with water if it occurs. For detailed guidance, the Report on Guidelines for the handling of cytotoxic drugs should be consulted: *Pharmaceutical Journal*, 1983, **233**: 230.

Great care must also be taken to avoid extravasation or leakage during intravenous injection, as severe local damage may occur. Extravasation can largely be avoided by a good injection technique, and careful choice of injection site with an adequate venous blood flow. A further injection of 10 ml or so of saline should be made after the drug has been injected. During an intravenous injection, the patient should be asked repeatedly about any discomfort or pain at the injection site.

If extravasation occurs or is suspected, the injection should be stopped immediately, but the needle or cannula should not be withdrawn, but used to remove as much of the injection fluid as possible. It may be advisable to inject some normal saline to reduce the concentration of the drug in the perivenous tissues.

Folinic acid may be injected in cases of methotrexate extravasation, sodium bicarbonate injection 8.4% may be of value in extravasation caused by doxorubicin, epirubicin and mustine, and the use of

---

Nursing points about cytotoxic drugs

(a) Four main types: alkylating agents, antimetabolites, cytotoxic antibiotics and vinca alkaloids.
(b) All (except bleomycin and vincristine) depress bone marrow activity, and regular blood counts are necessary.
(c) Severe nausea and vomiting are common side-effects.
(d) Nurses should refer to individual drugs and dosage schemes when advising patients about the side-effects of anticancer drugs, particularly about temporary hair loss.
(e) Many are skin irritants; care must be taken to avoid contact with cytotoxic drugs or solutions.

---

hyaluronidase has been suggested following the extravasation of the vinca alkaloids.

ALKYLATING AGENTS

The alkylating agents are a varied group of chemical substances which are non-specific, as they exert their lethal effects throughout the cell cycle. They readily form covalent bonds and react with bases in DNA, replacing hydrogen atoms with alkyl groups. This serves to cross-link or fragment the two strands of the double helix, so inhibiting RNA (ribonucleic acid), DNA and protein synthesis. As alkylating agents damage tumour cells regardless of whether the cell is actively dividing, they are more effective against slow-growing tumours. As this effect is not dissimilar from that induced by radiation, these drugs are sometimes called radiomimetics.

Busulphan §

Brand name: Myleran §
Busulphan is orally active, and has a selective depressive action on the bone marrow. It is used mainly in the treatment of chronic myeloid leukaemia, particularly in those patients who have become resistant to other forms of treatment.

Busulphan brings about a marked reduction in the excessive number of immature white cells, an increase in the haemoglobin level, and subjective improvement. It is given orally in doses of 2–4 mg daily initially, with maintenance doses of 0.5–2 mg daily. Close haematological control is essential at all times, as marked myelosuppression may occur, with loss of bone marrow function. Hyperpigmentation may occur in some patients.

Carmustine §

Brand name: BiCNU §
Carmustine is related to mustine, and is used as secondary therapy in Hodgkin's disease in combination with other drugs. It is also of value in multiple myeloma and some brain tumours. The dose is based on skin area, and an initial dose is 200 mg/m² by slow intravenous injection every 6 weeks. Rapid infusion may cause an intensive but transient flushing of the skin and conjunctiva. Subsequent doses depend on the haematological response.

Side-effects include nausea and vomiting, often dose-related, but the most severe side-effects are delayed myelosuppression and pulmonary toxicity.

Chlorambucil §

Brand name: Leukeran §
Chlorambucil is an orally active alkylating agent, used in chronic lymphocytic leukaemia, in the long-term treatment of Hodgkin's disease and various malignant lymphomas, as well as in combined therapy. The dose is 100–200 micrograms/kg daily for 6 weeks unless remission occurs earlier. Further suppressive treatment with lower doses of 100 micrograms/kg may be given daily, but a rest period is usually necessary between courses.

Side-effects Nausea, gastro-intestinal disturbances and severe rash may occur; the depression of the bone marrow is less severe than that of related drugs.

Cyclophosphamide §

Brand name: Endoxana §
Cyclophosphamide can be regarded as a pro-drug; following administration it is broken down by microsomal enzymes to release the active drug. Cyclophosphamide is used in the treatment of Hodgkin's disease, lymphosarcoma, carcinoma of the breast, lung and ovary, and in various leukaemias. It also has marked immunosuppressant properties.

Cyclophosphamide may be given orally, by slow intravenous injection or fast-running intravenous infusion, commencing with a daily dose of 100–300 mg with similar maintenance doses according to response.

Side-effects of cyclophosphamide are numerous and include nausea and haemorrhagic cystitis. The cystitis, which may be severe, is due to a locally toxic metabolite (acrolein), and can be reduced to some extent by a high fluid intake. It can be further controlled by the intravenous use of mesna (Uromitexan §), given at the same time as cyclophosphamide, as it reacts with the acrolein and reduces its urothelial toxicity. Further treatment may be given orally. The dose of mesna is based on the dose of the cytotoxic agent.

Estramustine §

Brand name: Estracyt §

Estramustine represents a combination of mustine with oestradiol but has an antimitotic action similar to that of the vinca alkaloids (p. 221). Following oral administration, it is concentrated in prostatic tissues and is used in the treatment of prostatic carcinoma. The initial dose is 560 mg daily between meals, followed by maintenance doses of 140 mg once or twice a day. It should not be taken with milk products.

Side-effects include nausea, angina and occasional gynaecomastia. Peptic ulcer, severe liver and cardiac disease are contra-indications.

Ifosfamide §

Brand name: Mitoxana §

Ifosfamide is a derivative of cyclophosphamide, with similar actions, uses and side-effects. It is given by intravenous infusion in total doses of $8–10 \, g/m^2$ in divided doses over 5 days. Ifosfamide may cause a dose-limiting haemorrhagic cystitis, and a high urinary output together with mesna given intravenously are essential. See p. 216.

Side-effects include nausea, renal damage and alopecia. Central nervous system toxicity may result in confusion and lethargy, which decline as therapy is withdrawn.

Lomustine §

Brand name: CCNU §

Lomustine is used in the treatment of brain and lung tumours, Hodgkin's disease and malignant melanoma. The dose based on skin area is $120–130 \, mg/m^2$ as a single oral dose every 6–8 weeks.

Side-effects include nausea and vomiting, followed by anorexia. The onset of bone marrow depression may be slow and its duration prolonged, and it may become irreversible after extended treatment.

Melphalan §

Brand name: Alkeran §

Melphalan represents a combination of mustine with an amino acid and the compound has the general cytotoxic properties of the nitrogen mustard group

and similar **side-effects**. It is used mainly in the treatment of myeloma, a condition characterized by an excessive formation of plasma cells by the bone marrow, which may erode bone and bring about skeletal changes. Melphalan suppresses such proliferation by a general depression of bone marrow activity, but repeated courses of treatment may be necessary to obtain the maximum response. It is given orally in doses of 150 micrograms/kg or more daily for 4–6 days, together with prednisone 40 mg daily, repeated at intervals of 6 weeks. It is also given intravenously in doses of $40 \, mg/m^2$.

Melphalan is also used by the regional perfusion technique in the treatment of localized malignant melanoma. By this method a large dose of the drug may be circulated through the tumour.

Mustine §

Mustine, once known as nitrogen mustard, was one of the first alkylating agents but is now little used. It has been given by a fast-running intravenous infusion in a dose of 400 mg/kg. It is highly irritant, and great care must be taken to avoid escape of the injection into the perivenous tissues or skin.

Thiotepa §

Thiotepa is used in the treatment of mammary and ovarian cancer, for superficial cancers of the bladder and to control pleural effusions. It has also been used by intrathecal injection in the control of malignant meningeal disease.

Thiotepa is less irritant than mustine, and may be given by intramuscular injection in divided doses of 15–30 mg three times a week for 2 weeks. A rest period of 6–8 weeks should elapse before a second course is given to allow the bone marrow activity to recover. For bladder instillation, a dose of 60 mg dissolved in 60 ml of water is used, and the solution should be retained for 2 hours.

For malignant pleural effusions, thiotepa has been given in doses of 10–60 mg by instillation at weekly intervals.

Side-effects are those common to most alkylating agents.

Treosulfan §

Treosulfan is used in the treatment of ovarian carcinoma, often to supplement surgery. It is given in oral doses of 250 mg four times a day for 1 month, followed by a similar rest period before therapy is resumed. **Side-effects** include nausea and vomiting, and alopecia may occur. Excessive doses may cause irreversible bone marrow depression.

ANTIMETABOLITES

The antimetabolites mimic the action of natural substances used for the synthesis of DNA. Most of this class are structural analogues of the purine and pyrimidine bases (adenine, guanine, cytosine and thymine) and either are substituted into DNA to produce a non-functional molecule, or else they inhibit the synthesis of DNA. Methotrexate is the exception in that it prevents cells from converting folic acid, which is required for DNA synthesis, from an inactive to an active form. They are phase-specific agents and are most active during the S-phase.

Cytarabine

Brand name: Cytosar §
Cytarabine, also known as cytosine arabinoside, interrupts cell replication by interfering with the synthesis of pyrimidine and inhibiting the action of DNA polymerase. It is used in acute myeloblastic leukaemia and other leukaemias in children and adults. By the nature of its action, it is a powerful depressant of bone marrow function and haematological control during treatment is essential.

Cytarabine is used in initial doses of 2–6 mg/kg daily for 7–10 days, given by intravenous injection, and subsequent doses are adjusted according to response. Intermittent therapy has also been used. Children tend to tolerate higher doses. Remission, once achieved, can be maintained by doses of 1–3 mg/kg given once weekly by subcutaneous or intramuscular injection. As with many other cytotoxic drugs, cytarabine may induce severe hyperuricaemia following the destruction of the nuclei of the neoplastic cells.

Fludarabine §

Brand name: Fludara §
Fludarabine is a fluorinated cytotoxic agent used in chronic lymphocytic leukaemia after other treatment has failed. Dose by intravenous infusion 25 mg/m^2 for 5 days a month.

Fluorouracil §

Fluorouracil inhibits cell division by blocking the enzyme synthesis of DNA. It is used mainly in the palliative treatment of breast and colorectal carcinoma, often in association with other drugs. It may be given orally in maintenance doses of 15 mg/kg weekly, or by intravenous injection and infusion. The dose is highly individual, but the total daily dose should not exceed 1 g. It is also used as a 5% cream (Efudix §) for superfical malignant skin lesions.

Side-effects include nausea, gastro-intestinal disturbance, leucopenia and thrombocytopenia and haemorrhage. Stomatitis requires immediate withdrawal of the drug.

Gemcitabine § ▼

Brand name: Gemzar § ▼
Gemcitabine is related to cytarabine, but is used in the treatment òf non-small cell lung cancer. It acts against several enzymes involved in DNA synthesis as well as inhibiting DNA repair mechanisms. Dose 1000 mg/m^2 by intravenous infusion once weekly for 3 weeks, repeated after a rest period of 1 week.

Side-effects include rash and transient flu-like symptoms.

Mercaptopurine §

Brand name: Puri-Nethol §
Mercaptopurine is related to adenine, a constituent of nucleic acid, and acts by interfering with the synthesis of nucleic acid and the development of the cancer cells. It has a valuable suppressive action in acute leukaemia and some cases of chronic myeloid leukaemia, particularly in children, but it is of no value in other malignant conditions.

Mercaptopurine is given orally in doses of 2.5 mg/kg daily, and there may be a time-lag of 3 weeks before any effect can be detected. It produces a remission of the disease of varying duration, but the response to a second course of treatment may be less satisfactory.

Side-effects include liver damage and hyperuricaemia. The dose should be reduced in patients receiving allopurinol as otherwise interference with the metabolism of mercaptopurine may occur.

Methotrexate §

Brand name: Matrex §
Methotrexate inhibits the dihydrofolate reductase enzyme system of folic acid, and pyrimidine synthesis, and so blocks further cell development. Methotrexate is used in the treatment of a variety of

neoplastic conditions, often as part of a multiple therapy scheme. Dosage varies accordingly.

It is given for maintenance therapy in acute lymphoblastic leukaemia in doses of 15–30 mg/m^2 once or twice weekly, orally or by intramuscular injection. More intensive treatment with higher doses has been used in the treatment of various lymphomas, but in association with folinic acid, a scheme referred to as Folinic Acid Rescue. Folinic acid (Leucovorin; Refolinon) suppresses some of the **side-effects** of methotrexate, particularly myelosuppression and mucositis, and treatment should be started 8–24 hours after beginning methotrexate therapy. It is given in divided doses up to a total of 120 mg over 24 hours by intramuscular or intravenous injection, followed by doses of 15 mg orally or by intramuscular injection 6-hourly for 48–72 hours. Blood counts, renal and liver function tests are essential during methotrexate therapy. Treatment with NSAIDs should be avoided, as they decrease the excretion of methotrexate and so increase its toxic effects. The use of methotrexate in rheumatoid arthritis is referred to on p. 209, and in psoriasis on p. 261.

Pentostatin § ▼

Brand name: Nipent § ▼
Pentostatin is an inhibitor of adenosine deaminase, an enzyme that is involved in the production of purines necessary for cell proliferation. It is used in hairy cell leukaemia in doses of 4 mg/m^2 by intravenous infusion under specialist supervision, with monitoring of the blood count.

Raltitrexed § ▼

Brand name: Tomudex § ▼
Raltitrexed is a specific inhibitor of thymidylate synthetase, a key enzyme in the formation of thymidine triphosphate, a nucleotide essential for DNA synthesis. It is used in the palliative treatment of colorectal cancer as an alternative to fluorouracil. Dose 3 mg/m^2 by intravenous infusion, repeated after 3 weeks.

Side-effects are gastro-intestinal disturbances, leucopenia, asthenia and fever.

Thioguanine §

Brand name: Lanvis §
Thioguanine has an action similar to that of mercaptopurine although its main use is in the treatment of

acute myeloid leukaemia and chronic granulocytic leukaemia. It is given in doses of 2–2.5 mg/kg daily for 5–20 days, followed by maintenance doses of 2 mg/kg daily according to response. Thioguanine is a powerful myelosuppressive drug, and close haemotological control is essential.

Cladribine § ▼

Brand name: Leustat § ▼
Cladribine is an antimetabolite used in hairy cell leukaemia. It is given as a single course of treatment in doses of 0.09 mg/kg daily for 7 days. **Side-effects** are numerous and myelosuppression may be severe.

CYTOTOXIC ANTIBIOTICS

Cytotoxic antibiotics (isolated from soil fungi) act by binding with DNA and so inhibiting further DNA and RNA synthesis. Some may act by inhibiting DNA-gyrase (topoisomerase II), the enzyme controlling the supercoiling of the long strands of DNA, as the activity of DNA-gyrase is markedly increased in proliferating cells. Some cytotoxic antibiotics also have radiomimetic properties, so combined radiotherapy should be avoided. The **side-effects** of cytotoxic antibiotics are similar to those of other anticancer drugs.

Aclarubicin §

Brand name: Aclacin §
Aclarubicin is an anthracycline antibiotic. It differs from doxorubicin in being less cardiotoxic, possibly because it is eliminated more rapidly. It is also less likely to cause alopecia. Aclarubicin is used mainly in relapsed acute non-lymphatic leukaemia (ANLL) and in patients resistant to other therapy, and is given in doses of 175–300 mg/m^2 by intravenous infusion over a period of 3–7 days. Maintenance doses of 25–100 mg/m^2 are given at intervals of 3–4 weeks according to the haematological response.

The cardiac efficiency should be monitored by ECG during treatment. Care is necessary as it is a tissue irritant.

Side-effects are nausea and vomiting, but leucopenia and thrombocytopenia may be dose-limiting.

Actinomycin D §

Brand name: Cosmegen §
Actinomycin D, also known as dactinomycin, is used mainly in the treatment of Wilm's tumour and

rhabdomyosarcoma. The standard adult dose is 500 micrograms by intravenous injection daily for 5 days. A second course may be given after an interval of 4 weeks. For children, doses of 15 micrograms/kg daily for 5 days have been given; alternatively a dose of 400–600 micrograms/m² body surface area may be injected daily for up to 5 days.

Actinomycin D is very irritant to the soft tissues and great care must be taken to avoid extravasation.

Side-effects, which may not be noted until a few days after a course of injections has stopped, include gastro-intestinal disturbances, general malaise, severe bone marrow depression, skin eruptions and stomatitis.

Bleomycin §

Bleomycin differs from other antibiotics as it is taken up selectively by certain tissues, particularly the skin, and is mainly used in the treatment of squamous cell skin cancers. It is also useful in Hodgkin's disease and other lymphomas, in chorio-carcinomas, mycosis fungoides and malignant effusions. It has the great advantage of not causing any significant depression of bone marrow activity, so the blood picture is not disturbed.

Bleomycin may be given by intramuscular or intravenous injection, and doses of 15–30 mg twice weekly have been used. Remissions in Hodgkin's disease have been maintained with weekly doses of 5 mg. In malignant effusions, a solution of 60 mg in 100 ml of saline is instilled after drainage.

The most serious **side-effect** is an occasional delayed progressive pulmonary fibrosis often associated with a total dose greater than 300 mg. Other side-effects include increased pigmentation of the skin and mucositis. Chill and fever and other hypersensitivity reactions may occur within a few hours.

Dactinomycin (*See Actinomycin D*)

Daunorubicin §

Brand name: Cerubidin §
Daunorubicin resembles doxorubicin, and is used mainly in acute myelogenous and lymphatic leukaemia. It is irritant, so is given by intravenous infusion in doses of 40–60 mg/m²; three doses on alternate days. A less irritant liposome formulation is DaunoXome §.

Doxorubicin §

Doxorubicin has wide applications in the treatment of neoplastic conditions, and it has been used with success in acute leukaemia, lymphomas, soft tissue and osteogenic neoplasms, and in breast and lung carcinomas. It may be used alone, or as part of a multiple drug regimen.

The dose of doxorubicin, given by a free-running intravenous infusion, is 60–75 mg/m² of body surface area, repeated at intervals of 3 weeks up to a total dose of not more than 500 mg/m². It has also been used for the treatment of papillary tumours of the bladder by the instillation of 100 ml of a solution containing 50 mg doxorubicin.

Side-effects are vomiting, buccal ulceration, myelodepression, tachycardia and alopecia, but the most serious side-effect, especially with higher doses, is cardiac myopathy that can lead to irreversible heart failure. Treatment should be carried out under ECG monitoring. Doxorubicin is largely excreted in the bile, and a raised bilirubin level indicates that dosage should be reduced. Epirubicin (Pharmorubicin §) is an analogue said to be less cardiotoxic.

Idarubicin §

Brand name: Zavedos §
Idarubicin has the action and uses of aclarubicin, and in ANLL it is given in doses of 30 mg/m² orally 3 days a week. It is also given by intravenous infusion in doses of 12 mg/m² daily for 3 days.

Mitomycin §

Mitomycin has a wide range of activity, but is used mainly in breast and upper gastro-intestinal cancer. It is given in doses of 10–20 mg/m² as a single dose by a fast-running intravenous infusion, repeated after 6–8 weeks. It has also been given in divided doses of 2 mg/m² daily for 5 days, repeated after a 2-day interval. Later doses are given when the leucocyte and platelet counts have returned to an acceptable level, as prolonged use may cause irreversible bone marrow damage. Mitomycin has also been used in bladder cancer by the instillation of a solution containing 10–40 mg. The **side-effects** include lung fibrosis, myelosuppression and renal damage.

Amsacrine §

Brand name: Amsidine §
Amsacrine is a synthetic drug, and is included here as it has an action similar to that of doxorubicin. It is used mainly in acute myeloid leukaemia, and is given by intravenous infusion as a solution

in 5% glucose, in doses of 90 mg/m^2 daily for 5 days, repeated at intervals of 2–3 weeks according to the response. Maintenance doses are about one-third of those needed to induce remission, and are given at intervals of 2–3 weeks, based on the blood count.

Side-effects are myelodepression, gastro-intestinal disturbances, mucositis and occasional epileptiform episodes. Amsacrine may cause hypokalaemia and cardiac irregularities, and monitoring of electrolytes may be necessary.

VINCA ALKALOIDS AND OTHER PLANT PRODUCTS

The vinca alkaloids, obtained from periwinkle, are antimitotics and inhibit cell division by binding to tubulin, inhibiting microtubule assembly, preventing spindle formation during mitosis, and arresting cell division at the metaphase. They are irritant substances, and should be handled with great care. Contact with the eyes may be severely irritant. They should never be given by intrathecal injection, as such use has resulted in fatal neurological damage.

Vincristine §

Brand name: Oncovin §
Vincristine is of importance in the management of acute leukaemias, malignant lymphomas, Wilm's tumour and rhabdomycosarcoma. It is given by intravenous injection at weekly intervals in doses of 50–150 micrograms/kg in children, but in adults a weekly dose of 25–75 micrograms/kg has been given. Doses must be adjusted to individual need and response to avoid toxicity.

Vincristine is exceptional in causing very little myelodepression, but neuromuscular damage may occur, with peripheral paraesthesia, which may be dose limiting and from which recovery is slow. Other **side-effects** include gastro-intestinal disturbances, constipation, weight loss, polyuria and alopecia.

Vinblastine §

Brand name: Velbe §
Vinblastine has the actions and uses of vincristine, but is used mainly in the treatment of generalized Hodgkin's disease and lymphosarcoma. It is given by intravenous injection as an initial dose of 100 micrograms/kg, increasing at weekly intervals

according to response up to a maximum dose of 500 micrograms/kg.

Vinblastine is less likely to cause neurotoxicity, but the bone marrow depression may be greater than with vincristine and close haematological control is essential.

Vindesine §

Brand name: Eldisine §
Vindesine has the general properties of the vinca alkaloids, and is used mainly in acute lymphoblastic leukaemia in children, particularly that resistant to other cytotoxic agents.

Vindesine is given by intravenous injection in initial doses of 3 mg/m^2, increased at weekly intervals by increments of 0.5 mg/m^2 up to 4–5 mg/m^2, adjusted at all times according to granulocyte and platelet counts.

Side-effects are similar to those of the other vinca alkaloids.

Vinorelbine § ▼

Brand name: Navelbine § ▼
Vinorelbine is a new semisynthetic vinca alkaloid used mainly in non-small cell lung cancer (NSCLC) and in relapsed or resistant advanced breast cancer. It is given in doses of 25–30 mg/m^2 weekly by intravenous infusion, after which the vein should be flushed with normal saline infusion.

The **side-effects** are those of the vinca alkaloids, but neutropenia may be severe, and close haematological control is necessary.

ASSOCIATED CYTOTOXIC DRUGS
Etoposide §

Brand name: Vepesid §
Etoposide is a semisynthetic derivative of the plant substance podophyllotoxin and inhibits DNA synthesis at the late S and G$_2$ phases. It is used in the treatment of lymphomas, small-cell carcinoma of the bronchi, and in some testicular carcinomas, sometimes in association with other cytotoxic drugs. Etoposide may be given initially by intravenous infusion in doses of 60–120 mg/m^2 daily for 5 days, repeated at intervals of 21 days. The oral dose is double that given by injection.

The drug is irritant, and care must be taken to avoid extravasation. **Side-effects** are myelodepression, nausea, vomiting and alopecia.

Taxanes

The taxanes are a small group of cytotoxic agents, of which the first was paclitaxel, obtained from the bark of the Pacific Yew. Some semisynthetic derivatives are also available. Like the vinca alkaloids, they are antimitotics, and are mainly used by specialists in the treatment of resistant cancers, often when platinum therapy has failed. They are toxic substances, and severe hypersensitivity is a frequent reaction. Careful premedication with a corticosteroid, together with an antihistamine and an H_2-receptor antagonist is essential. Docetaxol § (Taxere §) is used in resistant breast cancer, paclitaxel § (Taxol §) is given in ovarian and breast cancer. For details of dose, specialist literature should be consulted.

HORMONES, HORMONE ANTAGONISTS AND OTHER CYTOTOXIC DRUGS

Aminoglutethimide §

Brand name: Orimeten §
Aminoglutethimide is an enzyme inhibitor and blocks the production of steroids by the adrenal cortex. It also inhibits the conversion of androgens to oestrogens in the peripheral tissues. As an adrenal antagonist it is used in the treatment of post-menopausal metastatic breast cancer in doses of 250 mg twice daily for 1 week, later increased to four times a day. It is also used in advanced prostatic carcinoma. Much larger doses are given in Cushing's syndrome associated with malignancy. Because of its general inhibitory action on the adrenal cortex, it is essential to give supportive corticosteroid therapy during aminoglutethimide therapy.

Side-effects include drowsiness, drug fever and skin reactions. Aminoglutethimide has an enzyme induction effect on the liver, and the doses of some other drugs such as the oral anticoagulants may have to be increased.

Anastrozole § ▼

Brand name: Armidex § ▼
Anastrozole is a specific inhibitor of aromatase, the enzyme concerned in the conversion of androgens to oestrogens. It causes a drug-induced oestrogen deficiency and is used like aminoglutethimide in advanced breast cancer in postmenopausal women.

Side-effects are drowsiness, flushing and vaginal dryness.

Trilostane §

Brand name: Modrenal §
Trilostane resembles aminoglutethimide in being an adrenal antagonist, and in post-menopausal breast cancer it is given in doses of 240 mg daily, slowly increased up to a maximum of 240 mg four times a day.

Side-effects are diarrhoea and abdominal discomfort.

The use of trilostane in the treatment of Cushing's syndrome is referred to on p. 182.

Buserelin §

Brand name: Suprefact §
Buserelin is a synthetic analogue of gonadorelin, the gonadotrophin-releasing hormone of the hypothalamus (see p. 183). It is used in the treatment of metastatic prostatic carcinoma on the basis that it initially stimulates the release of the luteinizing hormone, and that stimulation results in a temporary increase in testosterone secretion by the testes. Following that initial stimulation, a secondary inhibition of luteinizing hormone occurs, with a subsequent inhibition of testosterone secretion, and relief of symptoms.

Buserelin is given initially by subcutaneous injection in doses of 500 micrograms 8-hourly for 7 days, after which doses of 100 micrograms are given by intranasal spray up to six times a day. It is also used in the treatment of endometriosis (p. 172).

A **side-effect** of buserelin is a temporary increase of tumour growth during the first 2–3 weeks of treatment, which may have the undesirable effect of causing pain and spinal cord compression (p. 172).

Cisplatin §

Cisplatin has an exceptional chemical structure, as it contains platinum bound up in an organic complex. It appears to have an action similar to that of the alkylating agents, and is used mainly in metastatic ovarian and testicular tumours, often as secondary therapy in association with other cytotoxic drugs in resistant conditions. It is given by intravenous injection in doses of 50–120 mg/m^2 every 3 or 4 weeks.

Side-effects include severe nausea and vomiting, ototoxicity, nephrotoxicity and myelosuppression.

Carboplatin (Paraplatin §) is a derivative of cisplatin, with which **side-effects** such as nausea and vomiting are less severe; the ototoxic and nephrotoxic effects are also reduced.

Crisantaspase §

Brand name: Erwinase §

Some malignant cells are unable to synthesize asparagine, and so utilize exogenous sources of that essential amino acid. The development of such cells can be prevented by crisantaspase, which is an enzyme that breaks down asparagine, and hinders further cell growth. It is used mainly to induce remission of acute lymphoblastic leukaemia in children, after pre-treatment with vincristine and prednisolone. It is given in doses of 200 units/kg by slow intravenous injection at intervals controlled by need and response.

Side-effects include anaphylactic reactions and hyperglycaemia, and skin tests for sensitivity with 2-unit doses should be carried out before treatment, and before re-treatment after an interval.

Cyproterone §

Brand name: Cyprostat §

Cyproterone blocks androgen receptors, and so has an anti-androgen action. It also has some direct inhibitory action on the production of testicular androgens. Cyproterone is used for the symptomatic treatment of metastatic prostatic carcinoma, often in association with other drugs such as buserelin. Dose 100 mg three times a day after food. Care is necessary in hepatic disease. Hepatotoxicity is a risk with extended treatment.

Flutamide §

Brand name: Drogenil §

Flutamide is an androgen-blocking agent, and inhibits the uptake of androgens by target organs. It is used for the treatment of advanced prostatic carcinoma in patients who have not responded to, or cannot tolerate other forms of anti-androgen therapy. It is usually given in association with a LHRH agonist such as goserelin. Flutamide is given in doses of 250 mg three times a day, preferably 3 days before LHRH therapy is commenced, in order to reduce the initial 'flare' response.

A frequent **side-effect** of flutamide is gynaecomastia, which may occur less often with combined goserelin treatment. Gastro-intestinal disturbances may occur, but liver dysfunction is a risk and periodic hepatic tests should be carried out if treatment is prolonged. An increase in the prothrombin time may occur in patients receiving warfarin, and adjustment of the dose of anticoagulant may be necessary.

Bicalutamide § (Casodex §) has similar actions and side-effects. Dose 50 mg daily.

Formestane §

Brand name: Lentaron §

Formestane, like anastrozole, specifically inhibits aromatase, the enzyme involved in the conversion of androgen to oestrogens. It binds irreversibly with the enzyme and oestrogen production is suspended until new enzyme is biosynthesized. Its cytostatic action is a result of oestrogen deficiency. It is used in advanced breast cancer in postmenopausal women, and is given in doses of 250 mg by deep intragluteal injection at intervals of 2 weeks.

Side-effects include flushes, rash, pruritus, pain and irritation at the injection site (which should be varied). Headache, dizziness and vaginal bleeding may also occur. Letrozole § ▼ (Femara §) has similar actions and side-effects. It is given in advanced postmenopausal cancer resistant to other anti-androgen treatment. Dose 2.5 mg daily.

Goserelin §

Brand name: Zoladex §

Goserelin is a synthetic analogue of gonadorelin (LHRH), the gonadotrophin-releasing hormone of the hypothalamus, and like buserelin, it is used in the treatment of prostatic carcinoma. Goserelin is given in a dose of 3.6 mg by the subcutaneous injection of an implant product from which the drug is slowly released at a rate that permits subsequent injections at intervals of 4 weeks.

Goserelin is used in similar doses for the treatment of advanced breast cancer in premenopausal women, as it inhibits oestrogen production by depression of LH secretion. Similar doses are given in endometriosis (p. 172).

Like buserelin, goserelin causes an initial rise in the plasma testosterone level, which may be associated with some increase in bone pain. Other **side-effects** are hot flushes and rash, but these are usually mild and transient. Triptorelin § ▼ (Decapeptyl sr §) has a similar action and use in prostatic carcinoma. Dose 4.2 mg by intramuscular injection every 28 days.

Leuprorelin § (dose: 3.75 mg monthly)

Brand name: Prostap SR §

Leuprorelin is a potent analogue of the gonadotrophic releasing hormones (GnRH) of the pituitary gland, which is ultimately concerned with the production of androgens (p. 182) and is used in the treatment of advanced prostatic cancer. Many such cancers are androgen-dependent, and medical treatment is with oestrogens that depress androgen activity. Oestrogen therapy has some undesirable side-effects, but a similar action can be achieved paradoxically by depressing GnRH activity with large doses of that hormone as leuprorelin. The initial effect of leuprorelin is to bring about a temporary rise in plasma testosterone and dihydrotestosterone levels, which causes an exacerbation of symptoms (the 'flare' effect), but the sustained action of the drug inhibits subsequent testosterone production which results in a chemical castration. In prostatic cancer, treatment with leuprorelin brings about symptomatic relief, a reduction in bone pain, and in many cases a regression of the cancer. Prostap SR is a sustained release product of leuprorelin, and is given as a dose of 3.75 mg by subcutaneous or intramuscular injection every 4 weeks. patients should be warned about the 'flare' effect, which can be reduced by giving an anti-androgen before and during the first 2–3 weeks of treatment. Other **side-effects** are sweating, flushing, impotence, oedema and fatigue.

OESTROGENS, PROGESTOGENS AND ANDROGENS

These have a selective action against some types of cancer, and are considered here as a group. Their other actions are referred to in Chapter 13.

Oestrogens

Oestrogens inhibit indirectly the production of androgens, and on that account they have been used in the treatment of prostatic cancer. Ethinyloestradiol is the main oestrogen in current use, and is given in doses of 3 mg daily, although other drugs are usually preferred. Polyestradiol § (Estradurin §) is given in prostatic cancer in doses of 80–160 mg monthly by deep intramuscular injection.

Fosfestrol § (dose: 120–360 mg daily)

Brand name: Honvan §
Fosfestrol is a pro-drug, but when activated in tissues rich in acid phosphatase, such as the prostate gland, stilboestrol is liberated locally, and systemic effects are correspondingly reduced. In prostatic cancer fosfestrol is given by slow intravenous injection in doses of 600–1200 mg daily for at least 5 days, with

maintenance doses of 300 mg up to four times a week. Oral maintenance doses are 240 mg three times a day for 7 days, slowly reduced to 120–360 mg daily.

Side-effects are nausea, fluid retention and thrombosis. Stilboestrol, the parent drug, is used less frequently because of its systemic side-effects, which include impotence and gynaecomastia.

Progestogens

Progestogens are alternative drugs used in breast cancer. They are generally well tolerated, but may cause nausea, fluid retention and weight gain.

Gestronol § (dose: 200–400 mg by injection)

Brand name: Depostat §
Gestronol is used in endometrial cancer in doses of 200–400 mg weekly by intramuscular injection. Dose in benign prostatic hypertrophy is 200–400 mg weekly.

Medroxyprogesterone § (dose: 100–500 mg daily)

Brand names: Farlutal §, Provera §
Medroxyprogesterone is used in endometrial, prostatic and renal cancer in doses of 100–500 mg daily orally, or 250 mg–1 g weekly by deep intramuscular injection. In breast cancer doses up to 1 g are given.

Megestrol § (dose: 40–320 mg daily)

Brand name: Megace §
Megestrol has the actions and uses of other progestogens. In breast cancer it is given in doses of 160 mg daily; in endometrial cancer 40–320 mg daily. Treatment should be continued for some weeks to assess the response.

Procarbazine §

Brand name: Natulan §
Procarbazine is used mainly as part of a multi-drug treatment of Hodgkin's disease and other lymphomas. It is given orally in doses of 50 mg initially, rising by 50 mg daily up to 300 mg daily in divided doses. Maintenance doses of 50–150 mg daily may then be given up to a total dose of at least 6 g. Regular blood counts are essential during procarbazine therapy. The mode of action is not yet known.

Side-effects are myelodepression, nausea and loss of appetite. The development of an allergic skin reaction is an indication for withdrawal of the drug. The taking of alcohol may cause a disulfiram like reaction (p. 10).

Tamoxifen §

Brand names: Nolvadex §, Tamofen §

Tamoxifen is a synthetic oestrogen antagonist, and acts as a cytotoxic agent by blocking receptor sites in oestrogen-dependent tumours. It is now regarded as a first-line drug in the treatment of all stages of breast cancer, and is given in doses of 10 mg twice a day, subsequently increased as required up to 20 mg twice a day. It was first used only in post-menopausal women with metastases, but it is now in use for premenopausal women with breast cancer. It may delay the development of metastases and prolong survival.

Side-effects are hot flushes, dizziness, vaginal bleeding and gastro-intestinal disturbances. Menstrual abnormalities occur with premenopausal patients. The drug may also cause some hypercalcaemia at the initial stages of treatment, especially when metastases are present. An increase in bone pain may precede the initial response, and nurses can help by encouraging patients to continue treatment. Tamoxifen markedly increases the activity of warfarin and related anticoagulants, and close control is necessary when tamoxifen is given to or withdrawn from patients receiving oral anticoagulants.

Toremifene § ▼ (Fareston §) has similar actions and uses, and is given in hormone-dependent post-menopausal breast cancer in doses of 60 mg daily. It may cause menstrual and endometrial changes that should be investigated.

Other cytotoxic drugs used less frequently include dacarbazine § (DTIC), hydroxyurea § (Hydrea §) and mitozantrone § (Novantrone §). The use of oestrogens in prostatic carcinoma is referred to briefly on p. 224.

IMMUNOSTIMULANTS (CYTOKINES)

Cytokines are peptides formed mainly in macrophages. They are important mediators of many cellular processes and functions, including the regulation of inflammatory and immune reactions. Two important groups are the interferons and the interleukins. Interleukin-2 has a cytotoxic action on certain solid tumours, and a recombinant form is aldesleukin (Proleukin §). It is given by intravenous infusion in metastatic renal cell carcinoma unresponsive to other treatment. It has marked toxic effects, as it causes capillary leakage leading to pulmonary oedema and hypotension. Other toxic effects are myelosuppression and CNS toxicity.

The interferons are glycoproteins, distinguished as interferon alpha and interferon beta, and are formed in response to viral and other stimuli. Recombinant forms of the interferons are now available, and interferon alpha (Intron A §, Roferon-A §, Viraferon § and Wellferon §) is used in chronic myeloid leukaemia, hairy cell leukaemia, as well as in hepatitis. They are being studied as a possible treatment of multiple sclerosis. Dosage schemes are complex, and specialist literature on both the interferons and aldesleukin should be consulted for further information. Immuno-suppressant drugs are referred to in Chapter 23.

RADIOPHARMACEUTICALS

Radioactive compounds have a limited place in the radiotherapy of some tumours, but they are more widely used as tracer compounds for the detection of malignancy. A more recent development is the tagging of monoclonal antibodies with radio-nucleotides. The following notes indicate the range of radiopharmaceuticals now available.

Radioactive materials are all potentially dangerous and great care must be taken in handling them. Care must also be taken with handling the patients' excreta.

Nursing points about radiopharmaceuticals

(a) Keep your distance, as the further you are away from a radiation source the smaller your dose (if you double your distance you half your dose).
(b) Store radioactive isotopes in shielded containers and use lead screens and aprons.
(c) Limit your time near radiation sources so as to lower your radiation dose.
(d) Ensure that radiation signs are visible wherever radioactive sources are in use.
(e) Wear film badges to monitor your own dose of radiation.
(f) Keep pregnant women and children away from where radioisotopes are being used.
(g) Strictly follow hospital regulations for the use and disposal of radioactive substances.
(h) Ensure patients and relatives are educated and reassured regarding the precautions.

Chromium-51

Chromium-51 is used as sodium chromate to label red cells in the circulation so as to measure the glomerular filtration rate and estimate the extent of gastro-intestinal bleeding.

Cobalt-57 and Cobalt-58

The metal cobalt forms part of the structure of vitamin B_{12}, so synthetic vitamin B_{12} containing cobalt-57 (cyanocobalamin 57Co) is used to measure the absorption of cyanocobalamin in the diagnosis of pernicious anaemia. A mixture of 57Co and 58Co is used to differentiate between failure of absorption because of the absence of the intrinsic factor (p. 144) and that due to poor ileal absorption.

Fluorine-18

Fluorine-18 is used in positron-emission tomography in the detection of malignant tumours.

Gallium-67

Gallium-67, as gallium citrate, is taken up and concentrated in some lymphatic tumours, and is used for tumour visualization by scanning techniques.

Gold-198

Gold-198 has been used as a colloidal suspension of metallic particles in the treatment of pleural and other malignant effusions.

Indium-111

Indium-111 as a complex with bleomycin and other substances has been used for tumour scanning, the localization of inflammatory lesions, and investigation of the lymphatic system.

Indium-113

Indium-113 is an isotope with a short half-life. It is used as a complex with mannitol and other substances for the scanning of the lungs and other organs.

Iodine-131

Iodine-131 is used as sodium iodide in the diagnosis of thyroid functions and treatment of thyrotoxicosis. As it is taken up selectively by the gland, large doses are sometimes used in the treatment of thyroid carcinoma. As iodinated serum albumin it is used in the determination of plasma volume.

Iron-59

Iron-59 is used as the ferric citrate in the determination of iron absorption and utilization. The amount absorbed can be measured by whole body radiation tests.

Phosphorus-32

As sodium phosphate, this isotope is taken up by rapidly growing tissues such as the bone marrow. It reduces the production of red cells and has been used in the treatment of polycythaemia vera. It is also used in diagnosis and location of tumours of the eye and brain.

Selenium-75

Selenium-75 as selemethionine is concentrated in the pancreas and parathyroid glands, and is used for the localization of tumours in those organs.

Technetium-99

This isotope is generated from the metal molybdenum. It has a half-life of about 6 hours, can be given in relatively high doses and is widely used. Following intravenous injection of the freshly prepared isotope, localization of tumours of the brain and many other tissues can be easily detected.

Xenon-133

This radioactive gas is used by intravenous injection as a solution in saline. It is rapidly excreted by the lungs, and is used to determine pulmonary function.

Yttrium-90

Yttrium is used as a suspension of colloidal yttrium silicate in the treatment of malignant ascites.

FURTHER READING

Adams L 1993 Managing chemotherapy-induced nausea and vomiting. Professional Nurse 9(2):91–94

Banks C 1991 Alleviating anticipatory vomiting. Nursing Times 87(16):42–43

Barnish L 1995 Tamoxifen: scientific basis, use and nursing implications. British Journal of Nursing 4(1):22–42

Cooley M, Davis L, Abrahm J 1994 Cisplatin: a clinical review. Part I – Current uses of cisplatin and administration guidelines. Cancer Nursing 17(3):173–184

Cooley M, Davis L, Abrahm J 1994 Cisplatin: a clinical review. Part II – Nursing assessment and management of side effects of cisplatin. Cancer Nursing 17(4):283–293

Coombes R C et al 1992 A new treatment for post-menopausal patients with breast cancer. European Journal of Cancer 28:1941–1945

Coukell A J, Spencer C M 1997 Polyethylene glycol-liposomal doxorubicin. Drugs 53(3):520–538

Furr B J A, Jordan V C 1984 The pharmacology and clinical use of tamoxifen. Pharmacology and Therapeutics 25:127–205

Hitchings R et al 1983 Working party report: Guidelines for handling cytotoxic drugs. Pharmaceutical Journal 233:230–231

Holmes S 1996 Making sense of cancer chemotherapy. Nursing Times 92(36):42–43

Jolivet J et al 1983 The pharmacology and clinical uses of methotrexate. New England Journal of Medicine 309:1094–1104

Lobert S 1992 Antimitotics in cancer chemotherapy. Cancer Nursing 15(1):22–33

Malik S, Waxman J 1992 Cytokines and cancer. British Medical Journal 305:265–266

Malpas J S 1993 Oncology. Postgraduate Medical Journal 69:85–94

Nieweg R M B et al 1994 Safe handling of antineoplastic drugs. Cancer Nursing 17(6):501–511

Robinson S 1993 Principles of chemotherapy. European Journal of Cancer Care 2:55–65

Ward U 1995 Biological therapy in the treatment of cancer. British Journal of Nursing 4(15):869–891

17

Allergy, antihistamines and anti-allergic drugs with a prophylactic action

ALLERGY

The immune system is a double-edged weapon, as although it protects against infection, it may occasionally over-react and so cause a hypersensitivity reaction. A common hypersensitivity reaction is the familiar allergic response such as hay fever, which in an extreme form may result in anaphylaxis which is potentially fatal. It is the result of an abnormal antigen–antibody response to a foreign substance, referred to as an allergen, which is usually but not necessarily protein in nature. Some common allergens are pollen, house dust, insect stings and some medicinal substances such as antibiotics. In sensitive individuals the allergen functions as an antigen and stimulates the formation of protective antibodies of the Class E(IgE) type (p. 277) which bind to specific receptors on the mast cells. As a result of re-exposure to the allergen, the antigen cross-bridges the IgE bound to the mast cell, and causes cell-wall breakdown, degradation of the mast-cell granules, and the release of histamine and other spasmogens (Fig. 17.1). The released histamine binds to histamine H_1-receptors on target cells, and brings about a number of physiological responses. In some cases these responses may be localized as erythema and urticaria, but as histamine is a powerful vasodilator and bronchoconstrictor, systemic responses include hypotension, bronchospasm and angioedema. It should be noted that in a few cases mast-cell degranulation may occur without immune system involvement (pseudo-allergy), and a hypersensitivy reaction may occur on the first exposure to the agent. Certain drugs may also act as pseudo-allergens.

Control of allergy

In order to control an allergic response, the chain reaction terminating in that response must be broken

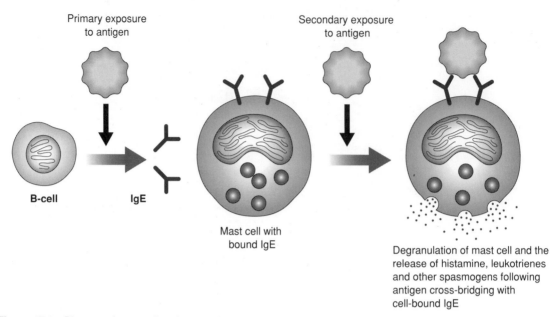

Primary exposure
to antigen

Secondary exposure
to antigen

B-cell

IgE

Mast cell with
bound IgE

Degranulation of mast cell and the
release of histamine, leukotrienes
and other spasmogens following
antigen cross-bridging with
cell-bound IgE

Figure 17.1   Diagram of mast-cell antigen–antibody response.

at some point. In the case of food allergy, avoidance of the food is the easy answer, but in practice may be very difficult. As only minute amounts of an allergen can stimulate an allergic reaction, traces may be present unknown to the consumer in some food products, and the unsuspected exposure to peanut products is an example. In hayfever and similar conditions, reliance is largely placed on symptomatic treatment with antihistamines. Anaphylaxis, on the other hand, is a medical emergency requiring immediate treatment with adrenaline (p. 90).

Occasionally the patient may be desensitized by a course of injections of weak solutions of the offending allergen. In some cases, as in hay fever when due to a clear sensitivity to grass pollens, desensitization with a grass pollen vaccine may be successful. When a number of allergens are involved desensitization is more difficult, and the results are usually less satisfactory. (Pharmalgen § is used for desensitization against bee and wasp stings.)

It is now recommended that desensitizing vaccines should only be used in seasonal allergic hay fever that has not responded to other treatment. Patients with asthma should not be so treated, as they are more susceptible to adverse reactions, the exception being patients hypersensitive to bee and wasp venoms, as reactions to such venoms may sometimes be lifethreatening. Desensitization should only be carried out where facilities for full cardiorespiratory resusci-

tation are immediately available. Anaphylaxis may occur within 30 minutes of the injection of the vaccine, bronchospasm may develop within 1 hour, and patients should be monitored accordingly (see p. 90).

Such immediate and anaphylactic reactions are classified as Type I (Table 17.1). In Type II reactions cell surface antigens stimulate B-lymphocytes to produce G and M class antibodies. These combine with the antigen, and the antigen–antibody complex brings about a subsequent lysis of cells as well as activating phagocytes. Examples of these membrane-reactive reactions are autoimmune thrombocytopenia, haemolytic anaemia and rhesus compatibility of the new-born, as well as the autoimmune haemolytic anaemia sometimes caused by methyldopa. Treatment is with glucocorticoids (p. 178) and immunoglobulins. Although the mechanism of action of the latter is not clear, it involves the suppression of antibody production and phagocyte activity. Human anti-D-immunoglobulin, for example, neutralizes the antibodies produced by rhesus-negative mothers to the fetal rhesus-positive blood cells which leak across the placenta during pregnancy.

In Type III or immune-complex hypersensitivity, the antigen–antibody complexes are formed as usual. These are normally removed rapidly by phagocytosis, but in Type III reactions they are deposited in the capillary beds and cause local inflammation and tissue damage. It occurs in serum sickness, where

Table 17.1 Gell and Coombs classification of hypersensitivity reactions

	Type I	Type II	Type III	Type IV
Other names	Immediate; acute; anaphylactic	Membrane reactive; antibody-mediated; cytotoxic	Immune complex; complex-mediated	Delayed; cell-mediated
Mediator	IgE Triggers mast-cell degranulation and release of chemical mediators	IgG/IgM Membrane bound antigen–antibody complex activates complement and macrophages	IgG/IgM Soluble antigen forms immune complexes and activates complement	T-cell T-cells release cytokines and recruit macrophages and lymphocytes
Timing of response	30 min	1–3 hours	1–3 hours	24–48 hours
Examples	Hay fever, 30% of asthma, urticaria, peanut and latex allergy	Thrombocytopenia, haemolytic anaemia, rhesus and blood transfusion incompatibility	Farmer's lung, infective endocarditis, glomerulonephritis, rheumatoid arthritis, serum sickness	Mantoux test, infective granulomas, granulomatous diseases, contact dermatitis, drug allergy, graft rejection
Drug therapy	Antihistamines, sodium cromoglycate, glucocorticoids, adrenaline	Glucocorticoids, immunoglobulins	Glucocorticoids	Glucocorticoids, immunosuppressants, immunoglobulins

the triggering antigen may be a drug. In Type IV, or delayed hypersensitivity reactions, antibody production is not involved, as the antigen stimulates T-lymphocytes to produce cytokines, a particular type of chemical messenger which attract and activate macrophages and lymphocytes. The macrophages in turn release lysosymes which cause damage and necrosis. Such sensitized cells produce more cytokines, and so the reaction escalates. Type IV reactions are commonly caused by certain micro-organisms such as those causing tuberculosis and leprosy, and form infective granulomas. Such reactions are also linked with graft rejection, contact dermatitis and some drug allergies. Suppression of such cell-mediated hypersensitivity reactions can be achieved with glucocorticoids, with more specific immunosuppressants such as cyclosporin, or some cytotoxic drugs. The use of monoclonal antibodies to human antigens is a new approach to the problem, and may have the advantages of increased selectivity with fewer side-effects.

ANTIHISTAMINES

These drugs are histamine antagonists, and act by binding to H_1-receptor sites, and so block the access of released histamine to the target receptors and inhibit the development of the allergic response.

Their action is therefore palliative and not curative, and treatment must be continued throughout the period of exposure to the offending allergen. (They do not block the action of histamine on gastric acid secretion; p. 148.) Nasal allergies and allergic rhinitis usually respond well to antihistamines, as do urticaria and other allergic skin reactions, drug allergies and insect bites, but they are of no value in asthma. The local use of antihistamines is no longer recommended, as paradoxically they have sometimes caused skin sensitization.

The presence of H_1-receptors in the central nervous system accounts for the main **side-effects** of most antihistamines which are drowsiness, dizziness and lassitude, and may be increased by alcohol. Patients should be warned accordingly about car-driving and other machine-related activities. Anticholinergic effects are dryness of the mouth, blurred vision and gastrointestinal disturbances. Older children usually tolerate antihistamines in suitable doses, but in young children they may have a central stimulant action and cause hyperpyrexia and epileptiform convulsions. Large doses may precipitate convulsions in epileptic patients. There is no antidote for antihistamine poisoning, and overdose may require removal of any unabsorbed drug from the stomach, and an injection of diazepam to control any convulsions.

Some of the newer or second generation antihistamines, such as astemizole and terfenadine, do not pass the blood–brain barrier as easily as the older drugs, and so have a reduced sedative action, but may be of less value in itching atopic eczema. On the other hand, in high doses they may cause ventricular arrhythmias, and the recommended doses should not be exceeded. See p. 233.

Nursing points about hay fever treatment

(a) First-line treatment is with antihistamines.
(b) Drowsiness is a common side-effect of which patients should be warned.
(c) Recommended doses of astemizole and terfenadine should not be exceeded.
(d) Sympathomimetic nasal decongestants are useful; use intermittently to avoid rebound congestion.
(e) Intranasal corticosteroids used prophylactically; useful when pollen count likely to be high and when symptoms not fully controlled by other means.
(f) The local treatment of allergic conjunctivitis is referred to in Chapter 20.

Other actions

Some antihistamines are useful for sedative premedication before surgery; others have anti-emetic properties, and are used in nausea, vomiting and travel sickness (p. 154) as well as in Meniere's disease. The following notes refer to a few individual antihistamines, and Table 17.2 indicates the wide range available.

Fexofenadine (Telfast) § ▼ is a new antihistamine for the symptomatic relief of chronic idiopathic urticaria.

Table 17.2 Antihistamines

Approved name	Brand name	Oral daily range
acrivastine[a]	Semprex	24 mg
astemizole[a]†	Hismanal, Pollon-Eze	10 mg
azatadine	Optimine	2–4 mg
brompheniramine	Dimotane	12–32 mg
cetirizine	Zirteck	10 mg
chlorpheniramine	Piriton	12–16 mg
clemastine	Tavegil	1–2 mg
cyproheptadine	Periactin	4–20 mg
fexofenadine[a]	Telfast	120 mg
loratadine	Clarityn	10 mg
mequitazine	Primalan	5–10 mg
phenindamine	Thephorin	100–200 mg
pheniramine	Daneral SA	75–150 mg
promethazine	Phenergan	25–50 mg
terfenadine[a]†	Triludan	60–120 mg
trimeprazine	Vallergan	30–100 mg

[a]Antihistamines with reduced sedative effects
†Dose not to be exceeded

Promethazine (dose: 25–75 mg daily)

Brand names: Phenergan; Sominex
Promethazine is a long-established antihistamine, widely used in the treatment of hay fever, urticaria, and other allergic conditions in doses of 10–25 mg three times a day. It may also be given as a single dose of 25–50 mg at night, and such a dose may be given when a simple sedative effect is required as in mild insomnia. It is also given by intramuscular or slow intravenous injection in the supportive treatment of anaphylactic emergencies and severe allergies, but great care is necessary to give intravenous injections slowly, and to avoid extravasation, as severe chemical irritation may result.

Promethazine also potentiates the action of some analgesic drugs and it has been given by injection with chlorpromazine and pethidine for pre-anaesthetic medication. The central effects of promethazine are also useful in the auxiliary treatment of parkinsonism.

Acrivastine § (dose: 24 mg daily)

Brand name: Semprex §
Acrivastine does not pass the blood–brain barrier easily, and so has reduced sedative potency. It also has little anticholinergic or antimuscarinic potency, and is less likely to cause dryness of the mouth, blurred vision, drowsiness or other **side-effects**. It is given in doses of 8 mg three times a day, but the onset of action is slow. It may have corresponding value in hay fever when taken for prophylaxis before an attack is anticipated. Acrivastine is not recommended for children under 12 years of age.

Astemizole (dose: 10 mg daily)

Brand name: Hismanal
Astemizole is an antihistamine with reduced sedative side-effects, as its penetration into the central nervous system is poor. It is used for the symptomatic treatment of allergic conditions generally, and is given in daily doses of 10 mg before food. In severe conditions, it may be given initially in single doses of up to 30 mg daily for not more than 7 days, after which the maximum dose of 10 mg daily must not be exceeded, as the drug has a long half-life.

Side-effects High doses may cause cardiotoxic arrhythmias, and combined treatment with macrolide antibiotics, antipsychotics, antidepressants and anti-arrhythmic drugs should also be avoided. See terfenadine, p. 233.

Chlorpheniramine (dose: 12–24 mg daily)

Brand name: Piriton

Chlorpheniramine is effective in doses of 4 mg three or four times a day. Proportionate doses may be given to children from the age of 1–2 years. Chlorpheniramine is the preferred antihistamine for allergic emergencies, and is then given by intramuscular or slow intravenous injection in doses of 10–20 mg after an injection of adrenaline solution (1–1000) in a dose of 0.5–1 ml (see p. 90).

Cyproheptadine (dose: 8–32 mg daily)

Brand name: Periactin

Some allergic conditions may be associated with the release of serotonin as well as histamine. Cyproheptadine has both antihistaminic and antiserotonin properties, and so may be more effective in allergic conditions not responding completely to conventional antihistamines. Dose 4 mg three to four times a day. Similar doses have been given in refractory migraine. Cyproheptadine may cause weight gain, and it has been used as an appetite stimulant.

Phenindamine (dose: 100–150 mg daily)

Brand name: Thephorin

Phenindamine is one of the older antihistamines, but is exceptional in having a mild central stimulant action. It is given in doses of 25–50 mg up to three times a day.

Terfenadine (dose: 120 mg daily)

Brand name: Triludan

Terfenadine has the general properties of the antihistamines, and is used in the symptomatic treatment of allergic conditions, including hay fever and urticaria. It is given in doses of 60 mg twice a day, or as a single morning dose of 120 mg.

Like astemizole, terfenadine is less likely to cause sedation than older antihistamines, and in standard doses it is well tolerated, with few **side-effects**. In high doses, particularly when given with certain other drugs, it may prolong the QT interval with a consequent risk of inducing ventricular arrhythmias. Terfenadine is metabolized in the liver, and hepatic impairment, or use with drugs that inhibit hepatic metabolism, may lead to a rise in the plasma level of terfenadine (as with astemizole) and a similar risk potential. Combined therapy with macrolide antibiotics, anti-arrhythmics, antidepressants, antipsychotics, diuretics and oral antifungal drugs is therefore contra-indicated.

Trimeprazine § (dose: 30–100 mg daily)

Brand name: Vallergan §

Trimeprazine is an antihistamine with sedative properties. It is used in the treatment of pruritus and related conditions in doses of 10 mg three times a day, up to a maximum of 100 mg daily. Trimeprazine is also used as a pre-operative sedative for children in doses of 2–4 mg/kg.

ANTI-ALLERGIC DRUGS WITH A PROPHYLACTIC ACTION

Sodium cromoglycate† § (dose: 20 mg four times a day)

Brand names: Cromogen §, Intal §

In the prophylactic treatment of allergic conditions, particularly asthma and bronchitis, antihistamines are of little value and a drug is required that prevents the release of histamine and other spasmogens, not one that acts as an antagonist at a later stage. A drug of that type is sodium cromoglycate. Although its mode of action is not yet fully understood, it has a stabilizing influence on mast cells, and so prevents their breakdown and in consequence inhibits the release of spasmogens. By the nature of its action it cannot affect the response to released spasmogens, and so is of no value in acute conditions.

Sodium cromoglycate is used prophylactically in the control of allergic asthma, in the prevention of exercise-induced asthma and in the prophylaxis of allergic rhinitis. As it is not absorbed when given orally, it is administered by the inhalation of the powder from a 'spin-inhaler'. Each dose of 20 mg is contained in a capsule, and the dose is released for inhalation as it is placed in the inhaler. It is often used with a 'spacer' device to improve the efficacy of the inhalation. As some patients may experience transient bronchospasm after inhalation of the powder, pre-treatment with an inhalation of salbutamol is often given.

Sodium cromoglycate may also be inhaled from a metered dose aerosol delivering 5 mg per puff in doses of 40–80 mg daily. For the prevention of exercise-induced asthma, sodium cromoglycate is given as a single dose half an hour before the anticipated exercise. All patients should be given full instruction in the proper use of sodium cromoglycate inhalation products if the optimum response is to be obtained, and regular use to maintain prophylaxis is essential.

---

†Sodium cromoglycate is not an antihistamine, but is included here because of its value as a prophylactic in hayfever.

Sodium cromoglycate is largely free from **side-effects**, but cough, irritation of the throat and transient bronchospasm may occur. Initially the treatment should be continued for 1 month, but the drug should then be withdrawn if the response is inadequate or absent.

Sodium cromoglycate is also given orally as Nalcrom § for the treatment of food allergies in doses of 200 mg four times a day, as it appears to have a stabilizing effect on the local inflammatory reaction in the gastro-intestinal tract. The use of sodium cromoglycate (Rynacrom) as a nasal spray for the prophylaxis of seasonal rhinitis is referred to briefly below. It is also used as Opticrom § in allergic conjunctivitis (p. 252).

Ketotifen § (dose: 2–4 mg daily)

Brand name: Zaditen §

Ketotifen has an action similar to that of sodium cromoglycate in stabilizing mast-cell membrane. It has the advantage of being active orally, and in the prophylactic treatment of asthma it is given in doses of 1 mg twice daily initially, increasing to 2 mg twice daily if necessary. The onset of action is slow, and some weeks may elapse before full protection is obtained. Ketotifen is of no value in acute asthma.

Side-effects Ketotifen may cause drowsiness, dry mouth and sedation, and potentiate the effects of alcohol, and patients should be warned accordingly about car driving.

Nedocromil § (dose: 8–16 mg daily)

Brand name: Tilade §

Nedocromil is used like sodium cromoglycate in the prophylactic treatment of asthma. It is considered that as reversible obstructive airway disease is associated with bronchial inflammation, the prevention and reduction of such inflammation could reduce the symptoms of the disease. Nedocromil has some of the required anti-inflammatory properties, as it inhibits the release of histamine, leukotrienes and other mediators of inflammation in the bronchial tract, and as pulmonary function improves, the frequency of asthmatic attacks is reduced.

Nedocromil is given by oral aerosol inhalation in doses of 4 mg (two puffs), usually twice daily, but up to four times a day if necessary. A response should be obtained within 1 week. It is of no value in the treatment of acute asthma.

Side-effects are transient headache and nausea.

Seasonal rhinitis

Seasonal rhinitis, commonly known as hay fever, is an allergic reaction in sensitive subjects that follows exposure to plant pollens. It is frequently treated with antihistamines and mild nasal decongestants as sprays or drops, which often give rapid but transient symptomatic relief. Severe nasal congestion may be less easily relieved, and such treatment is of no value in prophylaxis. Those individuals who are known to be subject to hay fever can be treated prophylactically with locally applied corticosteroids or sodium cromoglycate, but the patient must be well motivated to obtain the best response. It is necessary to commence treatment at least 2–3 weeks before hay fever attacks are anticipated, as it may take time for protection to develop, and treatment must be continued regularly for some months, or even longer. The products in use are given in Table 17.3.

Table 17.3 Products used for seasonal rhinitis

Approved name	Brand name	Product
azelastine	Rhinolast	Spray 0.1%
beclomethasone	Beconase	Spray 50 micrograms
betamethasone	Betnesol	Drops 0.1%
	Vista-Methasone	Drops 0.1%
budesonide	Rhinocort	Spray 100 micrograms
flunisolide	Syntaris	Spray 25 micrograms
fluticasone	Flixonase	Spray 50 micrograms
ipratropium	Rinatec	Spray 20 micrograms
sodium cromoglycate	Rynacrom	Spray 4%
xylometazoline	Otrivine	Spray and drops 0.1%

Dexa-Rhinospray is a mixed product containing dexamethazone, tramazoline and neomycin.

FURTHER READING

Brydon M J 1993 Management and treatment of seasonal rhinitis. Professional Nurse 8(10):662–666

Campbell J 1997 Anaphylaxis. Professional Nurse 12(6):429–432

Committee on Safety of Medicines 1993 Current problems in pharmacovigilance 19:7

Fisher M 1995 Treatment of acute anaphylaxis. British Medical Journal 311:751–753

McKenzie S 1994 Drugs used to control asthma. British Journal of Nursing 3(17):872–880

Patten B C, Holt J A 1992 When your patient is allergic. American Journal of Nursing 92(9):58–61

Ryhal B T, Fletcher M P 1991 The second generation antihistamines. Postgraduate Medicine 89(6):87–99

Sampford H 1996 Managing peanut allergy. British Medical Journal 312:1050–1051

18

Respiratory stimulants, expectorants and mucolytics

ASTHMA AND RESPIRATORY DRUGS

ASTHMA

Chronic obstructive airways disease is a term used to describe conditions in which there is chronic limitation of airflow in the lungs. Flow is reduced either because outflow pressure is lowered following a loss of the elastic recoil of the lungs, as is seen in emphysema, or because airway resistance is increased by narrowing of the large airways, which occurs in bronchitis, or of the small airways in the case of asthma. Chronic bronchitis is a functional disorder in which there is mucus hypersecretion with mucous gland hyperplasia. Many patients with chronic bronchitis have an asthmatic condition as well as emphysema.

Asthma is a common disorder affecting 10% of children and 5% of adults and is triggered by a variety of factors including allergy to house dust mites, upper respiratory tract infection, exertion, psychological stress, as well as drugs such as aspirin and some beta-blockers. During an asthma attack the small airways become reversibly obstructed by a combination of bronchospasm, inflammation and oedema, and mucus plugging, making breathing, especially expiration, very difficult.

Bronchial smooth muscle has β_2-adrenoceptors and if these are stimulated they cause muscle relaxation and bronchodilation. By using selective sympathomimetic drugs which are specific for these receptors, i.e. β_2-agonists, bronchodilation can be achieved without stimulating the β_1-receptors in the heart muscle. Salbutamol is an example of such a selective agonist, although it does possess some residual β_1-adrenoceptor activity and may cause cardiac disturbances such as tachycardia in sensitive patients. Such disturbances are less likely to occur when the drug is given by oral inhalation from a metered-dose, pressurized aerosol.

This inhalation method is the preferred method of administration, as the drug is delivered directly to the bronchi, and is effective more rapidly and with fewer side-effects, *provided* the aerosol is operated correctly. Some breath-actuated spacing devices and nebulizers are also available that enable a larger amount of the drug to reach the lungs. The spacers are also useful for patients who have difficulties in using metered-dose products, especially children. Powered-jet nebulizers also permit a larger dose to be given, but their use requires training and supervision.

Patients often require repeated instructions in the use of metered-dose aerosols, and nurses can play an important part in such inhalation therapy by emphasizing the importance of synchronizing breathing with inhalation, as well as warning against excessive use (see Fig. 1.3, p. 13). Failure to respond initially to inhalation therapy is more likely to be due to faulty technique than drug failure, whereas a failure to respond after previous control has been achieved should be investigated, as it may indicate that a deterioration of the airway disease has occurred that requires alternative therapy.

Table 18.1 indicates the different types of drugs used in the treatment of asthma.

Nursing points about bronchodilators
(a) Two main types – β_2-adrenoceptor stimulants and antimuscarinics (anticholinergics).
(b) Some are given by inhalation and patients should be given detailed instructions on the use of inhaler devices.
(c) Bronchodilators with a long action are not suitable for the treatment of acute attacks.
(d) Hypokalaemia is a potential risk with β_2-adrenoceptor stimulants, and may be increased by combined therapy. Plasma potassium levels should be monitored in severe asthma.

Salbutamol § (dose: 8–16 mg daily orally; 100–200 micrograms by oral inhalation as required; 500 micrograms by intramuscular injection)

Brand names: Salbulin §, Ventodisks §, Ventolin §, Volmax §

Salbutamol is a sympathomimetic agent with a selective stimulant action on the β_2-adrenoceptors and it is one of the most widely used drugs for the treatment of reversible airways disease generally. It is also effective in preventing exercise-induced bronchospasm.

Salbutamol may be given orally in doses of 4 mg three or four times a day, reduced to 2 mg for elderly patients, but for the rapid relief of acute bronchospasm it is given by oral inhalation from a pressurized aerosol in doses of 100–200 micrograms (1–2 puffs) as required. Such inhalation doses may also be given for the prophylaxis of exercise-induced bronchospasm or for maintenance therapy in acute conditions. The drug may also be administered by the inhalation of a powder from inhalation capsules, and some sustained-release oral products are available that are useful in the treatment of nocturnal asthma. In severe acute bronchospasm, salbutamol may be given by subcutaneous or intramuscular injection in doses of 500 micrograms, repeated 4-hourly as required; by slow intravenous injection in doses of 250 micrograms; or by intravenous infusion in doses of 5–20 micrograms/ minute according to need, together with corticosteroid therapy.

In status asthmaticus and severe conditions, salbutamol is sometimes given by the inhalation of a nebulized solution, delivered as a mist in oxygen-enriched air (to prevent hypoxaemia) from an intermittent, positive-pressure ventilator. Such ventilator treatment requires strict control, as the dose varies from 2.5 to 5 mg or more 4-hourly, or 1–2 mg

Table 18.1 Drugs used in asthma therapy

Drug group	Type of action
β_2-adrenoceptor agonists, e.g. salbutamol	Bronchodilator – relaxes bronchial smooth muscle
Xanthines, e.g. aminophylline	Bronchodilator – relaxes bronchial smooth muscle
Muscarinic antagonists, e.g. ipratropium	Bronchodilator – inhibits bronchoconstrictive effects of vagus nerve activity
Glucocorticosteroids, e.g. beclomethasone (see p. 178)	Anti-inflammatory – reduces bronchial oedema and mucus production
Mast cell stabilizers, e.g. sodium cromoglycate (see p. 233)	Inhibits release of inflammatory mediators, including histamine
LTD_4 antagonists (see p. 204)	Blocks the effect of leukotrienes which are powerful bronchoconstrictors
5-lipoxygenase inhibitors (see p. 204)	Inhibits the formation of leukotrienes which are powerful bronchoconstrictors

hourly, doses much larger than those given by aerosol inhalation.

Side-effects Salbutamol is usually well tolerated, but fine tremor, tension headache and tachycardia may occur, although the latter is less common with aerosol inhalation. Caution is necessary in hypertension, ischaemic heart disease and hyperthyroidism. Hypokalaemia is a potential risk with salbutamol, as with other β_2-adrenoceptors, especially in severe asthma, and may be increased by theophylline, diuretics and corticosteroids. It is now recommended that plasma potassium levels should be monitored in severe asthma.

The salbutamol derivative salmeterol § (Serevent §) has a longer action, and in doses of 50 micrograms by inhalation is suitable for twice daily maintenance treatment.

The use of salbutamol to prevent premature labour is referred to on p. 171.

Terbutaline § (dose: 7.5–15 mg daily orally; 250–500 micrograms by oral inhalation as required; 250–500 micrograms by injection)

Brand names: Bricanyl §, Monovent §

Terbutaline is a sympathomimetic agent with the actions, uses and **side-effects** of salbutamol. In reversible airways disease it is given in doses of 5 mg two or three times a day; for the control of intermittent bronchospasm and for the prophylaxis of exercise-induced conditions, terbutaline may be given by aerosol in doses of 250–500 micrograms (1–2 puffs) 4-hourly as needed. In the maintenance treatment of chronic obstructive airways conditions, the total daily inhalation dose should not exceed 2 mg (8 puffs).

In acute and severe obstructive states, terbutaline is given by subcutaneous, intramuscular or slow intravenous injection in doses of 250–500 micrograms up to four times a day. Alternatively, it may be given by continuous intravenous infusion in doses of 1.5–5 micrograms/minute according to need and response, together with supportive oxygen therapy to avoid hypoxia. As with salbutamol, in severe and acute conditions terbutaline may also be given by the inhalation of a nebulized solution. Bambuterol § (Bambec §) is a terbutaline pro-drug. It has similar actions and uses, but a more prolonged effect. It is given as a single dose of 10–20 mg at night.

Terbutaline is sometimes used as a myometrial relaxant in the control of premature labour (p. 171).

Orciprenaline § (dose: 40–80 mg daily orally; 750–1500 micrograms by oral inhalation)

Brand name: Alupent §

Orciprenaline has the bronchodilator properties of salbutamol, but it has a less selective action on the β_2-adrenoceptors, and is more likely to cause tachycardia. In reversible obstructive airways disease it is given orally in doses of 20 mg four times a day or by aerosol inhalation in doses of 750–1500 micrograms (1–2 puffs), up to a maximum of 12 puffs a day.

Side-effects of orciprenaline are similar to those of related drugs, but tremor, palpitations and cardiac irregularities are more common.

Bambuterol § (Bambec §), eformoterol § (Foradil §), fenoterol § (Berotec §), reproterol § (Bronchodil §), tulobuterol § (Respacal §) and rimiterol § (Pulmadil §) represent other selective β_2-adrenoceptor stimulants (agonists) with the action, uses and side-effects of salbutamol. Care should always be taken not to exceed the prescribed dose.

Ephedrine § (dose: 45–180 mg daily)

Ephedrine is a plant alkaloid with bronchodilator properties, but is now replaced by salbutamol and related drugs. It has been used in bronchospasm in doses of 15–60 mg three times a day. It has some central stimulant properties, and **side-effects** are insomnia, restlessness and tachycardia. It may cause retention of urine in prostatic hypertrophy.

OTHER BRONCHODILATORS USED IN BRONCHOSPASM

Ipratropium § (dose: 20–40 micrograms initially by aerosol inhalation)

Brand name: Atrovent §

Ipratropium is used mainly in the treatment of chronic bronchitis and related conditions of airways obstruction in patients no longer responding to bronchodilators of the salbutamol type. It is given by aerosol inhalation as a single dose of 20–40 micrograms (2–4 puffs) initially, followed by doses of 40–80 micrograms three or four times a day. Combivent § is an aerosol product providing doses of ipratropium 20 micrograms and salbutamol 100 micrograms.

Dry mouth is an occasional **side-effect** and care is necessary in prostatic hypertrophy. Ipratropium is sometimes given by inhalation of a nebulized solution, but it has occasionally caused a paradoxical bronchoconstriction, and such treatment requires close hospital supervision. Oxitropium § (Oxivent §) is an anticholinergic agent with similar properties used as a metered-dose inhaler in doses of 200 micrograms (two puffs) two or three times a day.

Aminophylline (dose: 300–1200 mg daily)

Aminophylline and the closely related theophylline are included here as they have a relaxant effect on smooth muscle and are used in the relief of bronchospasm and to stimulate respiration. In the treatment of reversible airways disease, aminophylline is given orally in doses of 100–300 mg up to four times a day after food, but in practice the gastric irritant effects often prevent the administration of adequate doses.

In severe conditions such as acute bronchial asthma and status asthmaticus, aminophylline may be given by *slow* intravenous injection in doses of 250–500 mg over 20 minutes, followed if necessary by doses of 500 micrograms/kg/hour. Intramuscular injections are painful and are not recommended. The plasma concentrations of theophylline/aminophylline should be monitored, as the therapeutic window (p.7) is narrow. Optimum level is 10–20 mg/litre.

Side-effects include gastrointestinal irritation with nausea and vomiting, headache, insomnia and confusion.

In general, the oral dosage of aminophylline and theophylline is complicated by individual variations in absorption and metabolism of the drug, with variations in response. These difficulties can be reduced to some extent by the use of long-acting oral preparations such as Phyllocontin Continus, Lasma, Neulin SA, Slo-phyllin, Theo-Dur and Uniphyllin Continus. These preparations of theophylline may provide an effective plasma level over 12 hours. Choline theophyl-linate (Choledyl), dose 100–400 mg up to four times a day after food, is a derivative said to be better tolerated than the parent drug.

Caution. The long-acting products should not be regarded as interchangeable, and a patient stabilized on one preparation should not be transferred to another without good cause, as variations in the plasma level of theophylline may occur.

RESPIRATORY STIMULANTS (ANALEPTICS)

The exact mode of action of these drugs in unknown. They appear to work on the brainstem and spinal cord, producing exaggerated reflex excitability and an increase in activity of the respiratory and vaso-motor centres. In larger doses they stimulate the motor cortex as well, causing convulsions. Their activity depends on adequate oxygenation, and may be reduced in severe hypoxaemia. Their use in modern medicine is limited to ventilatory failure due to chronic obstructive airways disease and postoperative respiratory distress, and then only under expert supervision in hospital with physiotherapy support. They are of no use in acute asthma, nor in respiratory depression due to drug overdose where a specific antagonist such as naloxone (p. 53) should be used. Doxapram is the only respiratory stimulant in current use, as older drugs such as ethamivan and nikethamide are not now available.

Doxapram § (dose: 1–1.5 mg/kg intravenously)

Brand name: Dopram §

Doxapram is a short-acting respiratory stimulant used mainly in postoperative respiratory depression. It is given by intravenous injection in doses of 1–1.5 mg/kg, repeated at hourly intervals as required. It is also given by intravenous infusion in doses of 2–3 mg/minute.

DRUGS USED IN THE RESPIRATORY DISTRESS SYNDROME

Neonatal respiratory distress syndrome (RSD) is caused by a deficiency of surfactant, the lecithin-rich lipid secreted by Type II pneumocytes which lowers surface tension in the alveoli, allowing normal lung expansion on inspiration. Surfactant deficiency means that the alveoli collapse, with resulting hypoxia and damage to alveolar and endothelial lining cells. In neonates weighing less than 1000 g the mortality rate is 50%.

RDS can be relieved by the use of pulmonary surfactant products obtained either from animal lung or synthetically. They are given by endotracheal tube in newborn babies who are receiving mechanical ventilation, preferably within eight hours of birth. Continuous monitoring of the arterial oxygenation and heart rate are necessary, as rapid change may occur. Care must be taken to avoid blocking of the endotracheal tube by mucus. Dosage and details of administration vary with the product used, and the manufacturer's data sheet should be studied. The following are available:

Beractant §; Survanta §; Colfosceril §; Exosuf §; Poractants; Curosurf § pumactants; Alec §.

Prevention of RDS can be assisted by administering corticosteroids to mothers about to deliver prematurely, as this stimulates surfactant production in the fetus.

As well as reducing alveolar surface tension, surfactant appears to have a variety of other actions. It stabilizes bronchioles and small airways, inhibits pulmonary oedema formation, lowers the viscosity and elasticity of mucus, improves ciliary action, relaxes smooth muscle, and has anti-inflammatory and antibacterial properties. As a result of these actions its use is being considered in meconium aspiration syndrome, cystic fibrosis, adult respiratory distress syndrome, pneumonia, lung transplantation, asthma and chronic bronchitis.

EXPECTORANTS AND MUCOLYTICS

Sputum is an abnormal, viscous secretion that is produced by the lower respiratory tract. It consists mainly of mucus, a proteinaceous material composed of mucopolysaccharide. In addition, sputum contains deoxyribonucleic acid (DNA) derived from the breakdown of mucosal cells, leukocytes and bacteria, which gives sputum its tenacious properties.

Expectorants are drugs that increase the amount of sputum and reduce the viscosity of bronchial secretions. The increase in the amount of sputum stimulates the cough reflex and the decrease in viscosity makes removal by ciliary action easier. Although they have been shown to be effective in vitro their clinical efficacy is unproved. They are, however, frequently prescribed or bought over the counter.

Mucolytic agents decrease sputum viscosity either by breaking down the polysaccharide fibres which make up mucus or by breaking down the DNA molecules. Again, their value has been questioned, and the use of steam inhalations, with or without a volatile inhalant such as benzoin or menthol, is probably just as useful. Alternatively, water or saline solutions can be nebulized and used to hydrate respiratory secretions.

Many proprietary cough remedies contain a variety of constituents, including an antihistamine, cough suppressants and bronchodilators. Some such products contain pseudoephedrine, and may cause hallucinations when given to young children. Any such reaction is an indication for withdrawal of the drug or a careful adjustment of dose.

Cough suppressants, represented by codeine and pholcodine, act centrally by a depressant effect on the cough centre, and are used mainly for the relief of useless cough, as Codeine Linctus (15 mg/5 ml) and Pholcodine linctus (5 mg/5 ml). They have the disadvantage of causing constipation.

Carbocisteine § (dose: 1.5 g daily)

Brand name: Mucodyne §

Carbocisteine reduces the viscosity of bronchial secretions, and so facilitates expectoration. It is said to produce a sputum with more normal characteristics, and is given in a variety of respiratory tract disorders requiring a reduction in sputum viscosity. Carbocisteine is given initially in doses of 750 mg three times a day, later reduced to doses of 500 mg three times a day. Children's doses are 20 mg/kg daily.

Side-effects are gastrointestinal irritation and rash.

Dornase alfa § ▼ (dose: 2500 units daily by inhalation)

Brand name: Pulmozyme §

A development in the treatment of cystic fibrosis is the use of a recombinant form of human deoxyribonuclease (rhDNase). The illness is associated with the formation of viscous purulent secretions in the airways, which reduce lung efficiency and exacerbate infection. Leukocytes accumulate in response to infection, and the viscous sputum contains large amounts of DNA released from degenerating leukocytes. Such extracellular DNA can be broken down with a reduction in sputum viscosity by dornase alfa, given by daily inhalation in doses of 2500 units by a suitable compressed air nebulizer. Continuous daily inhalation is necessary, as the improvement in pulmonary function brought about by the inhalation of dornase alfa subsides rapidly if treatment is withdrawn. As dornase alfa is an enzyme product, it should be refrigerator stored, and used as the supplied solution and not mixed with any other drugs. **Side-effects** are few, but some pharyngitis and hoarseness of the voice have been reported.

Ipecacuanha

Ipecacuanha is the root of a South American plant and the principal active constituent is the alkaloid emetine. In small doses it increases bronchial secretion and it is used in the treatment of cough where sputum is tough and scanty. Ipecacuanha is often used in association with alkalis such as ammonium bicarbonate, which are also said to liquefy bronchial secretions, and Ammonia and Ipecacuanha Mixture is a familiar expectorant cough mixture containing these traditional drugs. Large doses of ipecacuanha have an emetic action (p. 310).

Methylcysteine (dose: 300–800 mg daily)

Brand name: Visclair

Methylcysteine has the actions and uses of carbocisteine, and is given in doses of 100–200 mg three or four times a day. For long-term prophylactic treatment during winter, alternate day administration is recommended.

Benzoin

Gum benzoin is a natural balsamic resin and is the main constituent of that time-honoured remedy known as Friar's Balsam, which is still widely used as an inhalation for the treatment of bronchitis (p. 12).

Potassium iodide (dose: 250–500 mg)

Potassium iodide has a traditional place with other expectorants in cough mixtures and in preparations for bronchitis but is now used less frequently.

FURTHER READING

Barrington K J, Finer N N 1997 Care of near term infants with respiratory failure. British Medical Journal 315:1215–1218

Hopkins S J 1995 Advances in the treatment of cystic fibrosis. Nursing Times 91:40–41

Khammash et al 1993 Surfactant therapy in full-term neonates with severe respiratory failure. Paediatrics 92(1):135–139

Ranasinha C et al 1993 Efficacy and safety of short-term administration of aerolised recombinant human DNase (rhDNase) in adults with stable stage cystic fibrosis. Lancet 342:199–202

19

Neuromuscular blocking agents and other muscle relaxants

Skeletal or striped muscle differs from smooth muscle both anatomically and physiologically. Although acetylcholine is liberated at the nerve-endings of both types of muscle, it acts on different receptors, as those on skeletal muscle are of the nicotinic type and those on smooth muscle are of the muscarinic type. In consequence, different blocking agents are required to act on different receptors. Thus atropine, an antimuscarinic, relaxes smooth muscle but has no action on skeletal muscle, where a blocking agent is required to act on the neuromuscular or myoneural junction.

Such neuromuscular blocking agents are of two types, the non-depolarizing and the depolarizing agents. The former, represented by atracurium, act by competing with acetylcholine for receptor sites on the motor end-plate (p. 88), and reduce the ability of that plate to respond to acetylcholine. As they are competitive agents, their action can be reversed by drugs such as neostigmine that act as anti-cholinesterases and so permit the accumulation of acetylcholine at the end-plate.

The depolarizing agents (e.g. suxamethonium) block the ability of the end-plate to initiate muscle contraction. They act on receptors on that plate and trigger the opening of ionic channels, allowing an influx of charged sodium ions that depolarize the muscle fibre. That in turn initiates an action potential followed by muscle relaxation. The duration of action is brief, as activity is soon restored as the blocking agent is hydrolized by plasma cholinesterases.

Both types of neuromuscular blocking agents are widely used in surgery, as by their action adequate muscle relaxation can be obtained with relatively light levels of anaesthesia. However, assisted or controlled respiration is necessary until the effects of the relaxant have worn off and muscle function is restored.

NON-DEPOLARIZING OR COMPETITIVE MUSCLE RELAXANTS

Tubarine, obtained from a South American arrow poison, was the first muscle relaxant to be used in surgery, but it has now been replaced by a range of synthetic drugs which differ mainly in the duration of their relaxant action. Their action can be reversed if necessary, to shorten the duration of action or offset any respiratory depression, by the intravenous injection of neostigmine in doses of 1–3 mg, followed if necessary by a second dose after 20–30 minutes. Such doses may cause **side-effects** such as bradycardia and excessive salivation, so neostigmine must be given *after* atropine in a dose of 600 micrograms– 1.2 mg by intravenous injection.

Atracurium §

Brand name: Tracrium §
Atracurium is a widely used non-depolarizing muscle relaxant with a duration of action over 15 to 35 minutes. Unlike related drugs, the duration of activity is independent of urinary excretion or enzymatic metabolism, as the drug decomposes spontaneously at body temperature with the formation of inert breakdown products. Atracurium is therefore of value when renal or hepatic impairment is present, as repeated doses do not have a cumulative effect. The initial intravenous dose is 300–600 micrograms/kg body weight; supplementary doses are 100–200 micrograms/kg as required.

The drug is also given by continuous intravenous infusion in doses of 5–10 micrograms/kg/minute for long operative procedures. The relaxant action is increased by halothane and aminoglycoside antibiotics.

Atracurium should not be mixed with thiopentone in the same syringe, as rapid inactivation and loss of relaxant action will result.

Cisatracurium § (Nimbex §) is a closely related drug, but it lacks the histamine-releasing properties of the non-depolarizing muscle relaxants, and is less likely to cause cardiovascular **side-effects**.

Gallamine triethiodide §

Brand name: Flaxedil §
Gallamine is a synthetic relaxant that is now used less frequently. The average adult dose of gallamine is 80–120 mg intravenously; relaxation occurs within 2 minutes, continues for about 20 minutes, and can be maintained by a second dose of 40–60 mg.

Gallamine should be used with care in hyper-

tension and cardiac conditions where its tachycardial **side-effects** are undesirable.

Mivacurium §

Brand name: Mivacron §
Mivacurium is a non-depolarizing short-acting muscle relaxant with the action and uses of atracurium. It is given intravenously in doses of 70–150 micrograms/kg over 5–15 seconds to facilitate intubation, followed by maintenance doses of 8–10 micrograms/kg/minute by intravenous infusion. A slow initial injection rate up to 60 seconds is advisable in asthmatic patients and those with heart disease, as histamine release may follow the rapid injection of mivacurium.

Pancuronium bromide §

Brand name: Pavulon §
Pancuronium is given in doses of 50–100 micrograms/ kg intravenously, followed by doses of 10–20 micrograms/kg as required. There is little risk of blood pressure changes, and pancuronium is sometimes preferred when maintenance of cardiac output is of importance.

Vecuronium §

Brand name: Norcuron §
Vecuronium has a short to medium duration of action. It is given in initial intravenous doses of 80–100 micrograms/kg, with supplementary doses of 30–50 micrograms/kg. As with related compounds, the action is increased by a wide range of other drugs, including inhalation and intravenous anaesthetics, aminoglycoside antibiotics and beta-adrenergic blocking agents. Cardiovascular **side-effects** are uncommon, and spontaneous recovery is rapid. Rocuronium § (Esmeron §) is a newer muscle relaxant with similar actions and uses.

Nursing points about muscle relaxants used in anaesthesia

(a) Two types, depolarizing and non-depolarizing. Suxamethonium is the only example of the latter, and has a brief action.
(b) Depolarizing muscle relaxants have a longer action; some have side-effects associated with histamine release.
(c) The action of depolarizing agents can be reversed by neostigmine, which must be preceded by atropine.
(d) Patients given a muscle relaxant must have assisted or controlled respiration until the relaxant has been metabolized or antagonized.

DEPOLARIZING MUSCLE RELAXANTS

The depolarizing muscle relaxants are characterized by their brief action, although an extended effect can be obtained by repeated doses. Unlike the non-depolarizing relaxants, the action cannot be reversed by neostigmine and recovery is spontaneous.

Suxamethonium §

Brand names: Anectine §, Scoline §
Suxamethonium, also known as succinylcholine, is a depolarizing muscle relaxant that acts by simulating the action of acetylcholine on the motor end-plate that initiates muscle relaxation, but it evokes a longer response as it escapes the extremely rapid enzymatic breakdown of acetylcholine that normally occurs. When given by intravenous injection in doses of 20–100 mg, it induces a rapid relaxation of muscle, from which spontaneous recovery takes place after 5 minutes.

Suxamethonium is of value in procedures in which merely a brief relaxation is required, such as the passing of an endotracheal tube, but an extended action can be obtained by giving further doses of 2–5 mg/minute by intravenous infusion.

Suxamethonium causes an initial painful muscle fibrillation (with muscle pain after recovery), and it should be given after anaesthesia has been induced by an intravenous anaesthetic such as thiopentone.

The action of suxamethonium may be intensified by other drugs such as aminoglycoside antibiotics, and narcotic analgesics, and the bradycardia induced by the drug may be increased by halothane and cyclopropane (but not by thiopentone); premedication with atropine may be indicated. In a few patients who have a reduced ability to metabolize the drug, suxamethonium may have an exceptionally long action, with marked apnoea, requiring extended assisted respiration.

It is contra-indicated in severely injured patients, in severe eye injuries, in burned patients and in severe hepatic disease.

SKELETAL MUSCLE RELAXANTS

It is convenient to consider here some muscle relaxants that are used in spastic conditions and the relief of muscle spasm. Unlike the relaxants used in surgery, most drugs in the group act on the central nervous system, and not by neuromuscular blockade.

Nursing points about skeletal muscle relaxants
(a) Most act via the central nervous system.
(b) Dantrolene differs in acting directly on skeletal muscle.
(c) Botulinum toxin is used to control blepharospasm by localized muscle paralysis.

Baclofen § (dose: 15–100 mg daily)

Brand name: Lioresal §
Baclofen is an antispastic agent that acts at the spinal level, probably by stimulating GABA receptors. It gives relief in muscle spasticity associated with multiple sclerosis, tumours of the cord and similar conditions as well as spasticity of voluntary muscle due to cerebrovascular accidents or traumatic injuries. It has little effect on muscle power, so that relief of spasticity is not accompanied by a corresponding increase in muscular function, although the mobility of the patient may be improved.

Baclofen is given initially in doses of 5 mg three times a day, after food, with subsequent doses slowly increased according to response up to a maximum of 100 mg daily. Careful adjustment of dose is essential, especially in the elderly, to minimize muscle weakness in any unaffected limbs.

In severe chronic spasticity not responding to oral therapy, baclofen has been given in specialist centres by intrathecal injection in doses ranging from 10 to 1200 micrograms.

Side-effects include nausea, drowsiness, fatigue and confusion. Care is necessary in psychiatric illness, epilepsy and cardiovascular disease. Abrupt withdrawal of baclofen should be avoided, as visual hallucinations and convulsions may be precipitated.

Dantrolene § (dose: 50–400 mg daily)

Brand name: Dantrium §
Dantrolene acts by blocking the muscle contraction response at a site beyond the myoneural junction, probably by interfering with the release of calcium ions from the sarcoplasmic reticulum, and so is largely free from side-effects on the central nervous system. It is used mainly in severe spastic conditions of voluntary muscle associated with stroke, spinal cord injury, cerebral palsy and multiple sclerosis, and is given in initial doses of 25 mg daily, slowly increased to a maximum of 100 mg four times a day. Careful adjustment of dose to response

is necessary, and although for many patients a dose of 75 mg three times a day is the optimum, response to treatment may be slow, and if the drug is ineffective after 6 weeks, it should be withdrawn.

Nausea and fatigue are usually transient **side-effects**. Dantrolene is potentially hepatotoxic, and liver function tests are necessary before and during treatment. Care is necessary in obstructive pulmonary disease and myocardial impairment

As dantrolene has some central activity, patients should be warned not to drive until dose and response have been stabilized. The use of dantrolene in the treatment of malignant hyperthermia is referred to on p. 22.

Diazepam § (dose: 2–15 mg daily)

Brand name: Valium §

Diazepam, widely used in psychiatry (p. 32) also has a muscle relaxant action that appears to be mediated by the GABA receptors (p. 19). It is used in a variety of conditions associated with muscle spasm, in cerebral spasticity, and to control the spasms of tetanus and relieve status asthmaticus.

Diazepam is given orally in muscle spasm in doses of 2–5 mg three times a day, but in cerebral spastic conditions up to 60 mg daily in divided doses may be necessary. In acute conditions, diazepam may be given by deep intramuscular injection (from which absorption may be erratic) or by slow intravenous injection in doses of 10 mg, repeated after 4 hours. In the treatment of tetanus, a dose of 100–300-micrograms/kg is given by slow intravenous injection at intervals of 1–4 hours as required, or by continuous intravenous infusion in doses of 3–10 mg/kg over 24 hours. In status epilepticus, diazepam is given by slow intravenous injection in doses of 10–20 mg, repeated according to need, or by intravenous infusion up to a maximum of 3 mg/kg over 24 hours. It is also given rectally as a solution in doses of 10 mg, repeated if necessary.

Side-effects of diazepam include drowsiness, dizziness and occasional confusion, but intravenous injections may cause not only hypotension but also severe respiratory depression requiring the support of mechanical ventilation. Intravenous injections may also cause a local thrombophlebitis.

Related benzodiazepines (p. 32) represented by chlorodiazepoxide also have muscle relaxant properties that are useful in muscular–skeletal disorders, especially when an emotional component is present.

OTHER RELAXANTS

Mild muscle relaxants used in muscle spasm include carisoprodol § (Carisoma §) dose 1.5 g daily; methocarbamol § (Robaxin §) dose 6 g daily; and meprobamate § (Equanil §), dose 1.2 g daily. Some of these mild relaxants are included in various mixed preparations with a mild analgesic such as paracetamol.

Quinine § is given for nocturnal leg cramps in doses of 200–300 mg at night, but if there is no improvement after 4 weeks, treatment should be abandoned. If effective, a rest period should be taken after 3 months to assess the need for further treatment. Quinine overdose requires prompt and expert treatment. See p. 314.

Drugs used in the relief of tremor, chorea, tics and other muscle movements include propranolol (p. 111), primidone (p. 43) and benzhexol (p. 98). Tetrabenazine § (Nitoman §) is used mainly in Huntington's chorea in doses of 12.5 mg twice daily, increased to 25 mg three times a day if required. Piracetam § ▼ (Nootropil § ▼) is used in the adjunctive treatment of cortical myoclonus. It is given in initial doses of 2.4 g three times a day, increased as required at intervals of 3–4 days up to a maximum of 20 g daily.

Botulinum A haemagglutinin complex §

Brand names: Botox §, Dysport §

This toxin-complex is a muscle relaxant of an unusual type and very limited use, as it is a preparation of *Clostridium botulinum Type A* toxin. That toxin, which is the cause of botulism, blocks the release of acetylcholine by binding irreversibly with the motor end-plate, and causes death by respiratory failure. Yet very small doses of the toxin-complex can produce a localized muscle paralysis, and it is used by experts in the treatment of blepharospasm. This condition is characterized by repeated blinking with local irritation and photophobia, leading to uncontrollable closure of the eyelid. The toxin-complex, when injected into the appropriate muscles of the eye, produces a localized muscle weakness and relief of spasm. The onset of action is slow, and is not fully developed for 1–2 weeks, but relief is sustained for 2–3 months. Further injections are required at 8-week intervals, as muscle function returns as new nerve end-plates are slowly formed. The toxin-complex has also been used in the treatment of torticollis.

Side-effects are linked mainly with the spread of action to facial muscles. As the toxin-complex is a biological product, its use carries the potential risk of anaphylaxis.

Note: Botox and Dysport are not identical products and are not interchangeable.

FURTHER READING

Bruton-Maree N 1989 Neuromuscular blocking drugs. Journal of Neuroscience Nursing 21(3):198–200

Dickens M D 1995 Pharmacology of neuromuscular blockade: interactions and implications for concurrent drug therapies. Critical Care Nursing 18(2):1–12

Kaji D M 1976 Prevention of muscle cramps with quinine sulphate. Lancet 11:66–67.

Smith H 1995 The effects of botulin toxin on ocular tissue. Nursing Times 91(4):41–43

20

Drugs used in ophthalmology

The drugs used in ophthalmology fall into two main groups: (a) those applied locally, and (b) those used systemically. It should be noted that with some drugs used as eye-drops, some systemic drug absorption may occur occasionally via the conjunctival vessels, or via the nasal mucosa after drainage through the tear ducts, but such absorption may be reduced if minimal quantities of the eye-drops are used.

MYDRIATICS AND CYCLOPLEGICS

Mydriatics are drugs that dilate the pupil; cyclo-plegics are those that paralyse the ciliary muscle and prevent accommodation for near vision. Some drugs have both effects.

Pupil size is controlled by circularly and radially arranged smooth muscles which in turn are controlled by the sympathetic and the parasympathetic nervous systems; the former dilates the pupil, the latter constricts it. So to dilate the pupil for retinoscopy, two different types of drugs can be used, either sympathetic agonists (sympathomimetics) such as phenylephrine, or parasympathetic antagonists (antimuscarinics/anticholinergics) of which atropine is the most important (Fig. 20.1). Atropine §, used as eye-drops 1%, has a powerful and extended mydriatic action. It is best avoided in the elderly, as there is then a risk of precipitating an attack of acute closed-angle glaucoma, and the synthetic agent cyclopentolate § (Mydrilate §, 0.5%) or tropicamide § (Mydriacil §, 0.5%) may be preferred. Homatropine § (1%) has a similar but more rapid and shorter action, as the mydriatic effects fade after about 24 hours. Phenylephrine (1–10%) is also used, sometimes in conjunction with atropine.

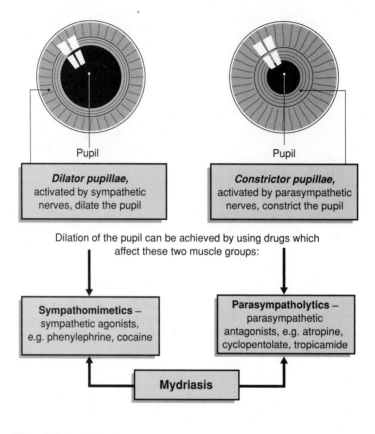

Figure 20.1 Mydriasis.

MIOTICS AND GLAUCOMA

Miotics are drugs that constrict the pupil, and as with mydriatics, two types of drug can be used for that purpose: the sympathetic antagonists and parasympathetic agonists. As well as affecting the iris, some drugs may also cause contraction of the ciliary muscle. The main use of miotics is in the treatment of simple glaucoma, but they can also be used to reverse mydriasis.

Glaucoma is usually an insidious disease characterized by a raised intra-ocular pressure due to a reduction in the normal drainage of the aqueous humour from the anterior chamber of the eye. If the high pressure is sustained it causes damage to the optic nerve and retina, and may lead to blindness unless treated by drugs that increase the drainage of aqueous humour and/or reduce its production (Fig. 20.2). The aqueous humour drains through the trabecular meshwork of the eye into the Canal of Schlemm,

and contraction of the ciliary muscle opens up the drainage channels in that meshwork and so promotes the outflow of the aqueous humour. A drug with that action is pilocarpine nitrate §. It is used as 1% eye-drops, and has an action lasting 3–4 hours. An alternative to eye-drops is the long-acting device Ocusert §, which has a pilocarpine reservoir. The device is placed in the conjunctival sac and is replaced weekly. Care in positioning the device is essential. The alkaloid physostigmine § (eserine) is another anticholinesterase that has been used as a miotic as eye-drops 0.5%.

Adrenaline § (epinephrine) also reduces intraocular pressure by the double action of promoting the drainage of aqueous humour and decreasing its rate of production, but standard solutions are too irritant for use as eye-drops. Less irritant adrenaline products are Eppy (1%) and Simplene § (0.5%). Dipivefrine § (Propine § 0.1%) is a pro-drug, it passes readily into the anterior chamber and is there converted to adrenaline. Adrenaline eye-drops are contra-indicated in closed-angle glaucoma as they have a mydriatic action.

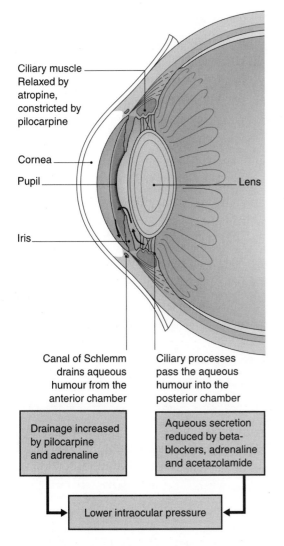

Ciliary muscle
Relaxed by
atropine,
constricted by
pilocarpine

Cornea

Pupil

Lens

Iris

Canal of Schlemm
drains aqueous
humour from the
anterior chamber

Ciliary processes
pass the aqueous
humour into the
posterior chamber

Drainage increased
by pilocarpine
and adrenaline

Aqueous secretion
reduced by beta-
blockers, adrenaline
and acetazolamide

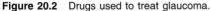

Lower intraocular pressure

Figure 20.2   Drugs used to treat glaucoma.

The antihypertensive agent guanethidine (p. 121) is also used as eye-drops in glaucoma, as it increases and prolongs the action of adrenaline, probably by blocking its uptake in the tissues. It is used as the mixed product Ganda §, which contains guanethidine 1% and adrenaline 0.2%. The prolonged use of guanethidine may cause conjunctival fibrosis, and eye examinations should be carried out every 6 months.

The beta-blockers are also used locally in the treatment of chronic simple glaucoma. They act by reducing the rate of formation of the aqueous humour, and are used as eye-drops twice a day. They include betaxolol 0.5% § (Betoptic §), carteolol 1% (Teoptic §), metipranolol 0.1% and timolol 0.25% (Timoptol §)

and Glaucol § 0.25% and 0.5%. Levobunolol 0.5% (Betagan §) has a longer action, and once-a-day use is often adequate.

Some systemic absorption may occur when beta-blockers are used as eye-drops, and the Committee on Safety of Medicines has advised that such drugs, even those said to be cardioselective, should not be used for patients with asthma or a history of obstructive airways disease unless no other treatment is available. If so used, the risk of drug-induced bronchospasm should be borne in mind. Caution is also necessary in patients with cardiac disturbances.

A different type of treatment is the use of inhibitors of the enzyme carbonic anhydrase such as the old acetazolamide § (Diamox §). It inhibits the formation of bicarbonate, which in turn reduces sodium ion transport and the production of aqueous humour. Acetazolamide is given orally in doses of 250 mg two to four times a day, and in doses of 250–500 mg by intravenous injection in the preoperative treatment of closed-angle glaucoma.

Side-effects   include paraesthesia, hypokalaemia and drowsiness. Dorzolamide § (Trusopt §) has a similar action but is used locally, either alone as eye-drops (2%) three times a day, or twice daily when used in conjunction with a beta-blocker.

Patients resistant to or not responding to other therapy may be treated with the new prostaglandin analogue latanoprost § (Xalatan §). It promotes uveoscleral outflow, and in open-angle glaucoma it is used to lower the intra-ocular pressure as eye-drops (0.005%) one drop daily. Latanoprost may increase the amount of brown pigment in the iris, and nurses should warn patients to report any change in the colour of the eye.

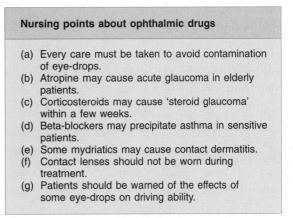

Nursing points about ophthalmic drugs

(a) Every care must be taken to avoid contamination of eye-drops.
(b) Atropine may cause acute glaucoma in elderly patients.
(c) Corticosteroids may cause 'steroid glaucoma' within a few weeks.
(d) Beta-blockers may precipitate asthma in sensitive patients.
(e) Some mydriatics may cause contact dermatitis.
(f) Contact lenses should not be worn during treatment.
(g) Patients should be warned of the effects of some eye-drops on driving ability.

(Some drugs used as eye-drops are available as single-use pre-sterilized products referred to as Minims.)

ANAESTHETICS

Cocaine, as a 2% solution, was once widely used as a local anaesthetic in ophthalmology, but the synthetic agents amethocaine § (0.5%), lignocaine § (2–4%), oxbuprocaine § (Benoxinate, 0.4% §) and proxymetacaine (Ophthaine 0.5% §) are now preferred. Proxymetacaine causes less initial stinging, and is correspondingly more suitable for children. Eye ointments should be used 3–4 times a day, but only at night when used together with eye-drops. Eye-drops should be used every 2 hours or even more frequently, then slowly reduced according to response, then maintained for 48 hours after healing.

ANTIBACTERIAL DRUGS

Some antibiotics, particularly those seldom used systemically, are of value when used locally in ophthalmic infections. Chloramphenicol § is used as eye-drops (0.5%) and ointment (1%), and other antibiotics with a wide range of activity include neomycin drops 0.5% § and framycetin 0.5% § (Soframycin §). Gentamicin 0.3% § (Garamycin §, Genticin §) and tobramycin 0.3% § (Tobralex §) are effective against *Pseudomonas aeruginosa*. Propamidine 0.1% § (Brolene §) and fusidic acid 1% (Fucithalmic §) are used in staphylococcal conjunctivitis. Chlortetracycline is also used locally as ointment 1%, and is effective in the treatment of trachoma. Ofloxacin 0.3% § (Exocin §) and ciprofloxacin 0.3% § (Ciloxan §) are synthetics used in ocular infections such as conjunctivitis.

ANTIVIRAL DRUGS

The herpes virus may occasionally cause a superficial, punctate keratitis of the eye, which in severe cases may develop into a dendritic corneal ulcer. Aciclovir (Zovirax), referred to on p. 80, is the only antiviral agent in current use for the treatment of such ulcers. It is used as a 3% ointment to be applied to the eye five times a day, and continued for at least three days after complete healing has occurred.

CORTICOSTEROIDS AND OTHER ANTI-INFLAMMATORY AGENTS

Corticosteroids are used in ophthalmology for the treatment of various non-infective inflammatory conditions such as keratitis, uveitis, scleritis and in post-operative ocular inflammation. For local use hydrocortisone as drops or ointment (1%) or prednisolone (Predsol 0.5% §) or dexamethasone (Maxidex 0.1% §) or fluorometholone (FML 0.1% §) and betamethasone (Betnesol 0.1% §) are effective, but frequent use of the drops is necessary.

The local use of steroids requires care and they should not be used in dendritic ulcer or undiagnosed 'red eye' as such inflammation may be linked with the herpes simplex virus. It should be noted that in some patients, a rise in intra-ocular pressure and the development of a 'steroid glaucoma' with irreversible damage may follow the use of corticosteroid eye-drops. The condition may also occur after prolonged high-dose oral therapy with a corticosteroid.

Some non-steroidal anti-inflammatory drugs used in the treatment of allergic conjunctivitis are sodium cromoglycate Hay-Crom, Opticrom (0.1%), referred to on p. 234, levocabastine (0.05%), lodoxamide § (Alomide 0.1%) and nedocromil (Rapitil 2%).

MISCELLANEOUS OPHTHALMIC PRODUCTS

Acetylcholine § (Miochol 1% §) is used in cataract surgery when rapid miosis is required; diclofenac (Voltarol Ophtha 0.1% §) and flurbiprofen § (Ocufen 0.03% §) are useful when the inhibition of intra-operative miosis is required during cataract surgery. Apraclonidine § (Iopidine 1% §) is used to prevent the postoperative rise of intra-ocular pressure that may occur after laser ophthalmic surgery. It is given as one drop of the solution 1 hour before laser treatment and one drop immediately postoperatively. Ketorolac § (Acular §) is used in ocular surgery as an anti-inflammatory agent.

Reduced tear production resulting in chronic soreness of the eyes often occurs in rheumatoid arthritis, and products for tear deficiency include eye-drops of acetylcysteine 5% (Ilube §), hypromellose 0.3% (Isopto, Tears Naturale), and polyvinyl alcohol 1% (Hypotears).

Lime burns

Lime (calcium oxide) has caustic properties, and as it is used in the building trade lime burns of the eye are not uncommon. Immediate irrigation is essential, if possible with trisodium edetate solution 0.4%. Trisodium edetate (Limclair) is a chelating agent, and dissolves metallic salts and removes them from the tissues as a soluble complex.

Corneal staining

It is occasionally necessary to determine the nature and extent of damage to the corneal epithelium, and this can be done by staining with fluorescein solution (2%). Fluorescein is a dye, and any areas of the cornea that have become denuded of epithelium by abrasions or ulcers, even if quite invisible to the naked eye, take up the dye, and are stained green. The undamaged epithelium remains unstained. Bengal rose solution (1%) is used in the same way, but the solution is irritant and the prior use of a local anaesthetic is advisable.

Fluorescein has been given by intravenous injection as a 5% solution to facilitate examination of the retinal vessels. Such use is not without risk, as sudden collapse has occurred after intravenous fluorescein, and resuscitation facilities should be available.

Eye-drops and sterility

Infections of the eye are always potentially serious, particularly when due to *Pseudomonas aeruginosa*. As a precautionary measure, eye-drops are supplied as sterile solutions, but the possibility of subsequent contamination during use remains an ever-present risk. It has been recommended that eye-drop bottles should not be supplied complete with dropper, and that a separate sterile disposable dropper should be used for each application of the drops.

As an extension of this safety measure, pre-filled single-use eye-droppers are in use as 'Minims' products, but the range of drugs so available is limited.

OCULAR REACTIONS TO DRUGS

It should be noted that certain drugs can cause adverse ocular reactions, and atropine, framycetin and neomycin may cause a drug-induced conjunctivitis. Eye ointments generally tend to cause more irritation than eye-drops, and the prolonged use of ointments in conditions such as chronic blepharitis should be avoided. Chlorpromazine and some related drugs may bring about a slate-blue discoloration of the eye lids, and the conjunctiva may develop a golden-brown pigmentation. Associated deposits of melanin in the cornea may cause blurred vision. Latanoprost may cause pigmentation of the iris. Chloroquine in full doses has been known to result in corneal opacity and pigmentation, but such reactions are usually reversible when treatment is stopped. Retinopathy, on the other hand, although uncommon, is progressive and correspondingly serious.

Occasionally, deposits of a dark pigment (adrenochrome) may occur following the use of adrenaline drops in glaucoma. The use of local corticosteroids in dendritic ulcers may permit the spread of such ulcers. These steroids can increase intraocular pressure, particularly in patients with chronic open-angle glaucoma. They may also cause lens opacity. Visual disturbances have followed the use of nalidixic acid.

FURTHER READING

Butcher J M, Austin M, McGalliard J et al 1994 Bilateral cataracts and glaucoma induced by long term use of steroid eye drops. British Medical Journal 309:43

Doona M, Walsh J B 1995 Use of chloramphenicol as topical eye medication: time to call a halt? British Medical Journal 310:1217–1218

Goldstein J 1987 Contact lens care products: uses and actions of ingredients. Journal of Ophthalmic Nursing and Technology 6(2):70–72

Goldstein J 1987 Pharmacology of ophthalmic drugs: anesthetics, mydriatics and cycloplegics and ocular hypotensives. Journal of Ophthalmic Nursing and Technology 6(4):146–150

Goldstein J 1987 Pharmacology of ophthalmic drugs: anti-inflammatory & anti-infective agents, part 2. Journal of Ophthalmic Nursing and Technology 6(5):193–197

Goldstein J 1987 Pharmacology of ophthalmic drugs: ocular decongestants, ocular lubricants and miscellaneous agents, part 3. Journal of Ophthalmic Nursing and Technology 6(6):238–241

Kelly J S 1994 Topical ophthalmic drug administration: a practical guide. British Journal of Nursing 3(10):518–520

Morlet N, Kelly M 1996 Improving drop administration by patients. Journal of Ophthalmic Nursing and Technology 15(2):60–64

O'Brien T P, Reynolds L A 1995 Basic ocular pharmacotherapy. Journal of Ophthalmic Nursing and Technology 14(4):160–164

Smith H 1995 The effects of botulinum toxin on ocular tissue. Nursing Times 91(4):41–43

21

Drugs used in some skin disorders

The skin is the largest organ of the body, as in adults it has an area of about 2 square metres. It has two layers, the epidermis and the dermis, and has a variety of functions including protection against trauma and infection, the regulation of body temperature, the synthesis of vitamin D and the excretion of certain waste products. The skin is exposed to the environment and the variety of substances in it, ranging from chemical pollutants to cosmetics. Many environmental factors can cause skin damage, but which of those factors is the cause of a particular skin disorder is often very difficult to find. However, a baffling dermatitis may clear readily when the offending substance is traced and can be removed from the environment, as for example nickel dermatitis from a wristwatch.

Many drugs used for skin disorders are applied as topical preparations, but their action may be modified or influenced by the base in which the drug is incorporated. The following brief survey of some dermatological formulations may be useful.

Dermatological product forms

Ointments   are a common form of skin medication, and two main types may be distinguished; the greasy ointments containing soft paraffin, which tend to retain skin moisture and are useful in dry lesions, and the non-greasy ointments that contain emulsifying waxes as in Emulsifying Ointment, often used as vehicles for locally acting drugs.

Pastes   are stiff ointments containing a high proportion of zinc oxide and starch in a soft paraffin base. They are used as protective applications, mainly to limited areas, such as those occurring in psoriasis and chronic eczema, but they may also be used more extensively on inflamed and excoriated areas. Pastes should be applied thickly and liberally, and additional applications should be made without attempting to remove paste previously applied.

Creams are soft, water-containing products prepared either from an emulsifying wax, as Aqueous Cream, or from a lanolin or wool alcohol base, as Oily Cream. They are of value in cooling, softening and humidifying the skin, but it is worth noting that on occasion, lanolin-containing products can themselves cause a skin reaction.

Lotions are aqueous solutions or suspensions of locally acting drugs; a common example is calamine lotion.

ANTIBIOTICS

Skin infections can often be treated systemically, but some superficial infections may be controlled by topical application. The antibiotics used in these local-use products should not be those that are also used systemically, bacterial resistance develops following local use, the value of systemically acting antibiotics will not be lost.

Neomycin § and the closely related framycetin § is too toxic for systemic use, but it has a wide range of activity and is present in some products for topical use in superficial bacterial infections such as impetigo, sycosis barbae and burns. It may cause sensitization, so prolonged local application should be avoided.

Gentamicin § is also present in some creams and ointments, and with the above warning in mind, may be useful in local infections due to *Pseudomonas* and related organisms. Fusidic acid (Fucidin §) is of value in staphylococcal skin infections, and chlortetracycline is sometimes used locally in the treatment of impetigo. The antibacterial metronidazole is also used locally (see p. 258).

Table 21.1 Antifungal preparations

Approved name (of main constituent)	Brand name
amorolfine	Loceryl
amphotericin	Fungilin
clotrimazole	Canestan, Masnoderm
econazole	Ecostatin, Pevaryl
ketoconazole	Nizoral
metronidazole	Metrogel
miconazole	Daktarin
nystatin	Nystan
sulconazole	Exelderm
terbinafine	Lamisil
tioconazole	Trosyl
zinc undecenoate	Mycota

Mupirocin § is an antibiotic unrelated to any others in current use, and is effective against a wide range of pathogens associated with skin infections. Its main use is the prevention of colonization by *methicillin-resistant Staphylococcus aureus* (MRSA). It is used as Bactroban §, an ointment containing 2% of mupirocin in a water-miscible base. It should not be used continuously for more than 10 days. Bactroban Nasal is used for the elimination of the nasal carriage of staphylococci.

Antifungal agents

Many antifungal preparations are available for the local treatment of fungal infections of the skin and nails such as candidiasis and some forms of ringworm (tinia). They vary from time-honoured drugs such as benzoic and salicylic acid (present in Whitfield's Ointment) to antibiotics represented by natamycin and nystatin, organic compounds such as the imidazoles, and metallic salts such as zinc undecenoate. They may be used as ointments, creams, lotions, sprays, paints or dusting powders. They are too numerous to refer to individually, but Table 21.1 indicates the range available. The use of griseofulvin and terbinafine orally in the treatment of ringworm of the skin and nails is referred to in Chapter 5, together with other antifungal agents that are taken orally for either systemic or superficial fungal infections.

CORTICOSTEROIDS

Corticosteroids have a suppressive action on inflammatory processes, and so are used in inflammatory skin conditions such as severe eczema, psoriasis, resistant dermatoses and similar conditions. They are also of value in allergic contact dermatitis due to some environmental factors. However, it should be remembered that when used as the sole agent, subsequent withdrawal may result in a return of the condition, so the underlying cause must be found and treated accordingly. A further disadvantage is that the corticosteroids have no antibacterial properties, so any local infection that may be present will remain unchecked, and may spread if not treated adequately.

Topically applied corticosteroids may also be absorbed from the skin in amounts sufficient to have undesirable systemic effects, including a depression of the pituitary–adrenal axis, a risk that is increased if an occlusive dressing is also used. Normally, local corticosteroid therapy should be commenced with a product containing a weak steroid (see Table 21.2), especially if treatment is likely to be prolonged. In severe conditions it may be necessary to begin treatment with a more potent corticosteroid, but a change to a weaker product should be made as soon as possible. The amount of a topical product to be applied is measured in 'fingertip' units of about 0.5 g (see Fig. 21.1).

Table 21.2 gives a general indication of the relative potency of some available products, but it does not include mixed products containing antibiotics. It should be noted that in preparations for local use, a derivative of the systemically active form of the corticosteroid may be used, as some derivatives have a more powerful local action. Hydrocortisone, for example, is considered to have a 'low' local activity whereas hydrocortisone butyrate (Locoid) is regarded as 'potent'.

In order to keep Table 21.2 simple, only the name of the basic drug is given. The local activity may sometimes be increased by auxiliary substances such as urea. Urea is considered to increase skin penetration, and hydrocortisone with urea is placed in

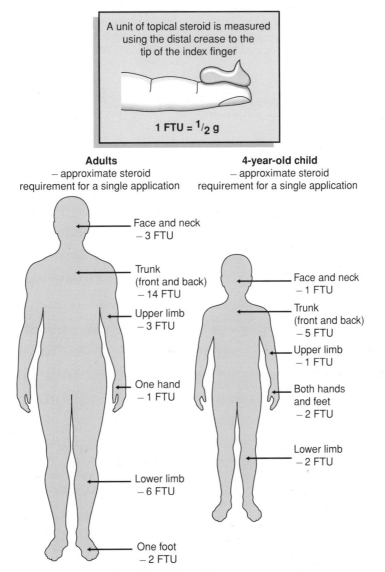

Figure 21.1 Application of topical steroids.

Table 21.2 Corticosteroids for local use

Approved name	Strength	Brand name	Potency
hydrocortisone	1%	Efcortelan (and many others)	Low
alclometasone	0.05%	Modrasone	
clobetasone[a]	0.05%	Eumovate	Medium
flurandrenolone	0.0125%	Haelan	
hydrocortisone	1% + urea	Alphaderm; Calmurid HC	
beclomethasone[a]	0.025%	Propaderm	Potent
betamethasone[a]	0.1%	Betnovate	
desoxymethasone	0.25%	Stiedex	
diflucortolone[a]	0.1%	Nerisone	
fluclorolone	0.025%	Topilar	
fluocinolone[a]	0.025%	Synalar	
fluocinonide	0.05%	Metosyn	
fluticasone	0.05%	Cutivate	
hydrocortisone[a]	0.1%	Locoid	
mometasone	0.1%	Elocon	
triamcinolone[a]	0.1%	Adcortyl	
clobetasol[a]	0.05%	Dermovate	
diflucortolone[a]	0.3%	Nerisone Forte	very potent
halcinonide	0.1%	Halciderm	

[a] Indicates those preparations containing a derivative with increased local activity.

the 'medium' potency group. Topical corticosteroids are mainly used in severe eczema, psoriasis, resistant dermatoses and neurodermatoses, and are also of value in other inflammatory skin conditions. They are also useful in the control of allergic contact dermatitis.

Side-effects include acne, thinning of the skin, mild pigmentation and increased hair growth.

ACNE

Acne vulgaris, which most commonly affects adolescents, is characterized by excessive sebaceous secretions, often in response to strong androgenic stimulation, together with hypercornification of the ducts of the glands. The sebaceous glands become blocked with sebum plugs, causing blackheads and pustules. Secondary infection may cause severe inflammation and scarring. Treatment is with keratolytics, antibacterials, or retinoids.

Keratolytics are abrasive peeling agents which remove superficial keratinized cells and help to clear blocked follicles. They form the first line of treatment and include preparations of sulphur, salicylic acid, and benzoyl peroxide. An alternative treatment is the use of Brasivol which contains particles of aluminium oxide in a detergent base. It is an abrasive agent designed to remove the superficial keratin layer mechanically.

Propionibacterium acnes and *Staphylococcus aureus* are frequently present in the sebum plugs, although their involvement in the pathology of acne is not clear. However, antibacterials can clear the condition. Benzoyl peroxide is an antibacterial agent used in a wide range of proprietary products, often as a 10% cream or lotion, but the response to treatment is slow. Azelaic acid § (Skinoren §) has a bacteriostatic action and is used as a 20% cream in mild to moderate acne. It is applied to the skin once or twice a day, but prolonged action up to a maximum of 6 months may be required. Zineryt § is an erythromycin–zinc acetate complex used for the local treatment of acne vulgaris, while metronidazole § is used as a 0.075% gel in acute acne rosacae, a chronic form of acne in adults that is characterized by telangiectasis, particularly of the nose. A prolonged course of tetracycline therapy is often given in refractory acne. Papulex gel is a new product for acne and contains 4% of nicotinamide, which has some anti-inflammatory properties.

A different type of product is Dianette § which contains cyproterone and ethinyloestradiol. It is essentially an anti-androgen product intended for use in females with severe acne refractory to prolonged treatment with antibiotics.

Retinoids

The retinoids are a small group of potent drugs used in the treatment of acne. They are derivatives of vitamin A, and appear to promote the formation of a less cohesive epidermal layer, as well as reducing the production of sebum. When applied locally they produce an erythematous reaction with eventual peeling. Response to treatment may be slow initially, and associated with a mild local exacerbation of inflammation. Isotretinion is exceptional in being used both locally and orally.

Adapalene § ▼

Brand name: Differin Gel § ▼

Adapalene is used in mild–moderate acne as a 0.1% gel, applied thinly once daily at night. It is not recommended for severe acne, or for use on large areas. Avoid contact with the eyes, nose and mouth, or use together with peeling agents. Local irritation is a **side-effect**; treatment should be stopped if severe.

Isotretinoin §

Brand names: Isotrex §, Roaccutane §

Isotretinoin is a potent retinoid that is used both locally and orally. It is used locally as Isotrex gel (0.05%), applied sparingly once or twice for 6–8 weeks. The gel should not be used near the eyes, mouth or on damaged skin, and exposure to ultraviolet light should be avoided. (Isotrexin also contains erythromycin.)

Isotretinoin is also given orally as Roaccutane in doses of 500 micrograms/kg daily with food for 4 weeks initially, and when the response is good, treatment is continued for 8–12 weeks. Occasionally doses up to 1 mg/kg daily may be required. It is intended for use in severe acne that has failed to respond to other local treatment or to systemic therapy with an antibacterial agent. It is also used in postmenopausal acne, as such acne in later life is often resistant to other therapy.

Isotretinoin given systemically is a potent drug with many **side-effects**, and specialist literature should be consulted. It is also a teratogenic agent, and pregnancy must be avoided before, during and for at least one month after treatment. The combined use of tetracyclines and high doses of vitamin A should also be avoided.

Nursing points about acne treatment

Aims of treatment are to prevent scarring, reduce duration and limit psychological stress. Response to treatment is often slow, and cooperation of the patient with the treatment is necessary.
The choice of product is wide, and selection depends on the severity of the condition.

Mild acne
Benzoyl peroxide preparations (2.5–5%), apply once daily
Azaleic acid cream (20%)
Clindamycin lotion (1%)
Erythromycin solution (2%) } apply once or twice daily
Tetracycline solution (2%)
Tretinoin cream (0.025%)

Moderate acne
Local preparations as above
Oral treatment with
  doxycycline 50 mg once a day
  erythromycin 250 mg
  tetracycline 250 mg } three times a day

Severe acne
High-dose antibiotics
  cyproterone 2 mg with ethinyloestradiol
  35 micrograms
  isotretinoin 500 micrograms/kg–1 mg/kg daily

Tretinoin

Brand name: Retin-A §

Tretinoin is used as a cream (0.025%), gel (0.01%) or lotion (0.025%) applied thinly once or twice a day. The lotion is suitable for use when large areas of the skin are involved. As with all retinoids for local use, contact with the eyes, mouth and nose should be avoided, as well as exposure to peeling agents or ultraviolet light.

Side-effects include local irritation and erythema.

PRURITUS

Pruritus is thought to be associated in some way with histamine release, yet no specific treatment has yet been found for this distressing itching condition. It is said that itching does not occur without an underlying cause, but identifying the cause can be very difficult. The many diseases associated with pruritus include obstructive jaundice, cirrhosis, diabetes and some malignant conditions; many drugs can also cause pruritus, and if possible drugs should be withdrawn when searching for the origin of pruritus (which may also be due to threadworms). Scratching should be discouraged, as although it often gives temporary relief, it may make the condition worse, cause tissue damage and increase the risk of infection.

It was long thought that itching was due to a low-level stimulation of pain receptors, but recently it has been suggested that there are some very small nerves in the body that respond slowly to histamine, but are insensitive to pain. That would explain to some extent why analgesics are of no value in pruritus; in fact morphine can cause itching.

At present treatment is with soothing applications such as calamine lotion, although crotamiton (Eurax) is said to be more effective. Local anaesthetic preparations, of which many are available, may also give some relief. On the basis that itching is linked with histamine release, antihistamine creams are also used. Such creams give some symptomatic relief, but they are intended for short-term use only, as such products may themselves cause skin sensitization.

The oral treatment of itching skin conditions is with trimeprazine § (alimemazine) (Vallergan §) in doses of 10 mg two or three times a day, rising in severe itching up to 100 mg daily. Cholestyramine/

colestyramine (Questran §) is used in the severe pruritus associated with jaundice and biliary obstruction.

PSORIASIS

Psoriasis is a chronic skin condition affecting 2–3% of the population. It occurs equally in both men and women, develops at any age, and the cause is unknown, although there is often a family history. In this condition, the process of epidermal cell production, keratinization, and migration to the cornified layer of the skin takes 4–5 days instead of the normal 3–4 weeks. Psoriasis presents as well demarcated red lesions on elbows, knees and scalp, but can involve any part of the body. The lesions are associated with inflammation, thickening and silvery scaling. Treatment is suppressive, not curative, and remissions and relapses may occur unexpectedly, although attacks may be precipitated by factors such as stress and some drugs, for example beta-blockers, chloroquine, lithium and NSAIDs.

Treatment of mild psoriasis is with emollients to reduce scaling and keep skin moist, and topical anti-inflammatory corticosteroids are of value in the short-term control of small lesions, and for use on the face and in the flexures where dithranol cannot be used. In more severe psoriasis dithranol, an anti-mitotic, is the treatment of choice. If dithranol is not tolerated coal tar products are the traditional treatment, but the response is often disappointing and patient compliance poor. In the hospital control of severe refractory or extensive psoriasis, methotrexate and cyclosporin have been used. Newer treatments include the vitamin D analogues calcipotriol and tacalcitol which regulate cell differentiation and cell proliferation, retinoids which inhibit epithelial keratinization leading to desquamation followed by a more normal epithialization, and photochemotherapy employing the photosensitizer methoxsalen and ultraviolet light.

Acitretin § (dose: 25–50 mg daily)

Brand name: Neotigason §
Acitretin is a derivative of vitamin A with a marked action on keratinizing epithelial cells. It is used in severe and extensive psoriasis resistant to other treatment, but it is a powerful drug for use only under expert supervision. It is teratogenic even in therapeutic doses, and that action must be considered carefully before acitretin is given to a female patient of child-bearing age, and these patients should avoid preg-

nancy for at least 2 years after such therapy. Acitretin is given in oral doses of 25 mg daily, subsequently adjusted according to response up to 50 mg daily. The drug has many **side-effects**, and specialist literature should be consulted for details.

Calcipotriol §

Brand name: Dovonex §
Calcipotriol is a vitamin D derivative and represents a different approach to the treatment of psoriasis. Human keratinocytes have vitamin D receptors, and some vitamin D derivatives are known to decrease the proliferation of such cells. Calcipotriol has a similar action with the advantage of having reduced hypercalcaemic effects, and it is now widely used for topical application as a cream or ointment containing 0.005% of the drug. It is used mainly in mild to moderate plaque psoriasis, including extensive lesions, and the cream or ointment should be applied to the affected areas twice daily up to a maximum weekly use of 100 g, but for no longer than 6 weeks. Calcipotriol has few **side-effects**, although some local irritation may occur and any elevation of the serum calcium level, which is uncommon with standard therapy, subsides rapidly when treatment is discontinued. Tacalcitol § ▼ (Curatoderm § ▼) is another vitamin D analogue used in plaque psoriasis as a 0.4% ointment, to be applied at night.

Cyclosporin § (dose: 2.5–5 mg/kg daily)

Brand names: Neoral §, Sandimmun §
Cyclosporin is an immunosuppressant (p. 209) and on the basis that psoriasis is due to some immunological abnormality, it is used orally in the short-term treatment of severe psoriasis resistant to conventional therapy. Cyclosporin is given initially in doses of 1.25 mg/kg twice daily, increased if the response is good to a maximum dose of 5 mg/kg daily. The treatment period should not exceed 8 weeks. The mode of action of cyclosporin is not clear, but it may inhibit the excessive production of epithelial cells by suppressing T-lymphocyte activity in the epidermis. Cyclosporin should be used under expert supervision, as it has many **side-effects**, and for details specialist literature should be consulted.

Dithranol

Brand names: Dithrocream, Micanol
Dithranol is a synthetic drug used solely for the treatment of psoriasis as it has some peripheral

cytotoxic action. It has some local irritant properties, and may cause a burning sensation when applied to the skin. As some patients are exceptionally sensitive to dithranol, a preliminary test for sensitivity should be carried out on a small area of the skin with a low-strength preparation (0.1%) to assess tolerance. Dithranol is often used as a Dithranol Paste (dithranol 0.1% in Zinc and Salicylic Acid Paste), and the strength of dithranol is slowly increased up to 1% according to response.

Treatment is often based on short-term contact, in which a 0.5% preparation is applied to the lesion for 15 minutes. The dithranol preparation is then washed off in an emollient bath. The application is repeated daily, but the exposure time is increased by 15 minutes each day, up to a maximum exposure time, if tolerated, of 1 hour daily. The concentration of dithranol in the application is then increased to 1%, but the exposure time is reduced to 15 minutes, and gradually increased as before. If irritation or burning occurs, treatment should be suspended for 48 hours, and recommenced with a lower strength preparation. In some cases, a dithranol strength of up to 5% may be tolerated. Dithranol paste is sometimes used after a slight erythema has been produced by previous exposure to ultraviolet radiation (Ingram's method).

Care must be taken to apply dithranol preparations to the psoriatic lesions only, as normal skin is highly susceptible to irritation by the drug, and concentrations as low as 0.05% can cause erythema, especially on fair skin. Patients should be warned to wash the hands thoroughly after using a dithranol preparation, to avoid any eye contact, and advised that dithranol can stain clothing and other fabrics.

Cade oil

Cade oil is obtained by the destructive distillation of juniper wood. It is a time-honoured treatment for psoriasis and survives as a constituent of some proprietary remedies.

Coal tar

Crude coal tar has long been used in the treatment of psoriasis, especially for patients unable to tolerate dithranol. It is used as Zinc and Coal Tar Paste, or as ointments containing 10–20% of coal tar, but such preparations may be cosmetically unacceptable to some patients. Some proprietary products, containing coal tar extracts are less objectionable, but may be less effective. An alcoholic solution of coal tar is present in some shampoo products for the treatment of psoriasis of the scalp. Coal Tar has some sensitizing properties, so small amounts of a low-strength product should be used initially to assess the response. Official preparations include Calamine and Coal Tar Ointment, Coal Tar and Salicylic Acid Ointment, Coal Tar Paste and Zinc/Coal Tar Paste.

Methotrexate § (dose: 10–25 mg weekly)

Brand name: Matrex §
Methotrexate is a cytotoxic agent (p. 218) that is occasionally used in severe psoriasis not responding to other treatment. It is given orally in doses of 10–25 mg once weekly according to response, but it has many and severe **side-effects**, and should be used only under specialist supervision. Blood counts are essential as suppression of haemopoiesis may occur without warning. Liver function tests must also be carried out. Pulmonary toxicity may occur in rheumatoid arthritis, and methotrexate toxicity generally may be increased by aspirin or any other NSAID, and patients should be warned of the risks of self-medication.

Tazarotene §

Brand name: Zorac §
Tazarotene is a new retinoid for the local treatment of mild to moderate plaque psoriasis. It is used as a 0.05–0.1% gel, applied once daily at night to the affected areas only. Treatment for up to 12 weeks may be required.

Side-effects are pruritus, erythema and burning. Excessive exposure to ultraviolet light during treatment should be avoided.

SOME OTHER DERMATOLOGICAL PRODUCTS

Aluminium acetate

Weak solutions of aluminium acetate have mild astringent and anti-inflammatory properties and are used in dermatitis and suppurating wounds. Strong solutions (10–20%) are used in hyperhydrosis as antiperspirants, but such strong solutions can be irritant.

Calamine

Calamine is a pink form of zinc carbonate, and has long been employed in association with zinc oxide as Calamine Lotion. It has a mildly astringent action on the skin, and is widely employed for the temporary relief of various forms of dermatitis. The lotion is also useful in the relief of sunburn.

Dimethicone

Dimethicone is a water-repellent silicone product, and is used in a wide range of barrier cream preparations as a protective against skin irritants, for the prevention of pressure sores and napkin rash, and colostomy discharge. Siopel represents one of the proprietary products containing dimethicone now available.

Formaldehyde and glutaraldehyde

These related compounds are used mainly as sterilizing agents, but they also have applications in the treatment of warts. Formaldehyde is used for plantar warts as a 3% solution or as a gel presentation (Veracur). Glutaraldehyde is applied as a 10% solution (Glutarol) or a gel form as Verucasep. These preparations are not suitable for the treatment of facial warts.

Gamolenic acid

Brand names: Epogam §, Efamast §
Gamolenic acid, which is present in evening primrose oil, is a prostaglandin precursor. It is used in the symptomatic treatment of atopic eczema in doses of 160–240 mg twice a day; half doses are given for children. Its use in the treatment of mastalgia is referred to on p. 173.

Ichthammol

Ichthammol is a thick black liquid with mild tar-like properties. It has a traditional reputation as a mild antiseptic and skin stimulant, and is present in many products for the treatment of mild chronic eczematous conditions.

Minoxidil

Brand name: Regaine
Minoxidil has been found to have some stimulant effect on hair growth, and is used for the treatment of male pattern baldness (alopecia androgenetica). It is supplied as 2% solution (Regaine) of which 1 ml should be applied to the affected areas of the scalp twice daily. Extended treatment is usually necessary, but treatment should be discontinued if there is no response after 1 year. Local itching is an occasional **side-effect**. Potential systemic effects are possible from the nature of the drug (p. 123).

Podophyllum

An irritant plant resin with some antimitotic properties. When dissolved in Compound Benzoin Tincture, it is used as a paint (15%) for the treatment of ano-genital and plantar warts. It is strongly irritant to normal skin and mucous membranes and should be washed off after 6 hours. Podophyllotoxin, the active principle, is available as a less irritant 0.5% solution (Condyline §, Warticon §) for the treatment of penile warts.

Resorcin

Also known as resorcinol, resorcin has exfoliative and keratolytic properties, and is a constituent of many preparations used as mild peeling agents in the treatment of acne.

Salicylic acid

Salicylic acid has a long established reputation as a mild keratolytic agent for softening and removing the horny layers of the skin. As Salicylic Acid Lotion or Ointment (2%) it is also used in various eczematous and psoriatic conditions, and is present in many preparations used for acne. Strong ointments and plasters are used to facilitate the reduction in size or removal of corns.

Selenium sulphide

Brand name: Selsun
This compound is used almost exclusively for the treatment of dandruff and seborrhoeic dermatitis of the scalp. It is available as a 2.5% suspension, and 5–10 ml are used as a shampoo, with a time of application of about 5 minutes. After thorough rinsing of the hair, further applications can be made at weekly or twice-weekly intervals according to the response.

Sulphur

Sulphur, like resorcin, has mild antiseptic and peeling properties. Both are present in Eskamel.

Zinc oxide

Zinc oxide is a heavy white powder, widely used in dermatology as zinc cream, ointment and paste, and also as calamine lotion. It has a soothing and protective action in eczema and many other excoriated skin conditions.

SKIN PARASITICIDES

The most common parasitic infection of the skin in the industrialized world is scabies, caused by the mite *Sarcoptes scabiei*. The female parasite burrows in the epidermis laying her eggs, and the characteristic itch is due to a hypersensitivity reaction to the mites and their eggs. The infestation is transmitted by close personal contact and the incubation time is 3 weeks. The soft skin of the flexures, digital webs, perineum and axilla are most affected.

Pediculosis is caused by the head louse *Pediculus humanus capitis*, the body louse *Pediculus humanus corporis*, or the crab louse *Phthirius pubis*. These arthropods feed on the host's blood and their bite causes intense itching, the scratching of which can result in impetigo. Apart from these inconveniences, these parasites also transmit two of the major epidemic diseases, namely typhus and relapsing fever.

The following drugs are in use but resistance has been noted in recent years and it is now recommended that different parasiticides should be used in rotation to obtain the optimum response.

Benzyl benzoate

Benzyl benzoate is used for scabies as a 25% emulsion applied to the entire body except the scalp. The application is repeated the following day, and removed a day later by washing. All members of the household should be treated. For pediculosis, the application should be made to the affected areas, and repeated as necessary. The application may be irritant, and so is not recommended for children.

Carbaryl

Brand names: Carylderm, Clinicide, Derbac, Suleo
Carbaryl is used as a 0.5% alcoholic lotion for the treatment of pediculosis. It is applied to the affected areas, and after 12 hours is removed by washing. The treatment is repeated if required after 1 week. Care should be taken to avoid contact of the drug with the eyes, and asthmatic patients may find the vapour of the lotion disturbing.

Crotamiton

Brand name: Eurax
Crotamiton has antipruritic properties, but it is also said to be effective in scabies. It is applied like benzyl benzoate.

Malathion

Brand names: Derbac-M, Prioderm, Suleo-M
Malathion is an organophosphorus insecticide that is widely used in pediculosis, particularly in children, as it is effective against both insects and eggs. It is applied to the scalp or other affected areas as a 0.5% lotion, which is allowed to dry and washed off 12 hours later. Treatment is repeated twice at intervals of 3 days. With prolonged treatment there is a potential but slight risk of organophosphorus toxicity.

Permethrin (Lyclear) and phenothrin (Full Marks) are pyrethrin derivatives that function as insect neurotoxins. They are used by local application and are effective against head lice and their eggs.

SUNSCREEN PREPARATIONS

Exposure to strong sunlight results in transient erythema due to the release of histamine-like substances from the damaged superficial cells. Further exposure leads to tanning as melanin in the basal cells migrates to the superficial cells to provide some protection from further exposure. Ultraviolet light of the wavelength 310–400 nanometers (UVA) is mainly responsible for the erythema of sunburn, whilst wavelengths of 290–320 (UVB) results in tanning. An individual's sensitivity to sunlight is expressed as the minimal erythema dose (MED), which is the exposure time which will result in a just perceptible skin redness after 24 hours. Sensitivity to sunlight may be increased by a variety of drugs, including amiodarone, chlorpromazine, NSAIDs, quinolones, tetracyclines, thiazides and tricyclic antidepressants.

Sunscreen preparations are of two types, those that contain titanium dioxide and zinc oxide and which scatter the ultraviolet light, and those containing UVL-absorbing compounds. They do not give complete protection, but their activity is expressed as a sun protection factor (SPF). Products with a low SPF give little protection against sunburn and permit tanning, whereas products with a high SPF, up to 15 or more, offer greater protection against burning.

Available products include Coppertone (UVB-SPF 23), Piz Buin (UVB-SPF 20), RoC (UVB-SPF 16), Spectroban (UVB-SPF 25), Sun E 45 (UVB-SPF 25) and Uvistat (UVB-SPF 15–30).

Commonsense methods to reduce over-exposure to sunlight include not sunbathing between noon and 2 p.m. when the sun is strongest, wearing protective clothing, especially hats, and the frequent re-application of sunscreen products. Chronic exposure to ultraviolet light leads to ageing of the skin, and may result in the development of skin cancers, the incidence of which has increased dramatically in recent years. These are of three main types, the most common being the slow growing basal cell carcinoma

(rodent ulcer) which presents as a firm raised nodule, often with central ulceration and a raised pearly edge which may show numerous telangiectatic vessels. The patient may give a history of repeated ulceration and healing. Squamous cell carcinoma grows more quickly and may present as an irregular plaque or hard lump, with a rough hyperkeratotic surface. Malignant melanoma is the most dangerous as it grows rapidly and spreads. It starts as an enlarging mole which has developed irregular edges, and become deeper and varied in colour. There may also be increased irritation, bleeding and ulceration. Medical advice should be sought if any mole shows any signs of change as it may be a melanoma.

FURTHER READING

Bowman J 1994 More than skin deep. Nursing Times 90(23):43–46

Donald S 1995 Atopic childhood eczema. Nursing Standard 10(9):33–39

Ferner R E, Moss C 1996 Minocycline for acne. British Medical Journal 312:138

Hutchison P, Berth-Jones J 1991 Calcipotriol: a better treatment for psoriasis? Prescriber 5:21–22

Lassus A et al 1987 Treatment of severe psoriasis with etretin (acitretin). British Journal of Dermatology 117:333–341

Perkins P 1996 The management of eczema in adults. Nursing Standard 10(35):49–53

Richards C 1995 The effects of psoriasis and its treatment: part 1. Nursing Times 91(21):38–39

Richards C 1995 Topical and systemic treatment of psoriasis: part 2. Nursing Times 91(25):38–39

Venables J 1995 The management and treatment of eczema. Nursing Standard 9(44):25–28

Weinstein G D 1996 Tazarotene: a new retinoid for the local treatment of psoriasis. British Journal of Dermatology 135:32–36 (suppl 49)

22

Anthelmintics, antimalarials and drugs used in tropical diseases

WORMS AND ANTHELMINTICS

The worms which have selected man as their unwitting host rarely cause severe disease but in some areas they can cause a great amount of chronic ill health. Infestation with parasitic worms is the most common disease in the world, and social conditions in some areas are such that infestation is almost impossible to prevent. Paradoxically, some irrigation schemes to increase soil fertility may bring about an extension of infestation by providing more favourable conditions for the development of certain parasites.

Human parasitic helminths or worms can be divided into three main groups: the nematodes, which include roundworms, hookworms, whipworms, threadworms and filariae; cestodes or tapeworms; and trematodes or flukes. The life cycle of many of these parasites is very complex, and an intermediate host may be involved before development from egg to mature worm in the human host can occur.

Roundworms (*Ascaris lumbricoides*)

Infestation with roundworm is most common in tropical and subtropical countries, but it also occurs in temperate climates and is contracted by eating or drinking contaminated food, particularly raw vegetables, salads and water. The adult roundworm inhabits the small intestine, and may cause abdominal pain and diarrhoea, and if present in large numbers may cause small bowel obstruction. Allergic symptoms are common, and migrating larvae that reach the lungs may cause pneumonia-like symptoms.

Less common is toxocariasis, an infestation of *Toxocara canis*, a roundworm that normally matures in the intestines of dogs and cats. It occurs mainly in young children as a result of contact with dog and cat faeces. The larvae are unable to complete their development in the human body, but their presence is characterized by persistent eosinophilia with hepatomegalia and fever. Invasion of the eye can cause blindness, and larvae in the CNS may cause epileptiform convulsions. For treatment see mebendazole (p. 267) and piperazine (p. 268).

Hookworms

This is a general term for the intestinal blood-sucking parasites, the main species being *Ancylostoma duodenale* and *Necator americanus*. The eggs hatch in the soil and the larvae have the ability to penetrate human skin, where they may cause a local reaction. They enter the veins, and eventually migrate to the alimentary tract, where they attach and feed on the host's blood. They cause abdominal pain and general debility, and in heavy infestations severe anaemia may develop. If reinfection can be avoided, the condition may be self-limiting, as the life-span of the parasite is short. For treatment see mebendazole (p. 267).

Creeping eruption or cutaneous larva migrans is caused by the dog/cat hookworm *Ancylostoma braziliense*, contracted by contact with infected faeces. The larva burrows in the epidermis and causes a winding trail of thread-like inflammation. For treatment see thiabendazole (p. 268).

Threadworm or pinworm (*Enterobius vermicularis*)

This is the most common of the intestinal worms, especially in children. Infestation occurs by transfer of the eggs to the mouth from bedding or toys, and after development the adult female worms (8–13 mm in length) emerge from the anus at night and lay eggs on the skin. The itching response leads to scratching of the skin and reinfection. For treatment see mebendazole (p. 267) and piperazine (p. 268).

Whipworm (*Trichocephalus trichiuris*)

Whipworm infestation is common in warm humid countries, and is often associated with hookworm. Heavy infestation may cause abdominal pain and intestinal blood loss. Treatment is as for threadworm.

Tapeworms

Tapeworms have long, flattened bodies that in some species may be several metres in length. The most common are the beef tapeworm (*Taenia saginata*), the pig tapeworm (*Taenia solium*), and the fish tapeworm (*Diphyllobothrium latum*). Infestation occurs as a result of eating undercooked food containing the larvae of the worm. The head or scolex of the worm has suckers by which it obtains food from the intestinal wall. For cure the head must be detached from its hold and excreted; the mere separation of the body of the worm from the head results in the re-growth of the worm. For treatment see niclosamide (p. 267) and prazinquantel (p. 268).

Hydatid disease is due to the presence in the body of the larval cysts of *Echinococcus granulosus*, a tapeworm found in dogs. The larvae do not develop into adults in the human host, but the cysts, which may occur in the liver, lung and brain, may become quite large and cause pressure symptoms.

Blood flukes (trematodes)

Blood flukes or schistosomes are non-segmented flat worms, and are the cause of schistosomiasis or bilharzia, common in Egypt and some parts of Asia. In water, the eggs develop into larvae (*miracidia*), and then enter a secondary host, a snail. Further development leads to the later release of free-swimming *cercariae*, which are capable of penetrating the human skin, after which they reach the bloodstream and mature to adults. The flukes of *Schistosoma haematobium* are found mainly in the veins of the bladder, whereas *S. japonicum* and *S. mansoni* occur in the veins of the bowel. The eggs erode the vein wall and so reach the bladder or colon and are subsequently excreted. They cause haematuria, and gastrointestinal and liver ulceration. Repeated infestation with *S. haematobium* is the main cause of bladder cancer. For treatment see metriphonate (p. 267) and praziquantel (p. 268).

Filariae

The filariae are a large group of long, thread-like worms widely distributed in tropical and subtropical countries. The most important species are *Brugia malayi*, *Wuchereria bancrofti* and *Onchocerca volvulus*. Filariasis is contracted by the bite of a mosquito (*Brugia, Wuchereria*) or a Simulium blackfly (*Onchocerca*) carrying infected microscopic larvae (microfilariae).

With *Onchocerca*, the microfilariae usually remain in the skin, where they cause inflammatory reactions and severe itching, but they may also invade the eyes and cause 'river blindness'. With *Brugia* and *Wuchereria*, the microfilaria live in the circulation, but later migrate to the lymphatic tissues, where they cause inflammation, fibrosis, lymph node obstructiona and oedema, which after some years may result in elephantiasis. For treatment see diethylcarbamazepine and ivermectin below.

ANTHELMINTICS

Following the introduction of more specific anthelmintics, the treatment of worm infestation is now more effective, although the problem of mass treatment for parasitic worm eradication remains to be solved. Drug resistance has been reported in recent years, and a new threat is the transfer of some veterinary parasitic diseases to humans.

Albendazole § (dose: 800 mg daily)

Brand name: Eskazole §
Albendazole is chemically related to mebendazole and is of value in hydatid disease. It is given in doses of 400 mg twice a day for 28 days followed by a rest period of 14 days, before treatment is repeated for up to three cycles; similar doses as an adjunct to the surgical removal of hydatid cysts.

Side-effects include gastrointestinal disturbances, headache, rash and occasional alopecia. Blood counts and liver function tests should be carried out during treatment.

Diethylcarbamazine citrate §

Brand name: Hetrazan §
Diethylcarbamazine is one of the few compounds effective in the treatment of filariasis (except onchocerciasis). The dose is 1 mg/kg on the first day, increased over 3 days to 6 mg/kg daily in divided doses for 3 to 4 weeks. It induces rapid destruction of the microfilariae by the immune system of the body, but the death of the parasites often leads to a very severe allergic reaction, the Mazzotti reaction, with severe itching, rash, fever and hypotension.

Ivermectin §

Brand name: Mectizan §
Ivermectin has a selective action on the microfilariae of *Onchocerca volvulus* and it is now the preferred drug. Unlike diethylcarbamazine, it is well tolerated and is effective in onchocerciasis in a single dose of 150 micrograms/kg. It does not kill the adult worms

and treatment should be repeated annually until the adult worms die out, which may take years. Reactions such as itching and rash are mild and transient.

Levamisole §

Brand name: Ketrax §
Levamisole is highly effective against roundworm, and acts by paralysing the worm by a process of enzyme inhibition. It is considered by some to be the drug of choice, but although used abroad, paradoxically it is not marketed in the UK.

Levamisole is given as a single dose of 120–150 mg for adults, with doses for children based on 3 mg/kg. In hookworm, doses of 2.5–5 mg/kg daily for 2–3 days have been given. It is usually well tolerated, but care is necessary in severe hepatic and renal disease.

Mebendazole §

Brand name: Vermox §
Mebendazole is effective against threadworm, whipworm, roundworm and hookworm. For the treatment of threadworm infestation, a single dose of 100 mg is given, repeated after 2 or 3 weeks for all patients over the age of 2 years. For other worm infestations, doses of 100 mg twice a day for 2 or 3 days are necessary. Mebendazole is usually well tolerated but is not recommended for children under 2 years of age.

Metriphonate §

Brand name: Bilarcil §
Metriphonate is a cholinesterase inhibitor with a selective action against *Schistosoma haematobium*. It is given in doses of 7.5 mg/kg at intervals of 2 weeks for three doses.

Niclosamide §

Brand name: Yomesan §
Niclosamide is a widely used and effective drug against tapeworms. The adult dose is 2 g, taken in the morning after a light breakfast (tablets should be chewed or crushed and taken with fluid). A brisk purge should be given 2 hours later. Children of 2–6 years of age may be given half doses. The killed worms disintegrate, and there is no immediate proof of cure.

Side-effects are nausea, abdominal pain, pruritus and lightheadedness.

Piperazine

Piperazine is very effective for the expulsion of both roundworm and threadworm. For roundworm treatment in adults it is usually given as a single dose of 30 ml of an elixir (750 mg/5 ml); children of 1–3 years 10 ml, older children in single doses according to age. A second dose may be given after 2 weeks. It is well tolerated, but giddiness and nausea may occur. Caution is necessary in epilepsy and renal disease.

The drug paralyses the worms, and they are excreted in the faeces. As the worms are not killed, a purge may be necessary to ensure their expulsion before the effects of the drug wear off after about 5 hours.

In threadworm infestation a course of treatment for 1 week is given. Adults and children over 12 may be given 15 ml doses of the elixir once a day for 7 days; proportionate doses for children over 2 years. A second course may be given if required after an interval of a week. Threadworm infection is easily spread, and it is necessary to treat all members of a family at the same time to ensure eradication. Piperazine is well tolerated, but some nausea and giddiness may be experienced by a few patients on full doses. Pripsen is a mixed product containing piperazine 4 g together with a senna extract, and provides the anthelmintic and purge in a single dose.

Praziquantel §

Brand name: Biltricide §

Praziquantel is one of the most effective of schistosomicides available, as it is active against all human schistosomes and has few side-effects. It is given as a one-day treatment in two doses of 20 mg/kg, but against *Schistosoma japonicum* three doses of 30 mg/kg are necessary.

It may prove the drug of choice for mass treatment. It is also effective in tapeworm infestation in a single dose of 10–20 mg/kg.

Thiabendazole §

Brand name: Mintezol §

Thiabendazole is a wide-range anthelmintic, effective against *Strongyloides*, roundworm, threadworms, whipworms, guinea worm and 'creeping eruption'. It is sometimes useful against refractory hookworm. It is given in doses of 1.5 g twice daily with meals, continued for 2 or 3 days. In mixed threadworm infestation, a second course after 1 or 2 weeks may be required.

Side-effects are nausea, diarrhoea, dizziness and drowsiness. Hypersensitivity reactions with fever and rash may also occur.

ANTIMALARIALS AND OTHER DRUGS USED IN TROPICAL DISEASES

Malaria is a disease of tropical and sub-tropical countries, and causes more than two million deaths annually. Unfortunately, as a result of high speed travel from infected areas, and possibly from global warming, it now occurs in temperate climates, and treatment is increasingly difficult as drug resistance is now a problem.

Malaria is a febrile protozoal infection with a species of *Plasmodium*, either *P. vivax*, *P. malariae*, *P. ovale* or *P. falciparum*. *Plasmodium vivax* causes benign tertian malaria; *P. malariae* causes quartan malaria; *P. falciparum*, the most virulent form, causes malignant tertian malaria; and *P. ovale* causes ovale tertian malaria. *P. vivax* and *P. falciparum* infections take about 48 hours to develop, *P. ovale* about 50 hours, and *P. malariae* about 72 hours. Malignant tertian malaria is so-called because as well as causing the common chills and fever, the attacks may become fulminating, with cerebral disturbances, and may be fatal.

The life cycle of the malaria parasite is complex as the disease is transmitted by the bite of an infected female anopheline mosquito. In biting the victim, the mosquito injects *Plasmodium* sporozoites, which migrate to the liver and tissues where they mature after about 2 weeks into tissue schizonts (the exoerythrocyte stage). The mature schizonts rupture and release 10 000 to 40 000 merozoites, which reach the circulation and enter the erythrocytes. (Some may remain dormant in the liver and cause a relapse at a later date.) The merozoites in the red blood cells further divide to the point that the blood cells burst and release the new merozoites into the circulation, causing the typical malarial attack, which may recur at intervals as a new generation of merozoites is released. However, some merozoites mature in the erythrocytes and form male and female gametes. If these are ingested by a feeding anopheles mosquito, fertilization takes place with the formation of zygotes, which in turn invade the gut mucosa of the mosquito and develop into oocysts. The oocysts later develop into sporozoites that migrate to the salivary glands of the mosquito and are injected into the next victim, where the life cycle is repeated. Figure 22.1 indicates the general outline of the life cycle of the malarial parasites, and the points of attack of various drugs.

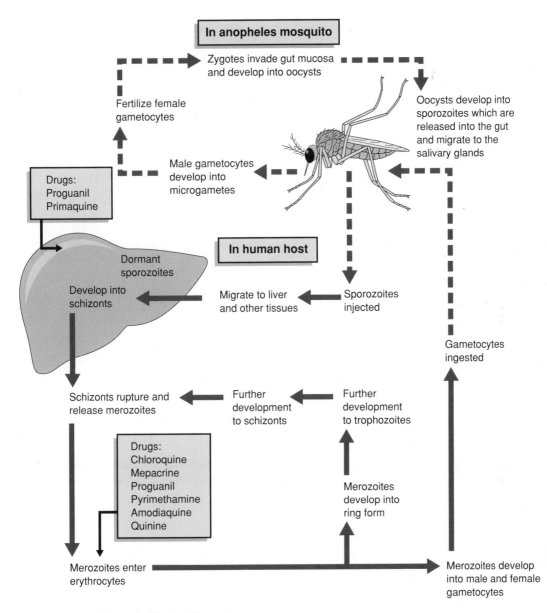

Figure 22.1   Life cycle of malarial parasites

Prophylaxis and treatment

So far, no vaccine against the malarial parasites has been developed (although DNA recombinant technology suggests that the problem may not be insoluble) and no drug has yet been found that will kill the sporozoites as injected by the mosquito. Treatment and prophylaxis are therefore directed against the organisms at a later stage of development. Drugs which act upon the parasites in the red blood cells are known as schizontocides, and those that attack the organisms in the tissues are referred to as tissue schizontocides.

The following notes refer to drugs in current use, but the prophylaxis and treatment of malaria is an increasingly difficult matter and expert advice should be sought. With the appearance of drug-resistant malaria, protection is increasingly difficult to achieve. Care is necessary even after return from a malarial area; any feverish illness occurring within 3 months of return could be malaria, and medical advice should be obtained immediately.

The mode of action of antimalarial drugs varies, as some inhibit the formation of folic acid required by the parasites, and others may interfere with the digestion of haemoglobin.

Chloroquine § (dose: 600 mg)

Brand names: Avloclor §, Nivaquine §
Chloroquine inhibits nucleic acid synthesis, and is used in the prophylaxis of malaria in areas where chloroquine resistance is not yet a problem, and in the treatment of benign tertian malaria. It is no longer recommended for falciparum malaria because of drug resistance. A standard dose is 600 mg initially, followed by 300 mg daily for 2 days. Chloroquine is usually well tolerated, but extended treatment may cause corneal opacity and pigment changes.

Halofantrine § ▼ (dose: 1.5 g)

Brand name: Halfan § ▼
Halofantrine has been used in chloroquine-resistant falciparum and vivax malaria, but the high risk of cardiac irregularities and arrhythmias has severely limited its value. It is given as three doses of 500 mg at 6-hourly intervals on an empty stomach, repeated after an interval of 1 week.

Mefloquine § (dose: 250 mg weekly)

Brand name: Lariam §
Mefloquine is used for the prophylaxis of drug-resistant malaria due to *Plasmodium falciparum* and chloroquine-resistant vivax malaria. For short-term prophylaxis extending over 3 months, mefloquine is given in doses of 250 mg weekly, starting 1–2 weeks before possible exposure to infection, and continuing for 4 weeks after leaving the area.

Side-effects are numerous and include gastro-intestinal disturbances, and dizziness and the drug should be withdrawn if any neuropsychiatric disturbances occur. Care is necessary in renal or hepatic impairment.

Primaquine § (dose: 15–60 mg daily)

Primaquine differs from most other antimalarials in acting upon the sporozoites in the liver and tissues, and on the gametocytes. It has little action on the erythrocytic forms of the parasites, and so is of no value alone in the treatment of acute malaria, but

given after a course of chloroquine, which kills off the erythrocytic stages, primaquine will promote the eradication of the remaining malarial parasites, and reduce the risk of relapse. It is used in the definitive treatment (radical cure) of benign tertian malaria in people returning from infected areas who are unlikely to be exposed to the risk of further infection. The dose is 15 mg of primaquine daily for 2–3 weeks weeks, after a standard course of chloroquine.

Quinine § (dose: 60–600 mg)

Quinine is of historical interest as the first effective drug for the treatment of malaria. It suppresses the development of the malarial parasites in the blood, but has no action against those in the tissues.

For some time it was virtually replaced by the synthetic antimalarials such as chloroquine, but the situation has changed markedly with the emergence of chloroquine-resistant strains of *Plasmodium falciparum*. In severe resistant malignant tertian malaria, quinine dihydrochloride, given by intravenous infusion is now the drug of choice. The standard dose is 10 mg/kg and three doses should be given at 8-hourly intervals.

In less severe infections quinine can be given orally in doses of 600 mg three times a day for 7 days. Following a course of treatment with quinine, it has been recommended that treatment should be concluded with a single dose of pyrimethamine 50–75 mg with sulfadoxine 1.5 g (equivalent to 3 tablets of Fansidar).

Suppressive treatment

In areas where malaria is common, re-infection may occur so easily after treatment that the prolonged use of a drug that will prevent development of the disease is essential. Chloroquine, already described and used mainly in the treatment of malarial attacks, is also used as a suppressive agent in weekly doses of 300 mg, but other useful prophylactic drugs are proguanil and pyrimethamine. Treatment should be commenced a week before possible exposure.

Proguanil § (dose: 100–300 mg daily)

Brand name: Paludrine §
Proguanil inhibits the development of the malarial parasites at several points, but in practice this action is too slow to be of value in the treatment of malaria attacks. Conversely, this slow action is of great advantage in suppressive treatment, and a daily dose of

200 mg will confer immunity on susceptible patients in some areas where malaria is common. In others, combined treatment with chloroquine 300 mg weekly may be necessary. Regular dosing is essential, as both *Plasmodium falciparum* and *Plasmodium vivax* may acquire a resistance to the drug if inadequate doses are given.

Pyrimethamine §

Brand name: Daraprim §

Pyrimethamine acts by interfering with the uptake of folic acid by the malarial organisms. Dapsone and sulphadoxine have a similar action but at a different stage of folic acid metabolism, and in practice pyrimethamine is always given in combination. Maloprim § contains pyrimethamine 12.5 mg together with dapsone 100 mg, and is used for prophylaxis in areas where there is a high risk of chloroquine-resistant falciparum malaria.

AMOEBIC DYSENTERY

Amoebic dysentery, also known as amoebiasis, is due to an infection with the protozon *Entamoeba histolytica*. It is mainly a tropical disease, and infection occurs when food or drink contaminated with the cyst form of the organism is ingested, or through symptomless human carriers. The cysts escape digestion in the stomach, but develop in the intestines and form trophozoites, which normally live on the mucosal surface as harmless commensals. Later, encysted forms develop and are passed in the faeces. Under certain and undefined conditions, the organism can become pathogenic and invade the intestinal mucosa, causing amoebic colitis, characterized by mucus, pus and blood in the stools. Complications include bowel perforation and peritonitis. The trophozoites may spread via the blood to reach the liver and cause hepatic abscess.

In some patients the disease runs a mild course, with apparent recovery. Some of these patients still harbour the cysts and may transmit the disease to others, and are referred to as 'carriers'.

Diloxanide furoate § (dose: 1.5 g daily)

Brand name: Furamide §

Diloxanide furoate has a specific action against *Entamoeba histolytica*, and is the preferred drug in the control of chronic infections and for the treatment of symptomless carriers of amoebic cysts. The standard adult dose of diloxanide is 500 mg three times a day for 10 days. It is also used after acute infections have been controlled to clear any remaining cysts from the intestines. Diloxanide is of no value in the treatment of hepatic amoe-biasis.

Side-effects are mild, but some flatulence, nausea and pruritus may occur.

Metronidazole § (dose: 1.2–2.4 g daily)

Brand name: Flagyl §

Metronidazole is the standard drug in the treatment of invasive amoebiasis, as it is effective at all sites of infection. In acute intestinal amoebiasis it is given in doses of 800 mg three times a day for 5 days, but in chronic conditions, and in amoebic liver abscess, doses of 400 mg three times a day are preferred. For symptomless carriers of the disease, doses of 400–800 mg three times a day for 5–10 days are given.

Tinidazole § (Fasigyn §, p. 72) has a similar action and use, and is given in doses of 1.5–2 g daily for 3–5 days.

LEISHMANIASIS

This tropical disease is due to *Leishmania*, protozoa transmitted by sandflies. They are intramacrophage parasites; *L. donovani* is found mainly in the liver and spleen, causing visceral leishmaniasis or kala-azar; *L. tropica* occurs in the skin, causing cutaneous leishmaniasis or oriental sore, and *L. brasiliensis* causes a progressive invasion of the mucocutaneous tissues of the nose and throat (espunda).

Sodium stibogluconate § (dose: 20 mg/kg daily by injection)

Brand name: Pentostam §

Sodium stibogluconate (sodium antimony gluconate) is the standard drug for the treatment of visceral and cutaneous leishmaniasis. It is given in doses of 20 mg/kg daily up to a maximum of 850 mg daily by intramuscular or intravenous injection. A further course may be given after a rest period. A 10-day dosage course is used in cutaneous leishmaniasis but it may cause very severe inflammation around the infected areas.

Anorexia, vomiting and diarrhoea are **side-effects**; cough and substernal pain may also occur, especially if the intravenous injection is given too quickly.

The form of kala-azar that occurs in the Sudan is resistant to antimony compounds, but may respond to pentamidine isethionate.

LEPROSY

This disease, although uncommon in the UK, may be seen more frequently as a consequence of air-travel from infected areas. It is caused by the Gram-positive organism *Mycobacterium leprae*, a close relative of the tubercle bacillus. It is spread by droplets, but the infectivity is low and it may be several years before the disease manifests itself.

Much of the pathology is attributable to the host immune response rather than to direct bacterial toxicity. In tuberculoid leprosy there is a marked cellular reaction, characterized by blotchy red lesions and damage to peripheral nerves, leading to loss of sensation, ulcers, muscle wasting and deformity. In lepromatous leprosy the tissue reaction is often slight or absent, and bacterial invasion of the mucous membranes may continue unchecked, resulting in extensive skin involvement with large numbers of the organisms in the infected areas. As the disease progresses, facial changes occur with the slow destruction of the bones of the nose and face.

As with tuberculosis, prolonged multi-drug treatment is required, usually with dapsone, clofazimine and rifampicin (p. 77). It should be noted that anaemia is frequent in leprosy, and the best response to treatment may not occur until the anaemia has been relieved.

Dapsone §

Dapsone acts indirectly by preventing the uptake of metabolites essential for the development of the leprosy bacillus. It is given in doses of 100 mg daily, with rifampicin 600 mg monthly, together with clofazimine 50 mg daily. Treatment with dapsone and other drugs must be prolonged up to 2 years or more.

Side-effects are allergic dermatitis, anorexia and anaemia. Neuropathy is a late complication of prolonged dapsone therapy.

Clofazimine §

Brand name: Lamprene §
Clofazimine is given in doses varying from 50 mg daily to 100 mg three times a week, but long-term treatment in association with other drugs is necessary. For lepra reactions doses of 300 mg daily for 3 months may be required. As it has some anti-inflammatory properties, it may give relief from the pain in swollen nerves that may occur in tuberculoid leprosy. Following absorption, the drug is deposited in the subcutaneous fat and slowly released.

It may cause a red pigmentation of the skin, and the lesions may acquire a bluish-black colour that may persist for some months after the course of treatment has ended.

TRYPANOSOMIASIS

This disease, also known as African sleeping sickness, is due to the presence in the blood of a flagellate parasite, either *Trypanosoma gambiense* or *Trypanosoma rhodesiense*. These parasites are transmitted from infected animals by the bite of the tsetse fly. The disease is characterized by a prolonged intermittent febrile condition, followed by a slow progressive mental and physical deterioration, ending in coma and death. The range of effective drugs is very limited, and early treatment is necessary.

Pentamidine isethionate § (dose: 4 mg/kg daily by injection)

Brand name: Pentacarinat §
Pentamidine is effective in the early stages of trypanosomiasis, but as it cannot cross the blood–brain barrier it is of much less value once the central nervous system has been invaded by the parasites. It is given by deep intramuscular or intravenous infusion in doses of 4 mg/kg daily or on alternate days, up to a total of ten injections. The course is repeated after a rest period of some weeks. For prophylaxis, a dose of 300 mg may be given every 6 months.

Pentamidine is also used in the treatment of *Pneumocystis carinii* pneumonia, sometimes referred to as pneumocystosis. The organism is a common cause of pneumonia in immunocompromised patients and in AIDS, and for treatment the standard dose of pentamidine should be given daily for 14 days. Pentamidine has also been used in the treatment of leishmaniasis.

Pentamidine has many and serious **side-effects**, including hypotension, hypoglycaemia, blood disorders and arrhythmias. The blood pressure should be monitored during administration of pentamidine, and regularly during treatment.

Suramin § (dose: 1 g weekly)

Suramin, once known as Antrypol, resembles pentamidine in its general properties and is most effective in the early stages of trypanosomiasis. After an initial test dose of 200 mg, doses of 20 mg/kg (up to 1 g) by slow intravenous injection are given at weekly intervals for 5 weeks. In the later stages of the disease it may be used in association with tryparsamide.

Suramin may cause vomiting and paraesthesia but a serious **side-effect** is albuminuria, and urine tests should be carried out during treatment. It is contra-indicated in renal disease.

Melarsoprol § (dose: 3.6 mg/kg intravenously)

Melarsoprol is an arsenical trypanocide that is effective in all stages of trypanosomiasis, but it is used mainly in the later stages of the disease in which the parasites have invaded the CSF. It is given by intravenous injection in doses of 3.6 mg/kg up to a maximum of 200 mg daily for 3 days, and repeated after a rest period of 7–10 days.

Side-effects are common and may be severe, and include hypersensitivity reactions. Another severe reaction, which has proved fatal, is a reactive encephalopathy, characterized by tremor, convulsions and coma, which is thought to be a Herxheimer reaction caused by antigens released from dead trypanosomes.

FURTHER READING

Ablon G R, Rosen T 1995 Helminthic skin infections: growing hazard in a shrinking world. Consultant May:631–639

Bradley D J, Warhurst D C 1995 Malaria prophylaxis: guidelines for travellers from Britain. British Medical Journal 310:709–714

Hay J, Dutton G N 1995 Toxoplasma and the eye. British Medical Journal 310:1021–1022

Kain K C 1993 Antimalarial chemotherapy in the age of drug resistance. Current Opinion in Infectious Diseases 6:803–811

Kerr-Muir M G 1994 *Toxocara canis* and human health. British Medical Journal 309:5–6

Mackenzie C D 1993 Anthelmintic therapy: current approaches and challenges. Current Opinion in Infectious Diseases 6:812–823

23

Immunology, immunoglobulins and vaccination

IMMUNOLOGY

The immune system is a protective one as it is concerned with the recognition and disposal of foreign matter that enters the body, usually invading and infection-causing micro-organisms, but now including life-saving organ-transplants. Resistance to such infection may be natural or innate, or acquired as the result of an adaptive immune response.

The adaptive immune system has two components, the B- and T-lymphocytes, the former evoking what is termed the humoral response, the latter referring to a cell-mediated response. Both B- and T-cells are produced in large numbers in the bone marrow, each with different surface receptors, and produce antibodies capable of responding to a particular antigen. Antigens are substances, usually protein in nature, that react with a specific antibody. Occasionally small metallic molecules can function as antigens, as may the individual's own body cells (autoantigens).

When activated by an antigen, B-cells appear in the lymph nodes and differentiate into plasma cells which secrete large amounts of antibodies (also known as immunoglobulins) that target the triggering antigens for destruction elsewhere in the immune system. Memory cells are also produced that do not secrete antibodies, but on re-exposure to the specific antigen at a later date they develop rapidly into antibody-producing cells.

The T-cells, which complete their development in the thymus gland, are similarly specific for a particular antigen, and after activation they proliferate and produce clones of specialized cells. Differentiated as helper T-cells they influence the production of antibodies by B-cells and stimulate other parts of the immune system, suppressor T-cells which produce cytokines that depress B-cell activity, and cytotoxic T-cells that act on cancer cells and virally infected cells, as well as memory cells (Fig. 23.1).

Acquired adaptive immunity

Acquired adaptive immunity may be natural or induced artificially. Natural immunity follows recovery from infection, and the degree and duration of such immunity varies with the type of the invading organism. Thus the recovery from diphtheria is followed by a high and prolonged degree of immunity, whereas the immunity following recovery from tetanus is brief and of low intensity. Acquired immunity is the result of the rapid production of antibodies by antigen-stimulated memory cells, and the response is so prompt that if the infection is mild, it may be symptomless, and the individual may not be aware that re-infection has occurred.

Active immunity may also be achieved artificially by vaccines, which are usually given by injection. Vaccines are antigen-containing preparations of living but attenuated or non-virulent strains of the organism against which immunity is desired. Alternatively, they may be preparations of chemically modified or inactivated organisms or their toxins or toxoids, the latter being toxins which have been deprived of some of their harmful properties, such as Tetanus Toxoid.

Passive acquired adaptive immunity

Passive immunity, like active immunity, can be natural or artificially acquired, and occurs when antibodies are transferred from one person to another. Natural passive immunity is acquired, for example, during pregnancy, when maternal antibodies cross the placenta and pass into the baby's blood, so giving the baby temporary protection against infection. In artificial passive immunity, products containing antibodies are given by injection. Such products were originally obtained from the blood of immunized horses, but reliance is now placed on selected human serum products containing various antibodies (immunoglobulins). With these human immunoglobulin preparations reactions are uncommon, but if an animal product is used, an initial test dose should be given to detect possible sensitivity.

Passive immunity with products such as diphtheria and tetanus antitoxins can be very effective and sometimes life-saving, but the protection thus obtained is short-lived and lasts only a few weeks.

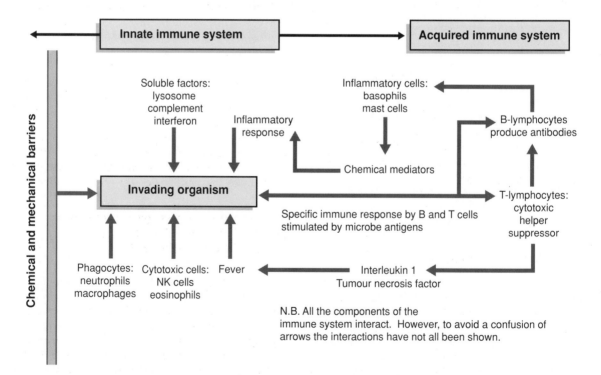

Figure 23.1 Components of the immune system.

Monoclonal antibodies

It is now possible to produce some specific antibodies by genetic engineering techniques that can target certain antigens more selectively, and such antibody therapy may prove to be an alternative to immunosuppressive drugs. There are also indications that monoclonal antibody therapy may be of value in a wide range of other disorders such as rheumatoid arthritis, psoriasis and systemic lupus erythematosus. The potential of such therapy is of considerable interest.

Immunoglobulins

Immunoglobulins (antibodies) are Y-shaped proteins with two main functions. The arms of the Y (the FAB fragments) are the recognition sites for the inactivation of specific antigens, and the tail of the Y (the Fc fragment) activates some of the defence systems of the body mediated via the B-lymphocytes. They markedly improve the effectiveness of the host response, and appear to neutralize the action of viruses by preventing the attachment of the virus particle to the host cell membrane.

The immunoglobulins have been classified as five groups, IgA, IgD, IgE, IgG and IgM. IgG is the most abundant, and is the major line of defence against infection in the first weeks of life. IgA protects the mucous membranes, and IgE is attached to mast cells. Cross-linkage of IgE with an antigen causes degranulation of the mast cell and release of histamine (p. 230). The level of IgE also rises in helminth infestation, and may play some part in the defence system against such parasites. IgM is the first immunoglobulin to be produced after antigen stimulation, and acts as a receptor on the surface of B-cells. IgD is also concerned with B-cell activation. The whole immune system is a very complex one, and Figure 23.1 gives a simplified indication of certain factors in that system and their different points of attack and interaction.

Auto-immune disorders

The immune system of the body recognizes the natural proteins of the body as such, but occasionally chemical compounds may couple with body proteins, and the new complex will be regarded as a foreign protein, leading to the formation of auto-antibodies and provoking an auto-immune reaction. Contact dermatitis and some forms of hypersensitivity to drugs are examples of such auto-immune reactions,

as is photosensitivity. The latter is a physically induced reaction, as ultraviolet light damages skin protein, and that damaged protein is not recognized as a normal body protein and so provokes an allergic reaction. Systemic lupus erythematosus, rheumatoid arthritis and some forms of haemolytic anaemia are also thought to be auto-immune disorders. Less frequently, a single organ may be involved, as in Hashimoto's thyroiditis.

Human normal immunoglobulin injection (HNIG) §

Brand names: Kabiglobulin §, Gammabulin §
This product is a fraction of pooled adult plasma obtained from at least 1000 individuals, and contains antibodies against mumps, measles, rubella, hepatitis and other common viral infections.

It is used by intramuscular injection to confer temporary protection on children who are unlikely to have developed adequate antibodies of their own. Specific human immunoglobulins obtained from the plasma of immunized individuals, or from patients recovering from an infection are also available for protection against tetanus, rabies, hepatitis B and varicella-zoster.

Human anti-D (Rho) § immunoglobulin is used to prevent a rhesus-negative mother from forming antibodies to fetal rhesus-positive blood cells that may pass into the maternal circulation. Such antibodies could produce haemolytic disease in subsequent children. The injection must be given within 72 hours of birth. The usual dose to the mother is 250–500 units by intramuscular injection. It is sometimes given in doses of 250 units.

For replacement therapy in hypogamma-globulinaemia, human normal immunoglobulin (HNIG) for *intravenous* injection is also available as Alphaglobin, Gamimune-N §, and Sandoglobulin §.

IMMUNOSUPPRESSION AND TRANSPLANT SURGERY

It has long been known that the body can recognize foreign tissues, and that grafts and transplant organs are rejected by the cell-mediated immunological response. As some cytotoxic agents are now used as immunosuppressants in transplant surgery, it is convenient to refer briefly to such drugs here. By the nature of their action, these drugs also depress the immune defences against infection and malignancy, so the treatment of immunocompromised patients is both difficult and complicated.

Azathioprine §

Brand names: Imuran §, Azamune §

Azathioprine is a derivative of mercaptopurine and has similar cytotoxic properties, but it is mainly used as an immunosuppressant in organ transplant surgery to reduce the risks of rejection of the organ and facilitate its acceptance and survival. It is given in doses that vary from 1 to 5 mg/kg daily, adjusted to individual requirements, and also depending on the use of other therapy such as the corticosteroids. It is sometimes given intravenously, but such use requires care as the solution is very irritant.

Careful control of treatment is essential as myelodepression may be severe. Other **side-effects** are hypersensitivity reactions, interstitial nephritis and liver damage.

Cyclosporin §

Brand names: Neoral §, Sandimmum §

Cyclosporin is a fungal metabolite and the discovery of its immunological properties added a new dimension to transplant surgery. It acts by inhibiting the proliferation of lymphocytes that is stimulated by the introduction of transplant tissues and it also inhibits the production of regulatory lymphokines such as interleukin-2. It does not depress haematopoiesis or the activity of phagocytes.

Cyclosporin is highly effective in organ transplantation generally, and in the control of graft-versus-host disease, and is given as a dose of 10–15 mg/kg some hours before transplantation, and continued at that level daily for 1–2 weeks. The dose is then slowly reduced by 2 mg/kg at intervals to a maintenance dose level of 6–8 mg/kg daily. The unpleasant taste can be disguised to some extent by giving the drug mixed with cold fruit juice or other liquid immediately before use. Cyclosporin may also be given by intravenous injection in doses of 3–5 mg/kg daily when oral therapy is not possible.

Side-effects include a dose-related rise in serum creatinine and urea (so kidney function should be monitored), hypertension and hepatotoxicity, hypertrichosis and tremor. A burning sensation in the hands and feet may occur during the first week of therapy, but unlike other immunosuppressive drugs cyclosporin is virtually free from myelotoxicity.

Mycophenylate mofetil § ▼

Brand name: Cellcept § ▼

Mycophenylate mofetil is a pro-drug that is metabolized to mycophenolic acid. That metabolite has an immunosuppressant action similar to but more selective than that of azathioprine. It is used prophylactically together with cyclosporin and corticosteroids in suppressing renal transplant rejection. It reduces the risks of acute rejection as well as the risks of opportunistic infections, although the incidence of leucopenia may be increased. It is given in doses of 1 g twice daily, starting within 72 hours of operation. The capsules should be taken with water on an empty stomach. Specialist literature should be consulted about **side-effects** and precautions. Full blood counts are necessary for months.

Tacrolimus § ▼

Brand name: Prograf § ▼

Tacrolimus is a macrolide derivative with the immunosuppressant actions and uses of cyclosporin. It appears to inhibit cytotoxic lymphocytes, the white cells thought to be responsible for the rejection of grafted organs. It also inhibits T-cell activation and T-helper cell proliferation. It is used as a primary immunosuppressive agent in liver and kidney transplantation where there is a risk of resistance to other immunosuppressive agents. Dose 50–100 micrograms/ kg twice a day, or by intravenous infusion over 24 hours. Cardiac hypertrophy and myopathy have been reported as **side-effects**, and specialist literature should be consulted.

IMMUNOSTIMULANTS

Immunostimulants such as the interferons are of increasing importance. Interferon alfa (Intron-A §, Roferon-A §, Viraferon §) is used in the treatment of leukaemia, lymphoma and some solid tumours, interferon beta-1a (Avonex §) and interferon beta-1b (Betaferon §) are used in multiple sclerosis, and interferon gamma-1b is indicated in chronic granulomatous disease.

Multiple sclerosis is a demyelinating disease of the central nervous system in which the immune system is over-active. The cause is unknown, but the disease is associated with increased T-cell proliferation and T-suppressor cell function is correspondingly low. Interferon beta-1b promotes the restoration of T-suppressor cell function and the inhibition of excessive T-cell proliferation. It is mainly of value in reducing the frequency and severity of the exacerbations of the disease, but the recurrence and remission of symptoms varies considerably from patient to patient. Specialist literature should be consulted for dosage and side-effects.

DIAGNOSTIC PRODUCTS

In a few cases, serological products are available which can be used to detect those individuals who lack a natural immunity.

Schick test

This test is occasionally used to detect susceptibility to diphtheria, and is carried out by the intradermal injection of 0.2 ml of a weak solution of diphtheria toxin. A positive reaction is shown by the development of a red area 10–50 mm in diameter. A negative response is not an absolute test of immunity as young children are rarely immune, and the test is used mainly for older children and young adults.

BCG tuberculin test

BCG vaccine is a live attenuated strain derived from *Mycobacterium bovis* which when given by intradermal injection, stimulates the development of a localized hypersensitivity to *M. tuberculosis*. A positive reaction is the development of a papule within 2–6 weeks which progresses to a benign ulcer of about 10 mm in diameter which heals after a few weeks.

A positive reaction indicates that the individual has been infected at some time with the tubercle bacillus, but it does not distinguish between past infection and present disease, except in young children. A positive reaction in a young child is an indication of an active infection that requires immediate treatment. In adults the diagnostic value of a positive test is of much less significance, but a reaction in a person known to have been a non-reactor is an indication of a new infection.

VACCINES (INCLUDING TOXOIDS) FOR ACTIVE IMMUNIZATION OR PROPHYLAXIS §

The following list of immunological products includes some that are available only from designated laboratories.

Immunological products are quickly inactivated unless properly stored, and as a general rule they should be refrigerator-stored between 2 and 8°C, unless advised otherwise. They should not be allowed to freeze. Vaccines are often suspensions, and should be well shaken immediately before use to ensure that the proper dose is injected.

Anthrax vaccine. Dose: 0.5 ml by intramuscular or deep subcutaneous injection, repeated at intervals of 3 weeks for three doses, with a final injection after 6 months. Reinforcing doses of 0.5 ml should be given at yearly intervals.

Bacillus Calmette–Guerin vaccine (BCG). Dose: 0.1 ml as a single intradermal prophylactic injection against tuberculosis. A vaccine prepared from isoniazid-resistant organisms is also available, as well as a special *percutaneous* preparation. The vaccine may lead to keloid formation in some skin areas, and the injection site should be chosen with the cosmetic result in mind. In the Mantoux test for the diagnosis of tuberculosis, a solution of 10 units of Tuberculin Purified Protein Derivative (PPD) is given by intradermal injection. A positive reaction is an area of palpable induration of 6 mm or more, often surrounded by erythema. The result should be read after 72 hours.

Botulism antitoxin. Dose for prophylaxis 20 ml by intramuscular injection as soon as possible after exposure; repeated doses by intravenous infusion.

Cholera vaccine. Dose: 0.5 ml initially by deep subcutaneous or intramuscular injection. It is now rarely used, as the protection is poor and it is no longer required for foreign travel.

Diphtheria vaccine. Adsorbed vaccine. Dose: 0.5 ml by intramuscular or deep subcutaneous injection, followed by three further doses at intervals of 4 weeks. Now usually given as the triple vaccine (diphtheria, tetanus and pertussis).

Hepatitis A vaccine. A vaccine containing inactivated hepatitis A virus grown in human cells. It is given by intramuscular injection, preferably in the deltoid area, as an initial dose of 1 ml, the second dose six months later.

Hepatitis B vaccine. A vaccine prepared from inactivated hepatitis B virus antigen, and obtained from yeast cells by recombinant DNA technology. It is given in doses of 1 ml by intramuscular injection, the second 1 month after the first, and the third 6 months after the initial dose.

Influenza vaccine. Dose: 0.5 ml by deep subcutaneous or intramuscular injection. The virus strains are grown in chick embryo, and the vaccine is contra-indicated in those hypersensitive to eggs or feathers.

Measles vaccine. Now replaced by MMR vaccine.

MMR vaccine. A combined measles, mumps and rubella vaccine, given routinely to children before primary school. Dose: 0.5 ml by intramuscular or subcutaneous injection. It may cause a febrile reaction, and is contra-indicated in egg allergy. It is not suitable for prophylaxis after exposure to mumps and rubella, as the onset of immunity is too slow.

Meningococcal polysaccharide vaccine. Contains one or more of the polysaccharide antigens of *Neisseria meningitidis* A and C. It is used in those countries where the risk of meningitis is high. Dose: 0.5 ml by deep subcutaneous or intramuscular injection.

Mumps vaccine. A live attenuated virus vaccine that induces protective antibodies in most non-immune individuals. Dose: 0.5 ml by subcutaneous injection. Not intended for children under 1 year of age. Contra-indicated in hypersensitivity to eggs or feathers. *Brand name:* Mumpsvax.

Pertussis vaccine. Dose: 0.5 ml by deep subcutaneous or intramuscular injection, repeated after 4 weeks and again after 6 months. It should not be given to children with a history of convulsions. Encephalopathy is a rare complication. It is often given as diphtheria, tetanus and pertussis vaccine.

Pneumococcal vaccine. Contains a mixture of the polysaccharide capsular antigens of *Streptococcus pneumoniae*. Dose: 0.5 ml by deep subcutaneous or intramuscular injection. Used when the risk of pneumococcal pneumonia is high, as with patients following splenectomy. Hypersensitivity reactions may occur, and re-vaccination is not recommended.

Poliomyelitis vaccine (inactivated). Dose: 0.5 ml by subcutaneous or intramuscular injection, followed by a second dose after 4–6 weeks, and a third dose after 8–12 months. The oral vaccine is preferred.

Poliomyelitis vaccine (oral). It contains three virus types. In infants the first dose should be given at the age of 6 months, the second dose 6–8 weeks later, and the third dose after 4–6 months.

Rabies vaccine. A human rabies vaccine is available for prophylaxis and treatment.

Rubella vaccine. Dose: 0.5 ml by deep subcutaneous injection. If rubella (German measles) is contracted in early pregnancy, there is a risk of damage to the fetus. Rubella vaccine should be given to all girls between the ages of 11 and 14 years, and to other females at risk, provided that they are not pregnant.

Tetanus vaccine (tetanus toxoid). Dose: 0.5–1 ml by deep subcutaneous or intramuscular injection, repeated after intervals of 6–12 weeks and 4–6 months.

Typhoid vaccine. Typhoid vaccine (Typhim VR) is prepared from the capsular polysaccharides of the organisms, and is given as a single dose of 0.5 ml by deep subcutaneous or intramuscular injection. Subsequent doses can be given at 3-year intervals when exposure is continuous. A live oral vaccine (Vivotif) is given as capsules, one to be taken daily on alternate days for three doses. Protection may persist for 3 years. (*Note:* Capsules should be refrigerator-stored.)

Table 23.1 Vaccination schemes (vaccination against smallpox is no longer used).

Age	Vaccine	Interval
During the first year of life	Diphtheria, tetanus, pertussis and oral polio vaccine (three doses); *Haemophilus* vaccine	The first dose should be given 2 months after birth, the second and third at monthly intervals
1–2 years	Measles, mumps and rubella vaccine; *Haemophilus* vaccine	
School entry	Diphtheria, tetanus and oral polio vaccine; measles, mumps, rubella vaccine if not already given	
10 and 13 years	BCG vaccine Rubella vaccine	For tuberculin-negative children All girls of this age group should receive rubella vaccine; an interval of 3 weeks should elapse between rubella and BCG vaccination
15–19 years Adults	Polio vaccine (oral) Tetanus vaccine Reinforcing doses of polio vaccine Rubella vaccine for susceptible women of child-bearing age	

Yellow fever vaccine. Dose: 0.5 ml by subcutaneous injection. Immunity persists for at least 10 years.

Note: The so-called desensitizing vaccines, used in the treatment of certain allergic conditions, are not true vaccines. They are weak solutions of various protein products known to be associated with allergic reactions, and are referred to on p. 230.

Vaccination schemes

Vaccination schemes have been designed to give protection during childhood and beyond against many common infections. A standard scheme is outlined in Table 23.1.

FURTHER READING

Anon 1995 New drugs. Tacrolimus (Prograf): a new choice to prevent organ rejection. American Journal of Nursing 95(4):55–56
Beardsley T 1995 Better than a cure. Scientific American Jan.:88–95
Bedford H, Moreton J 1997 Childhood immunisation. Nursing Standard 11(28):49–56
Cochrane S 1997 Care of patients undergoing immunoglobulin therapy. Nursing Standard 11(41):44–46
Cook R 1997 Adult immunisation. Nursing Standard 11(29):50–55
Cook R 1997 Influenza vaccination. Nursing Standard 12(1):49–56
Kahn B D 1989 Cyclosporin. New England Journal of Medicine 321:1725–1738

Lake K D, Kilkenny J M 1992 The pharmacokinetics and pharmacodynamics of immunosuppressive agents. Critical Care Nursing Clinics of North America 4(2):205–221
Leeming J 1995 Risks and benefits. Nursing Standard 9(34):22–23
Llewelyn M B, Hawkins R E, Russell S J 1992 Discovery of antibodies. British Medical Journal 305:1269–1272
Mollnes T E, Harboe M 1996 Clinical immunology. British Medical Journal 312:1465–1469
O'Donnell M, Parmenter K L 1996 Transplant medications. Critical Care Nursing Clinics of North America 8(3):253–271
Russell S J, Llewelyn M B, Hawkins R E 1992 Principles of antibody therapy. British Medical Journal 305:1424–1429

24

The vitamins

Experiments during the early part of the present century showed that artificial diets containing adequate amounts of protein, fats, carbohydrates, minerals and water could not maintain growth and health. Some other factors present in normal diets were necessary, and these factors are now well known as vitamins.

They differ widely in their chemical nature, and although the exact function of some vitamins is still obscure, they are closely concerned with various enzyme systems of the body. When first discovered they were identified by letters, but many have since been synthesized and are referred to by their chemical names. Reference will be made mainly to vitamins A, B, C, D, E and K. Vitamins C and E are exceptional, as they are also anti-oxidants and oppose the actions of reactive oxygen free radicals that are generated in the body and cause damage to DNA and other biomolecules. Endogenous anti-oxidants cannot provide an adequate defence against such radicals and inhibit such damage, so diet-derived anti-oxidants are necessary for the maintenance of health.

VITAMIN DEFICIENCY

A good mixed diet provides adequate amounts of vitamins so vitamin supplements are normally unnecessary, and are of no value as 'tonics'. Restricted diets, or defective absorption or utilization of food result in vitamin deficiencies which lead to a number of recognizable conditions (Table 24.1) and require the administration of the appropriate vitamins.

Deficiencies may occur in alcoholics, food faddists, and in the elderly on poor diets, and also when natural demands for vitamins are increased, as in

Table 24.1 Vitamins

Vitamin	Some deficiency symptoms	Some effects of overdose
Vitamin A[a] (retinol)	Night blindness, drying of mucous membranes, uncommon in the UK	Rash, pruritus, liver disease
Vitamin B_1 (thiamine) (aneurine)	Beri-beri, polyneuritis, uncommon in the UK	
Vitamin B_2 (riboflavine)	Cracking of corners of the mouth, uncommon in the UK	
Vitamin B_3 (nicotinamide)	Pellagra, a syndrome of dermatitis, diarrhoea and delirium, uncommon in UK	Peptic ulcer, hypotension, pruritus Hepatotoxicity
Vitamin B_6 (pyridoxine)	Polyneuritis, uncommon in the UK	Peripheral neuropathy
Vitamin B_{12} (cyanocobalamin)	Pernicious anaemia	
Vitamin C (ascorbic acid)	Scurvy, easy bruising	Oxalate stones in susceptible individuals
Vitamin D[a] (calciferol) (cholecalciferol)	Rickets, osteomalacia, common in steatorrhoea	Hypercalcaemia, renal calcinosis, hypertension
Vitamin E[a] (tocopherol)	Unknown	Potentiation of oral anticoagulants
Vitamin K_1,[a] (phytomenadione)	Prolonged bleeding, easy bruising	Haemolytic anaemia

[a] Fat-soluble vitamins.

fevers, pregnancy and metabolic disorders such as diabetes. A deficiency of vitamin B_{12} invariably develops after total gastrectomy and may also occur in vegans (total vegetarians). Drugs which have a bactericidal action on the organisms normally present in the intestines, such as some oral antibiotics, may also indirectly cause a vitamin deficiency. In such circumstances relatively small doses of vitamins are adequate to rectify the deficiency, but in certain unrelated conditions some vitamins are given in large doses, and should then be regarded as therapeutic agents and not as dietary supplements and in overdose may have toxic side-effects (Table 24.1).

Vitamins present in food can be divided into two classes, the fat-soluble and the water-soluble vitamins. The fat-soluble vitamins include vitamins A, D, E and K; the water-soluble vitamins are represented by vitamins B and C. As many vitamins are now made synthetically, and water-soluble derivatives are often available, this distinction between fat-soluble and water-soluble vitamins has become less important.

VITAMIN A

Vitamin A (retinol) (prophylactic dose: 4000 units; therapeutic dose: 50 000 units daily)

Vitamin A may be present in various foods as such, or as the closely related compound carotene, from which the vitamin can be formed in the body. Dietary sources of the vitamin include milk, butter, carrots and green vegetables, and vitamin A deficiency is uncommon. Fish liver oils contain large amounts together with vitamin D. Vitamin A deficiency is rare in the UK.

Vitamin A is concerned with the growth and maintenance of the epithelial tissues, as well as with normal vision, as it plays an essential part in the formation of the visual purple. A deficiency may

---

Nursing points about vitamins

(a) Used in specific deficiency states, most of which are uncommon in the UK.
(b) Usually unnecessary if a good mixed diet is taken.
(c) Of no value as 'tonics'.
(d) Excessive doses of vitamins A and D have toxic effects.
(e) Treatment of pernicious anaemia with vitamin B_{12} is for life.

lead to night blindness and, if prolonged, to a keratinized condition of the cornea (xerophthalmia) which cannot be relieved by subsequent treatment with vitamin A.

The chief value of vitamin A is in deficiency states such as coeliac disease and sprue, or where absorption has been reduced by the excessive use of liquid paraffin as a laxative. It may be given as capsules of halibut liver oil, containing 4000 units, as cod liver oil or as the synthetic vitamin. In severe deficiency states vitamin A can be given by deep intramuscular injection in doses of 150 000 units monthly. In liver disease doses of 100 000 units are given every 2–4 months. Overdose causes toxic effects such as rough skin, enlargement of the liver and serum calcium disturbance. Care is necessary to avoid overdose with vitamin A supplements in pregnancy, as high levels of the vitamin may cause birth defects. Liver products should also be avoided.

VITAMIN B GROUP

This group or complex includes several water-soluble vitamins that usually occur together in various foods and are concerned with the metabolism of proteins, fats and carbohydrates. The term 'vitamin B' was originally applied to what was thought to be a single substance, distinguished later as vitamins B_1, B_2, B_6, B_{12} etc. Since then more specific names have been introduced. Deficiency rarely occurs singly, and administration of all the main vitamins of the group is usually advisable. With the exception of vitamin B_{12}, vitamin B deficiency is rare in the UK.

Thiamine (prophylactic dose: 2–10 mg daily; therapeutic dose in severe deficiency: 200–300 mg daily by intramuscular injection)

Brand name: Benerva
Thiamine, also known as vitamin B_1 and aneurine, is essential for the utilization of carbohydrates and the nutrition of nerve cells. It is present in egg, liver, yeast and wheatgerm, but is now made synthetically. Severe deficiency, which is uncommon in the UK, results in beri-beri, a condition characterized by peripheral neuritis, cardiac enlargement, oedema and mental disturbances. Nausea and vomiting occur during the early stages of thiamine deficiency, and thus lead to further losses of the vitamin. In such conditions, thiamine is given in doses that may

vary from 25 to 300 mg daily according to the severity of the deficiency, and doses of 200–300 mg may also be given daily by intramuscular injection.

Thiamine is also given in the treatment of the various manifestations of polyneuritis, in gastrointestinal disorders, and during the administration of wide-range antibiotics. In alcoholism and severe deficiency states, large doses of thiamine are usually given by intramuscular or slow intravenous injection in association with other vitamins of the B group, and with vitamin C in products such as *Pabrinex*. Severe allergic reactions may occur during or soon after thiamine injections, and anaphylactic therapy must be immediately available.

Riboflavine (prophylactic dose: 1–4 mg daily; therapeutic dose: 5–10 mg daily)

A deficiency of riboflavine (vitamin B_2) results in a syndrome characterized by cracking of the lips and of the skin at the corners of the mouth (angular stomatitis), photophobia and other visual disturbances. Treatment with a mixed vitamin B preparation is usually required.

Nicotinic acid (prophylactic dose: 15–30 mg daily; therapeutic dose: 50–250 mg daily)

Nicotinic acid is present in liver, yeast and unpolished rice but it is now made synthetically. Lack of nicotinic acid, often associated with a maize-rich diet, results in the deficiency disease known as pellagra, characterized by diarrhoea, dermatitis and dementia. These symptoms, as well as the mental confusion, respond rapidly to nicotinic acid and associated vitamins.

Nicotinic acid also has vasodilatory properties, and has been used in Meniere's disease, peripheral vascular disorders and chilblains (p. 125) and as a blood-lipid lowering agent (p. 129).

Nicotinamide is closely related to nicotinic acid, and is used in pellagra and other deficiency states when the vasodilator action of the acid is not desired.

Pyridoxine (vitamin B_6) (dose: 50–150 mg daily)

Brand name: Benadon
Pyridoxine is concerned with the metabolism of proteins, amino acids and fats, and is present in a wide variety of foods. Deficiency results in peripheral neuritis, which although uncommon, may arise during treatment with isoniazid as well as in sideroblastic

anaemia. Pyridoxine has been used empirically in the nausea of pregnancy, in irradiation sickness and alcoholism, and in premenstrual syndrome, but not with marked success. Pyridoxine may reduce the response to levodopa in Parkinson's disease.

Cyanocobalamin (vitamin B₁₂) § (dose: 1 mg by injection)

Brand name: Cytamen §

Cyanocobalamin is the anti-anaemia factor, and its use in pernicious anaemia is discussed on p. 143. It has virtually been replaced by hydroxocobalamin.

VITAMIN C

Ascorbic acid (therapeutic dose: 200–600 mg daily; prophylactic dose: 25–75 mg daily)

Brand name: Redoxon

Ascorbic acid is the water-soluble vitamin present in oranges and other citrus fruits, blackcurrants and green vegetables. It is essential for the development of collagen, cartilage and bone, and is concerned in haemoglobin formation and tissue repair. Mild deficiency states may occur during pregnancy and in patients on restricted diets, and chronic marginal deficiency of vitamin C, especially in the elderly, may be more common than is normally suspected.

Severe vitamin C deficiency, now uncommon, causes scurvy, characterized by subcutaneous haemorrhages. Infantile scurvy may sometimes occur in bottle-fed infants. Vitamin C requirements are increased during infections and following trauma, and the drug has been given to promote wound healing. Very large doses have been used in the treatment of the common cold, but the response is not impressive.

VITAMIN D

Calciferol (vitamin D₂ [therapeutic dose: 5000–50 000 units (125 micrograms– 1.25 mg) daily; prophylactic dose: not more than 800 units (20 micrograms) daily]

The term vitamin D includes several related substances, of which calciferol, also known as ergocalciferol (vitamin D₂), is the most important. Vitamin D is found mainly in dairy products, and it is also formed as cholecalciferol, vitamin D₃, in the body by the action of sunlight on the skin. Although fish liver oils are a rich source, calciferol is now prepared synthetically. It is an essential factor in the absorption of calcium and phosphorus from the gastrointestinal tract, and thus in the formation of bone. See Fig. 24.1.

In children, a deficiency of calciferol results in rickets, a disease characterized by weak bones, bowed

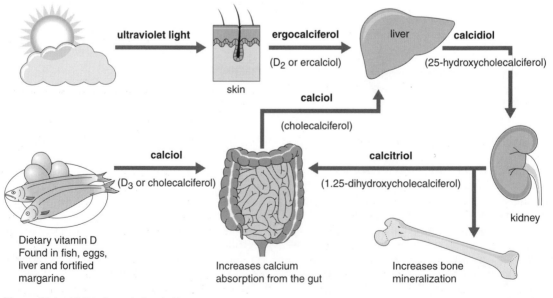

Figure 24.1 Metabolism of vitamin D.

legs and deformities of the chest. In confirmed rickets in children, the standard treatment is a daily dose of 1000–1500 units of calciferol, but occasionally a single dose of 300 000 units is given by intramuscular injection. Calciferol is also used in certain other conditions associated with calcium deficiency as in coeliac disease, and in the low blood calcium due to parathyroid deficiency. (The use of some vitamin D derivatives in psoriasis is referred to in Chapter 21.)

In general, the vitamins are well tolerated even in very large doses, but calciferol is the main exception, as **toxic effects** may follow the prolonged administration of high doses. Thirst, drowsiness and gastrointestinal disturbances, which may be severe, are among the symptoms of overdosage, and continued administration may result in the release of calcium from bone and its storage in the tissues, kidneys and arterial vessels, causing renal damage and hypertension.

Alfacalcidol § (dose: 0.25–5 micrograms daily) (hydroxycholecalciferol)

Brand names: Alfa D §, One-Alpha §
The action of calciferol is mediated by its conversion in the kidneys and liver to the much more potent hydroxylated metabolite calcitriol (Fig. 20.1). In renal impairment that conversion may be incomplete, and the response to calciferol less satisfactory. Alfacalcidol is a calciferol derivative which bypasses the renal stage of vitamin D metabolism and is converted in the liver to the final and most active metabolite calcitriol (dihydroxyvitamin D$_3$).

Alfacalcidol is indicated in a variety of conditions associated with disturbances in the biosynthesis of calcitriol, including renal osteodystrophy, osteomalacia, vitamin D resistance and hypoparathyroidism. The response to alfacalcidol is prompt and more controllable than that of slower-acting forms of vitamin D. It is given initially in doses of 1 microgram daily (half doses for the elderly) subsequently adjusted according to response as shown by changes in the plasma calcium levels, with maintenance doses of 0.25–1 micrograms daily. In severe conditions, similar doses may be given by intravenous injection. Absorption may be impaired by aluminium-based antacids, and the risks of hypercalcaemia are increased in patients taking thiazide diuretics or any calcium-containing products. The main **side-effect** is hypercalcaemia, which requires withdrawal of treatment, after which the normal plasma calcium level returns in about a week, when treatment can be resumed with half doses.

Calcitriol § (dose: 0.5–1 microgram daily)

Brand name: Rocaltrol §
Calcitriol (dihydroxyvitamin D$_3$) is the metabolite derived from calciferol formed in the liver, and is characterized by its high potency. Like alfacalcidol, it is used to correct abonormalites of calcium and phosphate metabolism, mainly when such abnormalities are associated with chronic renal failure as in renal osteodystrophy and proven postmenopausal osteoporosis. Calcitriol reduces the associated hypocalcaemia, and relieves the symptoms of bone disease.

The initial dose is 250 nanograms daily or on alternate days, slowly increased as required by increments of 250 nanograms at intervals of 3–4 weeks. Calcitriol is also used by intravenous injection as Calciject in the treatment of hypocalcaemia in dialysis patients. Dose 500 nanograms three times a week according to need. As with alfacalcidol, dosage requires careful and continued control.

Dihydrotachysterol § (dose: 250 micrograms–2 mg)

Brand name: AT10 §
Dihydrotachysterol is related to calciferol, but it has an action resembling that of the parathyroid hormone. It increases the absorption of calcium, and is used together with calcium gluconate in the hypocalcaemia due to parathyroid deficiency. It is given initially in doses of 750 micrograms daily, but maintenance doses vary from 250 micrograms to 1 mg or more, adjusted to the serum calcium levels. Excessive doses lead to decalcification of bone, hypercalcaemia and renal damage.

VITAMIN E

Tocopherol (dose: 10–200 mg daily)

Brand name: Ephynal
Tocopherol, also known as vitamin E, is an antioxidant present in wheatgerm, soyabean, lettuce and other green leaves, but the synthetic drug is referred to as alpha tocopherol. The vitamin has some general action on the metabolism of fats, carbohydrates and proteins but a deficiency is not followed by any clear symptoms. Tocopherol has been used empirically in muscular dystrophy, angina, Dupuytren's contracture, vascular disease and in certain anaemias in children, and for malabsorption in cystic fibrosis. In

general, the response to tocopherol treatment is variable and often disappointing.

MIXED VITAMIN PRODUCTS

Many mixed vitamin products are available, often containing mineral supplements. These mixtures are mainly of value in the treatment of deficiencies due to restricted diets but have no 'tonic' properties. A few are useful during the prenatal period, but their value in other conditions where full diets are available is problematical.

Some polyvitamin preparations are represented by Abidec, Dalivit and Forceval.

VITAMIN K

Vitamin K is essential for the formation of pro-thrombin in the liver, as well as the production of accessory factors essential for the functioning of the blood-clotting system (p. 133). Lack of vitamin K leads to hypoprothrombinaemia, or deficiency of prothrombin, resulting in delayed clotting of the blood and, if severe, to spontaneous haemorrhage.

The natural vitamin, which is present in green vegetables and eggs and is formed in the intestines by bacteria, is fat-soluble, and bile is essential for its absorption. A deficiency may therefore arise, even during an adequate dietary intake, in such conditions as obstructive jaundice or coeliac disease.

Deficiency may also occur during treatment with anticoagulants, which reduce vitamin K metabolism, and with antibacterial drugs which interfere with vitamin K synthesis by intestinal bacteria. Salicylates and clofibrate may also decrease the availability of vitamin K. Synthetic water-soluble compounds with a similar but more controllable action are now used instead of the natural vitamin.

Menadiol (dose: 10–40 mg daily)

Menadiol sodium phosphate is a water-soluble ana-logue of vitamin K and is suitable for the treatment of most forms of hypoprothrombinaemia. It is also used for the prophylaxis of haemorrhagic conditions associated with obstructive jaundice, or following the prolonged administration of salicylates or other drugs that may extend the bleeding time. Menadiol is given orally in doses of 10–40 mg daily according to need. Care is necessary in G6PD deficiency (p. 146) as there is some risk of haemolysis.

Phytomenadione § (dose: 5–20 mg orally, or by slow intravenous injection)

Brand name: Konakion §

Phytomenadione is a natural form of vitamin K, and is also referred to as vitamin K_1. It is an essential co-factor in the hepatic synthesis of prothrombin and other clotting factors, and its physiological function is the maintenance of the normal level of prothrom-bin in the blood. Therapeutically it is used to counteract the haemorrhage that may occur during oral anticoagulant therapy with synthetic drugs. (It is not an antidote to heparin.) In such cases, phytomenadione acts more rapidly than the water-soluble synthetic drugs such as menadiol, and the action is more prolonged (p. 134).

In severe haemorrhage, an initial dose of 10–20 mg may be given by slow intravenous injection. The prothrombin level should be determined 3 hours later, and subsequent doses adjusted according to need. For less severe conditions, phytomenadione may be given orally in doses of 10 mg, or by intra-muscular injection. (Tablets should be chewed or allowed to dissolve in the mouth.)

In the prophylactic treatment of haemorrhagic disorders of the newborn, the drug may be given to the mother by intramuscular injection in doses of 1–5 mg before delivery. It may also be given to the baby as a single dose of 0.5–1 mg, especially if intracranial or other haemorrhage is anticipated.

Opinion is still divided on the safety and route of administration of vitamin K_1, and local practice should be followed.

FURTHER READING

Blair K A 1986 Vitamin supplementation and megadoses. Nurse Practioner 11(7):19–36

Dickerson J 1993 Ascorbic acid, zinc and wound healing. Journal of Wound Care 1(3):45–55

Halliwell B 1996 Antioxidants in human health and disease. Annual Review of Nutrition 16:33–50

Wald N J, Bower C 1995 Folic acid and the prevention of neural tube defects. British Medical Journal 310:1019–1020

Watson N J, Hutchinson C H, Atta H R 1995 Vitamin A deficiency and xerophthalmia in the United Kingdom. British Medical Journal 310:1050–1051

25

Fluid therapy and clinical nutrition

BODY WATER AND ELECTROLYTES

The metabolic processes of the body depend on adequate supplies of water and electrolytes. In adults, water accounts for about 60% of the body weight, divided into two main compartments: the intracellular and the extracellular spaces. The intracellular water is about 40% of the body weight, the extracellular fluid accounts for about 20%.

The electrolytes are the mineral constituents of body fluids, of which the chief are sodium, potassium, calcium and magnesium, present as chlorides, sulphates and bicarbonates. These metallic salts dissociate in solution and form ions; the metallic ions are positively charged and are termed cations, whereas the chloride and other non-metallic ions are negatively charged and are termed anions. Both the intracellular and extracellular fluids contain similar ions but in different proportions, as the intracellular fluid contains more potassium, but the extracellular fluid contains most of the sodium. That difference is maintained by the sodium–potassium–adenosine triphosphate pump system in the cell membrane (the $Na^+K^+ATPase$ pump), which controls the intercellular movement of sodium ions in exchange for potassium ions.

ELECTROLYTE BALANCE AND INTRAVENOUS INFUSION

In illness the normal electrolyte/fluid balance of the body may be disturbed by the internal redistribution of water, as for example in oedema where there is an excess of interstitial fluid, or by the marked loss of water and electrolytes by prolonged vomiting, severe diarrhoea or over-treatment with diuretics. In diabetic coma the loss of electrolytes, especially potassium, may lead to respiratory and circulatory collapse, requiring rapid restoration of both fluid and electrolyte balance. Several standard intravenous fluid and electrolyte solutions are in use (Table 25.1).

Nurses should ensure that intravenous infusion fluids are run at the required rate, and monitor both fluid input and output. The infusion drip-rate can be calculated from the following equation:

Drops per minute = total amount to be infused (ml) × drops per ml/time in minutes in which to be infused

The simple glucose and glucose/saline solutions are used mainly for fluid replacement and when there is some loss of sodium, but others are used to correct potassium and multiple electrolyte disturbances. The type and volume of the intravenous infusion used will depend on the individual patient's need and response, as overdose can occur with such solutions as with other drugs. In the elderly, fluid overload may be fatal.

Additions are sometimes made to intravenous infusion fluids, as by that means drugs that have a narrow therapeutic index or are too toxic to give as a bolus dose can be given by slow infusion, and so achieve a more steady blood level of the drug. However, the addition of drugs to infusion solutions is not without risk, and such additions should be made in the pharmacy under sterile conditions. When that is not possible, and nurses are called on to make such additions, a strict aseptic technique must be used to avoid bacterial contamination of the solution.

Nurses must also remember that no drug should be added to an infusion fluid unless it is known that all the constituents are compatible, and that no loss of potency will occur. Only one container should be prepared at a time, and it should be used as soon as possible. Drugs should never be added to infusion solutions of sodium bicarbonate, amino acids, mannitol or blood products, and only special additive products prepared for the purpose, should ever be added to intravenous fat emulsions.

Table 25.1 Intravenous infusion fluids

| Solution | Electrolyte content (mmol per litre) | | | | | | Notes on use |
	Na^+	K^+	Ca^{2+}	Cl^-	HCO_3^- or lactate	Energy content per litre KJ	
Normal plasma values	142	4.5	2.5	103	26		
Glucose 5%	–	–	–	–	–	840	Fluid and energy replacement
Glucose 4% & sodium chloride 0.18%	30	–	–	30	–	680	Fluid, energy and electrolyte replacement
Glucose 5% & sodium chloride 0.9%	150	–	–	150	–	840	Fluid, energy and electrolyte replacement
Hartmann's solution	131	5	2	111	29	–	Fluid and multiple electrolyte replacement
Mannitol 10%, 15%, 20%	–	–	–	–	–	–	Osmotic diuretic, contraindicated in congestive cardiac failure and pulmonary oedema
Potassium chloride 0.3% & glucose 5%	–	40	–	40	–	840	For correction of potassium deficiency after severe diarrhoea, vomiting, and diuretics
Potassium chloride 0.2%, glucose 4% & sodium chloride 0.9%	150	30	–	180	–	680	Wherever possible these solutions should be used in preference to adding stronger potassium chloride solution to other infusions
Potassium chloride 0.3%, and sodium chloride 0.9%	150	40	–	190	–	–	Wherever possible these solutions should be used in preference to adding stronger potassium chloride solution to other infusions
Ringer's solution	147	4	2	155	–	–	Fluid and electrolyte replacement
Sodium bicarbonate 1.26%	150	–	–	–	150	–	Treatment of metabolic acidosis. Stronger solutions (8.4%) are used in severe acidosis after cardiac arrest
Sodium chloride 0.9%	150	–	–	150	–	–	Fluid and electrolyte replacement. Stronger solutions are available to correct acute sodium loss while weaker ones are used for maintenance therapy in secondary dehydration
Sorbitol 30%	–	–	–	–	–	5040	An alternative energy source

Some infusion solutions must be protected from light to reduce the risk of inactivation, and any change in colour or development of cloudiness in an infusion fluid is an indication to stop the infusion, but the absence of any change in appearance is not an assurance that no loss of potency has occurred. Care must be taken to ensure thorough mixing of the additive before the infusion is commenced. An additional label should be placed on the container, indicating what additive and how much, the date of preparation, by whom it was prepared, and the name of the patient. In some cases, as with certain irritant drugs, the additive is not added to the bulk of the infusion fluid, but is injected into the tubing of a fast-running intravenous infusion, thus ensuring rapid dilution and a reduced risk of local irritation. With drugs that are unstable in dilute solution, such as some antibiotics, intermittent infusion can be used, in which the drug is dissolved in about 100 ml of infusion fluid and infused over about 30 minutes.

SUBCUTANEOUS INFUSION

Hyaluronidase §

Brand name: Hyalase §
In young children and the elderly, intravenous infusion may not be easy and an alternative is subcutaneous infusion facilitated by hyaluronidase, a process referred to as hypodermoclysis. Hyaluronidase is a mucolytic enzyme that when injected causes a temporary decrease in the viscosity of the mucoprotein present in tissue spaces, and so promotes fluid diffusion. The dose of 1500 units may be given into the injection site or added to 500–1000 ml of the fluid to be infused. The absorption rate is about 100 ml/hour. Hyaluronidase is also used to promote the absorption of local anaesthetics and the resorption of blood from haematomas.

BLOOD VOLUME EXPANDERS

When blood is lost, as in haematemesis, trauma and burns, both fluid and plasma proteins which maintain osmotic pressure are also lost. Both need to be replaced, otherwise the reduced osmotic pressure will result in the leakage of fluid into the interstitial space and cause oedema. Blood loss can be replaced by blood transfusion, but in an emergency certain other fluid products can be given to restore the osmotic pressure and draw fluid from the interstitial space

back into the blood vessels. Plasma may be given as Plasma Protein Solution, which contains 4–5% of protein, mainly as albumin, or as Human Albumin Solution. Albutein and Zenalb are proprietary products containing 20% albumin.

Blood volume expanders (plasma substitutes)

Plasma substitutes are macromolecular substances that in solution have some of the physical properties of plasma, and are given by intravenous infusion for short-term use to expand and maintain blood volume.

Dextran §

Brand names: Gentran 40 §; Gentran 70 §; Macrodex §; Rheomacrodex §
Dextran is a polysaccharide, and such compounds can be regarded as sugar molecules linked together to form large aggregate units; the physical properties are related to the size of the unit. Dextran 70 is used as a temporary plasma substitute in severe blood loss, but any blood cross-matching should be carried out before the dextran infusion is commenced. The standard solution contains 6% dextran in either 5% glucose or normal saline solution. Gentran 40 and Rheomacrodex are preparations of a lower molecular weight dextran that is eliminated from the circulation more rapidly than dextran 70, and is used mainly for improving peripheral blood flow in cases of intravascular aggregation of blood cells, and in lower limb ischaemia.

Other blood volume expanders

Polygeline (Haemaccel §, Gelofusine §) are solutions of modified gelatin that are used as blood volume expanders. Hespan § and eloHAES § are modified starch preparations with similar uses. With all these products, the risks of allergic reactions should be borne in mind.

ENTERAL AND INTRAVENOUS NUTRITION

In any state of insufficient food intake, whether from disease, surgery or trauma, or where the metabolic rate is raised, the body stores of fat will be used first to provide energy, and later lean muscle protein will be drawn upon. The latter results in a negative nitrogen balance, and as lean tissue contains 90% of the body potassium, a potassium loss may also develop. One method of providing energy and protein to meet such deficiencies is enteral nutrition. Such feeding is effective only with a functioning gastro-intestinal tract, and may then either supplement or replace normal nutrition, and many preparations for such feeding are now available. Most contain amino acids, carbohydrates, fats, vitamins and minerals, and Elemental and Enlive are representative products. They may be given via a nasogastric tube, percutaneous gastrostomy or a drip feed. Diarrhoea and electrolyte disturbances are the most common **side-effects**.

Intravenous nutrition

When the gut is non-functional because of illness or surgery, it is necessary to supply nutrients intravenously. Special solutions containing the amino acids essential for protein formation, together with glucose, are now available, and details of some products in use are given in Table 25.2. In severe burns and other cases of high energy demand, a higher calorific intake is necessary, and can be provided by a soya bean oil emulsion specially prepared for intravenous nutrition, available as Intralipid. It must be given alone, with the single exception of Vitilipid N, a vitamin additive specially formulated for use with Intralipid. Other additives may break down the fat emulsion.

An extension of the method is total parenteral nutrition (TPN), in which a solution containing all the required nutritional substances is infused via a central venous catheter. The solution is prepared daily in the hospital pharmacy and supplied in a 3 litre bag. Protein is supplied as a mixture of essential and nonessential amino acids, glucose as the source of energy, together with phosphate to promote glucose utilization. Fat emulsion, given separately, is a rich source of extra calories, although the maximum utilization of fats may take some days to develop, and checks may be necessary to confirm the clearance of fats from the plasma. The whole system requires careful control and for details of dose and technique involved the manufacturer's literature should be consulted.

Nursing points about intravenous nutrition

(a) Accurate monitoring of fluid balance is required.
(b) Regular observation, particularly for signs of infection.
(c) Check for hyperglycaemia by daily urinalysis.

Continuous ambulatory dialysis

Although outside the scope of this book, it should be noted that special solutions are available for continuous ambulatory peritoneal dialysis (CAPD). These solutions provide an alternative to haemodialysis for patients with end-stage renal failure. CAPD enables patients to live and be treated at home, and has extended the availability of dialysis to diabetic and elderly patients previously excluded for various reasons, such as infection risks, from haemodialysis.

Oral rehydration

Diarrhoeal diseases causing loss of fluid and electrolytes are said to account for over 3 million deaths world-wide. Treatment is basically replacement therapy, which in some underdeveloped countries may be very difficult to provide. However, the recognition that the oral administration of salt and water can be enhanced by the addition of glucose (which stimulates the transport system) has led to the introduction of Oral Rehydration Salts (ORS) preparations for the treatment of dehydration due to acute gastro-enteritis. ORS products contain sodium chloride, potassium chloride, sodium citrate and glu-

---

Table 25.2 Parenteral nutrients. This table lists some products used in hospitals. More than one solution may be required to give a satisfactory balance of fluid, nitrogen, energy and electrolytes. Vitamin supplements are also needed. Many of these nutrient solutions are expensive, and their value as routine postoperative therapy has been questioned.

Solution	Calorie source	Energy (kJ/litre)	Nitrogen (g/litre)	Electrolytes (mmol/litre)					Other constituents
				Na^+	K^+	Mg^{2+}	Acetate⁻	Cl⁻	
Aminoplasmal L 10	Amino acids		16.0	48	25	2.5	59	62	phosphate
Aminoplex 12	Amino acids		12.4	35	30	2.5	5	67	
Glucoplex 1000	Glucose	4200		50	30	2.5		67	zinc phosphate
Intralipid 10%	Soya bean oil, egg lecithin and glycerol	4600							phosphate
Synthamin 9			9.1	70	60	5	100	70	
Vamin 9	Glucose	1700	9.4	50	20	1.5	2.5	50	phosphate

cose; Diocalm, Dioralyte, Electrolade and Rehidrat are proprietary preparations of a similar composition. After reconstitution with water, these ORS solutions should be used within an hour of preparation or discarded, unless a refrigerator is available, when they can be stored for 24 hours.

FURTHER READING

Abdulla A, Keast J 1997 Hypodermoclysis as a means of rehydration. Nursing Times 93(27):54–55

Barber C, Masiello M 1996 Oral rehydration therapy. Topics in Emergency Medicine 18(3):21–26

Bloe C G 1990 Peritoneal dialysis. Professional Nurse 5(7):345–349

Finlay T 1989 Fluid balance in patients undergoing major gut surgery. Surgical Nurse Apr.:11–16

Finnegan S, Oldfield K 1989 When eating is impossible: TPN in maintaining nutritional status. Professional Nurse 4(6):271–275

Ireton-Jones C S, Robinson N 1995 Peripheral parenteral nutrition: indications and guidelines. Support Line 17(5):11–13

Kennedy J F 1997 Enteral feeding in the critically ill patient. Nursing Standard 11(33):39–43

Kohlhardt S R, Smith R C, Wright C R 1993 Peripheral versus central intravenous nutrition: comparison of two delivery systems. British Journal of Surgery 81:66–70

Liddle K 1995 Making sense of percutaneous endoscopic gastrostomy. Nursing Times 91(18):32–33

McVicar A, Clancy J 1997 Principles of intravenous fluid replacement. Professional Nurse Supplement 12(8):S6–S9

Raper S, Maynard N 1992 Feeding the critically ill patient. British Journal of Nursing 1(6):273–280

Taylor S J 1989 A guide to enteral feeding. Professional Nurse 4(4):195–200

Zerwekh J V 1997 Do dying patients really need IV fluids? American Journal of Nursing 97(3):26–31

26

Antiseptics and disinfectants

Definition

The terms antiseptic and disinfectant are often used loosely and interchangeably. Both either destroy or inhibit the growth of micro-organisms in the non-sporing state. Disinfectants tend to be used to treat inanimate materials as well as skin, while antiseptics tend to be used on broken skin and internal tissues. Antiseptics are usually less irritant than disinfectants, but both are poisonous and both are toxic to living cells, be they micro-organisms or body cells. To justify their use, particularly in wound management, it must be demonstrated that the damage done to the micro-organism by the antiseptic is greater than the damage done to the body tissue.

Evaluation of antiseptics

Antiseptics come in a variety of forms including solutions, ointments, creams, gels, powders, sprays and dressings (see Chapter 27 for the latter). They are used as antimicrobial agents (both to treat infection and for prophylaxis), cleansers, deodorizers, debriders and to promote moist wound healing.

The ideal antiseptic should kill a wide range of micro-organisms, be non-toxic to human tissue and not cause local or systemic sensitivity reactions. It should act rapidly, have a high degree of penetration, be effective over a wide range of dilutions and work efficiently, even in the presence of organic material, e.g. pus, blood. It should be inexpensive and have a long shelf life. Not surprisingly the ideal antiseptic does not exist, and each product has its own strengths and weaknesses, some being more effective against some groups of organisms than others.

If the antiseptic is to be used for wound cleansing, then because of the toxic effects on granulation tissue it should be used judiciously and sparingly. Sodium chloride is probably just as effective as a general wound cleansing agent as an antiseptic, with the benefits of being cheap, non-toxic and isotonic to body tissues. Its availability in spray cans (e.g. Irriclens) makes its use particularly easy, especially in the community setting.

PHENOLIC ANTISEPTICS

Phenol

Phenol is now only of historical interest, as it was introduced into medicine in 1867 as carbolic acid, and the remarkable results achieved by Lister and his followers in reducing postoperative infection paved the way to the present era of aseptic surgery. Phenol has been replaced for most purposes by more active and less toxic compounds, but it survives in some mouthwashes and similar preparations.

Chlorocresol

A more powerful but less soluble derivative of phenol, used mainly as a bacteriostat to preserve the sterility of injection solutions. When injections are supplied in multiple-dose containers (i.e. rubber-capped bottles), there is a risk that the unused contents may become contaminated by a faulty technique or the use of an unsterile needle. A preservative is therefore added to such solutions to inhibit bacterial growth, and chlorocresol is used for that purpose in a strength of 0.1–0.2%. Chlorocresol has been used in some instrument storage solutions.

Chlorhexidine (Hibitane)

Brand name: Hibitane

Chlorhexidine is a complex phenyl derivative with a powerful bactericidal action against a wide range of organisms that is retained even in very dilute solutions as well as in the presence of blood and other body fluids. But *Pseudomonas* and *Proteus* are resistant, and sterilized solutions should be used.

For general antiseptic purposes, chlorhexidine may be used as a 1–2000 solution; for bladder irrigation a 1–5000 solution is effective. For rapid pre-operative sterilization of the skin, a 1–200 solution in 70% alcohol is used.

An aerosol spray product for skin disinfection is also available, which contains a dye to indicate the area treated. Chlorhexidine cream (1%) is also used for obstetric and general antiseptic purposes. Hibicet

is a general-purpose antiseptic, and is supplied as a concentrate containing chlorhexidine (1.5%) and cetrimide (15%). Cetrimide has detergent properties, and Hibicet has the properties of both constituents and has a wide range of activity. Cetrimide is also present in various products used for napkin rash and mild abrasions.

Hexachlorophane

Hexachlorophane has a bacteriostatic action against many Gram-positive organisms, even in high dilution, but it is less active against Gram-negative organisms. It is used mainly in soaps and creams, as continued use reduces the bacterial flora in the skin and it is useful in reducing cross-infection. It is also used to prevent neonatal staphylococcal infection and is used after ligation of the cord, and after napkin changes. Hexachlorophane dusting powder (Ster-Zac) should not be applied to mucous membranes or large raw surfaces.

OTHER ANTISEPTICS

Alcohol

Alcohol in the form of methylated spirit has been used for many years as an antiseptic, particularly for skin preparation. Isopropyl alcohol has similar general properties and may be used both for pre-operative cleansing of the skin and for surgical instruments.

Chlorinated lime

Chlorinated lime, or bleaching powder, is a powerful germicide and deodorant and has been widely used for general disinfectant purposes and to disinfect excreta.

Eusol is a solution of chlorinated lime and boric acid containing the equivalent of about 0.25% chlorine. It is used as an antiseptic wound dressing or lotion, but the solution is unstable and should not be used if more than 2 weeks old. Although Eusol has been in use for many years, it is now considered to be irritant and may delay healing.

Formaldehyde (formalin)

Formaldehyde is a powerful but irritant germicide, used mainly as a 5% solution for the disinfection of apparatus and the preservation of specimens. Together with potassium permanganate it is used in the disinfection of rooms.

Povidone–iodine (Betadine)

Povidone–iodine is a loose combination of iodine with polyvinylpyrrolidine, from which the iodine is slowly released. It is used as a 1% solution for oral hygiene, and as a 10% solution in water or alcohol for skin preparation. It is also available as a dry powder spray product (Savlon).

Iodoform

Iodoform is a lemon-yellow powder with a marked odour and contains iodine in organic combination. It was once used as a wound dressing, but now survives only as the antiseptic constituent of BIPP (bismuth, iodoform and paraffin paste) occasionally used with gauze as a packing for sinuses and abscesses, and in Whitehead's Varnish.

OXIDIZING AGENTS

Hydrogen peroxide

Hydrogen peroxide (H_2O_2) is easily decomposed in the presence of oxidizable matter to yield oxygen and water. It is mainly used to treat infected cavities and dirty wounds, as the tissue enzymes cause a rapid release of oxygen, and the gas has the added mechanical action of loosening cell debris in the tissue crevices.

It is also used, when diluted with water, as an antiseptic mouth wash. Solutions of hydrogen peroxide are often described as '10 volume' or '20 volume' strength. The numbers refer to the volume of oxygen yielded by 1 volume of the solution.

Potassium permanganate

Potassium permanganate has powerful antiseptic and deodorizing properties and is used as a 1–10 000 solution for suppurating wounds and abscesses. It has also been used for bladder and vaginal irrigation. It may stain the skin, fabrics and utensils brown.

ANTISEPTIC DYES

Some synthetic dyes have antiseptic properties, but the use of such substances has declined as more active chemotherapeutic drugs have become available for the treatment of infections. The following substances are still in use, but to a steadily diminishing extent and their value is open to question.

Crystal violet (gentian violet)

A solution containing 0.5% of crystal violet is used occasionally for pre-operative skin preparation and marking, but it is not recommended for application to broken skin or mucous membranes.

Proflavine

Proflavine and acriflavine are orange-red dyes with a bacteriostatic action. They were once widely used as a 1–1000 lotion. Proflavine cream (0.1%) is a surviving preparation.

SILVER COMPOUNDS

Silver salts have powerful antiseptic properties, but very few have any therapeutic applications. Silver nitrate solution (1%) was once used extensively as eye-drops as a prophylactic against ophthalmia neonatorum, and in some parts of the USA its use is still mandatory. Solid silver nitrate is used as a caustic to destroy warts and occasionally to remove over-granulation tissue.

Silver sulphadiazine (Flamazine §) is used as a 1% cream for the treatment of infected leg ulcers, burns and pressure sores, especially those infected with *Pseudomonas aeruginosa*. The complex is slowly metabolized by tissue exudates, but if the cream is applied extensively, some of the free sulphadiazine may be absorbed systemically.

FURTHER READING

Farrow S, Toth B 1990 The place of EUSOL in wound management. Health Care Evaluation Unit: Bristol
Gilchrist B 1997 Should iodine be reconsidered for wound management? Journal of Wound Care 6:(3)148–150
Hamilton-Miller J M T, Shah S, Smith C 1993 Silver sulphadiazine: a re-assessment. Chemotherapy 39:405–409

Lawrence J C 1997 Wound irrigation. Journal of Wound Care 6(1):23–26
Morgan D 1993 Is there still a role for antiseptics? Journal of Tissue Viability 3(3):80–84
Williams C 1996 Irriclens: a sterile wound cleanser in an aerosol can. British Journal of Nursing 5(16):1008–1010

27

Wound dressings

WOUND HEALING

Wound healing is a complex response to tissue damage resulting from mechanical, chemical or thermal trauma. It can be described as a four-stage process which starts with the traumatic inflammatory stage, moves through the destructive and proliferative stages and ends with the maturational stage.

The traumatic inflammatory stage is the phase in which the trauma is inflicted, and which frequently results in bleeding. Vasoconstriction, the formation of a platelet plug and the clotting cascade serve to minimize blood loss. Following limitation of the bleeding there is then an increase in blood flow to the damaged tissue, bringing with it oxygen, nutrients and white blood cells. This increased blood flow results in the area becoming red and hot. Increased vascular permeability allows fluid to leak into the tissues and so dilutes toxins and causes oedema. The swelling causes pain, as do the prostaglandins that are formed in response to the trauma. The pain serves to limit movement and so encourages resting of the area, which in turn aids healing. Thus inflammation, recognized by the classic symptoms of redness, heat, swelling, pain and loss of function, is part of the healing process.

The traumatic inflammatory stage ends with the arrival of the neutrophils, followed after about 8 hours by the monocytes (or macrophages as they become). The white cells begin the destructive phase as they clear the wound of the debris of damaged tissue, blood clot, bacteria, and foreign material. The macrophages also attract fibroblasts to the area, stimulate the fibroblasts to divide, promote the synthesis of collagen, and secrete the angiogenesis factor (a substance which stimulates the growth of new blood vessels).

In the proliferative stage endothelial buds grow into space cleared by macrophages where there is a low oxygen tension, and form new blood vessels. The endothelial buds carry fibroblasts with them into the wound. The fibroblasts produce strands of collagen, a process which requires oxygen, energy, protein, vitamin C and zinc. The fibroblasts also produce a ground substance much of which is derived from leaked glycoproteins. This ground substance together with collagen and new capillaries is termed granulation tissue.

As well as repairing the dermis by forming granulation tissue, the epithelium also has to be replaced. The epithelial cells at the wound edge, and those around hair follicles and sweat glands, proliferate and migrate over the viable tissue under the eschar or scab.

The final phase of the wound healing process is the maturational stage. During this stage remodelling occurs as modified fibroblasts, called fibroclasts, break down and resynthesize the original disorganized collagen, converting it into an organized array of collagen fibres. Further lysis and resynthesis occurs until there is optimal orientation of the collagen fibres. Cross-linking and condensation result in maximum tensile strength after 3–12 months. The fibroblasts disappear when they are no longer required. The blood vessels supplying the area shrink back, resulting in a paler scar.

CHOOSING A DRESSING

The purpose of a wound dressing is to optimize or to enhance the healing process. Many traditional dressings, e.g. gauze, do not achieve this and do not promote the healing process. This has led to the development of interactive dressings which produce environments which optimize healing. Work is also going on to produce bio-active dressings which will make use of growth factors and so go one stage further and enhance healing.

The choice of dressings on the market is wide, with new versions coming out monthly, so trying to become familiar with all the available dressings is not realistic. Thus an attempt must be made to rationalize choice, particularly if nurses are to become skilled in using particular dressings and in evaluating their success. To aid this process an algorithm and formulary can be developed by a hospital or clinic which identifies a limited number of dressings required to meet the needs of their particular patients (see Fig. 27.1 for an example).

The list of requirements of a wound dressing can be quite extensive but can be simplified down to three essentials. Firstly, the dressing must be efficacious, i.e. it should optimize healing. Secondly, it should be cost-effective, and finally it should improve the patient's quality of life. These requirements will be satisfied only if the clinician fully assesses the wound to identify what is required and then chooses the appropriate type of dressing to meet those needs.

Note. The specific dressings listed below are only examples, not an exhaustive inventory. * = available on FP10.

Alginates

- Fibracol – calcium – sodium alginate and bovine collagen sheet
- Kaltostat* – non-woven fibrous mat or rope
- Kaltostat Fortex – thick calcium – sodium non-woven fibrous mat
- Kaltocarb – Kaltostat bonded to a layer of activated charcoal cloth
- Kaltogel* – calcium – sodium quick gelling alginate
- Sorbsan * – calcium alginate non-woven fibrous mat or rope
- Sorbsan Plus* – calcium alginate with absorbent viscose pad
- Sorbsan SA – calcium alginate island dressing
- Tegagel* – calcium alginate sheet

These seaweed-based dressing are designed for use on moderate to heavily exuding wounds. They are highly absorbent, absorbing 15–20 times their own weight of exudate. Because they are so absorbent their use should be evaluated regularly, as they have the potential to dry out the wound bed and so prevent moist wound healing. As they are available in both ropes and sheet form they can be used to pack cavities as well as to manage flat wound beds. Alginates can be used for infected wounds, when it is recommended that the infection is treated systemically with antibiotics and the dressing is changed daily.

The Drug Tariff categorizes alginates into Type I dressings which contain calcium alginate, e.g. Sorbsan, and Type II dressings which contain calcium–sodium alginate, e.g. Kaltostat. Some such as Sorbsan are rich in mannuronic acid and form soft flexible gels, while those such as Kaltostat which are rich in guluronic acid form firm gels. The main differences between these two formats is that when calcium alginates are irrigated with sodium chloride solution they dissolve, making removal of the dressing very easy. Calcium–sodium alginates do not dissolve. However, they do have haemostatic properties and are therefore useful in the management of bleeding wounds.

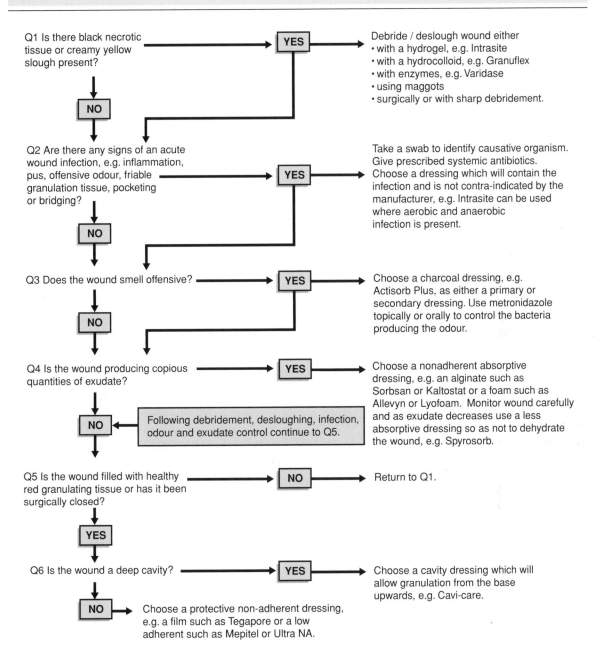

Figure 27.1 Wound management algorithm.

Charcoal dressings

- Actisorb Plus – activated charcoal cloth with 0.15% silver
- Carbonet – multi-layer dressing with a layer of woven activated charcoal

Infected wounds can sometimes produce extremely unpleasant odours, causing patients and carers much embarrassment and psychological distress. The main bacteria causing malodour are anaerobes, in particular the *Bacteroides* and *Clostridium perfringens*. Aerobic organisms, in particular *Pseudomonas spp.* and *Proteus mirabilis* can also cause wounds to smell. One way of controlling the odour is to use topical antibiotics, in particular metroniadazole gel. However, for palliative management of malodour, charcoal dressings can be used. These dressings contain activated charcoal which efficiently adsorbs gases and bacteria. The silver in Actisorb Plus acts as an antimicrobial, inhibiting the growth of the odour-producing bacteria.

Charcoal dressings are also available in combination with alginates and foams.

Enzyme products

- Varidase * – streptokinase 100 000 units with streptodornase 25 000 units

This is used for debriding wounds. Streptokinase facilitates fibrin and fibrinogen degradation while streptodornase liquefies deoxyribonucleic acid from the cell nuclei. Care has to be taken when making up the solution as vigorous shaking can denature the enzymes. Hard black necrotic tissue can be scored with a blade to facilitate penetration of the liquid or it can be injected carefully under the necrotic eschar. Alternatively, Varidase can be mixed with a hydrogel and applied to the wound. However, one study found that the combination of Varidase and hydrogel was no better than hydrogel on its own. Use of topical Varidase has been shown to increase antistreptokinase antibody titres. It should therefore be avoided in the elderly at risk of coronary artery disease.

Films – semi-permeable

- Arglaes – thin polyurethane membrane with controlled-release silver
- Bioclusive * – thin polyurethane membrane
- Opsite Flexigrid * – thin polyurethane membrane with wound grid assessment tool
- Tegaderm * – thin polyurethane membrane on a frame
- Tegaderm Plus – thin polyurethane membrane with iodine

These were the first interactive dressings developed. They are transparent, thin, adhesive-coated films. They are permeable to both water vapour and oxygen, but impermeable to micro-organisms. They are suitable as primary dressings for shallow wounds with minimal exudate, where they promote moist wound healing. If excess exudate does collect under the dressing it is possible, using a sterile syringe, to aspirate the fluid and then patch the hole with a small piece of film. They can also be used as secondary dressings to control loss of water vapour from wounds dressed with, for example, hydrogels and alginates. They are also used as prophylactic agents to protect fragile skin from friction damage.

They should not normally be used on infected wounds, and are not usually left on for more than 7 days.

Semi-permeable films are also available with the addition of antimicrobials which act as prophylaxis against bacteria, including methicillin resistant *Staphylococcus aureus*.

Film dressings are often used as dressings for peripheral and central intravenous catheters. However, their fluid handling properties are such that they provide a moist environment suitable for wound healing, which is not suitable for cannulas. These require a dry environment which inhibits bacterial proliferation. There are specially designed film dressings which are highly permeable to water vapour (about 3000 g/m^2/24 hours as against 700 g/m^2/24 hours for wound dressing) available to cover cannula sites, e.g. Opsite IV 3000.

Foams

- Allevyn * – polyurethane foam
- Allevyn Cavity Wound Dressing – polyurethane chips in a perforated membrane (circular/tubular)
- Allevyn Adhesive * – hydrocellular island dressing
- Cavi-care – two-part vulcanizing silicone foam
- Lyofoam * – polyurethane foam sheet
- Lyofoam Extra * – extra absorbent polyurethane foam sheet
- Lyofoam A – polyurethane foam island dressing
- Lyofoam C – polyurethane foam with activated carbon granules
- Flexipore – polyurethane foam
- Spyrosorb * – polyurethane foam

These are a diverse group of dressings. They are of variable absorbency and are suitable for exuding wounds. Most of them come in sheet form for use on flat wounds. However, Allevyn cavity comes in several sizes of circular and tubular forms which can be used for packing cavities, while Cavi-care is a two-part liquid which when mixed and poured into a wound rapidly sets, taking on the shape of the wound. As it goes into the wound as a liquid and then sets, Cavi-care must not be used with bottleneck wounds or those with tracking sinuses. The foam nature of this group of dressings means that they can cushion the wound, as well as providing thermal insulation. They can be used on infected wounds.

Hydrocolloids

- Aquacel – fibrous hydrocolloid in a non-woven pad or ribbon; very absorbent – 50% higher than alginates

- Biofilm – hydrocolloid sheet; gel-forming component also comes as a powder
- Comfeel Ulcer Dressing * – hydrocolloid sheet; gel-forming component also comes as a powder and a paste
- Comfeel Extra Absorbing Dressing – hydrocolloid sheet with calcium alginate
- Granuflex * – sheet; gel-forming component also comes as a paste
- Granuflex Extra Thin – low-profile hydrocolloid sheet
- Tegasorb * – hydrocolloid island dressing

These dressings are used as carriers for water-soluble topical drugs, e.g. metronidazole. They have a cooling effect at the skin surface and so can decrease pain at the wound site and are particularly useful in the management of radiotherapy burns. They have also been shown to soften, flatten and blanch scars and to reduce the formation of keloid and hypertrophic scars.

These are suspensions of semi-hydrated, hydrophilic, microgranules in various natural or synthetic polymers in an adhesive matrix. They are presented in the form of a flexible foam or film sheet covered with a layer of the hydrocolloid base and covered with a piece of release paper. In order to provide good adhesion the dressings should overlap the wound margins by about 2 cm. The base itself may also be available in the form of granules or paste which can be applied to the wound in conjunction with the sheet to increase the absorbency and flexibility of the system. Although they appear similar in appearance hydrocolloids differ markedly in performance and so cannot be freely interchanged.

Hydrocolloids are suitable for light to medium exuding wounds. A 10 × 10 cm dressing can absorb about 20 ml of exudate. They are permeable to water vapour but impermeable to exudate and microorganisms, giving them a role in the prevention of spread of infection. They promote autolysis and so are used a desloughing agents in necrotic and sloughy wounds. Hydrocolloids produce a wound environment with a low pH and so have been used as a treatment for wounds infected with *Pseudomonas*. They also produce hypoxic wound environments which promote angiogenesis and hence the formation of granulation tissue. However the low oxygen tension means that they are not suitable for wounds with anaerobic infections.

Hydrogels

- Cica-care–self-adhensive silicone gel sheet
- Granugel*–a combination of hydrogel and hydrocolloid
- Intrasite gel*–amorphous gel
- Nu-gel*–hydrogel with a alginate
- Spenco 2nd Skin–hydorogel sheet
- Sterigel*–amorphous gel
- Vigilon–hydrogel sheet dressing

These jelly-like dressings come in two forms, i.e. amorphous aqueous gels and transparent flexible sheets. These dressings have variable fluid handling properties and can both donate and absorb water. Their ability to donate water makes them very useful in rehydrating necrotic and sloughy tissue and in promoting autolysis. In granulating wounds they prevent desiccation and promote epithelialization. Their ability to absorb water means that they can be used on lightly to moderately exuding wounds without maceration. They generally need a secondary dressing to keep them in place.

Hydrogels can be used on infected wounds provided that they are covered with a non-occlusive secondary dressing and systemic antibiotics are given.

Hydropolymers

- Tielle* – foamed hydrogel island dressing

A hydropolymer is a non-particulate polymer or mixture of polymers. The polymers are hydrophilic and do not liquefy or break down, so they leave no particles in the wound, unlike hydrocolloids. Tielle, the only dressing in the group, is an island dressing with a multi-layered structure. It consists of a piece of highly absorbent foamed hydrogel located in the centre of a waterproof, polyurethane membrane coated with acrylic adhesive. A piece of non-woven wicking layer, which helps to disperse exudate throughout the dressing, is found between the foam and adhesive backing. The backing material allows evaporation of water vapour from the wound.

Tielle is suitable for low to moderately exuding, superficial wounds. It is highly conformable. The dressing does not require a secondary dressing, and as it is waterproof patients can shower and bath. It should not be used on clinically infected wounds without medical supervision. Tielle can be left on for up to 7 days.

Low adherent

- Inadine * – rayon gauze impregnated with 10% povidone–iodine ointment
- Melonin * – perforated film with absorbent fabric backing

- Mepital – fine mesh polyamide netting coated with silicone gel
- N/A * – knitted viscose sheet
- N/A Ultra* – siliconized knitted viscose sheet
- Paraffin gauze * – cotton and viscose fabric impregnated with white soft paraffin, e.g. Jelonet
- Medicated tulles * – as above with the addition of various antiseptics, e.g. chlorhexidine
- Release * – textured ethylene methylacrylate film sleeve with absorbent core
- Tegapore – woven polyamide net
- Tricotex * – knitted viscose sheet

These dressings are designed to cover and protect granulating wounds. However, they do not always live up to their title of low adherent and can stick to the wound, damaging the granulation tissue on removal. The reason dressings stick to the wound is two-fold. Firstly, because they are not occlusive the serum and wound exudate dries, forming a glue between the wound and the dressing. Secondly, capillary loops of the granulating tissue grow into the dressing anchoring it to the wound.

Adherence is least with the siliconized dressings and those which have pores large enough to allow the exudate to pass freely from the wound to a secondary dressing, e.g. Tegapore. They can be used on infected wounds and generally require a secondary dressing. Unless an appropriate secondary dressing is chosen they do not promote moist wound healing.

Some of the low-adherents contain antimicrobial substances, the value of which is debatable, as acquired resistance to some of them has been reported and the paraffin-based dressings do not release their antimicrobial constituent very effectively.

Polysaccharides

- Debrisan * – dextranomer beads or paste
- Iodosorb * – cadexomer iodine as a powder or ointment
- Iodoflex * – cadexomer iodine paste sandwiched in gauze

The forerunners of these dressings are honey and sugar paste, both of which have been used for centuries and are still being used. Both honey and sugar paste have an antibacterial effect because they are hygroscopic and hence dehydrate bacteria. Furthermore, honey also liberates hydrogen peroxide, and some types of honey contain antibacterial substances derived from the flowers visited by the bees. They are both useful for debriding and cleaning infected, dirty and malodorous wounds. For medical use honey must be obtained from specified pathogen-free hives, which have not been treated with drugs, and which are sited in areas where no pesticides are used, to ensure that infection and toxic materials are not introduced into the wound.

The commercially available polysaccharides are similarly used for cleaning and debriding sloughy or infected wounds. They are useful for lightly exuding wounds and can reduce local tissue oedema and control odour formation. Care must be taken with the iodine-based dressings, avoiding their use with patients with known iodine sensitivity or thyroid disease.

FURTHER READING

Bux M, Baig M K, Rodrigues E et al 1997 Antibody response to topical streptokinase. Journal of Wound Care 6(2):70–73

Hampson J P 1996 The use of metronidazole in the treatment of malodorous wounds. Journal of Wound Care 5(9):421–426

Martin S J, Corrado O J, Kay E A 1996 Enzymatic debridement for necrotic wounds. Journal of Wound Care 5(7):310–311

Morgan D A 1997 Formulary of wound management, 7th edn. Euromed Communications, Surrey

Thomas S 1990 Wound management and dressings. Pharmaceutical Press, London

Thomas S 1991 A comparative study of the properties of six hydrocolloid dressings. The Pharmaceutical Journal 247(6662):672–675

Thomas S 1994 Handbook of wound dressings. Macmillan, London

Williams C 1994 Tielle: a hydropolymer dressing. British Journal of Nursing 3(19):1029–1030

Williams C 1995 Mepitel. British Journal of Nursing 4(1):51–55

Willix D J, Molan P C, Harfoot C G 1992 A comparison of the sensitivity of wound-infecting species of bacteria to the antibacterial activity of manuka honey and other honey species. Journal of Applied Bacteriology 73:388–394

28

Diagnostic agents

This chapter includes notes on a few substances that are used clinically as aids to diagnosis, to evaluate certain body functions, to assess liability to infection or detect injury.

FUNCTIONAL TESTS

Bentiromide

Bentiromide is a derivative of aminobenzoic acid. It is metabolized in the gut by the pancreatic enzyme chymotrypsin to give the free acid, which is absorbed and excreted in the urine. On that account it is used as a test of pancreatic function by measuring the excretion of the drug after a dose of 500 mg. Fluorescein dilaurate has also been used for the same purpose.

Fluorescein

Fluorescein is used to detect corneal damage. See p. 253.

Indocyanine green (Cardio green)

When given by intravenous injection, indocyanine green is rapidly eliminated from the circulation, and is used to assess cardiac output and liver function. It is given in doses of 5 mg by a cardiac catheter, and the elimination is assessed photometrically.

Metyrapone

Metyrapone is used as a test of hypothalamo–pituitary function. See p. 182.

Pancreozymin

Pancreozymin is a polypeptide hormone used as a

pancreatic stimulant to assess the activity of the pancreas. It is also used in the diagnosis of biliary tract disorders. It is given by intravenous injection in doses of 1–2 units, often together with secretin.

Patent blue

Patent blue is used as a 2.5% solution by subcutaneous injection to visualize lymph vessels so that they can be injected with a contrast medium. It is given in a dose of 0.25 ml of the solution after dilution with saline or lignocaine solution.

Pentagastrin

Pentagastrin is a synthetic polypeptide that when given by injection simulates the action of natural gastrin. It is used to assess the secretory action of the stomach and is given in doses of 0.6 micrograms/kg by subcutaneous or intramuscular injection.

Phenolsulphonphthalein

Also known as phenol red, phenolsulphonphthalein has been used as a test of renal function. It is given in doses of 6 mg by intramuscular or intravenous injection, and the urine is collected later at intervals. The colour of the urine is then compared with that of a standard solution. Some 25% of the dye is normally excreted in 15 minutes and over 50% at the end of 1 hour, and any marked delay is an indication of the degree of renal dysfunction.

Rose Bengal

Rose Bengal is used to detect corneal damage. See p. 253.

Schick test

The Schick test is used to diagnose susceptibility to diphtheria and to detect those already immune who might react to an injection of diphtheria toxoid. In the test, 0.1–0.2 ml of diphtheria toxin solution is injected intradermally in one arm and an inert control solution into the other arm. A positive reaction is a red area about 10 mm or more in diameter appearing within 24 hours, and no reaction from the control injection.

Sodium aminohippurate

Sodium aminohippurate is given by intravenous injection for the measurement of renal plasma flow in doses to give a plasma concentration of 10–20 micrograms/ml.

Sulphan blue

Sulphan blue has been used to assess the state of the circulation in cases of burns and soft tissue trauma. It is given in doses of 0.25–0.5 ml/kg of a 6.2% solution by slow intravenous injection.

Sulphobromophthalein

This compound is a red dye, and following intravenous injection it is taken up by the liver and excreted in the bile. Normally most of the dye is removed from the blood within 30 minutes, and it has been used for assessing hepatic activity. The dose is 5 mg/kg body weight, given as a 5% solution by intravenous injection. Samples of blood are taken 45 minutes later and the amount of sulphobromophthalein present in the plasma, normally about 7%, is measured by comparison with standard solutions of the dye. It should not be used in patients with a history of allergy.

Tuberculin

The Mantoux test is used in the diagnosis of tuberculosis. See p. 279.

Xylose

Xylose is used to detect malabsorption from the stomach. It is given as a dose of 5 g or 25 g in 500 ml of water. The amount recovered from the urine after 5 hours is estimated, and a recovery of less than 16% is considered indicative of malabsorption, provided kidney function is not impaired.

X-RAY CONTRAST AGENTS

These are substances of high atomic weight which increase the absorption of X-rays as they pass through the body. As they are relatively opaque to X-rays, they appear as shadows on X-ray films and are invaluable in outlining various tissues. With the exception of barium sulphate, the substances used as contrast agents are almost invariably complex iodine-containing organic compounds.

Barium sulphate

Brand names: Baritop, Micropaque
Barium sulphate is a dense white powder, used for the visualization of the gastro-intestinal tract. It is

given as a suspension in water, orally or as an enema, according to the area to be examined, after previous fasting, etc., so that the gastro-intestinal tract is empty. When so used, barium sulphate forms a temporary coating of the alimentary tract, and abnormalities can be outlined and detected. Large doses varying from 100 to 250 g may be given, and it is important to obtain a complete and even coating of the mucosa as otherwise shallow ulcers and similar lesions may escape detection.

Iodine compounds

Iodine is highly opaque to X-rays, and the iodine compounds in use are derivatives of various organic acids. They fall into three groups: those used orally and concentrated in the gall bladder (for visualization of the biliary tract), those injected into the CSF to detect spinal cord damage, and those used intravenously. Of the latter, those agents in current use include those for outlining the vascular system (angiography), those for visualization of the urinary tract (urography) and those for examining the liver and bile ducts (choleocystography). Some compounds are suitable for more than one type of investigation.

A detailed consideration of contrast agents is beyond the scope of this book and specialist literature should be consulted.

29

The treatment of poisoning

All substances are poisons; there is no such thing as a non-poison. It is the amount that distinguishes a poison from a remedy.

(Paracelsus, 1493–1541)

The increasing use of potent drugs and industrial chemicals has increased the risks and incidence of poisoning. The term 'poison' is a relative one, as any chemical substance taken in excessive quantity (including water!) is toxic. It is a truism to say that unless a drug is capable of doing some harm it is unlikely to do much good, and that applies to medicinal drugs as well as herbal and other complementary/alternative medicines. Many people believe that because a remedy is 'natural' it is safe, but herbal and other remedies may contain sufficient pharmacologically active substances to cause poisoning. Opium, for example, is essentially a herbal medicine, and self-medication with comfrey leaves that were in fact digitalis leaves is not unknown.

READ THE LABEL!

Many cases of accidental poisoning are the result of careless handling or storage of drugs and chemicals, and every effort should be made to impress on patients, relatives and all users of potentially toxic substances the importance of keeping all such products (including household detergents) under proper control, and that applies to hospitals and nursing homes as well as the home.

With drugs, as with other things of potential danger as well as value, constant vigilance is the only safeguard. *No drug should ever be used from an unlabelled container*, neither should a product be used unless the label is clear and unambiguous, and conveys the required information.

BASIC PRINCIPLES OF TREATMENT OF POISONING

The primary aim of treatment is the maintenance of vital functions. The identification of the poison is often a secondary matter, as there are very few specific antidotes. Hospital admission is advisable as some poisonous substances have a delayed action that adds to the problems of treatment. A local National Poisons Information Centre should be consulted if necessary, particularly when industrial poisons are concerned.

It should be remembered that the successful treatment of poisoning does not end with the recovery of the patient. Attempts should be made to discover why the poison was taken in the first place, or if taken accidentally, to advise on better safety measures.

Immediate measures

A common cause of death in acute poisoning is the loss of the airway protective reflexes and consequent airway obstruction by the flaccid tongue. Immediate measures include the pulling forward of the tongue, removal of any dentures, and the insertion if available of an oropharyngeal airway. The patient should be turned to a left-side-head-down position to allow any secretion or vomit to drain out of the mouth, and so reduce the risk of pulmonary aspiration. If the poison has been inhaled, the patient should be removed immediately to fresh air.

Many poisons depress the respiration, and assisted ventilation by mouth-to-mouth or Ambu bag may be required; oxygen may also be necessary. Trained personnel should consider endotracheal intubation to maintain the airway and permit mechanical ventilation. Hypotension is also common in severe poisoning, and the patient's head should be kept down while other measures to support vital functions are being instituted. The use of pressor drugs or respiratory stimulants is not recommended.

Active treatment

Two measures of importance are the removal if possible of the poison from the body and treatment of the effects of the poison. If the poison has been swallowed, the removal of as much as possible of the poison from the stomach by emesis and gastric lavage should be considered, but the benefits must be weighed against the risks involved, the toxicity of the poison and the time since the poison was taken. Emesis can be induced without delay if the patient is conscious and the poison is not a corrosive agent or a petroleum product by giving Ipecacuanha Mixture (Paediatric) in a dose of 30 ml for an adult, 15 ml for children, or 10 ml for young children of 6–18 months, together with a glass of water. Making the patient move about sometimes stimulates the vomiting. A second dose may be given if necessary after 20 minutes. Other methods of inducing emesis such as mechanical pharyngeal stimulation or the use of salt and mustard are now regarded as ineffectual or dangerous.

While gastric lavage is being considered or prepared, activated charcoal should be given.

Activated charcoal has marked adsorptive properties, and is a first-line treatment of poisoning by many substances taken by mouth as it hinders their absorption. Repeated doses of 25–50 g or more can be given as a suspension in water. It has no other action, and is not itself absorbed. Although it should always be given as soon as possible after poisoning, repeated doses may promote further adsorption. Some drugs, for example, are excreted in part by the intestinal epithelium but are re-absorbed later. They can be retained in the gut by activated charcoal and excreted in the faeces.

Gastric lavage is a hospital procedure, but in many cases of poisoning it is not worthwhile unless carried out within a few hours. The main exception is when drugs that delay gastric transit have been taken, notably tricyclic antidepressants and other agents that have an antimuscarinic (anticholinergic) action. The main danger of gastric lavage is the risk of inhalation of stomach contents and pulmonary complications. It should not be carried out in cases of poisoning by corrosive agents or petroleum products. Lavage should be combined with the administration of activated charcoal.

The following is an outline of the gastric lavage procedure:

(1) protect the airway with a cuffed endotracheal tube if the patient is unconscious;
(2) pass the largest gastric tube available through the mouth or nose into the stomach;
(3) withdraw as much of the stomach contents as possible;
(4) pass 50 g or more of activated charcoal into the stomach;
(5) commence lavage with 300–500 ml of water

warmed to body temperature, withdraw and repeat until the returned fluid is free of toxic material;

(6) when appropriate further doses of activated charcoal may be given later to maintain the adsorptive action in the intestinal tract, and continued until charcoal appears in the faeces;

(7) a laxative may be given to maintain intestinal motility and promote the elimination of material not removed by lavage, such as iron tablets.

THE TREATMENT OF SOME SPECIFIC POISONS

Acids (strong)

Hydrochloric, nitric and sulphuric acids.

Symptoms. Burning of mouth and throat with oedema, blood-stained vomit, gastro-enteritis. May cause gastric injury more than oesophageal damage.

Treatment. Water or milk in quantity, wash skin, morphine for pain, arachis or olive oil as demulcents.

Alkalis

Ammonia (strong), potassium hydroxide (caustic potash), sodium hydroxide (caustic soda).

Symptoms. Oesophageal damage with penetration of tissues and liquefaction. Gastric perforation.

Treatment. No emetics, charcoal useless. Treat as acids above.

Amphetamines

Symptoms. Agitation, confusion, arrhythmias, hypertension, convulsions, hyperthermia.

Treatment. Gastric lavage, chlorpromazine i.m. or diazepam i.v. for marked excitement, supportive therapy. For severe hypertension phentolamine 5–10 mg i.v. or sodium nitroprusside 0.3 micrograms/kg/minute i.v.

Anticholinergics

Atropine, hyoscine (scopolamine), propantheline and related drugs. See Table 10.1, p. 152. Also belladonna/deadly nightshade.

Symptoms. Dryness of mouth, thirst, nausea and vomiting, blurred vision, confusion, arrhythmias, hypertension, hyperpyrexia, urinary retention, respiratory failure.

Treatment. Supportive therapy. Gastric aspiration and lavage. Neostigmine 0.25 mg subcutaneously

for peripheral effects. If marked central stimulation, give diazepam or short-acting barbiturate as necessary. Physostigmine 1–4 mg i.m. or i.v. will rapidly antagonize central complications (care with repeated doses).

Anticoagulants

Phenidione, warfarin and warfarin-type rodenticides.

Symptoms. Haematuria, haemoptysis, orange-yellow urine, extended prothrombin time.

Treatment. Gastric lavage, vitamin K_1 20 mg i.v. Blood transfusion.

Antidepressants

See Table 3.5., p. 35.

Symptoms. Dry mouth, dilated pupils, tachycardia, hypotension, ataxia, convulsions, urinary retention. Respiratory arrest may occur without warning. Renal failure and CNS toxicity more likely with amoxapine.

Treatment. Gastric lavage and charcoal. For convulsions give diazepam 10 mg i.v. or muscle relaxant. If QRS interval prolonged, give intravenous sodium bicarbonate to maintain arterial pH between 7.44 and 7.55.

Antihistamines

See Table 17.2, p. 232.

Symptoms. Drowsiness, flushed skin, tachycardia, hyperthermia, convulsions, coma. Hazardous arrhythmias have occurred with overdose of astemizole and terfenadine.

Treatment. Gastric lavage and charcoal. Diazepam 10 mg i.v. for convulsions. No emetics (risk of convulsions).

Aspirin

Symptoms. Nausea, vomiting, tinnitus, deafness, hyperventilation, hyperpyrexia. Respiratory alkalosis, metabolic acidosis, pulmonary oedema. Hypokalaemia may be severe.

Treatment. Gastric aspiration and lavage with repeated charcoal. Check the plasma salicylate level and if over 500 mg/l in adults or 350 mg/l in children and the elderly, alkalize the urine. Haemodialysis if level above 800 mg/l or 450 mg/l respectively, with intensive supportive therapy.

Benzodiazepines

See Table 2.1, p. 20 and Table 3.4, p. 32.

Symptoms. Drowsiness, tachycardia, hypotension, respiratory depression, coma.

Treatment. Gastric lavage and charcoal. Supportive therapy. Flumazenil (p. 20) reverses central effects, care in benzodiazepine addiction as it may precipitate acute withdrawal symptoms.

Bleaches

(1) Hypochlorite/household bleaches

Symptoms. Irritation of mouth and pharynx with oedema. Nausea and vomiting.

Treatment. Milk or water as soon as possible. Gastric lavage only when large amounts of concentrated solution have been swallowed.

(2) Oxalic acid

Symptoms as with hypochlorites. Hypocalcaemia may occur after absorption, causing twitching, tetany, convulsions and cardiac arrest.

Treatment. Gastric lavage with 10 g calcium lactate or gluconate to form insoluble calcium oxalate. Supportive therapy, control tetany with repeated intravenous calcium gluconate.

Carbon monoxide (including exhaust fumes)

Symptoms. Severe headache, nausea, vomiting, confusion, arrhythmias, hypotension, coma and respiratory failure.

Treatment. Immediate removal to fresh air. Take blood sample for carboxyhaemoglobin (COHb) assay. Oxygen immediately and continued until COHb level is below 5%. Hyperbaric oxygen if COHb level above 20%.

Cyanides

Potassium cyanide, prussic acid.

Symptoms. Exposure to cyanides can be rapidly fatal. Onset of headache, convulsions, coma, and collapse may be abrupt.

Treatment. Immediate treatment essential by breaking an ampoule of amyl nitrite under the patient's nose; repeat if necessary, maintain airway, give oxygen. Specific antidote is Kelocyanor (cobalt sodium edetate) 20 ml i.v., followed immediately by 50 ml of i.v. 50% glucose solution (repeat once if no recovery within 1–2 minutes), followed by slow i.v. injection of 25 ml of 50% sodium thiosulphate solution. Alternatively, 10 ml of 3% sodium nitrite solution i.v., followed by sodium thiosulphate as above. Gastric lavage and charcoal if cyanide has been taken orally. Kelocyanor is toxic except in cyanide poisoning, so care in diagnosis is important.

Digoxin and digitalis

Symptoms. Nausea, vomiting and diarrhoea are early symptoms, bradycardia, hypotension, visual disturbances, arrhythmias, hyperkalaemia in acute overdose, hypokalaemia in chronic overdose.

Treatment. Gastric lavage and charcoal, treat bradycardia with atropine 0.6 mg i.m. or i.v.; potassium chloride for hypokalaemia, lignocaine i.v. for arrhythmia. Specific antidote is Digibind i.v., 40 mg binds about 600 micrograms of digoxin within 30–40 minutes.

Ethylene glycol 'anti-freeze'

Symptoms. Burning sensation in the throat, followed by malaise, sweating and vomiting; vertigo, drowsiness, coma, profuse sweating, acidosis, oliguria, anuria or haematuria. Death occurs from uraemia.

Treatment. Gastric lavage with potassium permanganate solution 1–5000, repeated later; calcium gluconate intravenously. Treat for renal failure. Penicillin prophylactically.

Ferrous sulphate and other iron salts

Symptoms. Gastric pain, nausea, vomiting, haematemesis, bloody diarrhoea, tachycardia. Hours or days later, confusion, delirium, coma, respiratory and circulatory collapse.

Treatment. In mild poisoning give desferrioxamine 1 g i.m.; gastric lavage with desferrioxamine 2 g in 1 litre of water. In severe poisoning desferrioxamine i.v. in doses of 15 mg/kg hourly up to 6 g or more. Treat for shock. Measure serum iron 4 hours after ingestion. If X-ray shows iron tablets still in stomach after lavage, consider whole gut lavage. Treatment can be discontinued when urine loses pink/orange colour or serum iron returns to normal.

Lead

Symptoms variable and diagnosis difficult because of non-specific gastro-intestinal disturbances and non-specific neuromuscular dysfunction, delirium, coma.

Treatment. In severe poisoning consult National Poisons Unit. Give Ledclair (sodium calcium edetate) in doses up to 40 mg/kg by i.v. infusion twice daily for 5 days or more. Follow-up with penicillamine orally in doses of 1–2 g daily with food. Continue until urinary lead level below 500 micrograms/day.

Dimercaprol (BAL) sometimes used with Ledclair as adjunctive treatment in doses of 2.5 mg/kg i.m for 10 days.

Lithium

Poisoning due to reduced excretion may occur after prolonged lithium therapy, and may be linked with the use of diuretics.

Symptoms. Apathy, muscle twitching, tremor and diarrhoea. In severe poisoning, convulsions, renal failure and coma may occur, and are associated with a lithium plasma level of over 2 mmol/litre.

Treatment. Supportive, restoration of electrolyte balance, diazepam intravenously for convulsions. Forced diuresis and dialysis in renal failure.

Methyl alcohol (methanol, wood alcohol)

Symptoms. Nausea, vomiting, blurred vision, hyperventilation, acidosis, convulsions, coma. Blurred vision may result in blindness.

Treatment. Gastric aspiration and lavage, intensive supportive treatment. Ethyl alcohol orally or by i.v. injection as 10% solution to saturate alcohol dehydrogenase and so prevent the formation of toxic metabolites. Dose of alcohol depends on blood methanol concentration. Intravenous sodium lactate or bicarbonate for acidosis.

Morphine and other narcotic analgesics

(See p. 49.)

Symptoms. Headache, dizziness, pin-point pupils, respiratory and circulatory depression, pulmonary oedema.

Treatment. Gastric lavage, naloxone (Narcan) is a specific antidote given i.v. or by i.v. infusion in doses of 0.8–2 mg, repeated as needed at intervals of 1–2 minutes up to 10 mg. If respiration does not improve review diagnosis. Symptoms may return if naloxone treatment is withdrawn too quickly. May cause acute withdrawal symptoms in addicts.

Nicotine

Present in various horticultural pesticide products. It is one of the most toxic compounds and in severe poisoning death may occur in a few minutes owing to respiratory paralysis.

Symptoms. Giddiness, nausea, vomiting, diarrhoea, confusion, convulsions, respiratory depression and collapse.

Treatment. Gastric lavage with weak potassium permanganate solution; remove contaminated cloth-ing, wash skin. Oxygen, artificial respiration; atropine for bradycardia, intravenous diazepam for convulsions.

Organophosphate insecticides

These are very toxic as they act by inhibiting cholinesterases.

Symptoms. May be delayed following skin contact but include headache, constricted pupils, ataxia, muscle weakness, marked salivation, nausea, vomiting, diarrhoea, colic and convulsions. Bradycardia, hypotension, circulatory failure, bronchospasm, acute pulmonary oedema, respiratory failure.

Treatment. Gastric lavage if ingested. Toxic effects reversed by atropine 2 mg i.v. or i.m., repeated every 20–30 minutes until pupils dilate, skin becomes dry and flushed and bradycardia occurs. Pralodoxime is a reactivator of cholinesterase, but must be given within 24 hours in doses of 1 g, i.m. or i.v. infusion, repeated as necessary. Diazepam 10 mg i.v. to control convulsions.

Paracetamol

Symptoms. Vomiting, gastrointestinal haemorrhage, tachycardia, hypotension, liver damage, renal necrosis, hypoglycaemia. With a high blood level of paracetamol the capacity of the liver to metabolize the drug may be overwhelmed, and severe liver damage may occur very rapidly.

Treatment. Gastric lavage if overdose taken within 2–4 hours. Drugs such as acetylcysteine and methionine have a protective action, so treatment should be commenced within 15–30 hours of overdose if plasma paracetamol level greater than 200 mg/litre by the intravenous infusion of 150 mg/kg of acetylcysteine, followed by a further dose of 50 mg/kg over 4 hours, followed by a dose of 100 mg/kg infused over 16 hours. Methionine is also used within 10 hours (after emesis has been induced) in oral doses of 2.5 g 4-hourly for four doses. Give i.v. sodium bicarbonate for acidosis, and if haemolysis is severe, corticosteroids and blood transfusions may be necessary. Renal failure may require haemodialysis.

Patients taking anticonvulsants, rifampicin and alcohol, and those with glutathione deficiency (anorexics, poorly nourished, HIV positives) are more susceptible to paracetamol poisoning; treat if paracetamol plasma level is half the normal toxic level. Naloxone may also be necessary if the poisoning is due to co-proxamol (paracetamol with dextropropoxyphene) or similar products (see morphine).

Paraquat (pesticide)

Liquid form very toxic; taken up slowly by pulmonary alveolar cells, leading to cell necrosis and pulmonary fibrosis. Corrosive to skin and membranes.

Symptoms. Burning of mouth, nausea, vomiting, later painful buccal ulceration, days later progressive alveolitis and bronchiolitis.

Treatment. Gastric lavage with 300 ml of fuller's earth suspension 30%, leaving 300 ml in stomach. Activated charcoal 100 g if fuller's earth not available, magnesium sulphate purge. Intensive supportive therapy, consult National Poisons Information Centres. Splashes in eyes very irritant; irrigate and instil bactericidal eye-drops.

Petroleum products

Symptoms. Restlessness, coughing and choking of rapid onset, with nausea, vomiting and diarrhoea, drowsiness. Pulmonary congestion and convulsions after high doses, coma. Dyspnoea, cyanosis and pyrexia, especially if inhalation as well as ingestion has occurred; convulsions, coma.

Treatment. In mild cases no active measures need be taken. *No* gastric lavage (risk of inhalation). Antibiotics in full doses prophylactically to reduce the risks of bronchopneumonia. Mechanical ventilation in pulmonary oedema.

Phenol, creosote and related agents

Symptoms. Phenolic smell in breath and vomit. Burning pain in mouth and stomach which dulls later (local anaesthetic action). Diarrhoea with corrosive intestinal injury, convulsions, respiratory failure and liver damage. Absorption through skin, leaving painless white patches turning red-brown.

Treatment. Remove contaminated clothing; gastric lavage, charcoal and intensive supportive therapy.

Phenothiazines

See Table 3.2, p. 29

Symptoms. Restlessness, cardiac arrhythmias, oculogyric crises, hypotension, parkinsonism, hypothermia, convulsions, respiratory depression.

Treatment. Gastric lavage; intravenous diazepam 10 mg for convulsions, intravenous benztropine 2 mg for parkinsonism-like symptoms.

Quinine and quinidine

Symptoms. Tinnitus, vertigo, deafness, nausea and vomiting. Serious toxic effects are hypotension, cardiac arrhythmias, sudden loss of vision, convulsions and coma.

Treatment. Gastric lavage; intensive supportive therapy, ECG monitoring; isosorbide dinitrate in loss of sight following retinal artery spasm; possibly also stellate ganglion block. Forced diuresis of doubtful value.

Snake bite

Acute snake bite is rare in the UK.

Symptoms. Local swelling, pain and redness. (If no swelling within 2 hours bite unlikely to contain venom.) Agitation, vomiting, diarrhoea, respiratory failure and collapse.

Treatment. Do not suck or incise bite nor apply tourniquet. If swelling extends beyond near major joint, give two ampoules of Zagreb antivenom, diluted with sterile saline, by slow intravenous injection. Same dose for children. Risk of allergic reactions – adrenaline injection must be immediately available.

Thiazide diuretics

See Table 11.1, p. 164.

Symptoms Nausea, diarrhoea, polyuria, dehydration. Disturbances of electrolyte balance leading to hypochloraemia, hypokalaemia, metabolic acidosis, hyperglycaemia, hypotension. Renal and hepatic failure has occurred. May precipitate an acute attack of gout in gouty patients.

Treatment. Gastric aspiration and lavage, adequate fluid for rehydration. Supportive therapy. Monitor electrolytes and if necessary give supplementary salts to restore electrolyte balance.

POISONS INFORMATION CENTRES

Belfast (01232) 240503
Birmingham (0121) 507 5588/9
Cardiff (01222) 709901
Edinburgh (0131) 536 2300
Leeds (0113) 536 2300; (0113) 292 3547
London (0171) 635 9191
Newcastle (0191) 232 5131

FURTHER READING

Budden L, Vink R 1996 Paracetamol overdose: pathophysiology and nursing management. British Journal of Nursing 5(3):145–152

Davis J E 1991 A consideration not to be overlooked – Activated charcoal in acute drug overdoses. Professional Nurse 6(12):710–714

Hellman M G 1996 Pediatric poisonings. Emergency Medical Services. The Journal of Emergency Care, Rescue and Transportation 25(6):21–28

Krenzelok E P, Dunmire S M 1992 Acute poisoning emergencies. Postgraduate Medicine 91(2):179–186

Shepherd S M 1996 Plant exposures. Emergency Medical Services. The Journal of Emergency Care, Rescue and Transportation 25(6):39–45

30

Drugs and the Law

It has long been accepted that some legal control over the supply, storage and use of poisons is necessary, but with the extensive use of new and increasingly potent drugs, close control is more essential than ever.

In the UK the manufacture, distribution and use of all medicinal substances is now controlled by the Medicines Act 1968, which combined and replaced several earlier Acts. Some drugs are more liable to misuse than others and are controlled more rigidly by the Misuse of Drugs Act 1971.

THE MEDICINES ACT 1968

Before any drug can be marketed in the UK the manufacturer must supply the Committee on Safety of Medicines with detailed information on its safety and proposed use. Approval may then be given for clinical trials, and if the results are satisfactory a Product Licence may be granted. This licence allows the manufacturer to recommend the product only for those conditions for which the clinical trial results were accepted. It may therefore take several years from the discovery of a drug in the laboratory to the marketing of a medicinal product for clinical use.

The Act is also concerned with checking the premises and procedures used to manufacture medicines. This monitoring is carried out by the Medicines Inspectorate, and approval of premises and procedures is required for hospital pharmacy production units as well as commercial pharmaceutical factories and warehouses.

The distribution of medicines is also controlled and here the Act divides products into three categories:

1. General Sales List (GSL) items: a restricted range of simple medicines which may be sold by any retailer.

2. Pharmacy-only medicines (P): those items which may be sold to the public without prescription, but only from a registered pharmacy.
3. Prescription-only medicines (POM): those items which may be sold or supplied to the public in accordance with a prescription issued by a medical practitioner or dentist. This list includes most of the potent drugs in current use. It is now recognized that a number of products in this category, particularly those for local use, should be available without prescription. The range of Pharmacy-only (P) products is accordingly being increased from time to time. These three categories govern the supply of medicines directly to the public.

In hospital practice, differentiation into GSL, P and POM groups does not apply, as all medicines are regarded as being under control. All medicines stored on the ward should be in locked cupboards or trolleys and internal, external and reagent preparations should be stored separately. In addition, ward drug trolleys should be immobilized when not in use. A lockable drug refrigerator should also be used for the increasing range of drugs needing storage below 8°C. The keys to these receptacles should be kept on the person of the sister or nurse in charge of the ward, who is also the person responsible for checking and signing orders for pharmaceutical supplies, checking storage, and seeing that stock is rotated regularly to avoid having any out-of-date supplies.

THE MISUSE OF DRUGS ACT 1971

Drugs liable to misuse are controlled by the Misuse of Drugs Act 1971 and are usually termed 'Controlled Drugs' or 'CDs'. The Act totally prohibits the possession, supply, manufacture, import or export of Controlled Drugs except as allowed by regulations or by licence from the Secretary of State. The use of Controlled Drugs in medicine is permitted by the Misuse of Drugs Regulations 1985 which classifies drugs into five groups or schedules according to different levels of control. Schedule 1 includes drugs with no recognized medicinal use such as LSD and cannabis. They are not prescribable and any individual who requires such a drug for research must obtain a special licence from the Home Office. Schedule 2 drugs includes most of the opioids, e.g. morphine, heroin, methadone, the major stimulants such as amphetamines, and some analgesic injections, e.g. dihydrocodeine, pentazocine and codeine. Schedule 3 includes the less powerful stimulants such as benzphetamine, the barbiturates, except those used for intravenous anaesthesia, the appetite depressants diethylpropion and mazindol, meprobamate, phentermine and pentazocine. These drugs are less likely to be misused, but on rational grounds should not be freely available to the public. Both Schedule 2 and 3 drugs can be supplied only for a particular patient, whose name and address must be specified on the prescription, together with the dose to be taken. The prescription must be written in ink, the quantity to be supplied must be written in *both words and figures*, and it must be signed and dated *entirely* by the prescriber personally. (The future use of computor-prescribing may bring changes.) It is illegal to dispense any prescriptions for Controlled Drugs that do not give this essential information. The main difference between Schedule 2 and 3 drugs is that for the latter a Controlled Drugs Register is not required.

Schedule 4 refers to the benzodiazepine group of hypnotics and anxiolytics. Schedule 5 comprises controlled drugs such as codeine and morphine that are combined in such small amounts with non-toxic substances that misuse is both difficult and unlikely, e.g. Kaolin and Morphine Mixture. These drugs need no special storage or administration records other than the retention of invoices for at least 2 years, and may be obtained without a prescription.

HOSPITAL REGULATION

In hospitals, some relaxation of the strictly legal requirements is usually accepted, as the patient's own case sheet should supply the details of the patient's identity that the Act requires. Storage and record-keeping requirements are as stringent as those applying to Controlled Drugs generally. It should be noted that practitioners are prohibited from prescribing controlled drugs for addicts unless specifically licensed to do so.

Ward stocks of controlled drugs must be ordered in the special book supplied for the purpose, and the order must be signed by the Charge Nurse or deputy. The duplicate copies of the orders must be kept by the Charge Nurse for at least 2 years.

All supplies of the controlled drugs must be signed for when received, and stored away from other drugs in a special locked cupboard, or locked inner compartment of the drugs cupboard, and the key must be kept *on the person* of the Charge Nurse or deputy. No doctor has right of access to ward stocks of any drugs, as the responsibility for their storage and use rests with the nurse-in-charge.

A written record should be made of every amount of a controlled drug received by a ward, and a detailed record kept of each dose given. Records of the administration of these drugs should be signed by the nurse who gives the dose, as well as by the nurse who checks the drug and dose.

A running record of stocks of all controlled drugs should be kept, and any wastage or loss must be recorded immediately, countersigned and reported.

Table 30.1 indicates some of the Controlled Drugs of Schedules 2 and 3; in general, the restrictions apply to derivatives and preparations of the drugs concerned, but in order to simplify the list the names of many preparations have been omitted. Any such drug issued from a pharmacy must bear a label indicating that it is a Controlled Drug.

The strictly legal restrictions governing the use of controlled drugs should be regarded as the minimum, and in most hospitals a greater degree of control is exercised. The actual stock and the recorded stock of such drugs should be checked at frequent intervals, and any loss reported and investigated. Such a system reminds users of the need for care when dealing with potent drugs, and discourages misuse.

THE MEDICINES ACT, PART III

The control of medicinal substances generally has now been extended by the implementation of the Medicines Act, Part III. In effect, this increases the range of products not covered by other controls, so that any substance now in Part III can be sold only on prescription, and under the supervision of pharmacist.

These POM (prescription-only medicines) products include most medicines that few people would wish to buy without medical advice, and represents a further attempt to prevent the misuse of medicines. The list of medicines controlled in this way is too extensive to be given in this book, as it includes many drugs in current use. It is perhaps worthwhile mentioning that in many countries the control of drugs is much more lax than in the UK. In some parts of Europe, for example, antibiotics can be bought freely without prescription!

RESTRICTIONS ON PRESCRIBING

Since 1 April 1985, doctors have not been allowed to prescribe certain drugs under the National Health

Table 30.1   Some Controlled Drugs (Schedules 2 and 3)

alfentanil	morphine; its salts and preparations unless diluted below 0.2% morphine or its equivalent in a base from which the drug cannot be readily extracted
amphetamine	
barbiturates	
buprenorphine	
cocaine and its salts and preparations unless diluted below 0.1% cocaine in a base from which the drug cannot be readily extracted	MST Continus
	Narphen
	Omnopon
	Omnopon-Scopolamine
	Opium preparations unless diluted below 0.2% morphine in a base from which the drug cannot be readily extracted
codeine for injection	
Cyclimorph	
dexamphetamine	Palfium
dextromoramide	Pamergan preparations
diamorphine	papaveretum
diconal	pentazocine
dihydrocodeine for injection	pethidine
dipipanone	phenazocine
fentanyl	phenoperidine
heroin	Physeptone
levorphanol	Rapifen
methadone	Sevredol
	SRM-Rhotard
	Sublimaze
	Temgesic
	Thalamonal

Service. Restricted products include antacids, laxatives, mild analgesics, cough remedies, expectorants, tonics and vitamins.

In practice, many drugs will continue to be prescribable under the official or non-proprietary name, but not under a brand or proprietary name. Thus if a product such as 'Valium' is required, it must be prescribed as 'diazepam'. The prescribing of certain mixed products in that way is difficult, so some special non-proprietary names have been devised, under which those products can be supplied. See p. 342.

Many non-prescribable products (the so-called 'black list') are simple medicaments that can be easily purchased from any pharmacy; other more sophisticated products remain unprescribable.

NURSE PRESCRIBING

In 1986 the Cumberledge Report recommended that community nurses should be able to prescribe prescription-only medicines (POMs) from a limited list. The initial legislation – The Medicinal Products: Prescription by Nurses Act 1992 – enables nurses in the community to prescribe by identifying them as 'appropriate practitioners', and the Pharmaceutical Services Regulations of 1994 allow pharmacists to dispense medicines prescribed by nurses.

As the law stands, only district nurses, health visitors and midwives working in the community in designated pilot sites who have undergone special training can prescribe using a restricted Nurse Prescriber's Formulary. This means that the designated nurse makes a professional and independent assessment of the patient on the basis of which a free choice is made from the *Nurse Prescriber's Formulary* about the most appropriate drug or treatment. The opinion of a doctor is not required, and the nurse, who is wholly professional and legally accountable, signs the prescription form.

The government's 1996 White Paper on primary health care promises to extend the existing nurse prescribing, and is looking forward to full implementation of nurse prescribing by 1998. However, there is no provision in the present legislation to allow RGNs without a district nurse, health visitor or midwifery qualification to prescribe, so excluding hospital nurses and those based in GP practices and clinics.

The Medicines Act 1968 Section 58(2)b states that the supply of POMs does not require a prescription provided it is in accordance with written directives of a doctor or dentist. This allows nurses to administer against the written authorization of a doctor which is not patient specific, and hence has permitted the development of drug 'protocols' to enable experienced and competent specialist nurses to supply and administer POMs. The UKCC document Standards for the Administration of Medicines supports the concept of drug protocols and states 'where it is the wish of the professional staff concerned that practitioners in a particular setting be authorized to administer, on their own authority, certain medications, a local protocol has been agreed between medical practitioners, nurses and midwives and the pharmacist'. Nurses utilizing protocols are advised to ensure that they comply as closely as possible with current law (see Elliott Pennells 1997).

FURTHER READING

Elliott Pennels C J 1997 Nurse Prescribing. Professional Nurse 13(2):114–115
Elliott Pennels C J 1997 Protocols. Professional Nurse 13(2):115–117

Grimes J 1994 OTC Formulary. Macmillan
United Kingdom Central Council for Nursing, Midwifery and Health Visiting 1992 Standards for the Administration of Medicines. UKCC, London

Appendices

Appendix I: Table of drug interactions

Many drug reactions, although undesirable, are of little clinical significance, and occur in but a few patients. They are more likely to occur in those patients mostly at risk, such as the elderly, and others in whom renal and liver function may have deteriorated. In some cases, the potential risks can be anticipated, as the combined use of beta-blockers, antihypertensives and diuretics can be expected to have additive effects. The following table merely gives an indication of the very extensive range of possible drug interactions, which is constantly widening as new drugs are introduced. For detailed information a specialist book on drug interactions should be consulted. Nurses should report all drug reactions that they may observe without delay.

Drug	Drug	Possible effects of combination
acarbose	*see antidiabetics*	
ACE-inhibitors	antihypertensives	It should be assumed that the effects of ACE-inhibitors will be enhanced by any other drug with an antihypertensive action, including diuretics
	cyclosporin	Hyperkalaemia
	potassium sparing diuretics	Hyperkalaemia
	levodopa	Increased hypotensive action
	contraceptives	Hypotensive action antagonized
	chlorpromazine	Severe postural hypotension
alcohol	CNS depressants	Depressive action enhanced
	antibacterials	Disulfiram-like reaction with

Drug	Drug	Possible effects of combination
alcohol cont'd		cephamandole, metronidazole, noridazole and tinidazole
	oral anticoagulants	Effects enhanced
	antidiabetics	Effects enhanced by alcohol; flushing with chlorpropamide
	antihistamines	Sedative effects enhanced
	antihypertensives	Effects enhanced
	antipsychotics	Sedative effects enhanced
aminoglycosides	capreomycin cisplatin cyclosporin vancomycin	Increased risk of oto/nephrotoxicity
	loop diuretics	Muscle relaxant effects enhanced
amiodarone (has a long half-life; side-effects may be prolonged)	anticoagulants (oral) anti-arrhythmics beta-blockers calcium channel blockers	Anticoagulant effects increased Additive effects Increased risk of bradycardia
antidepressants (tricyclic)	anti-epileptics	Lower convulsive threshold
	antihypertensives	Hypotensive effects generally enhanced
	antihistamines	Sedative and anticholinergic effects increased
	central depressants	Sedative effects increased
antidiabetics	beta-blockers	Effects enhanced
	diuretics	Effects antagonized
beta-blockers	ACE-inhibitors	Hypotensive effects enhanced
	anti-arrhythmics	Increased risk of bradycardia
	antidepressants	Risk of arrhythmias with some
	antihypertensives	May increase risk of first-dose hypotension
	diuretics	May enhance hypotensive effects
	sympathomimetics	May enhance hypertension

Drug	Drug	Possible effects of combination
bromocriptine and cabergoline	sympathomimetics	Increase risks of toxicity
cimetidine	anti-arrhythmics	Increase plasma concentration
	beta-blockers	Increase plasma concentration
	oral anticoagulants	Effects enhanced
	antipsychotics	Effects enhanced
calcium channel blockers	anti-arrhythmics	Increase risk of bradycardia
	anti-epileptics	Effects may be reduced
	antihypertensives	Effects may be enhanced
	dixogin	Plasma concentration may be increased
	theophylline	Effects may be enhanced
corticosteroids	diuretics	Diuretic action antagonized
	anti-epileptics rifampicin	Increase metabolism and reduce effects of corticosteroid
cyclosporin	aminoglycosides co-trimoxazole amphotericin 4-quinolones	Increase risk of nephrotoxicity
	anti-epileptics rifampicin	Reduce plasma concentration of cyclosporin
	ketoconazole calcium channel blockers	Increase plasma concentration of cyclosporin
	progestogen grapefruit juice	May increase toxicity
	statins	Increase risk of myopathy
digoxin	amiodarone quinine quinidine calcium channel blockers erythromycin	Plasma concentration of digoxin increased
disopyramide	anti-arrhythmics	Increased myocardial depression
	diuretics	Risk of increased toxicity if hypokalaemia occurs

Drug	Drug	Possible effects of combination
disopyramide cont'd	anti-epileptics rifampicin	Plasma concentration of disopyramide reduced
	erythromycin	Plasma concentration of disopyramide increased
diuretics	NSAIDs	Increased risk of nephrotoxicity; diuretic effects antagonized
	aminoglycosides	Increased risk of ototoxicity
	vancomycin	Increased risk of hyperkalaemia with potassium-sparers
	antidiabetics	Hypoglycaemic effects antagonized
	antihypertensives	Hypotensive action enhanced
	corticosteroids	Increased risk of hypokalaemia
	carbenoxolone contraceptives	Diuretic action antagonized
ergotamine	beta-blockers	Peripheral vasoconstriction increased
erythromycin	oral anticoagulants	Effects of warfarin and nicoumalone increased
	cimetidine	Toxicity with deafness may increase
	cyclosporin	Plasma concentration of cyclosporin increased
	theophylline	Plasma concentration of theophylline increased
ethosuximide	anti-epileptics	Convulsive threshold lowered
	antidepressants antipsychotics	Toxicity increased without increase in anticonvulsant activity
flecainide	other anti-arrhythmics	Myocardial depression increased
	cimetidine	Increased plasma concentration of flecainide
fluconazole	anticoagulants	Effects of warfarin and nicoumalone enhanced

Drug	Drug	Possible effects of combination
fluvoxamine	anticoagulants	Effects of warfarin and nicoumalone enhanced
griseofulvin	oral anticoagulants	Effects of warfarin and nicoumalone reduced
heparin	aspirin dipyridamole	Anticoagulant effects increased
iron – oral	magnesium trisilicate tetracycline	Absorption of iron reduced
isoniazid	anti-epileptics	Metabolism of some anti-epileptics reduced with an enhanced effect
ketoconazole and similar antifungals	antacids anticholinergics	Reduce absorption
	oral anticoagulants	Effects of warfarin and nicoumalone enhanced
	anti-epileptics	Effect of phenytoin enhanced
	rifampicin	Reduces plasma concentration of antifungals
	cyclosporin	Plasma concentration of cyclosporin increased
lamotrigine	anti-epileptics	May increase toxicity
levodopa	MAOIs	Risk of hypertensive crisis
	benzodiazepines	Anxiolytic action antagonized
	antihypertensives	Hypotensive action enhanced
lignocaine	beta-blockers anti-arrhythmics	Myocardial depression increased
	diuretics	Effects of lignocaine antagonized
lithium	analgesics ACE-inhibitors	Reduce excretion and increase toxicity of lithium
	fluvoxamine fluoxetine	May cause tremor and convulsions
	diuretics anti-epileptics	May increase neurotoxicity

Drug	Drug	Possible effects of combination
MAOIs	tricyclic antidepressants	CNS stimulation and hypertension
	antidiabetics	Hypoglycaemic effects enhanced
	anti-epileptics	Lower convulsive threshold
	antihypertensives	Hypotensive effects enhanced
	sympathomimetics	Risks of hypertensive crisis
methotrexate	aspirin NSAIDs probenecid	Excretion of methotrexate reduced with increased toxicity
methyldopa	alcohol antidepressants beta-blockers calcium channel blockers diuretics nitrates NSAIDs	Enhance hypotensive effects
	corticosteroids contraceptives carbenoxolone	Antagonize hypotensive effects
metoclopramide	analgesics	Absorption increased
	opioid analgesics anticholinergics	Antagonize effects of metoclopramide on gastro-intestinal tract
	antipsychotics lithium	Increased risk of extrapyramidal effects
metronidazole	oral anticoagulants	Effects of warfarin and nicoumalone enhanced
	phenytoin	Metabolism of phenytoin inhibited
	cimetidine	Metabolism of metronidazole inhibited
	alcohol	Disulfiram-like reaction
muscle relaxants (atracurium and other non-depolarizing muscle relaxants)	aminoglycosides propranolol verapamil quinidine	Muscle relaxant effects enhanced
	neostigmine	Muscle relaxant effects antagonized
suxamethonium	cyclophosphamide thiotepa lithium	Muscle relaxant effects enhanced

Drug	Drug	Possible effects of combination
	digoxin	May cause arrhythmias
NSAIDs	ACE-inhibitors diuretics	Hypotensive effects antagonized; diuretic effects antagonized by NSAIDs and nephrotoxicity increased with risk of hyperkalaemia
	lithium	Excretion of lithium reduced
omeprazole	phenytoin	Anti-epileptic action enhanced;
	warfarin	anticoagulant action enhanced
phenindione	aspirin cholestyramine dipyridamole clofibrate	Anticoagulant effects increased
	contraceptives vitamin K	Anticoagulant effects antagonized
phenytoin	aspirin amiodarone metronidazole viloxazine ketoconazole cimetidine sulphinpyrazone	Plasma concentration of phenytoin increased
	contraceptives theophylline cyclosporin digoxin anticoagulants	Metabolism increased by phenytoin
	antidepressants	Convulsive threshold lowered
probenecid	indomethacin naproxen cephalosporins penicillins nalidixic acid aciclovir captopril zidovudine methotrexate	Excretion reduced and plasma concentrations increased by probenecid
procainamide	amiodarone	Procainamide plasma concentration increased
	cimetidine other anti-arrhythmics	Increased myocardial depression
quinidine	amiodarone cimetidine verapamil	Quinidine plasma concentration increased

Drug	Drug	Possible effects of combination
quinidine cont'd	diuretics	Toxicity increased in hyperkalaemia
	digoxin	Plasma concentrations of digoxin increased (reduce dose)
	oral anticoagulants	Effects of warfarin and nicoumalone increased
	phenobarbitone phenytoin primidone	Plasma quinidine concentration reduced
	muscle relaxants	Relaxant action increased
quinine	cimetidine	Plasma quinine concentration increased
	digoxin	Plasma digoxin concentration increased (reduce dose)
quinolones	antacids theophylline	Reduce absorption Plasma concentration of theophylline increased
	oral anticoagulants	Anticoagulant effects enhanced
retinoids	cytotoxics	May increase risks of hepatotoxicity
rifampicin	antacids	Absorption decreased; rifampicin increases the metabolism and reduces the plasma concentrations of a wide range of drugs
sucralfate	antacids tetracyline	Reduce activity of sucralfate
	warfarin phenytoin	Absorption decreased by sucralfate
sulphinpyrazone	aspirin	Action of sulphinpyrazone antagonized
	oral anticoagulants	Effects of warfarin and nicoumalone enhanced
	antidiabetics	Effects enhanced
	phenytoin	Plasma concentrations of phenytoin enhanced
	theophylline	Plasma concentration of theophylline reduced

Drug	Drug	Possible effects of combination
sympatho-mimetics	MAOIs	Risks of hypertensive crisis
	beta-blockers	Risks of severe hypertension
	corticosteroids	Risks in high doses of hypokalaemia
tamoxifen	oral anticoagulants	Anticoagulant effects may be markedly increased
theophylline	ciprofloxacin erythromycin diltiazem	Plasma theophylline levels increased
	verapamil viloxazine contraceptives cimetidine aminoglutethimide rifampicin carbamazepine phenobarbitone phenytoin primidone sulphinpyrazone	Plasma levels of theophylline reduced
	beta-blockers	May cause bronchospasm
thyroxine	oral anticoagulants	Effects of warfarin, phenindione, nicoumalone increased
	propranolol	Effects of propranolol reduced
	rifampicin carbamazepine phenobarbitone phenytoin primidone	Metabolism of thyroxine increased
topiramate	anti-epileptics	May enhance toxicity and increase interactions
valproate	antidepressants antipsychotics	Convulsive threshold lowered
	aspirin	Effects of valproate increased
	anticonvulsants	May increase toxicity and sedation
vancomycin	aminoglycosides	Increased risk of ototoxicity
	loop diuretics cephalosporins	Increased risk of nephrotoxicity
venlafaxine	MAOIs	Increase toxicity

Drug	Drug	Possible effects of combination
warfarin	analgesics (NSAIDs) allopurinol alcohol amiodarone chloral hydrate cimetidine clofibrates ketoconazole and related antifungals sulphinpyrazone tamoxifen	Anticoagulant effects increased, markedly by azapropazone
	many non-penicillin antibiotics rifamycins griseofulvin aminoglutethimide contraceptives sucralfate	Anticoagulant effects reduced

Appendix II: Approved and brand names of drugs

These lists do not include mixed products, the exceptions being the official names for certain approved preparations – see p. 342.)

Approved name	Proprietary name	Main action or indication
abciximab	Reopro	heparin adjunct
acamprosate	Campral	alcoholism
acarbose	Glucobay	diabetes
acebutolol	Sectral	hypertension
aceclofenac	Preservex	arthritis
acemetacin	Emflex	arthritis
acetazolamide	Diamox	glaucoma
acetylcholine	Miochol	cataract surgery
acetylcysteine	Parvolex	mucolytic, paracetamol overdose
acipimox	Olbetam	hyperlipidaemia
acitretin	Neotigason	psoriasis
aclarubicin	Aclacin	cytotoxic
acrivastine	Semprex	antihistamine
actinomycin D	Cosmegen	cytotoxic
aciclovir	Zovirax	antiviral
adapalene	Differin gel	acne
adenosine	Adenocor	anti-arrhythmic
albendazole	Eskazole	anthelmintic
alclometasone	Modrasone	topical corticosteroid
aldesleukin	Proleukin	cytotoxic
alendronic acid	Fosamax	osteoporosis
alfacalcidol	Alfa D, One-Alpha	vitamin D deficiency
alfentanil	Rapifen	narcotic analgesic

Approved name	Proprietary name	Main action or indication
alfuzosin	Xatral	prostatic hypertrophy
alglucerase	Ceridase	Gaucher's disease
allopurinol	Zyloric	gout
alprazolam	Xanax	antidepressant
alprostadil	Prostin VR	maintenance of ductus arteriosus in neonates
alteplase	Actilyse	fibrinolytic
altretamine	Hexalen	cytotoxic
alverine	Spasmonal	antispasmodic
amantadine	Symmetrel	parkinsonism
amifostine	Ethylol	cytoprotectant
amikacin	Amikin	antibiotic
amiloride	Midamor	diuretic
aminoglutethimide	Orimeten	cytotoxic
aminophylline	Pecram Phyllocontin	asthma
amiodarone	Cordarone X	anti-arrhythmic
amisulpride	Solian	antipsychotic
amitriptyline	Lentizol, Tryptizol	antidepressant
amlodipine	Istin	calcium antagonist
amorolfine	Loceryl	antifungal
amoxapine	Asendis	antidepressant
amoxycillin	Amoxil, Almodan	antibiotic
amphotericin	AmBisome, Amphocil	antifungal
amphotericin B	Abelcet, Fungilin, Fungizone	antifungal
ampicillin	Amfipen, Penbritin	antibiotic
amsacrine	Amsidine	cytotoxic
amylobarbitone	Amytal	hypnotic
anastrozole	Arimidex	cytotoxic
ancrod	Arvin	anticoagulant
anistreplase	Eminase	fibrinolytic
apomorphine	Britaject	parkinsonism
apraclonidine	Iopidine	cataract surgery
aprotinin	Trasylol	haemostatic
astemizole	Hismanal	antihistamine
atenolol	Tenormin	beta-blocker

Approved name	Proprietary name	Main action or indication
atorvastatin	Lipitor	hyperlipidaemia
atovaquone	Malarone	antimalarial
atracurium	Tracrium	muscle relaxant
auranofin	Ridaura	rheumatoid arthritis
azapropazone	Rheumox	antirheumatic
azatadine	Optimine	antihistamine
azathioprine	Azamune, Imuran	immunosuppressive
azelaic acid	Skinoren	acne
azelastine	Rhinolast	rhinitis
azithromycin	Zithromax	antibiotic
azlocillin	Securopen	antibiotic
aztreonam	Azactam	antibiotic
bacampicillin	Ambaxin	antibiotic
baclofen	Lioresal	muscle relaxant
balsalazide	Colazide	ulcerative colitis
bambuterol	Bambec	asthma
beclomethasone	Becotide	corticosteroid
beclomethasone	Propaderm	topical corticosteroid
bendrofluazide	Aprinox, Neo-Naclex	diuretic
benorylate	Benoral	analgesic
benperidol	Anquil	tranquillizer
benzhexol	Artane, Broflex	parkinsonism
benztropine	Cogentin	parkinsonism
benzylpenicillin	Crystapen	antibiotic
beractant	Survanta	neonatal respiratory distress
betahistine	Serc	Ménière's syndrome
betamethasone	Betnelan, Betnesol	corticosteroid
betamethasone	Betnovate	topical corticosteroid
betaxolol	Kerlone	beta-blocker
betaxolol	Beoptic	glaucoma
bethanechol	Myotonine	smooth muscle stimulant
bethanidine	Bendogen	hypertension
bezafibrate	Bezalip	hyperlipidaemia
bicalutamide	Casodex	cytotoxic
biperiden	Akineton	parkinsonism
bisacodyl	Dulcolax	laxative

Approved name	Proprietary name	Main action or indication
bismuth chelate	De-Noltab	peptic ulcer
bisoprolol	Emcor, Monocor	beta-blocker
botulinum toxin	Botox, Dysport	blepharospasm
bretylium tosylate	Bretylate	cardiac arrhythmias
brimonidine	Alphagan	glaucoma
bromazepam	Lexotan	anxiolytic
bromocriptine	Parlodel	lactation suppressant
brompheniramine	Dimotane	antihistamine
budesonide	Pulmicort, Rhinocort	rhinitis
bumetanide	Burinex	diuretic
bupivacaine	Marcain	anaesthetic
buprenorphine	Temgesic	analgesic
buserelin	Suprefact	prostatic carcinoma
buspirone	Buspar	anxiolytic
busulphan	Myleran	cytotoxic
butobarbitone	Soneryl	hypnotic
cabergoline	Dostinex	inhibition of lactation
cadexomer iodine	Iodosorb	leg ulcers
calcipotriol	Dovonex	psoriasis
calcitonin	Calcitare	hormone
calcitriol	Rocaltrol	vitamin D deficiency
candesartan	Amias	hypertension
canrenoate	Spiroctan-N	diuretic
capreomycin	Capastat	antibiotic
captopril	Acepril, Capoten	ACE-inhibitor
carbamazepine	Tegretol	epilepsy
carbaryl	Carylderm, Clinicide, Derbac	parasiticide
carbenoxolone	Bioral, Bioplex	mouth ulcers
carbimazole	Neo-Mercazole	thyrotoxicosis
carbocisteine	Mucodyne	mucolytic
carboplatin	Paraplatin	cytotoxic
carboprost	Hemabate	post-partum haemorrhage
carisoprodol	Carisoma	muscle relaxant
carmustine	BiCNU	cytotoxic
carteolol	Teoptic	glaucoma
carvedilol	Eucardic	beta-blocker

Approved name	Proprietary name	Main action or indication
cefaclor	Distaclor	antibiotic
cefadroxil	Baxan	antibiotic
cetamandole	Kefadol	antibiotic
cefixime	Suprax	antibiotic
cefodizime	Timecef	antibiotic
cefotaxime	Claforan	antibiotic
cefoxitin	Mefoxin	antibiotic
cefpirome	Cefrom	antibiotic
cefpodoxime	Orelox	antibiotic
cefrozil	Cefzil	antibiotic
ceftazidime	Fortum, Kefadim	antibiotic
ceftibuten	Cedax	antibiotic
ceftizoxime	Cefizox	antibiotic
ceftriaxone	Rocephin	antibiotic
cefuroxime	Zinacef, Zinnat	antibiotic
celiprolol	Celectol	beta-blocker
cephalexin	Ceporex, Keflex	antibiotic
cephazolin	Kefzol	antibiotic
cephradine	Velosef	antibiotic
cerivastatin	Lipobay	hyperlipidaemia
certoparin	Alphaparin	anticoagulant
cetirizine	Zirtek	antihistamine
chenodeoxycholic acid	Chendol, Chenofalk	gallstones
chloral hydrate	Noctec, Welldorm	hypnotic
chlorambucil	Leukeran	cytotoxic
chloramphenicol	Chloromycetin, Kemicetine	antibiotic
chlordiazepoxide	Librium, Tropium	tranquillizer
chlorhexidine	Hibitane	antiseptic
chlormethiazole	Heminevrin	hypnotic
chloroquine	Avloclor, Nivaquine	antimalarial
chlorothiazide	Saluric	diuretic
chlorpheniramine	Piriton	antihistamine
chlorpromazine	Largactil	tranquillizer
chlorpropamide	Diabinese	hypoglycaemic
chlortetracycline	Aureomycin	antibiotic
chlorthalidone	Hygroton	diuretic
cholestyramine	Questran	bile acid binder
choline theophyllinate	Choledyl	bronchospasm

Approved name	Proprietary name	Main action or indication	Approved name	Proprietary name	Main action or indication
chymotrypsin	Zonulysin	cataract surgery	co-codamol	Medocodone, Panadeine, Paracodol, Parake	analgesic
cidofovir	Vistide	CMV retinitis			
cilazapril	Vascase	ACE-inhibitor			
cimetidine	Galenemet, Tagamet	H_2-blocker	co-codaprin	Codis	analgesic
			co-dergocrine	Hydergine	dementia
cinnarizine	Stugeron	anti-emetic	co-dydramol	Paramol	analgesic
cinoxacin	Cinobac	antibiotic	co-fluampicil	Magnapen	antibiotic
ciprofibrate	Modalim	hyperlipidaemia	co-flumactone	Aldactide	diuretic
ciprofloxacin	Ciproxin	antibacterial	colestipol	Colestid	exchange resin
cisapride	Prepulsid	oesophageal reflux	colfosceril	Exosurf	neonatal respiratory distress
cisatracurium	Nimbex	muscle relaxant			
cisplatin	Neoplatin, Platosin	cytotoxic	colistin	Colomycin	antibiotic
			co-phenotrope	Lomotil	diarrhoea
citalopram	Cipramil	antidepressant	co-prenozide	Trasidrex	hypertension
cladribine	Leustat	cytotoxic	co-proxamol	Cosalgesic, Distalgesic, Paxalgesic	analgesic
clarithromycin	Klaricid	antibiotic			
clemastine	Tavegil	antihistamine			
clindamycin	Dalacin C	antibiotic	cortisone	Cortisyl	corticosteroid
clobazam	Frisium	anxiolytic	co-simalcite	Altacite plus	antacid
clobetasol	Dermovate	topical corticosteroid	co-tenidone	Tenoret 50, Tenoretic	hypertension
clobetasone	Eumovate	topical corticosteroid	co-triamterzide	Dyazide	diuretic
clodronate	Bonefos	hypercalcaemia of malignancy	co-trimoxazole	Bactrim, Chemotrim Septrin	antibacterial
clofazimine	Lamprene	antileprotic	crisantaspase	Erwinase	leukaemia
clofibrate	Atromid S	hyperlipidaemia	crotamiton	Eurax	antipruritic
clomiphene	Clomid, Serophene	infertility	cyanocobalamin	Cytacon, Cytamen	anti-anaemic
clomipramine	Anafranil	antidepressant	cyclizine	Marzine, Valoid	anti-emetic
clonazepam	Rivotril	epilepsy	cyclopenthiazide	Navidrex	diuretic
clonidine	Catapres, Dixarit	hypertension, migraine	cyclopentolate	Mydrilate	mydriatic
clopidogrel	Plavix	atherosclerosis	cyclophosphamide	Endoxana	cytotoxic
clorazepate	Tranxene	anxiolytic	cyclosporin	Sandimmun	immunosuppressant
clotrimazole	Canestan	antifungal	cyproheptadine	Periactin	antihistamine
cloxacillin	Orbenin	antibiotic	cyproterone	Androcur, Cyprostat	anti-androgen
clozapine	Clozaril	antipsychotic			
co-amilofruse	Frumil; Lasoride	diuretic	cytarabine	Alexan, Cytosar	cytotoxic
co-amilozide	Amilco, Moduret 25, Moduretic	diuretic	dacarbazine	DTIC	cytotoxic
			dactinomycin	Cosmogen	cytotoxic
co-amoxiclav	Augmentin	antibiotic	dalteparin	Fragmin	anticoagulant
co-beneldopa	Madopar	parkinsonism	danaparoid	Organan	anticoagulant
co-careldopa	Sinemet	parkinsonism	danazol	Danol	endometriosis

Approved name	Proprietary name	Main action or indication
dantrolene	Dantrium	muscle relaxant
daunorubicin	Cerubidin, DaunoXome	cytotoxic
demeclocycline	Ledermycin	antibiotic
desferrioxamine	Desferal	iron poisoning
desflurane	Suprane	inhalation anaesthetic
desipramine	Pertofran	antidepressant
desmopressin	DDAVP	diabetes insipidus
desoxymethasone	Stiedex	local corticosteroid
dexamethasone	Decadron	corticosteroid
dexamphetamine	Dexedrine	appetite suppressant
dextran	Gentran, Rheomacrodex	plasma substitute
dextromoramide	Palfium	analgesic
dextropropoxyphene	Doloxene	analgesic
diazepam	Diazemuls, Stesolid, Valium	anxiety; epilepsy
diazoxide	Eudemine	hypertension, hypoglycaemic
diclofenac	Motifene, Voltarol	antirheumatic
dicobalt edetate	Kelocyanor	cyanide poisoning
dicyclomine	Merbentyl	antispasmodic
didanosine	Videx	antiviral
diethylcarbamazine	Banocide	filariasis
diethylpropion	Tenuate	appetite suppressant
diflucortolone	Nerisone	topical corticosteroid
diflunisal	Dolobid	analgesic
digoxin	Lanoxin	heart failure
digoxin antibody	Digibind	digoxin overdose
dihydrocodeine	DF118	analgesic
dihydrotachysterol	AT10, Tachyrol	hypocalcaemia
diloxanide furoate	Furamide	amoebiasis
diltiazem	Adizem, Tildiem	calcium antagonist
dimenhydrinate	Dramamine	antihistamine
dinoprost	Prostin F2	uterine stimulant
dinoprostone	Prostin E2	uterine stimulant
diphenoxylate	Lomotil	diarrhoea
dipivefrine	Propine	glaucoma
dipyridamole	Persantin	vasodilator

Approved name	Proprietary name	Main action or indication
disodium etidronate	Didronel	Paget's disease
disodium pamidronate	Aredia	Paget's disease
disopyramide	Dirythmin-SA, Rythmodan	cardiac arrhythmias
distigmine	Ubretid	urinary retention
disulfiram	Antabuse	alcoholism
dobutamine	Dobutrex	cardiac stimulant
docetaxel	Taxotere	cytotoxic
docusate sodium	Dioctyl	laxative
domperidone	Motilium	anti-emetic
donepezil	Aricept	Alzheimer's disease
dopamine	Intropin	cardiac stimulant
dopexamine	Dopacard	cardiac surgery
dornase alfa	Pulmozyme	cystic fibrosis
dorzolamide	Trusopt	glaucoma
dothiepin	Prothiaden	antidepressant
doxapram	Dopram	respiratory stimulant
doxazosin	Cardura	hypertension
doxepin	Sinequan	antidepressant
doxorubicin	Caelyx	antibiotic
doxycycline	Nordox, Vibramycin	antibiotic
droperidol	Droleptan	neuroleptic
dydrogesterone	Duphaston	progestogen
econazole	Ecostatin, Pevaryl	antifungal
ecothiopate	Phospholine iodide	glaucoma
eformoterol	Foradil	bronchodilator
enalapril	Innovace	ACE-inhibitor
enflurane	Enthrane	inhalation anaesthetic
enoxaparin	Clexane	anticoagulant
enoximone	Perfan	heart failure
entacapone	Comtess	parkinsonism
epirubicin	Pharmorubicin	cytotoxic
epoprostenol	Flolan	bypass surgery
epoetin alfa epoetin beta	Eprex Recormon	anaemia in chronic renal failure
ergotamine	Lingraine	migraine
erythromycin	Erymax, Erythrocin, Ilotycin	antibiotic

Approved name	Proprietary name	Main action or indication	Approved name	Proprietary name	Main action or indication
erythropoietin	Eprex, Recormon	anaemia in chronic renal failure	flumazenil	Anexate	benzodiazepine antagonist
esmolol	Brevibloc	beta-blocker	flunisolide	Syntaris	corticosteroid
estramustine	Estracyt	cytotoxic	flunitrazepam	Rohypnol	hypnotic
ethacrynic acid	Edecrin	diuretic	fluocinolone	Synalar	topical corticosteroid
ethambutol	Myambutol	tuberculosis	fluocinonide	Metosyn	topical corticosteroid
ethamsylate	Dicynene	haemostatic			
ethosuximide	Emeside, Zarontin	anticonvulsant	fluocortolone	Ultralanum	topical corticosteroid
etidronate	Didronel	Paget's disease	fluorometholone	FML	topical corticosteroid
etodolac	Lodine	arthritis			
etomidate	Hypnomidate	i.v. anaesthetic	fluoxetine	Prozac	antidepressant
etoposide	Exelon, Vepesid	cytotoxic	flupenthixol	Depixol	schizophrenia
Factor VIIa	Novoseven	haemophilia A	fluphenazine	Modecate, Moditen	schizophrenia
Factor VIII	Kogenate Monoclate-P	haemophilia A	flurandrenolone	Haelan	topical corticosteroid
Factor IX	Mononine, Replenine	haemophilia B	flurazepam	Dalmane	hypnotic
			flurbiprofen	Froben	arthritis
famciclovir	Famvir	antiviral	flutamide	Drogenil	prostatic carcinoma
famotidine	Pepcid-PM	H_2-blocker	fluticasone	Cutivate	topical corticosteroid
felodipine	Plendil	hypertension			
fenbufen	Lederfen	antirheumatic	fluticasone	Flixonase	allergic rhinitis
fenofibrate	Lipantil	hyperlipidaemia	fluticasone	Flixotide	bronchodilator
fenoprofen	Fenopron, Progesic	arthritis	fluvastatin	Lescol	hyperlipidaemia
			fluvoxamine	Faverin	antidepressant
fenoterol	Berotec	asthma	folinic acid	Refolinon	methotrexate antidote
fentanyl	Durogesic, Sublimaze	analgesic patch	formestane	Lentaron	cytotoxic
fenticonazole	Lomexin	antifungal	foscarnet	Foscavir	antiviral
fexofenadine	Telfast	antihistamine	fosfestrol	Honvan	cytotoxic
filgrastim	Neupogen	neutropenia	fosfomycin	Monuril	urinary infections
finasteride	Proscar	prostatic hypertrophy	fosinopril	Staril	ACE-inhibitor
			framycetin	Soframycin	topical antibiotic
fish oil concentrate	Maxepa	hyperlipidaemia	frusemide	Lasix	diuretic
flavoxate	Urispas	antispasmodic	fusafungine	Locabiotal	antibiotic
flecainide	Tambocor	cardiac arrhythmias	gabapentin	Neurontin	epilepsy
flucloxacillin	Floxapen	antibiotic	gallamine	Flaxedil	muscle relaxant
fluconazole	Diflucan	antifungal	gammaglobulin	Kabiglobulin	hepatitis
flucytosine	Alcobon	antifungal	gamolenic acid	Epogam	eczema
fludarabine	Fludara	cytotoxic	ganciclovir	Cymevene	antiviral
fludrocortisone	Florinef	corticosteroid	gelatin	Gelofusine	blood volume expander

Approved name	Proprietary name	Main action or indication	Approved name	Proprietary name	Main action or indication
gemcitabine	Gemzar	cytotoxic	hydroxyurea	Hydrea	cytotoxic
gemfibrozil	Lopid	hyperlipidaemia	hydroxyzine	Atarax	tranquillizer
gentamicin	Cidomycin, Genticin	antibiotic	hyoscine butyl bromide	Buscopan	antispasmodic
gestrinone	Dimetriose	endometriosis	ibuprofen	Brufen, Fenbid	arthritis
gestronol	Depostat	endometrial carcinoma	idarubicin	Zavedos	cytotoxic
			idoxuridine	Herpid, Virudox	antiviral
glibenclamide	Daonil, Euglucon	hypoglycaemic	ifosfamide	Mitoxana	cytotoxic
			imipenem	Primaxin	antibiotic
gliclazide	Diamicron	hypoglycaemic	imipramine	Tofranil	antidepressant
glimepiride	Amaryl	hypoglycaemic	immunoglobulin G	Endobulin	antibody deficiency
glipizide	Glibenese, Minodiab	hypoglycaemic	indapamide	Natrilix	hypertension
gliquidone	Glurenorm	hypoglycaemic	indinavir	Crixivan	antiviral
glutaraldehyde	Glutarol	warts	indomethacin	Flexin, Indocid, Indomod	arthritis
glyceryl trinitrate	Sustac, Tridil	angina			
glycopyrronium	Robinul	antimuscarinic	indoramin	Baratol	beta-blocker
gonadorelin	Fertilol	infertility	indoramin	Doralese	prostatic hypertrophy
goserelin	Zoladex	prostatic carcinoma			
granisetron	Kytril	anti-emetic	inosine pranobex	Imunovir	antiviral
griseofulvin	Fulcin, Grisovin	antifungal	inositol nicotinate	Hexopal	vasodilator
guanethidine	Ismelin	hypertension	interferon	Intron, Roferon, Wellferon	leukaemia
guar gum	Guarem, Guarina	diabetes			
			ipratropium	Atrovent	bronchodilator
halcinonide	Halciderm	topical corticosteroid	irbisartan	Aprovel	hypertension
			irinotecan	Campto	cytotoxic
halofantrine	Halfan	antimalarial	iron-sorbitol	Jectofer	iron-deficiency anaemia
haloperidol	Dozic, Haldol, Serenace	schizophrenia			
			isocarboxazid	Marplan	antidepressant
halothane	Fluothane	anaesthetic	isoconazole	Travogyn	candidiasis
hetastarch	Elohes, Hespan	blood volume expander	isoniazid	Rimifon	tuberculosis
			isoprenaline	Saventrine	bronchospasm
hexamine hippurate	Hiprex	urinary antiseptic	isosorbide dinitrate	Cedocard, Isordil	angina
hyaluronic acid	Hyalgan	osteoarthritis			
hyaluronidase	Hyalase	enzyme	isosorbide mononitrate	Elantan, Monit	angina
hydralazine	Apresoline	hypertension	isotretinoin	Isotrex, Roaccutane	acne
hydrochlorothiazide	Hydrosaluric	diuretic			
hydrocortisone	Corlan, Efcortesol	corticosteroid	isradipine	Prescal	calcium antagonist
			itraconazole	Sporanox	antifungal
hydroflumethiazide	Hydrenox	diuretic	ivermectin	Mectizan	filariasis
hydromorphone	Palladone	opioid agonist	kanamycin	Kannasyn	antibiotic
hydroxocobalamin	Cobalin-H, Neo-Cytamen	anti-anaemic	ketamine	Ketalar	anaesthetic
			ketoconazole	Nizoral	antifungal
hydroxychloroquine	Plaquenil	antimalarial	ketoprofen	Alrheumat, Orudis	arthritis
hydroxyprogesterone	Proluton-Depot	progestogen			

Approved name	Proprietary name	Main action or indication
ketorolac	Toradol	analgesic
ketotifen	Zaditen	anti-asthmatic
labetalol	Labrocol, Trandate	beta-blocker
lacidipine	Motens	calcium antagonist
lactulose	Duphalac, Laxose	laxative
lamotrigine	Lamictal	epilepsy
lamivudine	Epiver	antiviral
lanreotide	Somatuline	acromegaly
lansoprazole	Zoton	peptic ulcer
latanoprost	Xalantan	glaucoma
lenograstim	Granocyte	neutropenia
lepuridin	Refludan	anticoagulant
lercandipine	Zanidip	hypertension
letrozole	Femara	cytotoxic
leucovorin	Isovorin	anticytoxic
leuprorelin	Prostap	prostatic carcinoma
levobunolol	Betagan	glaucoma
levocabastine	Livostin	allergic conjunctivitis
levofloxacin	Tavanic	antibacterial
lignocaine	Xylocaine	anaesthetic
lignocaine	Xylocard	cardiac arrhythmias
liothyronine	Tertroxin	thyroid deficiency
lisinopril	Carace, Zestril	ACE-inhibitor
lithium carbonate	Camcolit, Phasal	mania
lodoxamide	Alomide	allergic conjunctivitis
lofepramine	Gamanil	antidepressant
lofexidine	Britlofex	opioid withdrawal
lomustine	CCNU	cytotoxic
loperamide	Arret, Imodium	diarrhoea
loratadine	Clarityn	antihistamine
lorazepam	Ativan	tranquillizer
losartan	Cozaar	hypertension
loxapine	Loxapac	antipsychotic
lymecycline	Tetralysal	antibiotic
lypressin	Syntopressin	diabetes insipidus
lysuride	Revanil	parkinsonism
malathion	Derbac, Prioderm	parasiticide
maprotiline	Ludiomil	antidepressant
mebendazole	Vermox	anthelmintic
mebeverine	Colofac	antispasmodic
medroxyprogesterone	Provera	progestogen
mefenamic acid	Ponstan	arthritis
mefloquine	Larium	malaria
mefruside	Baycaron	diuretic
megestrol	Megace	cytotoxic
meloxicam	Mobic	osteoarthritis
melphalan	Alkeran	cytotoxic
meprobamate	Equanil	tranquillizer
meptazinol	Meptid	analgesic
mequitazine	Primalan	antihistamine
mercaptopurine	Puri-Nethol	cytotoxic
meropenem	Meropen	antibiotic
mesalazine	Asacol, Pentasa, Salofalk	ulcerative colitis
mesna	Uromitexan	urotoxicity due to cyclophosphamide
mesterolone	Pro-viron	androgen
metaraminol	Aramine	hypotension
metformin	Glucophage	hypoglycaemic
methadone	Physeptone	analgesic
methocarbamol	Robaxin	muscle relaxant
methohexitone	Brietal	anaesthetic
methotrexate	Maxtrex	cytotoxic
methotrimeprazine	Nozinan	pain in terminal cancer
methoxamine	Vasoxine	vasoconstrictor
methylcellulose	Celevac	laxative
methylcysteine	Visclair	mucolytic
methyldopa	Aldomet	hypertension
methylphenidate	Ritalin	hyperactivity
methylphenobarbitone	Prominal	epilepsy
methylprednisolone	Medrone	corticosteroid
methysergide	Deseril	migraine
metirosine	Demser	phaeochromocytoma
metoclopramide	Maxolon, Gastromax	anti-emetic
metolazone	Metenix, Xuret	diuretic
metoprolol	Betaloc, Lopresor	beta-blocker

Approved name	Proprietary name	Main action or indication
metronidazole	Flagyl, Zadstat	anaerobic infections, trichomoniasis
metyrapone	Metopirone	resistant oedema
mexiletine	Mexitil	cardiac arrhythmias
mianserin	Bolvidon, Norval	antidepressant
miconazole	Daktarin	antifungal
midazolam	Hypnovel	i.v. anaesthetic
mifepristone	Mifegyne	termination of pregnancy
milrinone	Primacor	severe heart failure
minocycline	Minocin	antibiotic
minoxidil	Loniten	hypertension
misoprostol	Cytotec	peptic ulcer
mitozantrone	Novantrone	cytotoxic
mivacurium	Mivacrom	muscle relaxant
mizolastine	Mizollen	rhinoconjunctivitis
moclobemide	Manerix	antidepressant
modafinil	Provigil	narcolepsy
moexipril	Perdix	hypertension
molgramostim	Leucomax	neutropenia
mometasone	Elocon	topical corticosteroid
moracizine	Ethmozine	anti-arrhythmic
monosulfiram	Tetmosol	scabies
moxonidine	Physiotens	hypertension
mupirocin	Bactroban	topical antibiotic
mycophenolate	CellCept	immuno-suppressant
nabilone	Cesamet	anti-emetic
nabumetone	Relifex	arthritis
nadolol	Corgard	beta-blocker
nafarelin	Synarel	endometriosis
naftidrofuryl	Praxilene	vasodilator
nalbuphine	Nubain	analgesic
nalidixic acid	Negram	urinary antiseptic
naloxone	Narcan	narcotic antagonist
naltrexone	Nalorex	opioid dependence
nanadrolone	Deca-Durabolin	anabolic steroid
naproxen	Synflex, Naprosyn	arthritis
naratriptan	Naramig	migraine

Approved name	Proprietary name	Main action or indication
nedocromil	Tilade	anti-asthmatic
nefopam	Acupan	analgesic
nefazodone	Dutonin	antidepressant
nelfinavir	Viracept	antiviral
neostigmine	Prostigmin	myasthenia
netilmicin	Netillin	antibiotic
nevirapine	Viramune	antiviral
nicardipine	Cardene	calcium antagonist
niclosamide	Yomesan	anthelmintic
nicorandil	Ikorel	angina
nicotinyl alcohol	Ronicol	vasodilator
nicoumalone	Sinthrome	anticoagulant
nifedepine	Adalat, Coracten, Nifensar	calcium antagonist
nimodipine	Nimotop	calcium antagonist
nisoldipine	Syscor	angina, hypertension
nitrazepam	Mogadon, Remnos, Somnite	hypnotic
nitrofurantoin	Furadantin, Macrodantin	urinary antiseptic
nizatidine	Axid, Zinga	H_2-blocker
noradrenaline	Levophed	hypotension
norethisterone	Primolut N, Menzol	progestogen
norfloxacin	Utinor	urinary tract infections
nortriptyline	Allegron	antidepressant
nystatin	Nystan	antifungal
octreotide	Sandostatin	carcinoid syndrome
oestradiol	Climaval	menopausal symptoms
ofloxacin	Exocin, Tarivid	antibacterial
olanzapine	Zyprexa	schizophrenia
olsalazine	Dipentum	ulcerative colitis
omeprazole	Losec	peptic ulcer
ondansetron	Zofran	anti-emetic
orciprenaline	Alupent	bronchodilator
orphenadrine	Biorphen, Disipal	parkinsonism
orlistat	Xenical	obesity
oxitropium	Oxivent	bronchodilator

Approved name	Proprietary name	Main action or indication
oxpentifylline	Trental	vasodilator
oxprenolol	Trasicor	beta-blocker
oxybutynin	Cystrin, Ditropan	urinary incontinence
oxypertine	Integrin	tranquillizer
oxytetracycline	Terramycin	antibiotic
paclitaxel	Taxol	cytotoxic
pamidronate	Aredia	hypercalcaemia of malignancy
pancuronium	Pavulon	muscle relaxant
pantoprazole	Protium	peptic ulcer
paroxetine	Seroxat	antidepressant
pemoline	Volital	cerebral stimulant
penciclovir	Vectavir	antiviral
penicillamine	Distamine, Pendramine	Wilson's disease
pentaerythritol tetranitrate	Mycardol	angina
pentamidine	Pentacarinat	leishmaniasis
pentastarch	Pentaspan	blood volume expander
pentazocine	Fortral	analgesic
pentostatin	Nipent	hairy-cell leukaemia
peppermint oil	Mintec	abdominal distension
pergolide	Celance	parkinsonism
pericyazine	Neulactil	schizophrenia
perindopril	Coversyl	ACE-inhibitor
permethrin	Lyclear	pediculocide
perphenazine	Fentazin	schizophrenia
phenazocine	Narphen	analgesic
phenelzine	Nardil	antidepressant
phenindamine	Thephorin	antihistamine
phenindione	Dindevan	anticoagulant
pheniramine	Daneral	antihistamine
phenoxybenzamine	Dibenyline	vasodilator
phentermine	Duromine,	appetite suppressant
phentolamine	Rogitine	phaeochromo-cytoma
phenylbutazone	Butacote	ankylosing spondylitis
phenytoin	Epanutin	epilepsy
phytomenadione	Konakion	hypoprothrombin-aemia

Approved name	Proprietary name	Main action or indication
pimozide	Orap	schizophrenia
pindolol	Visken	beta-blocker
piperacillin	Pipril	antibiotic
pipothiazine	Piportil	antipsychotic
piracetam	Nootropil	tics
pirbuterol	Exirel	bronchodilator
pirenzepine	Gastrozepin	peptic ulcer
piretanide	Arelix	diuretic
piroxicam	Feldene	antirheumatic
pivampicillin	Pondocillin	antibiotic
pizotifen	Sanomigran	migraine
podophyllotoxin	Condyline	penile warts
poldine	Nacton	antispasmodic
polyestradiol	Estradurin	prostatic carcinoma
polygeline	Haemaccel	blood volume expander
polystyrene resin	Resonium	hyperkalaemia
polythiazide	Nephril	diuretic
poractant	Curoserf	neonatal respiratory distress
pravastatin	Lipostat	hyperlipidaemia
prazosin	Hypovase	hypertension
prednisolone	Deltacortril, Deltastab, Precortisyl	corticosteroid
prilocaine	Citanest	anaesthetic
primidone	Mysoline	epilepsy
probenecid	Benemid	gout
procainamide	Pronestyl	cardiac arrhythmias
procarbazine	Natulan	cytotoxic
prochlorperazine	Stemetil	anti-emetic, vertigo
procyclidine	Arpicolin, Kemadrin	parkinsonism
proguanil	Paludrine	antimalarial
promazine	Sparine	tranquillizer
promethazine	Phenergan	antihistamine
promethazine theoclate	Avomine	anti-emetic
propafenone	Arythmol	cardiac arrhythmias
propantheline	Pro-Banthine	peptic ulcer
propiverine	Detrunorm	unstable bladder
propofol	Diprivan	i.v. anaesthetic
propranolol	Inderal	beta-blocker

Approved name	Proprietary name	Main action or indication
propyliodone	Dionosil	contrast agent
protriptyline	Concordin	antidepressant
provastatin	Lipostat	hyperlipidaemia
proxymetacaine	Ophthaine	corneal anaesthetic
pumactant	Alec	lung surfactant
pyrazinamide	Zinamide	tuberculosis
pyridostigmine	Mestinon	myasthenia
pyrimethamine	Daraprim	antimalarial
quetiapine	Seroquel	schizophrenia
quinagolide	Norprolac	hyperprolactinaemia
quinalbarbitone	Seconal	hypnotic
quinapril	Accupro	ACE-inhibitor
raloxitine	Evista	osteoporosis
raltitrexed	Tomudex	cytotoxic
ramipril	Tritace	ACE-inhibitor
ranitidine	Zantac	H_2-blocker
ranitidine bismuth citrate	Pylorid	peptic ulcer
razoxane	Razoxin	cytotoxic
reboxetine	Edronax	antidepressant
remifentanil	Ultiva	opioid agonist
reproterol	Bronchodil	bronchodilator
reteplase	Rapilysin	thrombolytic
rifabutin	Mycobutin	tuberculosis
rifampicin	Rifadin, Rimactane	tuberculosis
riluzole	Rilutek	motor neurone disease
rimiterol	Pulmadil	bronchodilator
risperidone	Risperdal	antipsychotic
ritodrine	Yutopar	premature labour
ritonavir	Norvir	antiviral
rivastigmine	Exelon	Alzheimer's disease
rizatriptan	Maxalt	migraine
rocuronium	Esmeron	muscle relaxant
ropinirole	Requip	parkinsonism
ropivacaine	Naropin	local anaesthetic
salbutamol	Ventolin	bronchospasm
salcatonin	Calsynar, Miacalcic	Paget's disease
salmeterol	Serevent	bronchospasm
saquinavir	Invirase	antiviral

Approved name	Proprietary name	Main action or indication
selegiline	Eldepryl Zelapar	parkinsonism
sermorelin	Geref	growth hormone
sertindole	Serdolect	schizophrenia
sertraline	Lustral	antidepressant
sevoflurane	–	anaesthetic
sildenafil	Viagra	impotence
silver sulphadiazine	Flamazine	antibacterial
simvastatin	Zocor	hyperlipidaemia
sodium acetrizoate	Diaginol	contrast agent
sodium aurothiomalate	Myocrisin	rheumatoid arthritis
sodium clodronate	Bonefos, Loron	hypercalcaemia of malignancy
sodium cromoglycate	Intal, Rynacrom	anti-allergic
sodium diatrizoate	Hypaque	contrast agent
sodium fusidate	Fucidin	antibiotic
sodium iothalamate	Conray	contrast agent
sodium ipodate	Biloptin	contrast agent
sodium iron edetate	Sytron	anti-anaemic
sodium metrizoate	Triosil	contrast agent
sodium stibogluconate	Pentostam	leishmaniasis
sodium valproate	Epilim	epilepsy
somatropin	Genotropin, Saizen	growth hormone
sotalol	Beta-Cardone, Sotacor	beta-blocker
spectinomycin	Trobicin	antibiotic
spironolactone	Aldactone, Spiroctan	diuretic
stanozolol	Stromba	anabolic steroid
stavudine	Zerit	antiviral
streptokinase	Kabikinase, Streptase	thrombosis
sucralfate	Antepsin	peptic ulcer
sulconazole	Exelderm	antifungal
sulfametopyrazine	Kelfizine	sulphonamide
sulindac	Clinoril	arthritis
sulphasalazine	Salazopyrin	ulcerative colitis
sulphinpyrazone	Anturan	gout
sulpiride	Dolmatil, Sulpitil	schizophrenia
sumatriptan	Imigran	migraine
suxamethonium	Anectine, Scoline	muscle relaxant

Approved name	Proprietary name	Main action or indication	Approved name	Proprietary name	Main action or indication
tacrolimus	Prograf	immunosuppressant	tocainide	Tonocard	cardiac arrhythmias
tamoxifen	Nolvadex, Tamofen	anti-oestrogen	tolazamide	Tolanase	hypoglycaemic
tamsulosin	Flomax	prostatic hypertrophy	tolbutamide	Rastinon	hypoglycaemic
			tolcapone	Tasmar	parkinsonism
tazarotene	Zorac	psoriasis	tolfenamic acid	Clotam	migraine
tazobactam	Tazocin	antibiotic	tolmetin	Tolectin	antirheumatic
teicoplanin	Targocid	antibiotic	tolterodine	Detrusitol	unstable bladder
temazepam	Normison	hypnotic	topiramate	Topamax	epilepsy
temocillin	Temopen	antibiotic	topotecan	Hycamtin	cytotoxic
tenoxicam	Mobilflex	arthritis	torasemide	Torem	diuretic
terazosin	Hytrin	hypertension	toremifene	Fareston	cytotoxic
terbinafine	Lamisil	antifungal	tramadol	Zamadol, Zydol	analgesic
terbutaline	Bricanyl, Monovent	bronchospasm	trandolapril	Gopten, Odrik	ACE-inhibitor
			tranexamic acid	Cyklokapron	antifibrinolytic
terfenadine	Triludan	antihistamine	tranylcypromine	Parnate	antidepressant
terlipressin	Glypressin	oesophageal bleeding	trazodone	Molipaxin	antidepressant
			treosulfan	—	cytotoxic
testosterone	Primoteston, Virormone	hypogonadism	tretinoin	Retin-A Vesanoid	acne antileukaemic
tetracosactrin	Synacthen	corticotrophin	triamcinolone	Adcortyl	corticosteroid
tetracycline	Achromycin	antibiotic	triamterene	Dytac	diuretic
theophylline	Nuelin	bronchodilator	tribavirin	Virazid	antiviral
thiabendazole	Mintezol	anthelmintic	triclofos	—	hypnotic
thiabutosine	Ciba 1906	anthelmintic	trientine	—	Wilson's disease
thioguanine	Lanvis	cytotoxic	trifluoperazine	Stelazine	tranquillizer
thiopentone	Intraval	i.v. anaesthetic	trilostane	Modrenal	aldosteronism
thioridazine	Melleril	tranquillizer	trimeprazine	Vallergan	antihistamine
thymoxamine	Opilon	vasodilator	trimethoprim	Trimopan	antibacterial
thyroxine	Eltroxin	thyroid deficiency	trimetrexate	Neutrexin	AIDS
tiagapine	Gabitril	anticonvulsant	trimipramine	Surmontil	antidepressant
tiaprofenic acid	Surgam	arthritis	triptorelin	Decapeptyl	cytotoxic
tibolone	Livial	menopausal symptoms	troglitazone	Romozin	insulin enhancer
			tropicamide	Mydriacyl	mydriatic
ticarcillin	Ticar, Timentin	antibiotic	tropisetron	Navoban	antin-emetic
tiludronic acid	Skelid	Paget's disease	tryptophan	Optimax	antidepressant
timolol	Blocadren, Betim	beta-blocker	tulobuterol	Respacal	bronchodilator
			urofollitrophin	Orgafol	infertility
tinidazole	Fasigyn	anaerobic infections	urokinase	Ukidan	hyphaemia; embolism
tinzaparin	Innohep, Logiparin	anticoagulant			
tioconazole	Trosyl	antifungal	ursodeoxycholic acid	Destolit	gallstones
tizanidine	Zanaflex	spasticity	valaciclivor	Valtrex	antiviral
tobramycin	Nebcin	antibiotic	valproate	Epilim	epilepsy

Approved name	Proprietary name	Main action or indication	Approved name	Proprietary name	Main action or indication
valproic acid	Convulex	epilepsy	vinorelbine	Navelbine	cytotoxic
valsartan	Diovan	hypertension	warfarin	Marevan	anticoagulant
vancomycin	Vancocin	antibiotic	xamoterol	Corwin	mild heart failure
vasopressin	Pitressin	diabetes insipidus	xipamide	Diurexan	diuretic
vecuronium	Norcuron	muscle relaxant	xylometazoline	Otrivine	nasal decongestant
venlafaxine	Efexor	antidepressant	zalcatabine	Hivid	HIV infections
verapamil	Cordilox, Univer	angina, hypertension	zidovudine	Retrovir	antiviral
vigabatrin	Sabril	anticonvulsant	zolmitriptan	Zomig	acute migraine
viloxazine	Vivalan	antidepressant	zolpidem	Stilnoct	hypnotic
vinblastine	Velbe	cytotoxic	zopiclone	Zimovane	hypnotic
vincristine	Oncovin	cytotoxic	zotepine	Zoleptil	schizophrenia
vindesine	Eldisine	cytotoxic	zuclopenthixol	Clopixol	schizophrenia

APPROVED NAMES OF MIXED PRODUCTS

Co-amilofruse: amiloride and frusemide (Frumil, Lasoride)
Co-amilozide: amiloride and hydrochlorothiazide (Amilco, Hypertane, Moduretic)
Co-amoxiclav: amoxycillin and clavulanic acid (Augmentin)
Co-beneldopa: levodopa and benserazide (Madopar)
Co-careldopa: levodopa and carbidopa (Sinemet)
Co-codamol: codeine and paracetamol (Paracodol)
Co-codaprin: codeine and aspirin (Codis)
Co-dydramol: dihydrocodeine and paracetamol (Paramol)
Co-fluampicil: ampicillin and flucloxacillin (Magnapen)
Co-flumactone: flumethiazide and spironolactone (Aldactide)
Co-phenotrope: diphenoxylate and atropine (Lomotil, Tropergen)
Co-prenozide: oxprenolol and cyclopenthiazide (Trasidex)
Co-proxamol: dextropropoxyhene and paracetamol (Cosalgesic, Distalgesic, Panalgesic)
Co-tenidone: atenolol and chlorthalidone (Tenoret, Tenoretic)
Co-triamterzide: triamterene and hydrochlorothiazide (Dyazide)
Co-trimoxazole: sulphamethoxazole and trimethoprim (Bactrim, Septrin)

Proprietary name	Approved name	Main action or indication
Abelcet	amphotericin	antifungal
Accupro	quinapril	ACE-inhibitor
Acepril	captopril	ACE-inhibitor
Achromycin	tetracycline	antibiotic
Aclacin	aclarubicin	cytotoxic
Actilyse	alteplase	fibrinolytic
Acupan	nefopam	analgesic
Adalat	nifedepine	calcium antagonist
Adcortyl	triamcinolone	topical corticosteroid
Adenocor	adenosine	anti-arrhythmic
Adipine	nifedipine	angina
Adizem	diltiazem	angina
Adriamycin	doxorubicin	antibiotic
Akineton	biperiden	parkinsonism
Alcobon	flucytosine	antifungal

Proprietary name	Approved name	Main action or indication
Aldactone	spironolactone	resistant oedema
Aldomet	methyldopa	hypertension
Alec	pumactant	lung surfactant
Alexan	cytarabine	cytotoxic
Alfa D	alfacalcidol	vitamin D deficiency
Alkeran	melphalan	cytotoxic
Allegron	nortriptyline	antidepressant
Aller-eze	clemastine	antihistamine
Almodan	amoxycillin	antibiotic
Alomide	iodoxamide	allergic conjunctivitis
Alphagan	brimonidine	glaucoma
Alphaparin	certoparin	anticoagulant
Alrheumat	ketoprofen	arthritis
Altacite plus	co-simalcite	antacid
Alupent	orciprenaline	bronchospasm
Amaryl	glimepiride	diabetes
Ambaxin	bacampicillin	antibiotic
AmBisome	amphotericin B	antifungal
Amfipen	ampicillin	antibiotic
Amias	candesartan	hypertension
Amikin	amikacin	antibiotic
Amoxil	amoxycillin	antibiotic
Amphocil	amphotericin B	antifungal
Amsidine	amsacrine	cytotoxic
Amytal	amylobarbitone	hypnotic
Anafranil	clomipramine	antidepressant
Androcur	cyproterone	anti-androgen
Anectine	suxamethonium	muscle relaxant
Anexate	flumazenil	benzodiazepine antagonist
Angilol	propranolol	beta-blocker
Anquil	benperidol	tranquillizer
Antabuse	disulfiram	alcoholism
Antepsin	sucralfate	peptic ulcer
Anturan	sulphinpyrazone	gout
Apresoline	hydralazine	hypertension
Aprinox	bendrofluazide	diuretic
Aprovel	irbisartan	hypertension
Apsifen	ibuprofen	arthritis
Aquadrate	urea	ichthyosis

Proprietary name	Approved name	Main action or indication
Aramine	metaraminol	vasoconstrictor
Aredia	disodium pamidronate	hypercalcaemia of malignancy
Aricept	donepezil	Alzheimer's disease
Arimidex	anastrozole	breast cancer
Arpicolin	procyclidine	parkinsonism
Arpimycin	erythromycin	antibiotic
Arret	loperamide	diarrhoea
Artane	benzhexol	parkinsonism
Arvin	ancrod	anticoagulant
Arythmol	propafenone	cardiac arrhythmias
Asacol	mesalazine	ulcerative colitis
Ascabiol	benzyl benzoate	scabies
Asendis	amoxapine	antidepressant
AT10	dihydrotachysterol	hypocalcaemia
Atarax	hydroxyzine	tranquillizer
Atensine	diazepam	tranquillizer
Ativan	lorazepam	tranquillizer
Atromid-S	clofibrate	hypercholesterol-aemia
Atrovent	ipratropium	bronchodilator
Aureomycin	chlortetracycline	topical antibiotic
Avloclor	chloroquine	antimalarial
Avomine	promethazine	anti-emetic
Axid	nizatidine	H_2-blocker
Azactam	aztreonam	antibiotic
Azamune	azathioprine	cytotoxic
Bactrim	co-trimoxazole	antimicrobial
Bactroban	mupirocin	topical antibiotic
Bambec	bambuterol	asthma
Banocide	diethylcarbamazine	filariasis
Baratol	indoramin	beta-blocker
Baxan	cefadroxil	antibiotic
Baycaron	mefruside	diuretic
Becloforte	beclomethasone	corticosteroid
Beconase	beclomethasone	rhinitis
Becotide	beclomethasone	corticosteroid
Bedranol SR	propranolol	beta-blocker
Bendogen	bethanidine	hypertension
Benemid	probenecid	gout
Benoral	benorylate	analgesic

Proprietary name	Approved name	Main action or indication
Benoxyl	benzyl peroxide	acne
Benzagel	benzyl peroxide	acne
Berkaprine	azathioprine	cytotoxic
Berkatens	verapamil	angina, hypertension
Berkmycen	oxytetracycline	antibiotic
Berkolol	propranolol	beta-blocker
Berkozide	bendrofluazide	diuretic
Berotec	fenoterol	bronchitis
Beta-Cardone	sotalol	beta-blocker
Betadine	povidone–iodine	antiseptic
Betagan	levobunolol	glaucoma
Betaloc	metapropolol	beta-blocker
Betim	timolol	beta-blocker
Betnelan	betamethasone	corticosteroid
Betnesol	betamethasone	corticosteroid
Betnovate	betamethasone	topical corticosteroid
Betoptic	betaxolol	glaucoma
Bezalip	bezafibrate	hyperlipidaemia
BiCNU	carmustine	cytotoxic
Biliodyl	phenobutiodil	contrast agent
Biloptin	sodium ipodate	contrast agent
Biltricide	praziquantel	anthelmintic
Bioplex	carbenoxolone	mouth ulcers
Bioral	carbenoxolone	mouth ulcers
Biorphen	orphenadrine	parkinsonism
Blocadren	timolol	beta-blocker
Bonefos	clodrinate	hypercalcaemia of malignancy
Botox	botulinum toxin	blepharospasm
Bretylate	bretylium	cardiac arrhythmias
Brevibloc	esmolol	beta-blocker
Bricanyl	terbutaline	bronchospasm
Brietal	methohexitone	anaesthetic
Britaject	apomorphine	parkinsonism
BritLofex	lofexidine	opioid withdrawal
Broflex	benzhexol	parkinsonism
Bronchodil	reproterol	bronchodilator
Brufen	ibuprofen	arthritis
Buccastem	prochlorperazine	vertigo
Burinex	bumetanide	diuretic

Proprietary name	Approved name	Main action or indication
Buscopan	hyoscine butyl bromide	antispasmodic
Buspar	buspirone	anxiolytic
Butacote	phenylbutazone	ankylosing spondylitis
Cacit	calcium carbonate	osteoporosis
Caelyx	doxorubicin	cytotoxic
Calabren	glibenclamide	hypoglycaemic
Calciparine	calcium heparin	anticoagulant
Calcisorb	sodium cellulose phosphate	hypercalciuria
Calcitare	calcitonin	Paget's disease
Calcium Resonium	exchange resin	hyperkalaemia
Calpol	paracetamol	analgesic
Calsynar	salcatonin	Paget's disease
Camcolit	lithium carbonate	mania
Campral	acamprosate	opioid antagonist
Campto	irinotecan	cytotoxic
Canestan	clotrimazole	antifungal
Capastat	capreomycin	tuberculosis
Caplenal	allopurinol	gout
Capoten	captopril	ACE-inhibitor
Caprin	aspirin	arthritis
Carace	lisinopril	ACE-inhibitor
Cardene	nicardipine	calcium antagonist
Cardilate	nifedipine	angina
Cardinol	propranolol	beta-blocker
Cardura	doxazosin	hypertension
Carisoma	carisprodol	muscle relaxant
Carylderm	carbaryl	parasiticide
Casodex	bicalutamide	cytotoxic
Catapres	clonidine	hypertension
Caverject	alprostadil	prostaglandin
CCNU	lomustine	cytotoxic
Cedocard	isosorbide dinitrate	angina
Cedax	ceftibuten	antibiotic
Cefrom	cefpirome	antibiotic
Cefzil	cefrozil	antibiotic
Celance	pergolide	parkinsonism
Celectol	celiprolol	beta-blocker
Celevac	methylcellulose	laxative

Proprietary name	Approved name	Main action or indication
CellCept	mycophenolate	immunosuppressant
Ceporex	cephalexin	antibiotic
Ceredase	alglucerase	Gaucher's disease
Cerubidin	daunorubicin	cytotoxic
Cesamet	nabilone	anti-emetic
Cetavlex	cetrimide	antiseptic
Chendol	chenodeoxycholic acid	gallstones
Chenofalk	chenodeoxycholic acid	gallstones
Chloromycetin	chloramphenicol	antibiotic
Choledyl	choline theophyllinate	bronchodilator
Ciba 1906	thiambutosine	leprosy
Cidomycin	gentamicin	antibiotic
Cilazapril	vascace	ACE-inhibitor
Ciloxan	ciprofloxacin	corneal ulcers
Cinobac	cinoxacin	antibiotic
Cipramil	citalopram	antidepressant
Ciproxin	ciprofloxacin	antibacterial
Citanest	prilocaine	anaesthetic
Claforan	cefotaxime	antibiotic
Clarityn	loratadine	antihistamine
Clexane	enoxaparin	anticoagulant
Climaval	oestradiol	menopausal symptoms
Clinicide	carbaryl	parasiticide
Clinoril	sulindac	arthritis
Cloburate	clobetasone	eye-drops
Clomid	clomiphene	gonadotrophin inhibitor
Clopixol	zuclopenthixol	schizophrenia
Clotam	tolfenamic acid	migraine
Clozaril	clozapine	antipsychotic
Cobalin-H	hydroxocobalamin	anti-anaemic
Cogentin	benztropine	parkinsonism
Colazide	balsalazide	ulcerative colitis
Colestid	colestipol	exchange resin
Colofac	mebeverine	antispasmodic
Colomycin	colistin	antibiotic
Colpermin	peppermint oil	antispasmodic
Comtess	entacapone	parkinsonism

Proprietary name	Approved name	Main action or indication
Concordin	protriptyline	antidepressant
Condyline	podophyllotoxin	penile warts
Conray	sodium iothalamate	contrast agent
Convulex	valproic acid	epilepsy
Coracten	nifedipine	calcium antagonist
Cordarone X	amiodarone	cardiac arrhythmias
Cordilox	verapamil	angina
Corgard	nadolol	beta-blocker
Corlan	hydrocortisone	local corticosteroid
Coro-Nitro	glycerol trinitrate	angina
Cortisyl	cortisone	corticosteroid
Corwin	xamoterol	mild heart failure
Cosmegen	dactinomycin	cytotoxic
Coversyl	perindopril	ACE-inhibitor
Cozaar	losartan	hypertension
Creon	pancreatin	cystic fibrosis
Crixiv	indinavir	antiviral
Crystapen	benzylpenicillin	antibiotic
Curatoderm	tacalcitol	psoriasis
Curoserf	poractant	neonatal respiratory distress
Cutivate	fluticasone	topical corticosteroid
Cyclogest	progesterone	premenstrual syndrome
Cyklokapron	tranexamic acid	antifibrinolytic
Cymevene	ganciclovir	antiviral
Cyprostat	cyproterone	prostatic carcinoma
Cystrin	oxybutynin	urinary spasm
Cytacon	cyanocobalamin	anti-anaemic
Cytamen	cyanocobalamin	anti-anaemic
Cytosar	cytarabine	cytotoxic
Cytotec	misoprostol	peptic ulcer
Daktarin	miconazole	antifungal
Dalacin C	clindamycin	antibiotic
Dalmane	flurazepam	hypnotic
Daneral-SA	pheniramine	antihistamine
Danol	danazol	endometriosis
Dantrium	dantrolene	muscle relaxant
Daonil	glibenclamide	hypoglycaemic
Daranide	dichlorphenamide	glaucoma
Daraprim	pyrimethamine	antimalarial

Proprietary name	Approved name	Main action or indication
DaunoXome	daunorubicin	cytotoxic
DDAVP	desmopressin	diabetes insipidus
Decadron	dexamethasone	corticosteroid
Deca-Durabolin	nandrolone	cytotoxic
De-Capeptyl SR	triptorelin	cytotoxic
Deltacortril	prednisolone	corticosteroid
Deltastab	prednisolone	corticosteroid
Demser	metirosine	phaeochromo-cytoma
De-Nol	bismuth chelate	peptic ulcer
De-Noltab	bismuth chelate	peptic ulcer
Depixol	flupenthixol	schizophrenia
Deponit	glyceryl trinitrate	angina
Depostat	gestronol	endometrial carcinoma
Derbac	carbaryl	parasiticide
Dermovate	clobetasol	topical corticosteroid
Deseril	methysergide	migraine
Desferal	desferrioxamine	iron poisoning
Destolit	ursodeoxycholic acid	gallstones
Detrunorm	propiverine	unstable bladder
Detrusitol	tolterodine	unstable bladder
Dexedrine	dexamphetamine	appetite depressant
DF-118	dihydrocodeine	analgesic
Diabinese	chlorpropamide	hypoglycaemic
Diaginol	sodium acetrizoate	contrast agent
Diamicron	glicazide	hypoglycaemic
Diamox	acetazolamide	glaucoma
Diazemuls	diazepam	anxiolytic
Dibenyline	phenoxybenzamine	vasodilator
Dicynene	ethamyslate	haemostatic
Didronel	disodium etidronate	Paget's disease
Differin	adapalene	acne
Diflucan	fluconazole	antifungal
Digibind	digoxin antibody	digoxin overdose
Dilzem	diltiazem	calcium antagonist
Dimetriose	gestrinone	endometriosis
Dimotane	brompheniramine	antihistamine
Dindevan	phenindione	anticoagulant
Dioctyl	docusate sodium	laxative

Proprietary name	Approved name	Main action or indication
Dionosil	propyliodone	contrast agent
Diovan	valsartan	hypertension
Dipentum	olsalazine	ulcerative colitis
Diprivan	propofol	i.v. anaesthetic
Dirythmin-SA	disopyramide	cardiac arrhythmias
Disipal	orphenadrine	parkinsonism
Distaclor	cefaclor	antibiotic
Distamine	penicillamine	Wilson's disease
Ditropan	oxybutynin	urinary spasm
Diurexan	xipamide	diuretic
Dixarit	clonidine	migraine
Dobutrex	dobutamine	cardiac stimulant
Dolmatil	sulpiride	schizophrenia
Dolobid	diflunisal	analgesic
Doloxene	dextropropoxyphene	analgesic
Domical	amitriptyline	antidepressant
Dopacard	dopexamine	cardiac surgery
Dopram	doxopram	respiratory stimulant
Doralese	indoramin	prostatic hypertrophy
Dostinex	cabergoline	inhibition of lactation
Dovonex	calcipotriol	psoriasis
Dozic	haloperidol	antipsychotic
Dramamine	dimenhydrinate	antihistamine
Drogenil	flutamide	prostatic carcinoma
Droleptan	droperidol	analgesic
DTIC	dacarbazine	cytotoxic
Dulcolax	bisacodyl	laxative
Duphalac	lactulose	laxative
Duphaston	dydrogestone	progestogen
Duragesic	fentanyl	analgesic patches
Duromine	phentermine	appetite suppressant
Dutonin	nefazodone	antidepressant
Dyazide	co-triamterzide	diuretic
Dyspamet	cimetidine	H_2-blocker
Dysport	botulinum toxin	blepharospasm
Dytac	triamterine	diuretic
Ebufac	ibuprofen	arthritis
Ecostatin	econazole	antifungal

Proprietary name	Approved name	Main action or indication
Edecrin	ethacrynic acid	diuretic
Edronax	reboxetine	antidepressant
Efalith	lithium succinate	seborrhoea
Efamast	gamolenic acid	mastalgia
Efcortelan	hydrocortisone	topical corticosteroid
Efexor	venlafaxine	antidepressant
Efudix	fluorouracil	cytotoxic
Elantan	isosorbide mononitrate	angina
Eldepryl	selegiline	parkinsonism
Eldisine	vindesine	cytotoxic
Elocon	mometasone	topical corticosteroid
Elohes	hetastarch	blood volume expander
Eltroxin	thyroxine	thyroid deficiency
Emblon	tamoxifen	anti-oestrogen
Emcor	bisoprolol	beta-blocker
Emeside	ethosuximide	anticonvulsant
Emflex	acemetacin	arthritis
Eminase	anistreplase	fibrinolytic
Endobulin	immunoglobulin G	antibody deficiency
Endoxana	cyclophosphamide	cytotoxic
Epanutin	phenytoin	anticonvulsant
Epilim	sodium valproate	anticonvulsant
Epivir	lamivudine	antiviral
Epogam	gamolenic acid	eczema
Eppy	adrenaline	glaucoma
Eprex	epoetin alpha	anaemia in chronic renal failure
Equanil	meprobamate	tranquillizer
Erwinase	crisantaspase	leukaemia
Erymax	erythromycin	antibiotic
Erythrocin	erythromycin	antibiotic
Eskazole	albendazole	anthelmintic
Esmeron	rocuronium	muscle relaxant
Estracyt	estramustine	cytotoxic
Estradurin	polyestradiol	prostatic carcinoma
Ethmozine	moracizine	anti-arrhythmic
Ethmozine	moracizine	anti-arrhythmic
Ethylol	amifostine	cytoprotectant
Eucardic	carvedilol	hypertension

Proprietary name	Approved name	Main action or indication
Eudemine	diazoxide	hypertension, hypoglycaemia
Euglucon	glibenclamide	hypoglycaemic
Eumovate	clobetasone	topical corticosteroid
Eurax	crotamiton	antipruritic
Evista	raloxifine	osteoporosis
Exelderm	sulconazole	antifungal
Exelon	rivastigmine	Alzheimer's disease
Exirel	pirbuterol	bronchodilator
Exocin	ofloxacin	antibacterial
Exosurf	colfosceril	neonatal respiratory distress
Fabrol	acetylcysteine	mucolytic
Famvir	famciclovir	antiviral
Fareston	toremifene	cytotoxic
Farlutal	medroxyproges-terone	progestogen
Fasigyn	tinidazole	anaerobic infections
Faverin	fluvoxamine	antidepressant
Feldene	piroxicam	arthritis
Femara	letrozole	cytotoxic
Femulen	ethynodiol	oral contraceptive
Fenbid	ibuprofen	arthritis
Fenopron	fenoprofen	arthritis
Fentazin	perphenazine	tranquillizer
Fertilol	gonadorelin	infertility
Flagyl	metronidazole	antimicrobial
Flamazine	silver sulphadiazine	antibacterial
Flaxedil	gallamine	muscle relaxant
Flexin	indomethacin	arthritis
Flixonase	fluticasone	allergic rhinitis
Flixotide	fluticasone	bronchodilator
Flolan	epoprostenol	preserving platelet function in bypass surgery
Flomax	tamsulosin	prostatic hypertrophy
Florinef	fludrocortisone	corticosteroid
Floxapen	flucloxacillin	antibiotic
Fluanxol	flupenthixol	antidepressant
Fludara	fludarabine	cytotoxic
Fluothane	halothane	inhalation anaesthetic

Proprietary name	Approved name	Main action or indication
FML	fluoromethalone	topical corticosteroid
Foradil	eformoteral	bronchodilator
Fortral	pentazocine	analgesic
Fortum	ceftazidime	antibiotic
Fosamax	alendronic acid	osteoporosis
Foscavir	foscarnet	antiviral
Fragmin	delteparin	anticoagulant
Framygen	framycetin	antibiotic
Frisium	clobazam	anxiolytic
Froben	flurbiprofen	antirheumatic
Frumil	co-amilofruse	diuretic
Fucidin	sodium fusidate	antibiotic
Fulcin	griseofulvin	antifungal
Fungilin	amphotericin B	antifungal
Fungizone	amphotericin B	antifungal
Furadantin	nitrofurantoin	urinary antiseptic
Furamide	diloxanide furoate	amoebiasis
Gabitril	tiagapine	anticonvulsant
Galcodine	codeine	antitussive
Galenamox	amoxycillin	antibiotic
Galenphol	pholcodine	antitussive
Gamanil	lofepramine	antidepressant
Garamycin	gentamicin	antibiotic
Gastromax	metaclopramide	anti-emetic
Galenamet	cimetidine	H_2-blocker
Gelofusine	gelatin	blood volume expander
Gemzar	gemcitabine	cytotoxic
Genotropin	somatrophin	growth hormone
Genticin	gentamicin	antibiotic
Gentran	dextran	plasma substitute
Geret	sermorelin	growth hormone
Gestanin	allyloestranol	progestogen
Glibenese	glipizide	hypoglycaemic
Glucobay	acarbose	diabetes
Glucophage	metformin	hypoglycaemic
Glurenorm	gliquidone	hypoglycaemic
Glypressin	terlipressin	oesophageal varices
Gopten	trandolapril	ACE-inhibitor
Granocyte	lenograstim	neutropenia
Grisovin	griseofulvin	antifungal

Proprietary name	Approved name	Main action or indication
Guarem	guar gum	diabetes
Guarina	guar gum	diabetes
Haelan	flurandrenolone	topical corticosteroid
Halciderm	halcinonide	topical corticosteroid
Haldol	haloperidol	schizophrenia
Halfan	halofantrine	antimalarial
Harmogen	oestrone	menopause
Hemabate	carboprost	post-partum haemorrhage
Heminevrin	chlormethiazole	psychosis, hypnotic
Hep-Flush	heparin	anticoagulant
Heplok	heparin	anticoagulant
Hepsal	heparin	anticoagulant
Herpid	idoxuridine	antiviral
Hespan	hetastarch	blood volume expander
Hetrazan	diethylcarbamazine	filariasis
Hexalen	altretamine	cytotoxic
Hexopal	inositol nicotinate	vasodilator
Hibitane	chlorhexidine	antiseptic
Hiprex	hexamine hippurate	urinary antiseptic
Hismanal	astemizole	antihistamine
Hivid	zalcatabine	antiviral
Honvan	fosfestrol	cytotoxic
Humatrope	somatrophin	growth hormone
Humegon	gonadotrophin	infertility
Hyalase	hyaluronidase	enzyme
Hyalgan	hyaluronic acid	osteoarthritis
Hycamtin	topotecan	cytotoxic
Hydergine	co-dergocrine	dementia
Hydrea	hydroxyurea	cytotoxic
Hydrenox	hydro flumethiazide	diuretic
Hydrocortistab	hydrocortisone	corticosteroid
Hydrocortisyl	hydrocortisone	corticosteroid
Hydrocortone	hydrocortisone	corticosteroid
HydroSaluric	hydrochlorothiazide	diuretic
Hygroton	chlorthalidone	diuretic
Hypnomidate	etomidate	i.v. anaesthetic
Hypnovel	midazolam	i.v. anaesthetic
Hypovase	prazosin	hypertension
Hytrin	terazocin	hypertension

Proprietary name	Approved name	Main action or indication
Ibular	ibuprofen	arthritis
Iduridin	idoxuridine	antiviral
Ikorel	nicorandil	angina
Ilosone	erythromycin	antibiotic
Imbrilon	indomethacin	arthritis
Imdur	isosorbide mononitrate	angina
Imigran	sumatriptan	migraine
Immunoprin	azathioprine	immunosuppressant
Imodium	loperamide	diarrhoea
Imtack	isosorbide dinitrate	angina
Imunovir	inosine pranobex	antiviral
Imuran	azathioprine	immunosuppressant
Inderal	propranolol	beta-blocker
Indocid	indomethacin	arthritis
Indolar	indomethacin	arthritis
Indomod	indomethacin	arthritis
Innohep	tinzaparin	anticoagulant
Innovace	enalapril	ACE-inhibitor
Inoven	ibuprofen	analgesic
Intal	sodium cromoglycate	asthma
Integrin	oxypertine	antipsychotic
Intraval	thiopentone	i.v. anaesthetic
Intron A	interferon	leukaemia
Invirase	saquinavir	antiviral
Iodosorb	cadexomer iodine	leg ulcers
Iopidine	apraclonidine	cataract surgery
Ipral	trimethaprim	antibacterial
Ismelin	guanethidine	hypertension
Ismo	isosorbide mononitrate	angina
Isoket	isosorbide dinitrate	angina
Isordil	isosorbide dinitrate	angina
Isotrate	isosorbide mononitrate	angina
Isotrex	isotretinoin	acne
Isovorin	leucovorin	anticytoxic
Istin	amlodipine	calcium antagonist
Jectofer	iron-sorbitol	iron deficiency anaemia
Kabiglobulin	gamm-aglobulin	hepatitis
Kabikinase	streptokinase	fibrinolytic

Proprietary name	Approved name	Main action or indication
Kannasyn	kanamycin	antibiotic
Kefadim	ceftazidime	antibiotic
Kefadol	cefamandole	antibiotic
Keflex	cephalexin	antibiotic
Kefzol	cephazolin	antibiotic
Kelfizine	sulphametopyrazine	sulphonamide
Kelocyanor	dicobalt edetate	cyanide poisoning
Kemadrin	procyclidine	parkinsonism
Kemicetine	chloromycetin	antibiotic
Kenalog	triamcinolone	corticosteroid
Kerlone	betaxolol	beta-blocker
Ketalar	ketamine	i.v. anaesthetic
Kinidin	quinidine	cardiac arrhythmias
Klaricid	clarithromycin	antibiotic
Kogenate	Factor VIII	haemophilia A
Konakion	phytomenadione	hypoprothrombin-aemia
Kytril	granisetron	anti-emetic
Lamictal	lamotrigine	epilepsy
Lamisil	terbinafine	antifungal
Lamprene	clofazimine	leprosy
Lanoxin	digoxin	heart failure
Lanvis	thioguanine	cytotoxic
Laraflex	naproxen	arthritis
Largactil	chlorpromazine	antipsychotic
Lariam	mefloquine	malaria
Larodopa	levodopa	parkinsonism
Lasix	frusemide	diuretic
Lasma	theophylline	bronchodilator
Laxoberal	sodium picosulphate	laxative
Lederfen	fenbufen	antirheumatic
Ledermycin	demeclocycline	antibiotic
Lederspan	triamcinolone	corticosteroid
Lentaron	formestane	cytoxic
Lentizol	amitriptyline	antidepressant
Lescol	fluvastatin	hyperlipidaemia
Leucomax	molgramostim	neutropenia
Leukeran	chlorambucil	cytotoxic
Leustat	cladribine	cytotoxic
Levophed	noradrenaline	vasoconstrictor
Lexotan	bromazepam	anxiolytic

Proprietary name	Approved name	Main action or indication
Librium	chlordiazepoxide	antipsychotic
Limclair	trisodium edetate	ocular lime burns
Lingraine	ergotamine	migraine
Lioresal	baclofen	muscle relaxant
Lipantil	fenofibrate	hyperlipidaemia
Lipitor	atorvastatin	hyperlipidaemia
Lipobay	cerivastatin	hyperlipidaemia
Lipostat	pravastatin	hyperlipidaemia
Liskonum	lithium carbonate	mania
Litarex	lithium citrate	mania
Livial	tibolone	menopausal symptoms
Livostin	levocabastine	allergic conjunctivitis
Locabiotal	fusafungine	antibiotic
Loceryl	amorolfine	antifungal
Lodine	etodolac	arthritis
Logiparin	tinzaparin	anticoagulant
Lomexin	fenticonazole	antifungal
Lomotil	diphenoxylate	diarrhoea
Loniten	minoxidil	hypertension
Lopid	gemfibrozil	hyperlipidaemia
Lopressor	metoprolol	beta-blocker
Loron	sodium clodronate	hypercalcaemia of malignancy
Losec	omeprazole	peptic ulcer
Loxapac	loxapine	antipsychotic
Ludiomil	maprotiline	antidepressant
Lustral	sertraline	antidepressant
Lyclear	permethrin	pediculocide
Macrobid	nitrofurantoin	urinary infections
Macrodantin	nitrofurantoin	urinary infections
Macrodex	dextran	plasma substitute
Madopar	co-beneldopa	parkinsonism
Magnapen	co-fluampicil	antibiotic
Manerix	moclobemide	antidepressant
Marcain	bupivacaine	anaesthetic
Marevan	warfarin	anticoagulant
Marplan	isocarboxazid	antidepressant
Maxalt	rizatriptan	migraine
Maxepa	fish oil concentrate	hyperlipidaemia
Maxolon	metoclopramide	anti-emetic

Proprietary name	Approved name	Main action or indication	Proprietary name	Approved name	Main action or indication
Maxtrex	methotrexate	cytotoxic	Monit	isosorbide mononitrate	angina
Mectizan	ivermectin	filariasis	Mono-Cedocard	isosorbide mononitrate	angina
Medrone	methylprednisolone	corticosteroid	Monoclate-P	Factor VIII	haemophilia A
Mefoxin	cefoxitin	antibiotic	Monocor	bisoprolol	beta-blocker
Megace	megestrol	cytotoxic	Mononine	Factor IX	haemophilia B
Melleril	thioridazine	tranquillizer	Monoparin	heparin	anticoagulant
Menzol	norethisterone	menorrhagia	Monotrim	trimethaprim	antibacterial
Meptid	meptazinol	analgesic	Monovent	terbutaline	asthma
Merbentyl	dicyclomine	antispasmodic	Monuril	fosfomycin	urinary infections
Meronem	meropenem	antibiotic	Motens	lacidipine	calcium antagonist
Mestinon	pyridostigmine	myasthenia	Motifene	diclofenac	antirheumatic
Metenix	metolazone	diuretic	Motilium	domperidone	anti-emetic
Metopirone	metyrapone	resistant oedema	Motrin	ibuprofen	arthritis
Metosyn	fluocinonide	corticosteroid	MST Continus	morphine	analgesic
Metrodin	urofollitrophin	infertility	Mucodyne	carbocisteine	mucolytic
Metrolyl	metronidazole	anaerobic infections	Multiparin	heparin	anticoagulant
Metrotop	metronidazole	topical deodorant	Myambutol	ethambutol	tuberculosis
Mexitil	mexiletene	cardiac arrhythmias	Mycardol	pentaerythritol	coronary dilator
Miacalcic	salcatonin	Paget's disease	Mycobutin	rifabutin	tuberculosis
Mifegyne	mifepristone	termination of pregnancy	Mydriacyl	tropicamide	mydriatic
Minitran	glyceryl trinitrate	angina	Mydrilate	cyclopentolate	mydriatic
Minocin	minocycline	antibiotic	Myleran	busulphan	cytotoxic
Minodiab	glipizide	hypoglycaemic	Myocrisin	sodium aurothiomalate	rheumatoid arthritis
Mintec	peppermint oil	abdominal distension	Myodil	iophendylate	contrast agent
Mintezol	thiabendazole	anthelmintic	Myotonine	bethanechol	cholinergic
Miochol	acetylcholine	cataract surgery	Mysoline	primidone	epilepsy
Mitoxana	ifosfamide	cytotoxic	Nacton	poldine	antispasmodic
Mivacron	mivacurium	muscle relaxant	Nalcrom	sodium cromoglycate	anti-allergic
Mizollen	mizolastine	rhinoconjunctivitis	Nalorex	naltrexone	opioid dependence
Mobic	meloxicam	osteoarthritis	Naprosyn	naproxen	arthritis
Mobiflex	tenoxicam	arthritis	Naramig	naratriptan	migraine
Modalim	ciprofibrate	hyperlipidaemia	Narcan	naloxone	narcotic antagonist
Modecate	fluphenazine	antipsychotic	Nardil	phenelzine	antidepressant
Moditen	fluphenazine	schizophrenia	Narphen	phenazocine	analgesic
Modrasone	alclometasone	topical corticosteroid	Natrilix	indapamide	hypertension
Modrenal	trilostane	adrenal cortex inhibitor	Natulan	procarbazine	cytotoxic
			Navelbine	vinorelbine	cytotoxic
Mogadon	nitrazepam	hypnotic	Navidrex	cyclopenthiazide	diuretic
Molipaxin	trazodone	antidepressant	Navoban	tropisetron	antin-emetic

Proprietary name	Approved name	Main action or indication
Nebcin	tobramycin	antibiotic
Negram	nalidixic acid	urinary antiseptic
Neo-Cytamen	hydroxocobalamin	anti-anaemic
Neo-Mercazole	carbimazole	thyrotoxicosis
Neo-Naclex	bendrofluazide	diuretic
Neoral	cyclosporin	immunosuppressant
Neotigason	acitretin	psoriasis
Nephril	polythiazide	diuretic
Nerisone	diflucortolone	corticosteroid
Netillin	netilmicin	antibiotic
Neulactil	pericyazine	schizophrenia
Neupogen	filgrastim	neutropenia
Neurontin	gabapentin	epilepsy
Neutrexin	trimetrexate	AIDS
Nifensar	nifedepine	calcium antagonist
Niferex	iron complex	anaemia
Nimbex	cisatracurium	muscle relaxant
Nimotop	nimodipine	subarachnoid haemorrhage
Nipent	pentostatin	hairy-cell leukaemia
Nitoman	tetrabenazine	chorea
Nitrocine	glyceryl trinitrate	angina
Nitro-Dur	glyceryl trinitrate	angina
Nitrolingual	glyceryl trinitrate	angina
Nitronal	glyceryl trinitrate	angina
Nivaquine	chloroquine	antimalarial
Nivemycin	neomycin	antibiotic
Nizoral	ketoconazole	antifungal
Noltam	tamoxifen	anti-oestrogen
Nolvadex	tamoxifen	anti-oestrogen
Nootropil	piracetam	tics
Norcuron	vecuronium	muscle relaxant
Norditropin	somatotrophin	growth hormone
Norflex	orphenadrine	muscle relaxant
Norprolac	quinagolide	hyperprolactinaemia
Norvir	ritonavir	antiviral
Novantrone	mitozantrone	cytotoxic
NovoSeven	Factor VIIa	haemophilia A
Nozinan	methotrimeprazine	pain in terminal cancer
Nubain	nalbuphine	analgesic
Nuelin	theophylline	bronchodilator
Nupercainal	cinchocaine	local anaesthetic
Nycopren	naproxen	arthritis
Nystan	nystatin	antifungal
Nytol	diphenhydramine	mild insomnia
Ocusert Pilo	pilocarpine	glaucoma
Odrik	trandolapril	calcium antagonist
Olbetam	acipimox	hyperlipidaemia
Omnopon	papaveretum	analgesic
Oncovin	vincristine	cytotoxic
One-Alpha	alfacalcidol	vitamin D deficiency
Operidine	phenoperidine	analgesic
Ophthaine	proxymetacaine	corneal anaesthetic
Opilon	thymoxamine	vasodilator
Opticrom	sodium cromoglycate	allergic conjunctivitis
Optimax	tryptophan	antidepressant
Optimine	azatadine	antihistamine
Orap	pimozide	schizophrenia
Orbenin	cloxacillin	antibiotic
Orelox	cefpodoxime	antibiotic
Orgafol	urofollitrophin	infertility
Orgaran	danaparoid	anticoagulant
Orimeten	aminoglutethimide	cytotoxic
Orudis	ketoprofen	arthritis
Oruvail	ketoprofen	arthritis
Otex	urea–hydrogen peroxide	ear-drops
Otrivine	xylometazoline	nasal decongestant
Oxivent	oxitropium	bronchodilator
Palfium	dextromoramide	analgesic
Palladone	hydromorphone	opioid agonist
Paludrine	proguanil	antimalarial
Panadol	paracetamol	analgesic
Paraplatin	carboplatin	cytotoxic
Parlodel	bromocriptine	lactation suppressant
Parnate	tranylcypromine	antidepressant
Paroven	oxyrutins	varicose states
Parvolex	acetylcysteine	paracetamol overdose
Pavulon	pancuronium	muscle relaxant
Pecram	aminophylline	bronchodilator

Proprietary name	Approved name	Main action or indication
Penbritin	ampicillin	antibiotic
Pendramine	penicillamine	Wilson's disease
Pentacarinat	pentamidine	leishmaniasis
Pentasa	mesalazine	ulcerative colitis
Pentaspan	pentastarch	blood volume expander
Pentostam	sodium stibogluconate	leishmaniasis
Pepcid	famotidine	H_2-blocker
Percutol	glyceryl trinitrate	angina
Perdix	moexipril	hypertension
Perfan	enoximone	heart failure
Pergonal	menotrophin	hypogonadism
Periactin	cyproheptadine	antihistamine
Persantin	dipyridamole	angina
Pertofran	desipramine	antidepressant
Pevaryl	econazole	antifungal
Pharmorubicin	epirubicin	cytotoxic
Phenergan	promethazine	antihistamine
Phyllocontin	aminophylline	bronchodilator
Physeptone	methadone	analgesic
Physiotens	moxonidine	hypertension
Picolax	sodium picosulphate	laxative
Piportil	pipothiazine	antipsychotic
Pipril	piperacillin	antibiotic
Piriton	chlorpheniramine	antihistamine
Pitressin	vasopressin	diabetes insipidus
Plaquenil	hydroxychloroquine	antimalarial
Plavix	clopidogrel	atherosclerosis
Plendil	felodipine	calcium antagonist
Pondocillin	pivampicillin	antibiotic
Ponstan	mefenamic acid	arthritis
Posiject	dobutamine	cardiac support
Potaba	potassium P-aminobenzoate	scleroderma
Praxilene	naftidrofuryl	vasodilator
Precortisyl	prednisolone	corticosteroid
Predsol	prednisolone	corticosteroid
Pregnyl	gonadotrophin	infertility
Premarin	oestrogen	menopause
Prepidil	dinoprostone	cervical ripening
Prepulsid	cisapride	oesophageal reflux

Proprietary name	Approved name	Main action or indication
Prescal	isradipine	calcium antagonist
Preservex	aceclofenac	arthritis
Priadel	lithium carbonate	mania
Primacor	milrinone	severe heart failure
Primalan	mequitazine	antihistamine
Primaxin	imipenem	antibiotic
Primolut N	norethisterone	progestogen
Primoteston	testosterone	hypogonadism
Pro-Banthine	propantheline	antispasmodic
Profasi	gonadatrophin	infertility
Progesic	fenoprofen	arthritis
Prograf	tacrolimus	immunosuppressant
Proleukin	aldesleukin	cytotoxic
Proluton-Depot	hydroxyprogesterone	progestogen
Prominal	methylphenobarbitone	epilepsy
Pronestyl	procainamide	cardiac arrhythmias
Propaderm	beclomethasone	topical corticosteroid
Propine	dipivefrin	glaucoma
Proscar	finasteride	prostatic hyperplasia
Prostap	leuprorelin	prostatic carcinoma
Prostin E2	dinoprostone	induction of labour
Prostin F2	dinoprost	uterine stimulant
Prostin VR	alprostadil	maintenance of ductus arteriosus in neonates
Prothiaden	dothiepin	antidepressant
Protium	pantoprazole	peptic ulcer
Provera	medroxyprogesterone	progestogen
Provigil	modofinil	narcolepsy
Pro-Viron	mesterolone	androgen deficiency
Prozac	fluoxetine	antidepressant
Pulmadil	rimiterol	bronchospasm
Pulmicort	budesonide	rhinitis
Pulmozyme	dornase alfa	cystic fibrosis
Puri-Nethol	mercaptopurine	cytotoxic
Pylorid	ranitidine bismuth citrate	peptic ulcer
Questran	cholestyramine	bile acid binder

Proprietary name	Approved name	Main action or indication
Rapifen	alfentanyl	narcotic analgesic
Rapilysin	reteplase	thrombolytic
Rapitil	nedocromil	ocular allergy
Rastinon	tolbutamide	hypoglycaemic
Razoxin	razoxane	cytotoxic
Recormon	epoetin beta	anaemia in chronic renal failure
Refludan	lepuridin	anticoagulant
Refolinon	folinic acid	methotrexate antidote
Regaine	minoxidil	baldness
Remnos	nitrazepam	hypnotic
Relifex	nabumetone	arthritis
Reo-Pro	abciximab	antiplatelet
Replenin	Factor IX	haemophilia B
Requip	ropinirole	parkinsonism
Resonium A	exchange resin	hyperkalaemia
Respacal	tolubuterol	bronchodilator
Restandol	testosterone	androgen deficiency
Retin-A	tretinoin	acne
Retrovir	zidovudine	antiviral
Revanil	lysuride	parkinsonism
Rheomacrodex	dextran	blood volume expander
Rheumox	azapropazone	arthritis
Rhinocort	budesonide	rhinitis
Rhinolast	azelastine	rhinitis
Ridaura	auranofin	rheumatoid arthritis
Rifadin	rifampicin	tuberculosis
Rifinah	rifampicin	tuberculosis
Rilutek	riluzole	motor neurone disease
Rimactane	rifampicin	tuberculosis
Rimifon	isoniazid	tuberculosis
Rinatec	ipratropium	rhinorrhoea
Risperdal	risperidone	antipsychotic
Ritalin	methylphenidate	hyperactivity
Rivotril	clonazepam	anticonvulsant
Roaccutane	isotretinoin	severe acne
Robaxin	methcarbamol	muscle relaxant
Rocaltrol	calcitriol	vitamin D deficiency

Proprietary name	Approved name	Main action or indication
Roccal	benzalkonium	antiseptic
Rocephin	ceftriaxone	antibiotic
Roferon-A	interferon	leukaemia
Rogitine	phentolamine	phaeochromo-cytoma
Rohypnol	flunitrazepam	hypnotic
Romozin	troglitazone	insulin enhancer
Ronicol	nicotinyl alcohol	vasodilator
Rosex	metronidazole	acne
Rynacrom	sodium cromoglycate	allergic rhinitis
Rythmodan	disopyramide	cardiac arrhythmias
Sabril	vigabatrin	anticonvulsant
Saizen	somatropin	growth hormone
Salamol	salbutamol	asthma
Salazopyrin	sulphasalazine	ulcerative colitis
Salbulin	salbutamol	bronchospasm
Salofalk	mesalazine	ulcerative colitis
Saluric	chlorothiazide	diuretic
Sandimmun	cyclosporin	immunosuppressant
Sandoglobulin	immunoglobulin	hepatitis
Sandostatin	octreotide	carcinoid syndrome
Sanomigran	pizotifen	migraine
Saventrine	isoprenaline	bronchospasm
Scoline	suxamethonium	muscle relaxant
Scopoderm TTS	hyoscine	motion sickness
Seconal	quinalbarbitone	hypnotic
Sectral	acebutolol	beta-blocker
Securon	verapamil	angina
Securopen	azlocillin	antibiotic
Selsun	selenium sulphide	dandruff
Semprex	acrivastine	antihistamine
Serc	betahistine	Ménière's syndrome
Serenace	haloperidol	schizophrenia
Serdolect	sertindole	schizophrenia
Serevent	salmeterol	bronchospasm
Serophene	clomiphene	infertility
Seroquel	quetiapine	schizophrenia
Seroxat	paroxetine	antidepressant
Sevredol	morphine	analgesic
Simplene	adrenaline	glaucoma
Sinequan	doxepin	antidepressant

Proprietary name	Approved name	Main action or indication
Sinthrome	nicoumalone	anticoagulant
Skelid	tiludronic acid	Paget's disease
Skinoren	azelaic acid	acne
Slo-Phyllin	theophylline	bronchodilator
Slow-Trasicor	oxprenolol	beta-blocker
Slozem	diltiazem	calcium antagonist
Soframycin	framycetin	antibiotic
Solian	amisulpride	antipsychotic
Solu-Cortef	hydrocortisone	corticosteroid
Solu-Medrone	methylprednisolone	corticosteroid
Somatuline	lanreotide	acromegaly
Sominex	promethazine	mild hypnotic
Soneryl	butobarbitone	hypnotic
Sorbid SA	isosorbide dinitrate	angina
Sorbitrate	isosorbide dinitrate	angina
Sotacor	sotalol	beta-blocker
Sparine	promazine	antipsychotic
Spasmonal	alverine	antispasmodic
Spiroctan	canrenoate	diuretic
Spirolone	spironolactone	diuretic
Sporanox	itraconazole	antifungal
Stafoxil	flucloxacillin	antibiotic
Staril	fosinopril	ACE-inhibitor
Stelazine	trifluoperazine	antipsychotic
Stemetil	prochlorperazine	anti-emetic
Stesolid	diazepam	anxiolytic
Stiedex	desoxymethasone	topical corticosteroid
Stiemycin	erythromycin	acne
Stilnoct	zolpidem	hypnotic
Streptase	streptokinase	fibrinolytic
Stromba	stanozolol	anabolic steroid
Stugeron	cinnarizine	anti-emetic
Sublimaze	fentanyl	analgesic
Sulpitil	sulpiride	schizophrenia
Suprane	desflurane	inhalation anaesthetic
Suprax	cefixime	antibiotic
Suprecur	buserelin	endometriosis
Suprefact	buserelin	prostatic carcinoma
Surgam	tiaprofenic acid	arthritis
Surmontil	trimipramine	antidepressant

Proprietary name	Approved name	Main action or indication
Survanta	beractant	neonatal respiratory distress
Suscard Buccal	glyceryl trinitrate	angina
Sustac	glyceryl trinitrate	angina
Sustamycin	tetracycline	antibiotic
Sustanon	testosterone	androgen deficiency
Symmetrel	amantadine	parkinsonism
Synacthen	tetracosactrin	corticotrophin
Synalar	fluocinolone	topical corticosteroid
Synarel	nafarelin	endometriosis
Synflex	naproxen	arthritis
Synkavit	menadiol	hypoprothrombin-aemia
Syntaris	flunisolide	local corticosteroid
Syntocinon	oxytocin	post-partum haemorrhage
Syntopressin	lypressin	diabetes insipidus
Syscor	nisoldipine	angina, hypertension
Sytron	sodium iron edetate	anti-anaemic
Tagamet	cimetidine	peptic ulcer
Tambocor	flecainide	cardiac arrhythmias
Tamofen	tamoxifen	anti-oestrogen
Targocid	teicoplanin	antibiotic
Tarivid	ofloxacin	urinary tract infections
Tasmar	tolcapone	parkinsonism
Tavegil	clemastine	antihistamine
Tavenic	levofloxacin	antibacterial
Taxol	paclitaxel	cytotoxic
Taxotere	docetaxel	cytotoxic
Tazocin	tazobactam	antibiotic
Telfast	fexofenadine	antihistamine
Tegretol	carbamazepine	anticonvulsant
Temgesic	buprenorphine	analgesic
Temopen	temocillin	antibiotic
Tenormin	atenolol	beta-blocker
Teoptic	carteolol	glaucoma
Terramycin	oxytetracycline	antibiotic
Tertroxin	liothyronine	thyroid deficiency
Tetmosol	monosulfiram	scabies

Proprietary name	Approved name	Main action or indication
Tetralysal	lymecycline	antibiotic
Theo-dur	theophylline	bronchospasm
Thephorin	phenindamine	antihistamine
Ticar	ticarcillin	antibiotic
Tilade	neocromil	asthma
Tilarin	nedocromil	allergic conjunctivitis
Tildiem	diltiazem	calcium antagonist
Tiloreth	erythromycin	antibiotic
Timecef	cefodizime	antibiotic
Timentin	ticarcillin	antibiotic
Timoptol	timolol	glaucoma
Tobralex	tobramycin	eye infections
Tofranil	imipramine	antidepressant
Tolanase	tolazamide	hypoglycaemic
Tolectin	tolmetin	antirheumatic
Tomudex	raltitrexed	cytotoxic
Topamax	topiramate	epilepsy
Tonocard	tocainide	cardiac arrhythmias
Topicycline	tetracycline	acne
Toradol	ketorolac	analgesic
Torem	torasemide	diuretic
Tracrium	atracurium	muscle relaxant
Tramake	tramadol	analgesic
Trandate	labetalol	beta-blocker
Transiderm-Nitro	glyceryl trinitrate	angina
Tranxene	clorazepate	anxiolytic
Trasicor	oxprenolol	beta-blocker
Trasidrex	co-prenozide	hypertension
Trasylol	aprotinin	pancreatitis
Travogyn	isoconazole	candidiasis
Traxam gel	felbinac	sprains
Trental	oxpentifylline	vasodilator
Triludan	terfenadine	antihistamine
Trimopan	trimethoprim	antibacterial
Tritace	ramipril	ACE-inhibitor
Trobicin	spectinomycin	antibiotic
Trosyl	tioconazole	antifungal
Trusopt	dorzolamide	glaucoma
Tryptizol	amitriptyline	antidepressant
Ukidan	urokinase	hyphaemia, embolism

Proprietary name	Approved name	Main action or indication
Ultiva	remifentanil	opioid agonist
Ultralanum	fluocortolone	topical corticosteroid
Uniparin	heparin	anticoagulant
Uniphyllin Continus	theophylline	bronchospasm
Univer	verapamil	hypertension, angina
Uriben	nalidixic acid	urinary tract infections
Urispas	flavoxate	cystitis
Uromitexan	mesna	urotoxicity due to cyclophosphamide
Ursofalk	ursodeoxycholic acid	gallstones
Utinor	norfloxacin	urinary tract infections
Utovlan	ethisterone	progestogen
Valium	diazepam	anxiolytic, muscle relaxant
Vallergan	trimeprazine	sedative, pruritus
Valoid	cyclizine	anti-emetic
Valtrex	valaciclovir	antiviral
Vancocin	vancomycin	antibiotic
Vascace	cilazapril	ACE-inhibitor
Vasoxine	methoxamine	acute hypotension
Vectavir	penciclovir	antiviral
Velbe	vinblastine	cytotoxic
Velosef	cephradine	antibiotic
Ventolin	salbutamol	bronchospasm
Vepesid	etoposide	cytotoxic
Vermox	mebendazole	anthelmintic
Vesanoid	tretinoin	leukaemia
Viagra	sildenafil	impotence
Vibramycin	doxycycline	antibiotic
Videx	didanosine	antiviral
Vidopen	ampicillin	antibiotic
Viracept	nelfinaver	antiviral
Viramune	nevirapine	antiviral
Virazid	tribavirin	antiviral
Virormone	testosterone	hypogonadism
Visclair	methylcysteine	mucolytic
Visken	pindolol	beta-blocker
Vistide	cidofovir	CMV retinitis

Proprietary name	Approved name	Main action or indication
Vivalan	viloxazine	antidepressant
Vividrin	sodium cromoglycate	allergic rhinitis
Volital	pemoline	hyperkinaesia
Volmax	salbutamol	bronchodilator
Volraman	diclofenac	arthritis
Voltarol	diclofenac	antirheumatic
Welldorm	chloral hydrate	hypnotic
Wellferon	interferon	leukaemia
Wellvone	atavaquone	antimalarial
Xalantan	latanoprost	glaucoma
Xanax	alprazolam	anxiolytic
Xatral	alfuzosin	prostatic hyperplasia
Xenical	ortistal	obesity
Xuret	metolazone	diuretic
Xylocaine	lignocaine	anaesthetic
Xylocard	lignocaine	cardiac arrhythmias
Yomesan	niclosamide	anthelmintic
Yutopar	ritodrine	premature labour
Zaditen	ketotifen	anti-asthmatic
Zadstat	metronidazole	trichomoniasis
Zamadol	tramadol	analgesic
Zanaflex	tizanidine	spasticity
Zanidip	lercandipine	hypertension
Zantac	ranitidine	H_2-blocker
Zarontin	ethosuximide	anticonvulsant

Proprietary name	Approved name	Main action or indication
Zavedos	idarubicin	cytotoxic
Zelapar	selegiline	parkinsonism
Zerit	stavudine	antiviral
Zestril	lisinopril	ACE-inhibitor
Zimovane	zopiclone	hypnotic
Zinacef	cefuroxime	antibiotic
Zinamide	pyrazinamide	tuberculosis
Zinga	nizatidine	peptic ulcer
Zinnat	cefuroxime	antibiotic
Zirtek	cetirizine	antihistamine
Zita	cimetidine	H_2-blocker
Zithromax	clarithromycin	antibiotic
Zocor	simvastatin	hyperlipidaemia
Zofran	ondansetron	anti-emetic
Zoladex	goserelin	prostatic carcinoma
Zomacton	somatropin	growth hormone
Zomig	zolmitriptan	acute migraine
Zonulysin	chymotrypsin	cataract surgery
Zorac	tazarotene	psoriasis
Zoton	lansoprazole	peptic ulcer
Zovirax	acyclovir	antiviral
Zumenon	oestradiol	menopausal symptoms
Zydol	tramodol	analgesic
Zyloric	allopurinol	gout
Zyprexa	olanzapine	schizophrenia

New products that have become available since Appendix II was prepared:

Basiliximab

Brand name: Simulect
A monoconal antibody which binds with the inter-leukin-2 receptor and inhibits T-cell proliferation. Used in prophylaxis of organ rejection. Dose is 20 mg just before transplantation and 20 mg 4 days after-wards, by intravenous infusion.

Cefrozil (dose: 500 mg daily)

Brand name: Cefzil
A new cephalosporin antibiotic with a wide range of activity.

Clopidogrel (dose: 75 mg daily)

Brand name: Plavix
A new platelet aggregation inhibitor for myocardial infarct and other arteriosclerotic events.

Entacapone

Brand name: Comtess
An adjunct to levodopa in parkinsonism. Dose is 200 mg with each dose of levodopa/levodopa inhibitor. Other treatment may need to be adjusted.

Grepafloxacin (dose: 400–600 mg daily)

Brand name: Raxar
A broad-spectrum quinolone antibacterial.

Hyaluronic acid

Brand name: Hyalgan
A new preparation for the sustained relief of pain of osteoarthritis of the knee. The dose is 20 mg by intra-articular injection once a week for 5 weeks.

Lanreotide

Brand name: Somatuline
A new inhibitor of peptide hormones for acromegaly. Dose is 30 mg by intramuscular injection at intervals of 14 days.

Lepuridin

Brand name: Refludan
A recombinant form of huridin for heparin-associated thrombocytopenia and thrombo-embolic disease. Dose is 0.15 mg/kg hourly by continuous intravenous infusion for 2–10 days.

Lercandipine (dose: 10–20 mg daily)

Brand name: Zanidip
A calcium channel blocking agent for hypertension.

Mizolastine (dose: 10 mg daily)

Brand name: Mizollen
A new antihistamine for seasonal allergic rhinocon-junctivitis.

Modafinil (dose: 200–400 mg daily)

Brand name: Provigil
A new central stimulant for the treatment of narcolepsy.

Montelukast (dose: 10 mg at night)

Brand name: Singulair
A leukotriene receptor antagonist used as add-on therapy in the treatment of asthma.

Nelfinavir (dose: 750 mg three times a day)

Brand name: Viracept
A protease inhibitor for the treatment of advanced HIV-I infections.

Nevirapine (dose: 200 mg daily initially)

Brand name: Viramune
An inhibitor of reverse transcriptase for HIV-I infections.

Orlistat (dose: 120 mg with each main meal)

Brand name: Xenical.
A new inhibitor of gastro-intestinal lipases for the treatment of obesity. Any antidiabetic treatment may need monitoring.

Propiverine (dose: 30–45 mg daily)

Brand name: Detrunorm
A new spasmolytic for urinary incontinence and unstable bladder conditions.

Rituximab (dose: 375 mg/m² once weekly by intravenousinfusion)

Brand name: Mabthera
A monoclonal antibody for the treatment of resistant stage III-IV follicular lymphoma.

Rivastigmine (dose: 3–12 mg daily)

Brand name: Exelon
A new acetylcholinesterase inhibitor for Alzheimer's disease.

Rizatriptan (dose: 10 mg, not more than two doses in 24 hours)

Brand name: Maxalt
A new serotonin receptor agonist for the treatment of migraine.

Sildenafil (dose: 50 mg 1 hour before intercourse, not more than 1 dose a day)

Brand name: Viagra
A phophodiesterse inhibitor that increases the blood flow in the penis, and used in impotence.

Tiagabine (dose: 10–45 mg daily)

Brand name: Gabitril
A new selective inhibitor of GABA uptake for add-on therapy in epilepsy. Contra-indicated in severe hepatic impairment.

Tolerodine (dose: 2–4 mg daily)

Brand name: Detrusitol
A new antimuscarinic agent for treatment of unstable bladder conditions.

Zotepine (dose: 75 mg daily up to 300 mg daily)

Brand name: Zoleptil
An antipsychotic agent with an action mediated via dopamine receptors and the inhibition of the re-uptake of noradrenaline. Dose in schizophrenia. Care is necessary in hepatic impairment.

Appendix III: Weights and measures

Metric system

Nanogram	= 0.001 microgram
Microgram (μg)	= 0.001 mg
Milligram (mg)	= 0.001 g
Centigram (cg)	= 0.01 g
Decigram (dg)	= 0.1 g
Gram (g)	= 1 g
Kilogram (kg)	= 1000 g

The common metric measures of volume are the millilitre (ml), which is almost identical with the cubic centimetre (cc), and the litre (1000 ml or cc).

The British National Formulary gives all doses and formulations in the metric system. The standard dose for mixtures is 10 ml, for linctuses and children's mixtures the dose is 5 ml. Special 5-ml medicine spoons are available, and the use of domestic teaspoons for measuring medicines should be abandoned.

Appendix IV: Abbreviations

Abbreviations sometimes used in prescriptions are:

a.c.	ante cibum	before food
aq.	aqua	water
b.d.	bis die	twice a day
c.	cum	with
et	et	and
mitt.	mitte	send
o.n.	omni nocte	every night
p.c.	post cibum	after food
p.r.n.	pro re nata	occasionally
q.d.	quater die	four times a day
q.q.h.	quarta quaque hora	every 4 hours
q.s.	quantum sufficiat	sufficient
s.o.s.	si opus sit	when necessary
stat.	statim	at once
t.d.s.	ter die sumendus	to be taken three times a day
t.i.d.	ter in die	three times a day
ung.	unguentum	ointment

Note: The abbreviations s.c., i.m., i.v. and i.v.f. refer to subcutaneous, intramuscular and intravenous injections, and intravenous infusions

Appendix V: Glossary

Active transport: An energy-requiring process that moves small chemicals, including drugs, across cell membranes.

Adrenoceptors: Receptors in cell membranes to which adrenaline and noradrenaline bind.

Agonists: Drugs that bind to a receptor, and initiate or increase a response.

Alkaloids: Basic organic substances produced by many plants. Many are pharmacologically active, such as atropine, morphine and quinine.

Amoebiasis: An infection of the intestines and liver by pathogenic forms of single-cell protozoa, particularly *Entamoeba histolytica*.

Anaemia: A deficiency of haemoglobin, the oxygen-carrying constituent of red blood cells. It may occur as a result of lack of iron, a deficiency of vitamin B_{12} (pernicious anaemia), or as a side-effect of some drugs.

Anaphylaxis: A state of severe shock, induced by an antigen–antibody reaction in the tissues. The reaction is linked with the release of spasmogens and inflammatory factors, and may cause severe bronchospasm and collapse.

Antagonists: Drugs that bind to cell receptors. They function mainly as blocking agents, and by preventing other substances from interacting with the receptors, they inhibit the normal response.

Anticholinergics: Drugs that block the action of the neurotransmitter acetylcholine.

Antimuscarinics: Drugs that block the action of the neurotransmitter acetylcholine at muscarinic receptors.

Antimycotics: Antifungal agents.

Antigens: Substances that stimulate the formation of antibodies.

Antipyretics: Drugs that lower the body temperature in feverish conditions.

Aplastic anaemia: A form of anaemia due to complete failure of the bone marrow.

Antitussives: Cough depressants and suppressants.

Ascariasis: Infestation with nematode worms.

Behçet's syndrome: a disease of unknown cause, with conjunctivitis, mouth and genital ulcers.

Beta-lactam: A nitrogen-containing ring that is an essential part of the penicillin and cephalosporin structure. Breakdown of the ring by enzymes results in loss of activity.

Beta-lactamases: Enzymes that can break the beta-lactam ring structure of penicillins. They are formed by some penicillin- and cephalosporin-resistant organisms.

Bioavailability: The proportion of a dose of a drug that reaches the circulation and affects the tissues.

Blocker: Drugs that block ion channels and stop them functioning. An alternative term for drugs which act as antagonists, e.g. β-blockers.

Blood dyscrasia: A developmental disorder of the blood.

Blood–brain barrier: The mechanism that inhibits the passage of materials from the blood into the brain tissue.

Bolus: A large initial dose of a drug, given to obtain a rapidly effective blood level.

Candidiasis: Infection with the fungus *Candida*. Also known as thrush and moniliasis.

Carbonic anhydrase: An enzyme that reversibly catalyses the combination of carbon dioxide and water to form carbonic acid.

Carcinoid syndrome: The result of a tumour of the appendix that may secrete large amounts of serotonin (5-HT) and cause diarrhoea.

Carriers: Proteins found in the cell membrane which utilize energy to 'pump' chemicals such as ions and amino acids across cell membranes against their concentration gradient.

Chelating agents: Substances that can combine with and inhibit the activity of certain ions, and promote their excretion as an inactive complex. Desferrioxamine is an example of a chelating agent.

Chemoreceptor trigger zone: An area of the brain sensitive to chemicals, which forms part of the vomiting reflex.

Cholinesterases: Enzymes that limit the action of acetylcholine by converting it to choline and acetic acid.

Cross-resistance: Some groups of antibacterial agents have a common basic structure; consequently a strain of organism that has become resistant to one member of a group may be resistant to others.

Cycloplegics: Drugs that paralyse the ciliary muscle in the eye, and so facilitate examination.

Cytotoxics: Drugs that have a destructive effect on cells, and are used in the treatment of cancer.

Cytochrome P450: A group of hepatic enzymes involved in the metabolism of chemicals within the body, including drugs.

Dependence: This can be physical or psychological, and means that a person's body has come to rely on a drug, which if removed will cause a variety of unpleasant symptoms.

Desensitization: The process by which very small amounts of a foreign protein are given, until it ceases to produce a noticeable immune reaction.

Dose level saturation: Occurs when the normal metabolic enzymes are overwhelmed. There is the danger that toxic metabolites can accumulate.

Double-blind trial: A method of examining the efficacy of a new drug, by which the response is compared with a similar drug or a placebo. The test is so arranged that neither the doctor nor the patient knows who is receiving the new drug and who is receiving the alternative until the end of the trial (unless some severe side-effect requires early investigation).

Down-regulation: Internalization of cellular receptors. Continuous exposure to a chemical such as a drug can result in the surface receptors being moved inside the cell, so that the cell is less sensitive to the particular chemical.

Endogenous: Operating within the organism.

Endorphins: A group of centrally acting neuropeptides that act on specific receptors concerned with the perception of pain. Analgesics of the morphine type appear to act as agonists at these receptors.

Endotoxins: Toxic protein products of bacterial metabolism that are stored in the bacterial cell wall and released after the cell breaks down. *See* Exotoxins.

Enteric coated: The application of an outer layer to a drug which prevents it from breaking down until it is in an alkaline environment.

Enterohepatic recirculation: The movement of a drug from the gut to the liver, via the portal circulation, and then back to the gut, via the bile.

Enzyme: A protein that functions as a catalyst, and controls the metabolic activities of cells. Its action is often highly specific.

Enzyme induction: The production of more cellular enzymes in response to stimulation by a drug.

Enzyme inhibition: Enzyme activity is reduced as a result of the toxic effects of a drug.

Erythropoiesis: The production of red blood cells.

Exogenous: Of external origin, as opposed to endogenous.

Exotoxins: Toxic products of bacterial metabolism that are released during cell growth, and may cause systemic infections. *See* Endotoxins.

Extrapyramidal side-effects: The extrapyramidal tracts of the central nervous system coordinate and control muscular contraction. Disturbances of that control by drugs may produce many side-effects, including tremor and rigidity.

Extravasation: The escape of fluid into surrounding tissues. Extravasation of an irritant drug given intravenously may cause severe damage.

False substrate: A drug that mimics the normal substrate of an enzyme or carrier, and 'fools' the enzyme or carrier into carrying out its normal function on the drug instead of on its normal substrate.

First-pass metabolism: Metabolism of a drug that occurs before it enters the systemic circulation, e.g. in the gut wall and liver.

Glycosides: Organic substances produced by many plants, consisting of a carbohydrate combined with an active principle, such as digoxin.

Gram-positive and Gram-negative: A method of staining, named after a Danish physician (1853–1938), which distinguishes between two main groups of bacteria. Gram-positive bacteria have a peptidoglycan-containing cell wall that takes up and retains the stain. Gram-negative organisms have a multi-layer cell wall containing lipoproteins, which does not retain the stain.

Half-life: The time taken for the concentration of a circulating drug to fall by half after absorption and distribution is complete.

Hypersensitivity: Through the development of adaptive immunity, i.e. activation of B- and T-cells, the body has become too sensitive to a foreign antigen for its own good.

Idiosyncrasy: When a patient exhibits a markedly unusual qualitative rather than quantitative response to a drug.

Immunoglobulin: Antibody. A protein produced by B-cells in response to stimulation with an antigen.

Inhibitor: A drug which interacts with an enzyme, and by binding to its active site prevents the enzyme from catalysing chemical reactions.

Ion channel: A protein in a cell membrane that allows the access of ions into the cell, down their concentration and electrochemical gradients.

Ligand: Any small molecule which binds to a receptor.

Liposome: An artificial, drug-containing lipid globule; a new drug transport system.

Metabolism: The sum of the physical and chemical changes that constantly take place in a living organism. It includes food and tissue breakdown (catabolism) and biosynthesis of proteins and other essential substances (anabolism).

MIC: Minimum inhibitory concentration. A measure of the activity of an antibiotic. The lower the MIC, the more potent the drug.

Miotics: Drugs that constrict the pupil.

Modulator: Drugs that either increase or decrease the likelihood of an ion channel opening, depending on the drug.

Mydriatics: Drugs that dilate the pupil.

Neuroleptic: Antipsychotic drugs. Used to be called major tranquillizers.

Opioids: Compounds with effects similar to morphine, and which are antagonized by naloxone.

Parasympathomimetic: Drugs that mimic the effects of the parasympathetic nervous system.

Parasympatholytic: Drugs that inhibit the effects of the parasympathetic nervous system.

Parenteral: Administration by a route other than through the digestive system, as by intramuscular or intravenous injection.

Partial agonist: Drugs that have both agonistic and antagonistic effects at receptors.

Penicillinases: Enzymes formed by certain bacteria, particularly staphylococci, that break down and inactivate penicillins.

Peptidoglycans: Polysaccharide–peptide complexes that are part of the structure of the bacterial cell wall.

Pharmacodynamics: The study of how drugs exert their effects on the body.

Pharmokinetics: The study of what the body does to a drug with time, i.e. the processes of absorption, distribution, metabolism and excretion.

Placebo: An inert substance. Placebo tablets and capsules are widely used to compare the pychological effects of a drug with its pharmacological effects during clinical trials.

Potency: Refers to the amount of drug required to evoke a given response. The more potent the drug, the lower the dose to get the same effect.

Pro-drug: An inactive drug that is metabolized in the body into active derivatives.

Receptors: Sites on and within cells with a specific structure and function, to which hormones and neurotransmitters bind to trigger a response. Drugs may also bind to receptors, and may increase or block the effects of the endogenous molecule.

Substrate: A chemical that undergoes change as a result of being acted on by an enzyme.

Sympathomimetic: Drugs that mimic the effects of the sympathetic nervous system.

Synergism: The working together of two agents. Synergistic drugs, when given together, have a greater effect than the sum of the drugs acting in isolation.

Tardive dyskinesia: The involuntary and repeated movements of muscles of the face and limbs. It commonly affects older patients who receive prolonged therapy with neuroleptic drugs.

Telengiectasia: The permanent dilatation of certain groups of superficial capillaries, especially of the nose.

Teratogenic: Capable of influencing fetal development and causing malformations.

Therapeutic window/index: The ratio between the dose of a drug required for a therapeutic effect and the dose required to bring about toxic effects. Drugs with a high therapeutic index are safest.

Titration: A method of quantitative analysis by which the unknown strength of a solution can be determined by the use of a standard solution. It is sometimes applied to the careful adjustment of dose necessary with certain drugs, where a small variation in dose may produce a rapid and marked change in response.

Tolerance: A reduced response to a drug, requiring an increase in dose in order to maintain the effect. It occurs following the prolonged use of benzodiazepines and narcotics.

Toxoids: Chemically modified toxins, in which the toxicity has been reduced or eliminated without loss of antigenicity.

Vaccine: Antigens that have been sufficiently altered to not produce disease, but are able to stimulate an adaptive immune response.

Zollinger–Ellison syndrome: Hypersecretion of gastric acid, due to excessive secretion of gastrin by a tumour of the pancreas, leading to severe ulceration of the gastrointestinal tract.

Index